OPERATIVE TECHNIQUES IN SHOULDER AND ELBOW SURGERY

OPERATIVE TECHNIQUES IN
FOOT AND ANKLE SURGERY

Editor: Mark E. Easley
Editor-In-Chief Sam W. Wiesel

OPERATIVE TECHNIQUES IN
PEDIATRIC ORTHOPAEDICS

Editor: John M. Flynn
Editor-in-Chief Sam W. Wiesel

OPERATIVE TECHNIQUES IN
ORTHOPAEDIC TRAUMA SURGERY

Editors: Paul Tornetta III
Gerald R. Williams
Matthew L. Ramsey
Thomas R. Hunt III
Editor-in-Chief Sam W. Wiesel

OPERATIVE TECHNIQUES IN
SPORTS MEDICINE SURGERY

Editor: Mark D. Miller
Editor-in-Chief Sam W. Wiesel

OPERATIVE TECHNIQUES IN
ADULT RECONSTRUCTION SURGERY

Editors: Jarvad Parvizi & Richard H. Rothman
Editor-in-Chief Sam W. Wiesel

OPERATIVE TECHNIQUES IN
HAND, WRIST, AND FOREARM SURGERY

Editors: Thomas R. Hunt III
Editor-in-Chief Sam W. Wiesel

OPERATIVE TECHNIQUES IN SHOULDER AND ELBOW SURGERY

EDITORS

Gerald R. Williams, MD

Professor of Orthopaedic Surgery
Chief, Shoulder and Elbow Service
The Rothman Institute
Jefferson Medical College, Thomas
Jefferson University
Philadelphia, Pennsylvania

Matthew L. Ramsey, MD

Shoulder and Elbow Service
The Rothman Institute
Associate Professor of Orthopaedic Surgery
Jefferson Medical College, Thomas
Jefferson University
Philadelphia, Pennsylvania

Sam W. Wiesel, MD

EDITOR-IN-CHIEF
Professor and Chair
Department of Orthopaedic Surgery
Georgetown University Medical School
Washington, DC

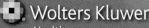
. Wolters Kluwer | Lippincott Williams & Wilkins
Health

Philadelphia · Baltimore · New York · London
Buenos Aires · Hong Kong · Sydney · Tokyo

Acquisitions Editor: Robert A. Hurley
Developmental Editor: Grace Caputo, Dovetail Content Solutions
Product Manager: Dave Murphy
Marketing Manager: Lisa Lawrence
Manufacturing Manager: Ben Rivera
Design Manager: Doug Smock
Compositor: Maryland Composition/ASI
Copyright 2011

Printed in China

Library of Congress Cataloging-in-Publication Data

Operative techniques in shoulder and elbow surgery / [edited by] Gerald R. Williams,
Matthew L. Ramsey ; Sam W. Wiesel, editor-in-chief.
    p. ; cm.
   Chapters derived from Operative techniques in orthopaedic surgery / editor-in-chief, Sam Wiesel. c2010.
   Includes bibliographical references and index.
   Summary: "Operative Techniques in Shoulder and Elbow Surgery contains the chapters on the shoulder and elbow from Sam W. Wiesel's Operative Techniques in Orthopaedic Surgery and provides full-color, step-by-step explanations of all operative procedures. Written by experts from leading institutions around the world, this superbly illustrated volume focuses on mastery of operative techniques and also provides a thorough understanding of how to select the best procedure, how to avoid complications, and what outcomes to expect. The user-friendly format is ideal for quick preoperative review of the steps of a procedure. Each procedure is broken down step by step, with full-color intraoperative photographs and drawings that demonstrate how to perform each technique. Extensive use of bulleted points and tables allows quick and easy reference. Each clinical problem is discussed in the same format: definition, anatomy, physical exams, pathogenesis, natural history, physical findings, imaging and diagnostic studies, differential diagnosis, non-operative management, surgical management, pearls and pitfalls, postoperative care, outcomes, and complications. To ensure that the material fully meets residents' needs, the text was reviewed by a Residency Advisory Board"--Provided by publisher.
   ISBN 978-1-4511-0264-2
   1. Shoulder--Surgery. 2. Elbow--Surgery. I. Williams, Gerald R., 1958- II.
Ramsey, Matthew L. III. Wiesel, Sam W. IV. Operative techniques in orthopaedic surgery.
   [DNLM: 1. Shoulder--surgery. 2. Elbow--surgery. 3. Orthopedic Procedures. WE 810]
   RD557.5.O637 2011
   617.5'72059--dc22
                        2010031580

To purchase additional copies of this book, call our customer service department at (800) 638-3030 or fax orders to (301) 223-2320. International customers should call (301) 223-2300.

Visit Lippincott Williams & Wilkins on the Internet at LWW.com. Lippincott Williams & Wilkins customer service representatives are available from 8:30 am to 6 pm, EST.

10 9 8 7 6 5 4 3 2 1

Dedication

To our wives, Robin and Nancy, and our children, Mark and Alexis and Chelsea, Alex, and Julia.

—GRW and MLR

CONTENTS

CONTRIBUTORS

Joseph A. Abboud, MD
Clinical Assistant Professor of Orthopaedic
  Surgery
University of Pennsylvania Health System
Philadelphia, Pennsylvania

Aymeric André, MD
Resident
Department of Plastic Surgery
University Hospital Rangueil
Paul-Sabatier University
Toulouse, France

Carl Basamania, MD, FACS
The Polyclinic First Hill
Seattle, Washington

Robert H. Bell, MD
Associate Professor of Orthopaedics
Crystal Clinic
Orthopaedic Surgeons, Inc.
Akron, Ohio

Ryan T. Bicknell, MD, MSc, FRCS(C)
Assistant Professor of Orthopaedic Surgery
Queen's University
Kingston General Hospital
Kingston, Ontario, Canada

Louis U. Bigliani, MD
Frank E. Stinchfield Professor and
  Chairman of Orthopedic Surgery
Columbia University
Director of the Orthopedic Surgery Service
New York-Presbyterian Hospital/Columbia
  University Medical Center
New York, New York

Theodore A. Blaine, MD
Associate Professor of Orthopaedic Surgery
Brown Alpert Medical School
Attending Orthopaedic Surgeon
Rhode Island Hospital
Providence, Rhode Island

Kamal I. Bohsali, MD
Attending Orthopaedic Surgeon, Shoulder
  and Elbow Reconstruction
Department of Orthopaedics
Memorial Hospital
St. Luke's Hospital
St. Vincent's Hospital
Jacksonville, Florida

Nicolas Bonnevialle, MD
Clinical Assistant in Orthopedic Surgery
Department of Orthopedics and
  Traumatology
University Hospital Purpan
Paul-Sabatier University
Toulouse, France

Christopher T. Born, MD
Professor of Orthopaedic Surgery
The Warren Alpert Medical School of
  Brown University
Rhode Island Hospital
Providence, Rhode Island

Joanna G. Branstetter, MD
Orthopaedic Surgeon
Madigan Army Medical Center
San Antonio, Texas

Juan Castellanos-Rosas, MD
Orthopaedic Surgeon
Department of Trauma Surgery
Hospital General Regional
Col Girasoles, Coyoacán, Mexico

Michael J. Codsi, MD
Department of Orthopaedic Surgery
The Everett Clinic
Everett, Washington

Mark S. Cohen, MD
Professor and Director
Section of Hand and Elbow Surgery
Rush University Medical Center
Chicago, Illinois

J. Dean Cole, MD
Medical Director
Florida Hospital Orthopaedic Institute
  Fracture Care Center
Orlando, Florida

Patrick M. Connor, MD
Clinical Faculty
Shoulder and Elbow Surgery, Sports
  Medicine, and Trauma
Department of Orthopaedic Surgery
Carolinas Medical Center
Charlotte, North Carolina

Allen Deutsch, MD
Clinical Assistant Professor
Department of Orthopaedic Surgery
Baylor College of Medicine
Kelsey-Seybold Clinic
Houston, Texas

Mark T. Dillon, MD
Fellow, Shoulder and Elbow Surgery
Department of Orthopaedic Surgery
University of Pennsylvania Presbyterian
  Medical Center
Philadelphia, Pennsylvania

Bassem Elhassan, MD
Assistant Professor of Orthopedics
Mayo Clinic
Rochester, Minnesota

Evan L. Flatow, MD
Professor of Orthopaedic Surgery
Mount Sinai Medical Center
New York, New York

Leesa M. Galatz, MD
Associate Professor
Department of Orthopaedic Surgery
Washington University School of Medicine
St. Louis, Missouri

Matthew J. Garberina, MD
Department of Orthopaedic Surgery
Summit Medical Group
Berkeley Heights, New Jersey

Charles L. Getz, MD
Assistant Professor of Orthopaedic Surgery
Thomas Jefferson University Hospital
Rothman Institute
Philadelphia, Pennsylvania

Filippos S. Giannoulis, MD
Department of Upper Extremity and
  Microsurgery
KAT Hospital
Athens, Greece

David L. Glaser, MD
Assistant Professor of Orthopaedic Surgery
University of Pennsylvania
Chief, Shoulder and Elbow Service
Penn Presbyterian Medical Center
Philadelphia, Pennsylvania

Andreas H. Gomoll, MD
Assistant Professor of Orthopaedic Surgery
Brigham and Women's Hospital
Harvard Medical School
Boston, Massachusetts

Thomas P. Goss, MD
Professor of Orthopaedic Surgery
Department of Orthopaedics and Physical
  Rehabilitation
University of Massachusetts Medical
  School
Worcester, Massachusetts

Andrew Green, MD
Associate Professor of Orthopaedic Surgery
Brown Alpert Medical School
Chief, Shoulder and Elbow Surgery
Rhode Island Hospital
Providence, Rhode Island

George Frederick Hatch III, MD
USC Orthopaedic Surgery Associates
Los Angeles, California

Laurence D. Higgins, MD
Associate Professor
Chief, Sports Medicine and Shoulder
  Service
Department of Orthopedic Surgery
Brigham & Women's Hospital
Boston, Massachusetts

Joseph P. Iannotti, MD, PhD
Maynard Madden Professor of
  Orthopaedic Surgery
Chairman, Orthopaedic and
  Rheumatologic Institute
The Cleveland Clinic
Cleveland, Ohio

ix

Asif M. Ilyas, MD
Director, Temple Hand Center
Assistant Professor, Orthopaedic Surgery
Temple University Hospital
Philadelphia, Pennsylvania

John M. Itamura, MD
Associate Professor
Department of Orthopaedic Surgery
University of Southern California
Keck School of Medicine
Los Angeles, California

Jesse B. Jupiter, MD
Hanstorg Wyss/AO Professor of
Orthopaedic Surgery
Harvard Medical School
Chief, Hand and Upper Limb Service
Massachusetts General Hospital
Boston, Massachusetts

Steven P. Kalandiak, MD
Assistant Professor of Clinical
Orthopaedics
University of Miami
Miami, Florida

**Srinath Kamineni, MBBCh, BSc(Hons),
FRCS-Orth**
Associate Professor of Elbow and Shoulder
Surgery
Professor of Bioengineering
Department of Sports, Orthopaedics, and
Trauma
Kentucky Clinic
University of Kentucky
Lexington, Kentucky

Leonid I. Katolik, MD
Philadelphia Hand Center
Philadelphia, Pennsylvania

Graham J. W. King, MD, MSc, FRCSC
Professor of Surgery
Division of Orthopaedic Surgery
University of Western Ontario
Hand and Upper Limb Centre
St. Joseph's Health Centre
London, Ontario, Canada

Raymond A. Klug, MD
Active Staff
Department of Orthopaedic Surgery
Los Alamitos Medical Center
Los Alamitos, Califonia

Thomas J. Kovack, DO
Department of Orthopaedic Surgery
Doctors Hospital
Hillard, Ohio

Sumant G. Krishnan, MD
Fellowship Director
Department of Shoulder Service
The Carrell Clinic
Dallas, Texas

John E. Kuhn, MD
Associate Professor
Chief of Shoulder Surgery
Department of Orthopaedics and
Rehabilitation
Vanderbilt University Medical Center
Nashville, Tennessee

Phillip Langer, MD, MS
Assistant Team Physician and Orthopedic
Surgeon
NFL Atlanta Falcons
NHL Atlanta Thrashers
Atlanta Sports Medicine & Orthopedic
Center
Atlanta, Georgia

Jonathan H. Lee, MD
Fellow in Adult Reconstruction
Department of Orthopaedic Surgery
Hospital for Special Surgery
New York, New York

William N. Levine, MD
Vice Chairman and Professor
Residency Director and Director of Sports
Medicine
Department of Orthopaedic Surgery
Columbia University Medical Center
New York, New York

Steven B. Lippitt, MD
Professor of Orthopaedic Surgery
Northeastern Ohio Universities College of
Medicine
Akron General Medical Center
Akron, Ohio

Bryan J. Loeffler, MD
Department of Orthopaedic Surgery
Carolinas Medical Center
Charlotte, North Carolina

John Lunn, FRCSI
Department of Orthopaedics
Hermitage Medical Clinic
Dublin, Ireland

Pierre Mansat, MD, PhD
Professor of Orthopedic Surgery
Department of Orthopedics and
Traumatology
University Hospital Purpan
Paul-Sabatier University
Toulouse, France

Frederick A. Matsen III, MD
Professor and Chair
Department of Orthopaedics and Sports
Medicine
University of Washington
Seattle, Washington

Jesse A. McCarron, MD
Associate Professor
Department of Orthopaedic Surgery
The Cleveland Clinic
Cleveland, Ohio

Michael D. McKee, MD, FRCS(c)
Professor
Division of Orthopaedics
Department of Surgery
University of Toronto
Toronto, Ontario, Canada

Mark A. Mighell, MD
Associate Director of Shoulder and Elbow
Fellowship
Florida Orthopaedic Institute
Associate Professor
Department of Upper Extremity Surgery
University of South Florida
Tampa, Florida

Steven Milos, MD
Department of Orthopaedics
Swedish American Hospital
Rockford, Illinois

Anthony Miniaci, MD, FRCSC
Professor of Surgery
Cleveland Clinic Lerner College of
Medicine
Director, Case Western Reserve University
Center
Head, Sports Medicine
Cleveland Clinic Sports Health Center
Orthopaedic and Rheumatologic Institute
Garfield Heights, Ohio

Anand M. Murthi, MD
Assistant Professor of Orthopaedics
Chief of Shoulder and Elbow Service
Department of Orthopaedics
University of Maryland School of Medicine
Baltimore, Maryland

Andrew S. Neviaser, MD
Resident
Department of Orthopaedic Surgery
Hospital for Special Surgery
New York, New York

Robert J. Neviaser, MD
Professor and Chairman
Department of Orthopaedic Surgery
George Washington University
Washington, District of Columbia

Daniel D. Noble, BA
Research Assistant
Crystal Clinic
Orthopaedic Surgeons, Inc.
Akron, Ohio

Jeffrey S. Noble, MD
Associate Professor of Orthopaedics
Crystal Clinic
Orthopaedic Surgeons, Inc.
Akron, Ohio

Brett D. Owens, MD
Assistant Professor
Department of Orthopaedic Surgery
Service
Keller Army Hospital
West Point, New York

Bradford O. Parsons, MD
Assistant Professor of Orthopaedic Surgery
Mount Sinai Medical Center
New York, New York

Jubin B. Payandeh, MD, FRCS(c)
Staff Surgeon
Department of Surgery
Big Thunder Orthopaedics
Thunder Bay, Ontario, Canada

Alexander H. Payatakes, MD
Assistant Professor
Hand and Wrist Service
Department of Orthopaedics
Penn State College of Medicine
Penn State Milton S. Hershey Medical
Center
Hershey, Pennsylvania

Matthew D. Pepe, MD
Sports Medicine Surgeon
The Rothman Institute
Voorhees, New Jersey

Matthew L. Ramsey, MD
Associate Professor of Orthopaedic Surgery
Rothman Institute Shoulder and Elbow
    Surgery
Thomas Jefferson University
Philadelphia, Pennsylvania

Michael A. Rauh, MD
Clinical Assistant Professor of Orthopaedic
    Surgery
State University of New York at Buffalo
Buffalo, New York

David Ring, MD, PhD
Associate Professor of Orthopaedic Surgery
Harvard Medical School
Department of Orthopaedic Surgery
Massachusetts General Hospital
Boston, Massachusetts

Robin R. Richards, MD, FRCSC
Professor
Department of Surgery
University of Toronto
Sunnybrook Health Sciences Center
Toronto, Ontario, Canada

Charles A. Rockwood, MD
Professor and Chairman Emeritus of
    Orthopaedics
The University of Texas Health Science
    Center at San Antonio
San Antonio, Texas

Anthony A. Romeo, MD
Associate Professor of Orthopaedic Surgery
Director, Section of Shoulder & Elbow
Rush University Medical Center
Chicago, Illinois

Yishai Rosenblatt, MD
Orthopaedic Surgeon
Hand and Upper Limb Surgeon
The Unit of Hand Surgery and
    Orthopaedic Surgery
Tel-Aviv Sourasky Medical Center
The Sackler Faculty of Medicine
Tel-Aviv University
Tel-Aviv, Israel

Joaquin Sanchez-Sotelo, MD, PhD
Associate Professor
Department of Orthopedic Surgery
Mayo Clinic
Rochester, Minnesota

Shadley C. Schiffern, MD
Attending Orthopaedic Surgeon
NorthEast Orthopedics, PA
Concord, North Carolina

Ryan W. Simovitch, MD
Shoulder and Elbow Service
Palm Beach Orthopaedic Institute
Palm Beach Gardens, Florida

Anshu Singh, MD
Shoulder and Elbow Surgeon
Kaiser Permanente
San Diego, California

Dean G. Sotereanos, MD
Professor of Orthopaedic Surgery
Drexel University College of Medicine
Allegheny General Hospital
Pittsburgh, Pennsylvania

Edwin E. Spencer, Jr., MD
Knoxville Orthopaedic Clinic
Knoxville, Tennessee

Jason A. Stein, MD
Assistant Professor
Department of Orthopaedics
University of Maryland
Baltimore, Maryland

Scott P. Steinmann, MD
Professor of Orthopaedics
Mayo Clinic
Rochester, Minnesota

Bradford S. Tucker, MD
Clinical Instructor
Department of Orthopaedic Surgery
Thomas Jefferson University Hospital
Egg Harbor Township, New Jersey

Gilles Walch, MD
Department of Shoulder Surgery
Centre Orthopédique Santy
Hopital Privé J Mermoz
Lyon, France

Jon J. P. Warner, MD
Chief, The Harvard Shoulder Service
Professor of Orthopaedics
Massachusetts General Hospital
Boston, Massachusetts

Brent B. Wiesel, MD
Chief, Shoulder Service
Department of Orthopaedic Surgery
Georgetown University Hospital
Washington, District of Columbia

Gerald R. Williams, MD
Professor of Orthopaedic Surgery
Chief, Shoulder and Elbow Service
The Rothman Institute
Jefferson Medical College
Philadelphia, Pennsylvania

Michael A. Wirth, MD
Professor of Orthopaedics
The Charles A. Rockwood, Jr., MD Chair
University of Texas Health Science Center
San Antonio, Texas

PREFACE

When a surgeon contemplates performing a procedure, there are three major questions to consider: Why is the surgery being done? When in the course of a disease process should it be performed? And, finally, what are the technical steps involved? The purpose of this text is to describe in a detailed, step-by-step manner the "how to do it" of the vast majority of orthopaedic procedures. The "why" and "when" are covered in outline form at the beginning of each procedure. However, it is assumed that the surgeon understands the basics of "why" and "when," and has made the definitive decision to undertake a specific case. This text is designed to review and make clear the detailed steps of the anticipated operation.

Operative Techniques in Shoulder and Elbow Surgery differs from other books because it is mainly visual. Each procedure is described in a systematic way that makes liberal use of focused, original artwork. It is hoped that the surgeon will be able to visualize each significant step of a procedure as it unfolds during a case.

Each chapter has been edited by a specialist who has specific expertise and experience in the discipline. It has taken a tremendous amount of work for each editor to enlist talented authors for each procedure and then review the final work. It has been very stimulating to work with all of these wonderful and talented people, and I am honored to have taken part in this rewarding experience.

Finally, I would like to thank everyone who has contributed to the development of this book. Specifically, Grace Caputo at Dovetail Content Solutions, and Dave Murphy and Eileen Wolfberg at Lippincott Williams & Wilkins, who have been very helpful and generous with their input. Special thanks, as well, goes to Bob Hurley at LWW, who has adeptly guided this textbook from original concept to publication.

SWW
January 1, 2010

RESIDENCY ADVISORY BOARD

The editors and the publisher would like to thank the resident reviewers who participated in the reviews of the manuscript and page proofs. Their detailed review and analysis was invaluable in helping to make certain this text meets the needs of residents today and in the future.

Daniel Galat, MD
Dr. Galat is a graduate of Ohio State University College of Medicine and the Mayo Clinic Department of Orthopedic Surgery residency program.
He is currently serving at Tenwek Hospital in Kenya as an orthopedic surgeon.

Lawrence V. Gulotta, MD
Fellow in Sports Medicine/Shoulder Surgery
Hospital for Special Surgery
New York, New York

Dara Chafik, MD, PhD
Southwest Shoulder, Elbow and Hand Center PC
Tuscon, Arizona

Gautam Yagnik, MD
Attending Physician
Orthopaedic Surgery
DRMC Sports Medicine
Dubois, Pennsylvania

Gregg T. Nicandri, M.D.
Assistant Professor
Department of Orthopaedics (SMD)
University of Rochester
School of Medicine and Dentistry
Rochester, New York

Catherine M. Robertson, MD
Assistant Clinical Professor
UCSD Orthopaedic Surgery—Sports Medicine
San Diego, California

Jonathan Schoenecker, MD
Assistant Professor
Departments of Orthopaedics, Pharmacology and Pediatrics
Vanderbilt University
Nashville, Tennessee

OPERATIVE TECHNIQUES IN SHOULDER AND ELBOW SURGERY

Chapter 1

Anatomy of the Shoulder and Elbow

Joseph A. Abboud, Matthew L. Ramsey, and Gerald R. Williams

OVERVIEW OF SHOULDER AND ELBOW SURGERY

- In order to diagnose and treat problems of the shoulder and elbow, one must fully understand the anatomy of the region and appreciate how this translates to functional derrangements.
- There is no line of demarcation between the shoulder and elbow regions. Pain in the arm may originate at the neck or shoulder and refer down the arm. Less often pain noted by patients at the elbow or forearm have local origin. If the slightest doubt exists as to the etiology of the pain, the patient is examined from neck to fingers.
- The upper extremity functions to position and move the hand in space. The upper extremities are attached to the body by the sternoclavicular joint. Otherwise, they are suspended from the neck and held fast to the torso by soft tissues (muscles and fascia).
    - The upper extremity gains leverage against the posterior aspect of the thorax by virtue of the broad, flat body of the scapula.
    - The elbow along the upper extremity is a complex modified hinge articulation. Unlike the shoulder, the elbow has a much more intrinsic stability based on its bony architecture. The primary purpose of the elbow is to position the hands in space. The elbow joint is perhaps the main joint responsible for communicating the actions of the hand to the trunk.
- The surgical management of major shoulder and elbow conditions has rapidly progressed over the last 30 years as our understanding of the pathoanatomy and biomechanics has greatly enhanced our ability to treat certain problems. Consequently, new surgical techniques have allowed the surgeon to more effectively treat many disorders.
    - Arthroscopic surgery in particular has significantly increased our ability to surgically manage conditions and reduce morbidity. The sports medicine portion of this textbook handles the arthroscopic management of shoulder and elbow disorders.
- The art of any surgery lies in the reconstruction of diseased or injured tissues with minimal additional destruction. Skillful handling of the soft tissues is the hallmark of all upper extremity surgery, including the shoulder and elbow. Knowledge of anatomy defines the precision and safety of surgery. Approaches to any joint in the body are developed on this foundation, with particular emphasis on the exploitation of internervous planes. Familiarity with the intricate anatomy and multiple approaches to the shoulder and elbow allows the surgeon to confidently embark on the repair or reconstruction of the injury or disorder of the joint.

ANATOMY OF THE SHOULDER

- The shoulder has the greatest mobility of any joint in the body and therefore the greatest predisposition to dislocation.
- This great range of motion is distributed to three diarthrodial joints: the glenohumeral, the acromioclavicular, and the sternoclavicular.
- The last two joints, in combination with the fascial spaces between the scapula and the chest, are known collectively as the scapulothoracic articulation.

OSTEOLOGY

Clavicle

- This is a relatively straight bone when viewed anteriorly, whereas in the transverse plane, it resembles an italic S (**FIG 1**).
- There are three bony impressions for ligament attachment to the clavicle:
    - On the medial side is an impression for the costoclavicular ligament, which at times may be a rhomboid fossa.
    - At the lateral end of the bone is the conoid tubercle.
    - Just lateral to the conoid tubercle is the trapezoid tubercle.
- Muscles that insert on the clavicle are the trapezius on the posterosuperior surface of the distal end and the subclavius muscle, which has an insertion on the inferior surface of the middle third of the clavicle.
- Functionally, the clavicle acts mainly as a point of muscle attachment.
    - Some of the literature suggests that with good repair of the muscle, the only functional consequences of surgical removal of the clavicle are with heavy overhead and that, therefore, its function as a strut is less important.
- Four muscles take origin from the clavicle: deltoid, pectoralis major, sternocleidomastoid, and sternohyoid.
- Important relations to the clavicle are the subclavian vein and artery and the brachial plexus posteriorly.

Scapula

- This is a thin sheet of bone that functions mainly as a site of muscle attachment (**FIG 2A**).
- It is thicker at its superior and inferior angles in its lateral border, where some of the more powerful muscles are attached.

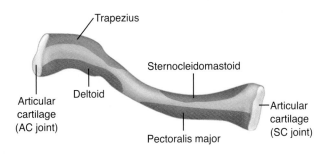

FIG 1 • The clavicle.

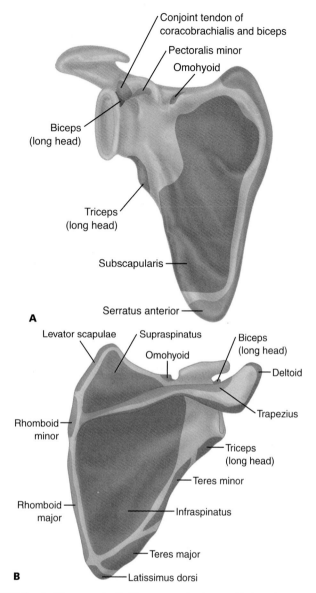

FIG 2 • A. The scapula. **B.** The supraspinatus and infraspinatus fossa.

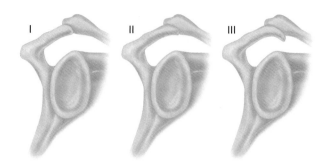

FIG 3 • Acromion morphologies.

■ It is also thick in forming its processes: coracoid, spine, acromion, and glenoid.

■ The coracoid process comes off the scapula at the upper base of the neck of the glenoid and passes anteriorly before hooking to a more lateral position.

  ■ Functions as the origin of the short head of the biceps and the coracobrachialis tendons

  ■ Serves as the insertion of the pectoralis minor muscle and the coracoacromial, coracohumeral, and coracoclavicular ligaments

■ The spine of the scapula functions as part of the insertion of the trapezius on the scapula as well as the origin of the posterior deltoid.

  ■ Also serves to suspend the acromion in the lateral and anterior directions to serve as a prominent lever arm for function of the deltoid

■ The posterior surface of the scapula and the presence of the spine create the supraspinatus and infraspinatus fossa (**FIG 2B**).

■ The acromion is the most studied process of the scapula because of the amount of pathology involving the acromion and the rotator cuff.

  ■ Three types of acromion morphologies have been defined by Bigliani and Morrison (**FIG 3**).

  ■ Type 1, with its flat surface, provided the least compromise of the supraspinatus outlet, whereas type 3, which has a hook, was associated with the highest rate of rotator cuff pathology in a series of cadaver dissections.

■ The glenoid articular surface is within 10 degrees of being perpendicular to the blade of the scapula, with the mean being 6 degrees of retroversion.

  ■ More caudad portions face more anteriorly than cephalad.

■ Three processes—the spine, the coracoid, and the glenoid—create two notches in the scapula.

  ■ Suprascapular notch is at the base of the coracoid.

  ■ Spinoglenoid, or greater scapular notch, is at the base of the spine.

■ Major ligaments that take origin from the scapula are:

  ■ Coracoclavicular

  ■ Coracoacromial

  ■ Acromioclavicular

  ■ Glenohumeral

  ■ Coracohumeral

■ Blood supply to the scapula derives from vessels in the muscles that take fleshy origin from the scapula.

  ■ Vessels cross these indirect insertions and communicate with bony vessels.

Humerus

■ The articular surface of the humerus at the shoulder is spheroid, with a radius of curvature of about 2.25 cm.

■ With the arm in the anatomic position (ie, with the epicondyles of the humerus in the coronal plane), the head of humerus has retroversion of about 30 degrees, with a wide range of normal values.

■ The intertubercular groove lies about 1 cm lateral to the midline of the humerus (**FIG 4**).

■ The axis of the humeral head crosses the greater tuberosity at about 9 mm posterior to the bicipital groove.

■ The lesser tuberosity lies directly anterior, and the greater tuberosity lines up on the lateral side.

  ■ The lesser tuberosity is the insertion for the subscapularis tendon.

  ■ The greater tuberosity bears the insertion of the supraspinatus, infraspinatus, and teres minor in a superior to inferior order.

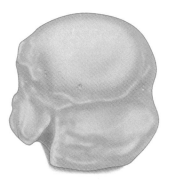

FIG 4 • The humerus.

▪ Greater and lesser tuberosities make up the boundaries of the intertubercular groove through which the long head of the biceps passes from its origin on the superior lip of the glenoid.
  ▪ The intertubercular groove has a peripheral roof referred to as the intertubercular ligament or the transverse humeral ligament, which has varying degrees of strength.
  ▪ In the coronal plane, the head–shaft angle is about 135 degrees.
  ▪ The space between the articular cartilage and the ligamentous and tendon attachments is referred to as the anatomic neck of the humerus.
  ▪ Below the level of the tuberosities, the humerus narrows in a region that is referred to as the surgical neck of the humerus because of the frequent occurrence of fractures at this level.

STERNOCLAVICULAR JOINT

▪ This is the only skeletal articulation between the upper limb and the axial skeleton.

Ligaments

▪ The major ligaments of the sternoclavicular joint are the anterior and posterior sternoclavicular ligaments.
▪ The most important ligament of this group, the posterior sternoclavicular ligament, is the strongest.

Blood Supply

▪ Blood supply of the sternoclavicular joint derives from the clavicular branch of the thoracoacromial artery, with additional contributions from the internal mammary and the suprascapular arteries.

Nerve Supply

▪ Arises from the nerve to the subclavius, with some contribution from the medial suprascapular artery

ACROMIOCLAVICULAR JOINT

▪ Only articulation between the clavicle and the scapula

Ligaments

▪ Ligaments about the acromioclavicular articulation are the trapezoid and the conoid ligaments (**FIG 5**).
  ▪ The anteroposterior stability of the acromioclavicular joint is controlled by the acromioclavicular ligaments, and the vertical stability is controlled by the coracoclavicular ligaments.

Blood Supply

▪ Blood supply derives mainly from the acromial artery, a branch of the deltoid artery of the thoracoacromial axis.

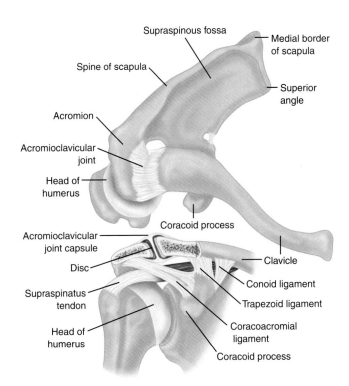

FIG 5 • Acromioclavicular joint.

▪ There are rich anastomoses between the thoracoacromial artery, suprascapular artery, and posterior humeral circumflex artery.
▪ The acromial artery comes on to the thoracoacromial axis anterior to the clavipectoral fascia and perforates back through the clavipectoral fascia to supply the joint.

Nerve Supply

▪ Innervation of the joint is supplied by the lateral pectoral, axillary, and suprascapular nerves.

SHOULDER LIGAMENTS: CAPSULOLIGAMENTOUS AND LABRAL ANATOMY (**FIG 6**)

Superior Glenohumeral Ligament (SGHL)

▪ Arises near the origin of the long head of the biceps brachii
▪ If the glenoid had the markings of a clock, with the 12-o'clock position superiorly and the 3-o'clock position anteriorly, the origin of the superior glenohumeral ligament would correspond to the area from the 12-o'clock to the 2-o'clock positions.
▪ SGHL runs inferiorly and laterally to insert on the humerus, superior to the lesser tuberosity.

Middle Glenohumeral Ligament (MGHL)

▪ Usually arises from the neck of the glenoid just inferior to the origin of the SGHL and inserts into the humerus just medial to the lesser tuberosity
▪ Presence of the MGHL most variable of any shoulder ligament

Inferior Glenohumeral Ligament (IGHL)

▪ Most important ligament for providing anterior and posterior shoulder stability
▪ IGHL has been described as having an anterior and posterior band, with an axillary pouch between the bands.

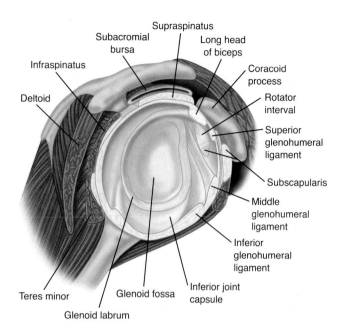

FIG 6 • Shoulder ligaments

▪ With abduction and external rotation, the anterior band fans out and the posterior band becomes cordlike.
▪ Likewise, with internal rotation, the posterior band fans out and the anterior band appears cordlike.
▪ Anterior band of the IGHL arises from various areas corresponding to the 2- to 4-o'clock positions on the glenoid.
▪ Insertion site of this ligament has two attachments, one to the glenoid labrum and the other directly to the anterior neck of the glenoid.
▪ Posterior band originates at the 7-o'clock to 9-o'clock positions.
▪ With the arm at the side, both the anterior and the posterior bands pass through a 90-degree arc and insert on the humerus.

Labrum

▪ Surrounds the periphery of the glenoid and is a site of attachment of the capsuloligamentous structures
▪ It is composed of dense fibrous connective tissue, with a small fibrocartilaginous transition zone at the anteroinferior attachment of the osseous glenoid rim.
▪ The labrum acts as a load-bearing structure for the humeral head and serves to increase the surface area of the glenoid.
▪ Howell and Galinat showed that the labrum deepened the glenoid socket by nearly 50%.
▪ Lippett and coworkers have shown that removal of the labrum decreases the joint's stability to sheer stress by 20%.
▪ Triangular cross-section of the labrum allows it to act as a chock-block to help prevent subluxation.

SCAPULOTHORACIC MUSCLES

Trapezius

▪ Largest and most superficial of scapulothoracic muscles
▪ Takes origin from spinous process of C7 through T12 vertebrae
▪ Insertion of the upper fibers is over the distal one third of the clavicle.

▪ Lower cervical and upper thoracic fibers of the trapezius have their insertion over the acromion and spinous scapula.
▪ Lower portion of the muscle takes insertion at the base of the scapular spine.
▪ Acts as a scapular retractor, with the upper fibers used mostly for elevation of the lateral angle
▪ Spinal accessory nerve is the motor supply.
▪ Arterial supply is derived from transverse cervical artery.

Rhomboids

▪ Similar in function to the midportion of the trapezius, with origin from the lower ligamentum nuchae, C7 and T1 for the rhomboid minor and T2 through T5 for the rhomboid major
▪ Rhomboid minor inserts on the posterior portion of the medial base of the spine of the scapula.
▪ Rhomboid major inserts to the posterior surface of the medial border, from where the minor leaves off down to the inferior angle of the scapula.
▪ Action of the rhomboids is retraction of the scapula, and because of their oblique course they also participate in elevation of the scapula.
▪ Innervation is the dorsal scapular nerve (C5), which may arise off the brachial plexus in common with the nerve to the subclavius or with the C5 branches of the long thoracic nerve.
▪ Dorsal scapular artery provides arterial supply to the muscles through their deep surfaces.

Levator Scapula and Serratus Anterior

▪ The levator scapula and the serratus anterior are often discussed together because of their close relationship anatomically and functionally.
▪ The levator scapula takes origin from the posterior tubercles of the transverse process from C1 through C3 and sometimes C4.
▪ Inserts on the superior angle of the scapula
▪ Acts to elevate the superior angle of the scapula
▪ In conjunction with the serratus anterior, produces upward rotation of the scapula
▪ Innervation is from the deep branches of C3 and C4.
▪ Serratus anterior takes origin from the ribs on the anterior lateral wall of the thoracic cage.
▪ Bounded medially by the ribs and intercostal muscles and laterally by the axillary space
▪ Protracts the scapula and participates in upward rotation of the scapula
▪ More active in flexion than in abduction because straight abduction requires some retraction of the scapula
▪ Absence of serratus activity, usually because of paralysis, produces a winging of the scapula with forward flexion of the arm and loss of strength in that motion.
▪ Innervation is supplied by the long thoracic nerve (C5, C6, and C7).
▪ Blood supply is from the lateral thoracic artery, with a large contribution from the thoracodorsal artery.

Pectoralis Minor

▪ Takes fleshy origin anteriorly on the chest wall, and second through fifth ribs, and has its insertion onto the base of the medial side of the coracoid

▪ Function is protraction of the scapula if the scapula is retracted and depression of the lateral angle or downward rotation of the scapula if the scapula is upwardly rotated.

▪ Innervation is from the medial pectoral nerve (C8 and T1).

▪ Blood supply is through the pectoral branch of the thoracoacromial artery.

GLENOHUMERAL MUSCLES (**FIG 7**)

Deltoid

▪ Largest and most important of the glenohumeral muscles, consisting of three major sections:

   ▪ Anterior deltoid takes origin off the lateral third of the clavicle, middle third of the deltoid takes origin off the acromion, and posterior deltoid takes origin from the spine of the scapula.

▪ The deltoid is supplied by the axillary nerve (C5 and C6), which enters the posterior portion of the shoulder through the quadrilateral space and innervates the teres minor in this position.

   ▪ Nerves to the posterior third of the deltoid enter the muscle very close to their exit from the quadrilateral space, traveling in the deltoid muscle along the medial and inferior borders of the posterior deltoid.

   ▪ Branch of the axillary nerve that supplies the anterior two thirds of the deltoid ascends superiorly and then travels anteriorly, about 2 inches inferior to the rim of the acromion.

▪ Vascular supply to the deltoid is largely derived from the posterior humeral circumflex artery, which travels with the axillary nerve through the quadrilateral space of the deep surface of the muscle.

   ▪ Deltoid is also supplied by the deltoid branch of the thoracoacromial artery.

Supraspinatus

▪ Lies on the superior portion of the scapula

▪ It takes origin from the supraspinatus fossa and overlying fascia and inserts into the greater tuberosity.

▪ Its tendinous insertion is in common with the infraspinatus posteriorly.

▪ It is active in any motion involving elevation.

▪ It exerts maximum effort at about 30 degrees of elevation.

▪ Innervation of the supraspinatus is supplied by the suprascapular nerve (C5, C6).

▪ Arterial supply is the suprascapular artery.

▪ Nerve comes through the suprascapular notch and is bound above by the transverse scapular ligament.

   ▪ Artery travels above this ligament.

▪ Suprascapular vessels and nerve supply the deep surface of the muscle.

Infraspinatus

▪ Second most active rotator cuff muscle

▪ Its tendinous insertion is in common with the supraspinatus anterosuperiorly and the teres minor inferiorly at the greater tuberosity.

▪ One of the two main external rotators of the humerus and accounts for as much as 60% of external rotation force

▪ Also functions as a depressor of the humeral head

▪ Even in a passive state, it is an important stabilizer against posterior subluxation.

▪ Innervated by the suprascapular nerve

▪ Blood supply is from two large branches of the suprascapular artery.

Teres Minor

▪ One of the few external rotators of the humerus

▪ It provides up to 45% of the external rotation force.

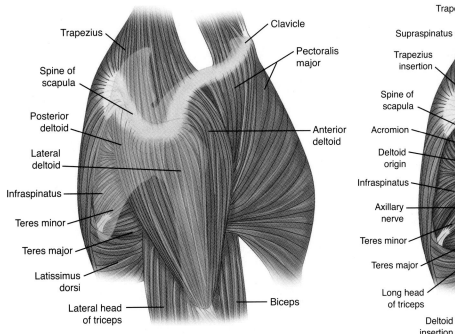

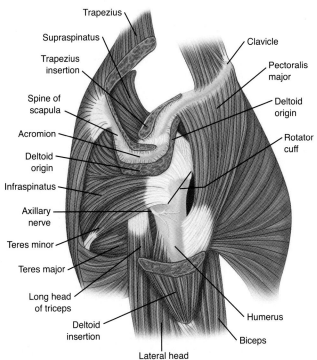

FIG 7 ▪ Glenohumeral muscles.

- It is important in controlling stability in the anterior direction.
- Innervated by the posterior branch of the axillary nerve (C5 and C6)
- Blood supply is derived from several vessels in the area, especially the posterior humeral scapular circumflex artery.

Subscapularis

- Makes up the anterior portion of the rotator cuff
- Takes origin from the subscapularis fossa, which covers most of the anterior surface of the scapula
- Its upper 60% inserts through a cartilaginous tendon into the lesser tuberosity of the humerus, and its lower 40% has a fleshy insertion into the humerus below the lesser tuberosity cupping the head and neck.
- Functions as an internal rotator and passive stabilizer to anterior subluxation and serves in its lower fibers to depress the humeral head
- Innervation usually supplied by two sources:
  - Upper subscapular nerve (C5) and lower subscapular nerves (C5 and C6)
  - Upper subscapular nerves usually come off the posterior cord.
- Blood supply originates from the axillary and subscapular arteries.

Teres Major

- Takes origin from the posterior surface of the scapula along the inferior portion of the lateral border
- It has a muscular origin and a common tendinous insertion with the latissimus dorsi into the humerus along the medial lip of the bicipital groove.
- In their course, both the latissimus dorsi and the teres major undergo a 180-degree spiral; thus, the formerly posterior surface of the muscle is represented by fibers on the anterior surface of the tendon.
- Function is internal rotation, adduction, and extension of the arm.
- Innervation is supplied by the lower subscapular nerve C5 and C6.
- Blood supply is derived from the subscapular artery.

Coracobrachialis

- Originates from the coracoid process, in common with and medial to the short head of the biceps, and inserts onto the anteromedial surface in the midportion of the humerus
- Action is flexion and adduction of the glenohumeral joint.
- Innervation supplied by small branches from the lateral cord and the musculocutaneous nerve
- Because the larger musculocutaneous nerve's entrance to the muscle may be situated as high as 1.5 cm from the tip of the coracoid to as low as 7 to 8 cm, it must be protected during certain types of repair.
- Major blood supply is usually off the axillary.

MULTIPLE JOINT MUSCLES

Pectoralis Major

- Consists of three portions:
  - Upper portion takes origin from the medial one half to two thirds of the clavicle and inserts along the lateral lip of the bicipital groove.

- Middle portion takes origin from the manubrium and upper two thirds of the body of the sternum and ribs 2 through 4.
  - It inserts directly behind the clavicular portion and maintains a parallel fiber arrangement.
  - Inferior portion of the pectoralis major takes origin from the distal body of the sternum, the fifth and sixth ribs, and the external oblique muscle fascia.
- Action
  - Clavicular portion participates somewhat in flexion with the anterior portion of the deltoid while the lower fibers are antagonistic.
  - Is active in internal rotation against resistance and will extend the shoulder from flexion until the neutral position is reached
  - Powerful adductor of the glenohumeral joint
- Innervation is supplied by two sources:
  - Lateral pectoral nerve (C5, C6, and C7) innervates the clavicular portion of the muscle.
  - Loop contribution from the lateral to the medial pectoral nerve carrying C7 fibers into the upper sternal portion
- Major blood supply derives from two sources:
  - The deltoid branch of the thoracoacromial artery supplies the clavicular portion and the pectoral artery supplies the sternocostal portion of the muscle.

Latissimus Dorsi

- Takes origin by the large and broad aponeurosis from the dorsal spines of T7 through L5, a portion of the sacrum, and the crest of the ilium
- Wraps around the teres major and inserts into the medial crest and floor of the bicipital or intertubercular groove
- Actions are inward rotation and abduction of the humerus, shoulder extension, and indirectly through its pull on the humerus downward rotation of the scapula.
- Innervation is through the thoracodorsal nerve (C6 and C7).
- Major blood supply is derived from the thoracodorsal artery.

Biceps Brachii

- There are two origins of the biceps muscle in the shoulder:
  - The long head takes origin from the bicipital tubercle at the superior rim of the glenoid.
  - The short head takes origin from the coracoid tip lateral.
- Has two distal tendinous insertions:
  - Lateral insertion is to the posterior part of the tuberosity of the radius
  - Medial insertion is aponeurotic (lacertus fibrosus), passing medially across and into the deep fascia of the muscles of the volar forearm.
- Loss of the long head attachment expresses itself mainly as loss of supination strength (20%), with a smaller loss (8%) of elbow flexion strength.
- Actions of the biceps are flexion and supination at the elbow.
- Main action is at the elbow rather than the shoulder.
- Innervation is supplied by branches of the musculocutaneous nerve (C5 and C6).
- Blood supply derives from a single large bicipital artery from the brachial artery (35%), multiple very small arteries (40%), or combination of two types.

Triceps Brachii

- Long head takes origin from the infraglenoid tubercle.
- Major action of the muscle is extension at the elbow.

■ Innervation is supplied by the radial nerve with root innervation C6 to C8.

■ Arterial supply is derived mainly from the profunda brachial artery and the superior ulnar collateral artery.

BRACHIAL PLEXUS

■ The standard brachial plexus is made up of distal distribution of the anterior rami of spinal nerve roots C5, C6, C7, C8, and T1. The plexus has contributions from C4 and T1 (**FIG 8**).

Trunks, Divisions, and Cords

■ The roots combine to form trunks: C5 and C6 form the superior trunk; C7 forms the middle trunk; and C8 and T1 form the inferior trunk.

■ The trunks then separate into anterior and posterior divisions.

■ The posterior divisions combine to form the posterior cord, the anterior division of the inferior trunk forms the medial cord, and the anterior division of the superior and middle trunks forms the lateral cord.

■ These cords give off the remaining largest number of the terminal nerves of the brachial plexus, and roots from the lateral and medial cords come together to form the median nerve.

■ The brachial plexus leaves the cervical spine and progresses into the arm through the interval between the anterior and middle scalene muscles.

■ The subclavian artery follows the same course. The plexus splits into cords at or before it passes below the clavicle.

■ As the cords enter the axilla, they become closely related to the axillary artery, attaining positions relative to the artery indicated by their names: lateral, posterior, and medial.

Terminal Branches

■ Plexus gives off some terminal branches above the clavicle.

■ The dorsal scapular nerve comes off C5 with some C4 fibers and penetrates the scalenus medius and the levator scapulae, sometimes contributing with C4 fibers to the latter.

■ The dorsal scapular nerve accompanies the deep branch of the transverse cervical artery or the dorsal scapular artery on the undersurface of the rhomboids and innervates them.

■ Rootlets of the nerves C5, C6, and C7 immediately adjacent to the intravertebral foramina contribute to the formation of the long thoracic nerve, which immediately passes between the middle and posterior scalene muscles or penetrates the middle scalene.

■ Next most proximal nerve is the suprascapular nerve.

    ■ It arises from the superolateral aspect of the upper trunk shortly after its formation at Erb's point.

■ The lateral cord generally contains fibers of C5, C6, and C7 and gives off three terminal branches:

    ■ Musculocutaneous
    ■ Lateral pectoral
    ■ Lateral root of the median nerve

■ Posterior cord supplies most of the innervations of the muscles of the shoulder, in this order:

    ■ Upper subscapularis, thoracodorsal, lower subscapular, axillary, and radial

■ Medial cord has five branches, in the following order:

    ■ Medial pectoral nerve, medial brachial cutaneous, medial antebrachial cutaneous, medial root of the median nerve, and ulnar nerve

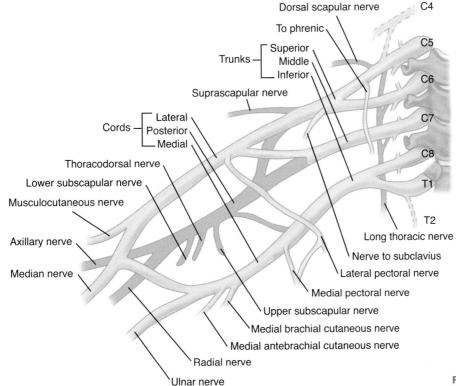

FIG 8 • The brachial plexus.

ARTERIES

Subclavian Artery

- Blood supply to limb begins with the subclavian artery, which ends at the lateral border of the first rib.
- Divided into three portions in relation to the insertion of the scalenus anterior muscle
- Vertebral artery takes origin in the first portion, and the costocervical trunk and thyrocervical trunk take origin in the second portion.
- There are usually no branches in the third portion of the artery.
- Two vessels encountered more frequently by the shoulder surgeon are the transverse cervical artery and the suprascapular artery.
  - Come off the thyrocervical trunk in 70% of dissections
  - In the remaining cases, they come off directly, or in common from the subclavian artery.

Axillary

- Is the continuation of the subclavian artery
- It begins at the lateral border of the first rib and continues along the inferior border of the latissimus dorsi, at which point it becomes the brachial artery.
- This artery is traditionally divided into three portions:
  - First portion is above the superior border of the pectoralis minor.
  - Second portion is deep to the pectoralis minor.
  - Third portion is distal to lateral border of the pectoralis minor.
- Usual number of branches for each of the three sections corresponds to the name of the section: one branch in the first portion, two in the second, and three in the third.
  - First section gives off the superior thoracic artery.
  - Second portion gives off the thoracoacromial artery and the lateral thoracic artery.
  - Third portion gives off the following:
    - Largest branch is the subscapular artery, and this is the largest branch of the axillary.
    - Next branch is the posterior humeral circumflex artery, and the third branch is the anterior humeral circumflex artery.
    - Anterior humeral circumflex artery is an important surgical landmark because it travels laterally at the inferior border of the subscapularis tendon, marking the border between the upper tendinous insertion of the subscapularis and the lower muscular insertion.

VEINS

Axillary Vein

- Begins at the inferior border of the latissimus dorsi as the continuation of the basilic vein, continues along the lateral border of the first rib, and becomes the subclavian vein

Cephalic

- Cephalic vein is the superficial vein in the arm that lies deep to the deep fascia after reaching the deltopectoral groove and finally pierces the clavipectoral fascia, emptying into the axillary vein.

ANATOMY OF THE ELBOW

OSTEOLOGY

Distal Humerus

- The distal humerus consists of two condyles, which form the articular surfaces of the trochlea and capitellum (**FIG 9A**).

Trochlea

- Hyperbolic, pulley-like surface that articulates with the semilunar notch of the ulna, covered by articular cartilage over an arc of 300 degrees
- Medial margin is large and projects more distally than does the lateral margin.
- The prominent medial and lateral margins are separated by a groove that courses in a helical manner from an anterolateral to the posteromedial direction.

Capitellum

- Capitellum is almost spheroidal in shape and is covered with hyaline cartilage, which is about 2 mm thick anteriorly.
- Posteromedial limit of the capitellum is marked by a prominent tubercle.
- A groove separates the capitellum from the trochlea, and the rim of the radial head articulates with this groove throughout the arc of flexion and during pronation and supination.

Joint Surface Orientation

- In the lateral plane, the orientation of the articular surface of the distal humerus is located anteriorly about 30 degrees with respect to the long axis of the humerus (**FIG 9B**).
- The center of the concentric arc formed by the trochlea and capitellum is on a line that is coplanar with the anterior and distal cortex of the humerus.
- In the transverse plane, the articular surface is rotated inwardly about 5 degrees, and in the frontal plane, it is tilted about 6 degrees in valgus (**FIG 9C**).

Epicondyles of Humerus

- Medial epicondyle serves as the source of attachment of the ulnar collateral ligament and the flexor pronator group of muscles.
- Lateral epicondyle is located just above the capitellum and is much less prominent than the medial epicondyle.
- The lateral collateral ligament and the supinator extensor muscle group originate from the flat, irregular surfaces of the lateral epicondyle.

Anterior Surface of Humerus

- Anteriorly, the radial and coronoid fossae accommodate the radial head and coronoid, respectively, during flexion.

Posterior Surface of Humerus

- Posteriorly, the olecranon fossa receives the tip of the olecranon in extension (**FIG 9D**).

Radius

- The proximal radius includes the radial head, which articulates with the capitellum and exhibits a cylindrical depression in the midportion to accommodate the capitellum.

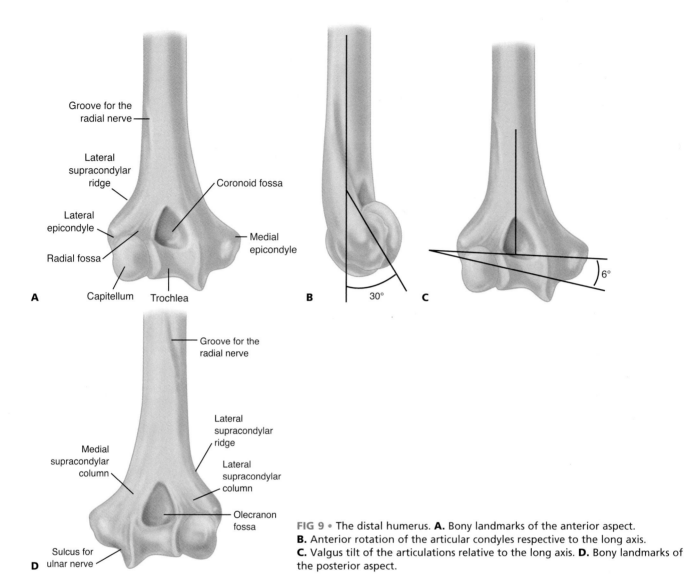

FIG 9 • The distal humerus. **A.** Bony landmarks of the anterior aspect. **B.** Anterior rotation of the articular condyles respective to the long axis. **C.** Valgus tilt of the articulations relative to the long axis. **D.** Bony landmarks of the posterior aspect.

▪ Hyaline cartilage covers the depression of the radial head. The outside circumference of the radial head articulates with the ulna at the lesser sigmoid notch.

▪ About 240 degrees of the circumference of the radial head is covered with cartilage. With the arm in neutral rotation, the anterolateral third of the circumference of the radial head is void of cartilage.

▪ This part of the radial head lacks subchondral bone, and thus is not as strong as the part that supports the articular cartilage.

▪ This part has been demonstrated to be the portion most often fractured.

▪ The disc-shaped head is held against the ulna by the annular ligament distal to the radial head.

▪ The head and neck of the radius are not colinear with the rest of the bone. The head and neck are offset by an angle of about 15 degrees with respect to the shaft of the radius opposite to the radial tuberosity (**FIG 10**).

▪ The neck of the radius is tapered, and the angular relationship between the head and neck has been implicated in the etiology of radial neck fractures.

Ulna

▪ The proximal ulna provides the major articulation of the elbow that is responsible for its inherent stability (**FIG 11A,B**).

▪ The broad, thick proximal aspect of the ulna consists of the greater sigmoid notch (incisura semilunaris), which articulates with the trochlea of the humerus.

▪ The sloped cortical surface of the coronoid process serves as the site of insertion of the brachialis muscle.

▪ The olecranon comprises the posterior portion of the articulation of the ulnohumeral joint and is the site of attachment for the triceps tendon.

▪ On the lateral aspect of the coronoid process, the lesser sigmoid or radial notch articulates with the radial head and is oriented roughly perpendicular to the long axis of the bone.

▪ On the lateral aspect of the proximal ulna, a tuberosity, the crista supinatoris, is the site of the insertion of the lateral ulnar collateral ligament (**FIG 11C**).

▪ This stabilizes the humeroulnar joint to resist varus and rotational stresses.

▪ The medial aspect of the coronoid process (sublime tubercle) serves as the site of attachment of the anterior bundle of the medial collateral ligament.

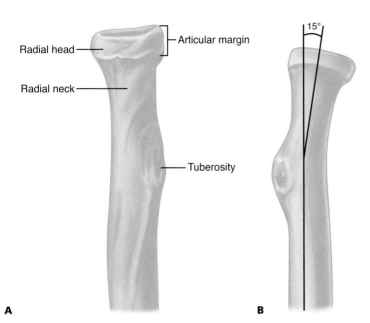

A

B

FIG 10 • The proximal radius. **A.** Bony landmarks. **B.** Angle of the radial neck relative to long axis.

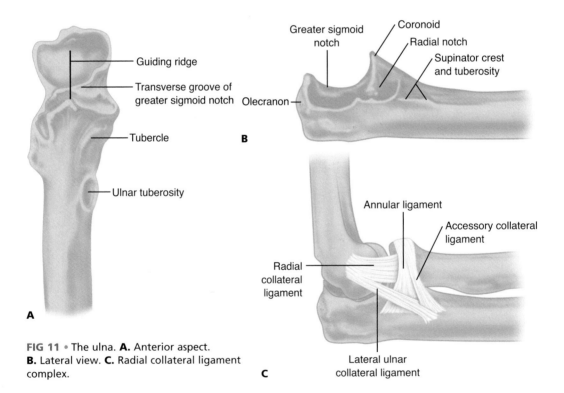

FIG 11 • The ulna. **A.** Anterior aspect. **B.** Lateral view. **C.** Radial collateral ligament complex.

SURVEY OF TOPICAL ANATOMY

Landmarks

Lateral Landmark

■ The tip of the olecranon, the lateral epicondyle, and the radial head form an equilateral triangle, providing an important landmark for entry into the elbow for such things as joint aspiration.

Flexion Crease

■ The flexion crease of the elbow is in line with the medial and lateral epicondyles. It is actually 1 to 2 cm proximal to the joint line when the elbow is extended.

Antecubital Fossa

■ Inverted triangular depression on the anterior aspect of the elbow that is just distal to the epicondyles

Topographical Regions of the Elbow and Corresponding Musculature

Lateral Margin of Antecubital Fossa

■ Extensor forearm musculature originates from the lateral epicondyle and has been termed the mobile wad.
■ This forms the lateral margin of the antecubital fossa and the lateral contour of the forearm and comprises the brachioradialis and the extensor carpi radialis longus and brevis muscles.

Medial Margin of the Antecubital Fossa

▪ Muscles making up the contour of the medial anterior forearm include the pronator teres, flexor carpi radialis, palmaris longus, and flexor carpi ulnaris.

Dorsum

▪ The dorsum of the forearm is contoured by the extensor musculature, consisting of the anconeus, extensor carpi ulnaris, extensor digitorum quinti, and extensor digitorum communis.

Cutaneous Innervation

Proximal Elbow

▪ Skin about the proximal elbow is innervated by the lower lateral cutaneous (C5, C6) and the medial cutaneous (radial nerve, C8, T1, and T2) nerves of the arm.

Forearm

▪ Forearm skin is innervated by the medial (C8, T1), lateral (musculocutaneous, C5, C6), and posterior (radial nerve, C6 through C8) cutaneous nerves of the forearm.

Elbow Joint Structure

Joint Articulation

▪ The elbow joint consists of two types of articulations:
▪ The ulnohumeral joint resembles a hinge (ginglymus), allowing flexion and extension.
▪ The radiohumeral and the proximal radioulnar joint allow actual rotation or pivoting type of motion.
▪ Because of this joint articulation, the elbow is classified as a trochoginglymoid joint and is one of the most congruent joints of the body.

Carrying Angle

▪ Angle formed by the long axis of the humerus and the ulna with the elbow fully extended
  ▪ In males, mean carrying angle is 11 to 14 degrees.
  ▪ In females, mean carrying angle 13 to 16 degrees.

Joint Capsule

▪ The anterior capsule inserts proximally above the coronoid and radial fossae.
▪ Distally, the capsule attaches to the anterior margin of the coronoid medially as well as to the annular ligament laterally.
▪ Posteriorly, the capsule attaches just above the olecranon fossa, distally along the supracondylar bony columns, and then down along the medial and lateral margins of the trochlea.
▪ Distally, the attachment is along the medial and lateral articular margin of the sigmoid notch; laterally, it occurs along the lateral aspect of the sigmoid notch and blends with the annular ligament.
▪ Normal capacity of the fully extended joint capsule is 25 to 30 mL.
▪ The joint capsule is innervated by branches from all major nerves crossing the joint, including contributions from the musculocutaneous nerve.

LIGAMENTS OF THE ELBOW

▪ Ligaments of the elbow consist of specialized thickening of the medial and lateral capsule that forms medial and lateral collateral ligament complexes.

Medial Collateral Ligament Complex

▪ The medial collateral ligament consists of three parts: anterior, posterior, and transverse segments.
▪ Anterior bundle is the most discrete component.
▪ The posterior portion, being a thickening of the posterior capsule, is well defined only in about 90 degrees of flexion.
▪ The transverse component appears to contribute a little or nothing to elbow stability.
▪ Clinically and experimentally, the anterior bundle is clearly the major portion of the medial ligament complex.

Lateral Collateral Ligament Complex

▪ Unlike the medial collateral ligament complex, with a rather consistent pattern, the lateral ligaments of the elbow joint are less discrete and some individual variation is common.
▪ Several components make up the lateral ligament complex: radial collateral ligament, the annular ligament, a variably present accessory lateral collateral ligament, and the lateral ulnar collateral ligament.

Lateral Ulnar Collateral Ligament

▪ This structure originates from the lateral epicondyle and blends with the fibers of the annular ligament, but arching superficial and distal to it.
▪ Insertion is through the tubercle of the crest of the supinator on the ulna.
▪ The function of this ligament is to provide stability to the ulnohumeral joint; it was shown to be deficient in posterolateral rotary instability of the joint.
▪ This ligament represents the primary lateral stabilizer of the elbow and is taut on flexion and extension.

Accessory Lateral Collateral Ligament

▪ Its function is to further stabilize the annular ligament during varus stress.

VESSELS

Brachial Artery and Its Branches

▪ The brachial artery descends in the arm, crossing in front of the intramuscular septum to lie anterior to the medial aspect of the brachialis muscle.
▪ The median nerve crosses in front of and medial to the artery at this point, near the middle of the arm. The artery continues distally at the medial margin of the biceps muscle and enters the antecubital space medial to the biceps tendon and lateral to the nerve.
▪ At the level of the radial head, it gives off its terminal branches, the ulnar and radial arteries, which continue into the forearm.

Radial Artery

▪ Usually the radial artery originates at the level of the radial head, emerges from the antecubital fossa between the brachioradialis and the pronator teres muscle, and continues down the forearm under the brachioradialis muscle.

Ulnar Artery

▪ The ulnar artery is the larger of the two terminal branches of the brachial artery.
▪ The artery traverses the pronator teres between its two heads and continues distally and medially behind the flexor digitorum superficialis muscle.

- It emerges medially to continue down the medial aspect of the forearm under the cover of the flexor carpi ulnaris.

NERVES

Musculocutaneous Nerve

- Originates from C5 through C8 nerve roots and is a continuation of the lateral cord
- Innervates the major elbow flexors and the biceps and brachialis and continues through the brachial fascia lateral to the biceps tendon, terminating as the lateral antebrachial cutaneous nerve
- Motor branch enters the biceps about 15 cm distal to the acromion; it enters the brachialis about 20 cm below the tip of the acromion.

Median Nerve

- Median nerve arises from C5 through C8 and T1 nerve roots.
- The nerve enters the anterior aspect of the brachium, crossing in front of the brachial artery as it passes across the intramuscular septum.
  - It follows a straight course into the medial aspect of the antecubital fossa, medial to the biceps tendon and the brachial artery.
  - It then passes under the bicipital aponeurosis.
  - There are no branches of the median nerve in the arm.
- The first motor branch is given to the pronator teres, through which it passes.
- In the antecubital fossa, a few small articular branches are given off before the motor branches to the pronator teres, the flexor carpi radialis, the palmaris longus, and the flexor digitorum superficialis.

Anterior Interosseous Nerve

- Arises from the median nerve near the inferior border of the pronator teres and travels along the anterior aspect of the interosseous membrane in the company of the anterior interosseous artery
- Innervates the flexor pollicis longus and the lateral portion of the flexor digitorum profundus

Radial Nerve

- Is a continuation of the posterior cord and originates from the C6, C7, and C8 nerve roots, with variable contributions of the C5 and T1 roots
- In the midportion of the arm, the nerve courses laterally just distal to the deltoid insertion to occupy the groove in the humerus that bears its name.
- It then emerges in a spiral path inferiorly and laterally to penetrate the lateral intramuscular septum.
- Before entering the anterior aspect of the arm, it gives off the motor branches to the medial and lateral heads of the triceps, accompanied by the deep branch of the brachial artery.
- After penetrating the lateral intramuscular septum in the distal third of the arm, it descends anterior to the lateral epicondyle behind the brachioradialis.
- It innervates the brachioradialis with a single branch to this muscle.
- In the antecubital space, the nerve divides into the superficial and deep branches. The superficial branch is the continuation of the radial nerve and extends into the forearm to innervate the mid-dorsal cutaneous aspect of the forearm.

- Motor branches of the radial nerve are given off to the triceps above the spiral groove, except for the branch to the medial head of the triceps, which originates at the entry to the spiral groove.
- This branch continues distally through the medial head to terminate as a muscular branch to the anconeus.
- In the antecubital space, the recurrent radial nerve curves around the posterolateral aspect of the radius, passing deep through supinator muscle, which it innervates. During its course through the supinator muscle, the nerve lies over the bare area, which is distal to and opposite to the radial tuberosity. The nerve is believed to be at risk at this site with fractures of the proximal radius. It emerges from the muscle as the posterior interosseous nerve, and the recurrent branch innervates the extensor digitorum minimi, the extensor carpi ulnaris, and occasionally the anconeus.
- The posterior interosseous nerve is accompanied by the posterior interosseous artery and sends further muscle branches distally to supply the abductor pollicis longus, the extensor pollicis longus, the extensor pollicis brevis, and the extensor indicis on the dorsum of the forearm.

Ulnar Nerve

- The ulnar nerve is derived from the medial cord of the brachial plexus from roots C8 and T1. In the mid-arm, it passes posteriorly through the medial intramuscular septum and continues distally along the medial margin of the triceps in the company of the superior ulnar collateral branch of the brachial artery and the ulnar collateral branch of the radial artery.
- There are no branches of this nerve in the brachium.
- The ulnar nerve may undergo compression as it passes behind the medial epicondyle, emerging into the forearm through the cubital tunnel.
- The roof of the cubital tunnel has been defined by a structure termed the cubital tunnel retinaculum.
- The first motor branch is the single nerve to the ulnar origin of the pronator and another one to the epicondylar head of the flexor carpi ulnaris. Distally, the nerve sends a motor branch to the ulnar half of the flexor digitorum profundus.
- Two cutaneous nerves arise from the ulnar nerve in the distal half of the forearm to innervate the skin of the wrist and the hand.

MUSCLES

Elbow Flexors

Biceps

- Covers the brachialis muscle in the distal arm and passes into the cubital fossa as the biceps tendon, which attaches to the posterior aspect of the radial tuberosity
- Bicipital aponeurosis or lacertus fibrosus is a broad, thin band of tissue that is a continuation of the anterior, medial, and distal muscle fascia. It runs obliquely to cover the median nerve and the brachial artery and inserts into the deep fascia of the forearm and possibly into the ulna as well.
- The biceps is a flexor of the elbow that has a large cross-sectional area but an intermediate mechanical advantage because it passes relatively close to the axis of rotation.
- In the pronated position, the biceps is a strong supinator of the forearm.

Brachialis

- Largest cross-sectional area of any of the elbow flexors but suffers from a poor mechanical advantage because it crosses so close to the axis of rotation
- Origin consists of the entire anterior distal half of the humerus, and it extends medially and laterally to the respective intermuscular septa.
- Crosses the anterior capsule, with some fibers inserting into the capsule that are said to help retract the capsule during elbow flexion
- Insertion of the brachialis is along the base of the coronoid and into the tuberosity of the ulna.
- More than 95% of the cross-sectional area is muscle tissue at the elbow joint, a relationship that may account for high incidence of trauma to this muscle with elbow dislocation.

Brachioradialis

- Has a lengthy origin along the lateral supracondylar column that extends proximally to the level of the junction of the middle and distal humerus
- Origin separates the lateral head of the triceps and the brachialis muscle
- Lateral border of the cubital fossa is formed by this muscle, which crosses the elbow joint with the greatest mechanical advantage of any elbow flexor. It progresses distally to insert into the base of the radial styloid.
- Protects and is innervated by radial nerve (C5 and C6) as it emerges from the spiral groove
- Major function is elbow flexion.

Extensor Carpi Radialis Longus

- Originates from the supracondylar bony column joint just below the origin of the brachioradialis
- As it continues into the midportion of the dorsum of the forearm, it becomes largely tendinous and inserts to the dorsal base of the second metacarpal.
- Innervated by the radial nerve
- Functions as wrist extensor, and possibly an elbow flexor

Extensor Carpi Radialis Brevis

- Originates from the lateral superior aspect of the lateral epicondyle
- Its origin is the most lateral of the extensor group and is covered by the extensor carpi radialis longus.
- This relationship is important as the most commonly implicated site of lateral epicondylitis.
- Extensor carpi radialis brevis shares the same extensor compartment as the longus as it crosses the wrist under the extensor retinaculum and inserts into the dorsal base of the third metacarpal.
- Function of the extensor carpi radialis brevis is pure wrist extension, with little or no radial or ulnar deviation.

Extensor Digitorum Communis

- Originating from the anterior distal aspect of the lateral epicondyle, the extensor digitorum communis accounts for most of the contour of the extensor surface of the forearm.
- Extends and abducts fingers
- Innervation is from the deep branch of the radial nerve, with contributions from the sixth through eighth cervical nerves.

Supinator

- This flat muscle is characterized by the virtual absence of tendinous tissue and has a complex origin and insertion.
- It originates from three sites above and below the elbow joint: the lateral anterior aspect of the lateral epicondyle; the lateral collateral ligament; and the proximal anterior crest of the ulna along the crista supinatoris, which is just anterior to the depression for the insertion of the anconeus.
- Form of the muscle is roughly that of a rhomboid as it runs obliquely, distally, and radially to wrap around and insert diffusely on the proximal radius, beginning lateral and proximal to the radial tuberosity and continuing distal to the insertion of the pronator teres at the junction of the proximal middle third of the radius.
- The radial nerve passes through the supinator to gain access to the extensor surface of the forearm.
  - This anatomic feature is clinically significant with regard to exposure of the lateral aspect of the elbow joint and the proximal radius and in certain entrapment syndromes.
- Functions as a supinator of the forearm, but it is a weaker supinator than the biceps.
  - Unlike the biceps, however, the effectiveness of the supinator is not altered by the position of the elbow flexion.
- Innervation is derived from the muscular branch given off by the radial nerve just before and during its course through the muscle.

Elbow Extensors

Triceps Brachii

- Comprises the entire musculature of the arm posteriorly
- Two of its three heads originate from the posterior aspect of the humerus.
- The long head has a discrete origin from the infraglenoid tuberosity of the scapula.
- The lateral head originates in a linear fashion from the proximal lateral intramuscular septum on the posterior surface of the humerus.
- The medial head originates from the entire distal half of the posteromedial surface of the humerus, bounded laterally by the radial groove and medially by the intramuscular septum.
- Each head originates distal to the other with progressively larger areas of origin.
- The long and lateral heads are superficial to the deep medial head, blending in the midline of the humerus to form a common muscle that then tapers into the triceps tendon and attaches to the tip of the olecranon with Sharpey fibers.
  - The tendon is usually separated from the olecranon by the subtendinous olecranon bursa.
- Innervated by the radial nerve, the long and lateral heads are supplied by branches that arise proximal to the entrance of the radial nerve into the groove.
  - The medial head is innervated distal to the groove with a branch that enters proximally and passes through the entire medial head to terminate by innervating the anconeus.

Anconeus

- This muscle has little tendinous tissue because it originates from a rather broad site on the posterior aspect of the lateral epicondyle and from the lateral triceps fascia and inserts into the lateral dorsal surface of the proximal ulna.

- Innervated by the terminal branch of the nerve to the medial head of the triceps
- Function of this muscle has been the subject of considerable speculation.
- Some suggest that the primary role is that of a joint stabilizer.
- Covers the lateral portion of the annular ligament and the radial head
- For the surgeon, the major significance of this muscle is its position as a key landmark in various lateral and posterolateral exposures, and it is used for some reconstructive procedures.

Flexor Pronator Muscle Group

Pronator Teres

- This is the most proximal of the flexor pronator group.
- There are usually two heads of origin; the larger arises from the anterosuperior aspect of the medial epicondyle and the second from the coronoid process of the ulna, which is absent in about 10% of individuals.
  - Two origins of the pronator muscle provide an arch through which the median nerve typically passes to gain access to the forearm.
  - This anatomic characteristic is a significant feature in the etiology of median nerve entrapment syndrome.
- The common muscle belly proceeds radially and distally under the brachioradialis, inserting at the junction of the proximal middle portion of the radius by a discrete broad tendinous insertion into a tuberosity on the lateral aspect of the bone.
- A strong pronator of the forearm, it also is considered a weak flexor of the elbow.
- Innervated by two motor branches from the median nerve

Flexor Carpi Radialis

- The flexor carpi radialis originates inferior to the origin of the pronator teres and the common flexor tendon at the anteroinferior aspect of the medial epicondyle.
- It continues distally and radially to the wrist, where it can be easily palpated before it inserts into the base of the second and sometimes third metacarpal.
- Chief function is as a wrist flexor
- Innervation is from one or two branches of the median nerve.

Palmaris Longus

- When present, it arises from the medial epicondyle and from the septa it shares with the flexor carpi radialis and flexor carpi ulnaris.

- It becomes tendinous in the proximal portion of the forearm and inserts into and becomes continuous with the palmar aponeurosis.
- Absent in about 10% of the extremities
- Innervated by a branch of the median nerve

Flexor Carpi Ulnaris

- Most posterior of the common flexor tendons originating from the medial epicondyle
- Second and largest source of origin is from the medial border of the coronoid and the proximal aspect of the ulna.
- Ulnar nerve enters and innervates the muscle between these two sites of origin with two or three motor branches given off just after the nerve has entered the muscle. The muscle continues distally to insert into the pisiform, where the tendon is easily palpable, because it serves as a wrist flexor and ulnar deviator.
- With an origin posterior to the axis of rotation, weak elbow extension may also be provided by the flexor carpi ulnaris.

Flexor Digitorum Superficialis

- The flexor digitorum superficialis muscle is deep to those originating from the common flexor tendon but superficial to the flexor digitorum profundus; thus it is considered the intermediate muscle layer.
- This broad muscle has a complex origin.
  - Medially, it arises from the medial epicondyle by way of the common flexor tendon and possibly from the ulnar collateral ligament and medial aspect of the coronoid.
  - The lateral head is smaller and thinner and arises from the proximal two thirds of the radius.
- The unique origin of the muscle forms a fibrous margin under which the median nerve and ulnar artery emerge as they exit from the cubital fossa.
- The muscle is innervated by the median nerve with branches that originate before the median nerve enters the pronator teres.
- Action of the flexor digitorum superficialis is flexion of the proximal interphalangeal joints.

Flexor Digitorum Profundus

- Originates from the proximal ulna distal to the elbow joint and is involved in flexion of the distal interphalangeal joints

Chapter 2

Surgical Approaches to the Shoulder and Elbow

Joseph A. Abboud, Matthew L. Ramsey, and Gerald R. Williams

SHOULDER APPROACHES

ANTERIOR APPROACH TO THE SHOULDER

Indications

- Surgical stabilization for recurrent dislocations
- Subscapularis and biceps tendon repair
- Shoulder arthroplasty
- Fracture fixation

Incisions

- Anterior shoulder can be approached through two different incisions.
- Anterior incision:
  - 10- to 15-cm incision along the deltopectoral interval (**FIG 1A**)
  - Incision begins just above the coracoid process and progresses toward the deltoid tuberosity.
- Axillary incision
  - Vertical incision 8 to 10 cm long (**FIG 1B**)
  - Incision begins inferior to the tip of the coracoid and progresses toward the anterior axillary fold.

Internervous Plane

- Deltoid muscle is supplied by the axillary nerve.
- Pectoralis major muscle is supplied by medial and lateral pectoral nerves.

Surgical Dissection

- Skin flaps are developed around the deltopectoral interval.
- The deltopectoral interval, with its cephalic vein, is identified.
- The deltopectoral interval is developed by retracting the pectoralis major medially and the deltoid laterally.
  - Vein may be retracted either medially or laterally.
  - We prefer to take it laterally, as fewer tributaries are disrupted.
- The lateral border of the conjoint tendon is identified and the short head of the biceps (supplied by the musculocutaneous nerve) and coracobrachialis (supplied by the musculocutaneous nerve) are displaced medially to allow access to the anterior aspect of the shoulder joint.
  - Simple medial retraction of the conjoined tendon may be enough for a procedure such as subscapularis repair or capsular repair.
  - If more exposure is necessary, the conjoint tendon can be detached with the tip of the coracoid process.
- The axillary artery is surrounded by cords of brachial plexus, which lie behind the pectoralis minor muscle.
  - To minimize risk for nerve injury, the arm should be kept adducted while work is being done around the coracoid process.
  - Remember, the musculocutaneous nerve enters the coracobrachialis on its medial side.

- Overly aggressive retraction can cause a neurapraxia of the musculocutaneous nerve.
- Behind the conjoined tendon of the coracobrachialis and the short head of biceps lies the subscapularis muscle.
- Externally rotating the arm brings the subscapularis further into the operative field.
  - This maneuver increases the distance between the subscapularis and axillary nerve as it disappears below the lower border of the muscle.
- Identifiable landmarks on the inferior border of the subscapularis are three small vessels (from the anterior humeral circumflex artery) that run transversely and often require ligation or cauterization.
  - These vessels run as a triad (often called the "three sisters"): a small artery with its two surrounding venae comitantes.
- The superior border of the subscapularis muscle blends in with the fibers of the supraspinatus muscle in the rotator interval (**FIG 1C**).
  - The tendon of the subscapularis is tagged with stay sutures.
  - There are various ways of taking down the subscapularis as per surgeon preference.
    - Some divide the subscapularis 1 to 2 cm from its insertion onto the lesser tuberosity.
    - Some detach this insertion with a small flake of bone using an osteotome.
- Inferior border of the subscapularis is the easiest location to allow separation between the subscapularis and capsule.
- The capsule is incised longitudinally to enter the joint wherever the selected repair must be performed.

ANTEROSUPERIOR APPROACH TO THE SHOULDER

Indications

- Rotator cuff repair
- Subacromial decompression of the shoulder
- Acromioclavicular reconstructions
- Greater tuberosity fractures
- Removal of calcific deposits from the subacromial bursa
- Reverse shoulder replacement

Incision

- An incision is made paralleling the lateral acromion that begins at the anterolateral corner of the acromion and ends just lateral to the tip of the coracoid (**FIG 2A**).

Internervous Plane

- The deltoid muscle is detached proximal to its nerve supply; therefore, there is no internervous plane with this approach.

Surgical Dissection

- The incision is deepened to the deep deltoid fascia.
- Subcutaneous flaps are raised.

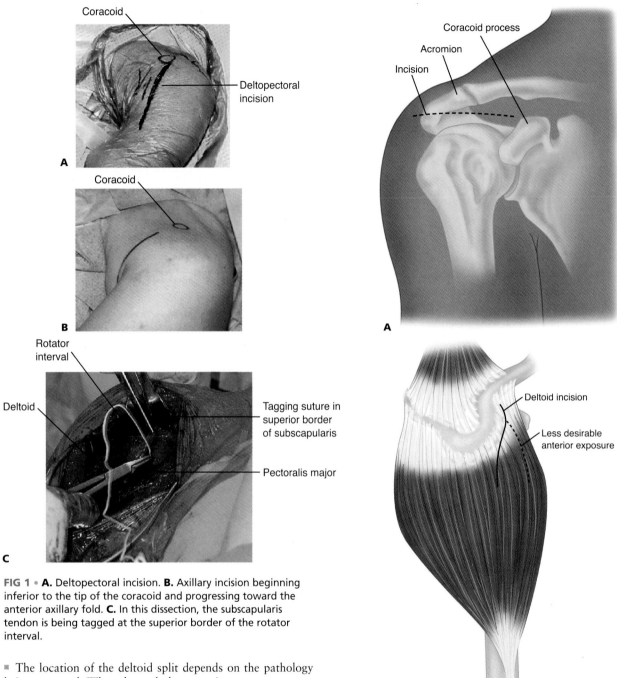

FIG 1 • **A.** Deltopectoral incision. **B.** Axillary incision beginning inferior to the tip of the coracoid and progressing toward the anterior axillary fold. **C.** In this dissection, the subscapularis tendon is being tagged at the superior border of the rotator interval.

FIG 2 • **A.** Anterosuperior approach to the shoulder. A transverse incision begins at the anterolateral corner of the acromion and ends just lateral to the coracoid. **B.** The posterior curve of the deltoid incision can be moved more posteriorly, as depicted here, to allow necessary exposure as dictated by the pathology.

- The location of the deltoid split depends on the pathology being managed. When the pathology requires more exposure, moving the deltoid split posteriorly will improve exposure (**FIG 2B**).
- Subperiosteally, the anterior deltoid is elevated from the acromion and the acromioclavicular joint. Continue the detachment by sharp dissection laterally to expose the anterior aspect of the acromion.
  - Bleeding will be encountered during this dissection as a result of the division of the acromial branch of the coracoacromial artery.
  - The surgeon should not detach more of the deltoid than is necessary.
- The deltoid split is extended 2 to 3 cm distal to the acromion.
  - Stay sutures are inserted in the apex of the split to prevent the muscle from inadvertently splitting distally during retraction and damaging the axillary nerve.

- The split edges of the deltoid muscle are retracted to reveal the underlying coracoacromial ligament.
- The coracoacromial ligament is detached from the acromion by sharp dissection.
- The supraspinatus tendon with its overlying subacromial bursa now can be visualized.
- The head of the humerus is rotated to expose different portions of the rotator cuff.

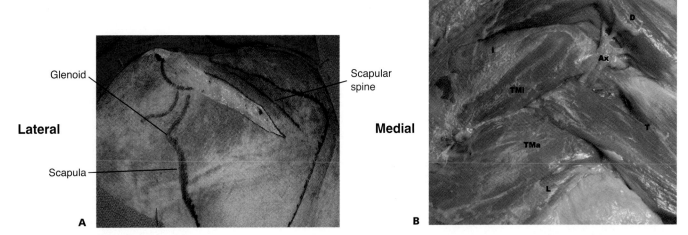

FIG 3 • **A.** Horizontal incision along the scapular spine allowing for the posterior approach to the shoulder. **B.** Cadaveric specimen depicting the internervous plane between the infraspinatus and teres minor as well as the axillary nerve in the quadrangular space. (**A**: From Goss TP. Glenoid fractures: open reduction and internal fixation. In: Widd, DA, ed. Master Techniques in Orthopaedic Surgery: Fractures, ed 2. Philadelphia: Lippincott Williams & Wilkins, 1998:3–17; **B**: Courtesy of Jesse A. McCarron, MD, Michael Codsi, MD, and Joseph P. Iannotti, MD.)

POSTERIOR APPROACH TO THE SHOULDER

Indications

- Repair in cases of recurrent posterior dislocation or subluxation of the shoulder
- Glenoid osteotomy
- Treatment of fractures of the scapular neck
- Treatment of posterior fracture and dislocations of the proximal humerus
- Spinoglenoid notch cyst drainage

Incision

- A horizontal incision is made along the scapular spine extending to the posterolateral corner of the acromion (**FIG 3A**)

Internervous Plane

- Between teres minor (axillary nerve) and infraspinatus (suprascapular nerve)
- The suprascapular nerve passes around the base of the spine of the scapula as it runs from the supraspinatus fossa to the infraspinatus fossa.

Surgical Dissection

- The origin of the deltoid is identified on the scapular spine. There are three ways to manage the deltoid during posterior exposures:
  - Detach the origin on the scapular spine
  - Split the deltoid muscle along the length of its fibers
  - Elevate the deltoid from the inferior margin
- The plane between the deltoid muscle and the underlying infraspinatus muscle is identified.
  - The plane is easier to locate at the lateral end of the incision.
- The internervous plane between the infraspinatus and teres minor muscles is identified (**FIG 3B**).
  - The axillary nerve runs longitudinally in the quadrangular space beneath the teres minor.
  - The posterior circumflex humeral artery runs with the axillary nerve in the quadrangular space between the inferior borders of the teres minor muscle.

- The infraspinatus is retracted superiorly and the teres minor inferiorly to reach the posterior regions of the glenoid cavity and the neck of the scapula.
- The posteroinferior corner of the shoulder joint capsule should be visible.

HUMERUS APPROACHES

ANTERIOR APPROACH TO THE HUMERUS

Indications

- Internal fixation of fractures of the humerus
- Management of humeral nonunions
- Osteotomy of the humerus

Incision

- A longitudinal incision is made over the tip of the coracoid process of the scapula; it runs distally and laterally in the line of the deltopectoral interval to the insertion of the deltoid muscle on the lateral aspect of the humerus, about halfway down its shaft.
- The incision should be continued distally as far as necessary, following the lateral border of the biceps muscle (**FIG 4A**).

Internervous Plane

- The anterior approach uses two different internervous planes.
- Proximally, the plane lies between the deltoid muscle (supplied by axillary nerve) and the pectoralis major muscle (supplied by medial and lateral pectoral nerves) (**FIG 4B**).
- Distally, the plane lies between the medial fibers of the brachialis muscle (musculocutaneous nerve) and the lateral fibers of the brachialis muscle (radial nerve) (**FIG 4C**).

Surgical Dissection

Proximal Humeral Shaft

- The deltopectoral interval is identified using the cephalic vein as a guide and the two muscles are separated, retracting the cephalic vein either medially with the pectoralis major or laterally with the deltoid.

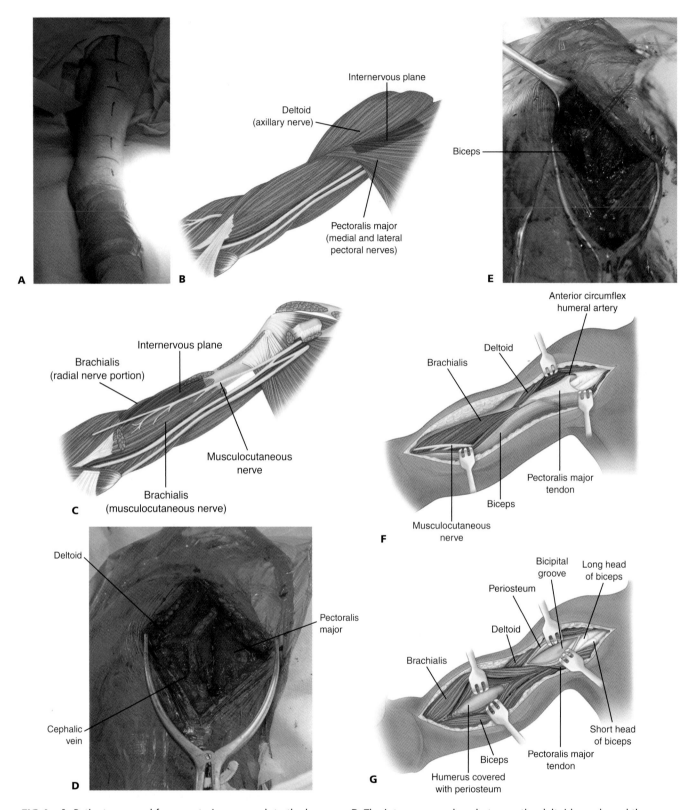

FIG 4 • A. Patient prepared for an anterior approach to the humerus. **B.** The internervous plane between the deltoid muscle and the pectoralis major muscle. **C.** Further distally, one can appreciate the internervous plane between the medial fibers of the brachialis (musculocutaneous nerve) medially and the lateral fibers of the brachialis (radial nerve) laterally. **D.** Deltopectoral incision: developing the interval between the deltoid and pectoralis major. The cephalic vein can be seen separating these two structures. **E.** With deeper dissection, the biceps tendon is seen running in the rotator interval. **F.** Further distal dissection reveals the musculocutaneous nerve passing along the medial border of the biceps muscle. **G.** To expose the distal third of the humerus, the fibers of the brachialis are split. Flexion of the elbow will relieve the tension off the brachialis, making the exposure easier. (**A**: Courtesy of Matthew J. Garberina, MD, and Charles L. Getz, MD.)

▪ The muscular interval is developed distally down to the insertion of the deltoid into the deltoid tuberosity and the insertion of the pectoralis major into the lateral lip of the bicipital groove (**FIG 4D,E**).

▪ To expose the bone fully, the surgeon may need to detach part or all of the insertion of pectoralis major muscle.

▪ The minimum amount of soft tissue should be detached to allow adequate visualization and reduction of the fracture.

▪ If further exposure is needed, the surgeon dissects medially in a subperiosteal manner to avoid damage to the radial nerve, which lies in the spiral groove of the humerus and crosses the back of the middle third of the bone in a medial to lateral direction.

Distal Humeral Shaft

▪ The surgeon identifies the muscular interval between the biceps brachii and brachialis.

▪ The interval is developed by retracting the biceps medially (**FIG 4F**).

▪ Beneath it lies the brachialis muscle, which covers the humeral shaft.

▪ The fibers of the brachialis are split longitudinally in the interval between the medial 2/3 and the lateral 1/3 to expose the periosteum on the anterior surface of the humeral shaft.

▪ The periosteum is incised longitudinally in line with the muscle dissection, and the brachialis is stripped off the anterior surface of the bone (**FIG 4G**).

▪ In the anterior compartment of the distal third of the arm, the radial nerve pierces the lateral intermuscular septum and lies between the brachioradialis and brachialis muscles.

POSTERIOR APPROACH TO THE HUMERUS

Indications

▪ Open reduction and internal fixation of a fracture of the humerus

▪ Treatment of nonunion

▪ Exploration of the radial nerve in the spiral groove

Incision

▪ A longitudinal incision is made in the midline of the posterior aspect of the arm, from 8 cm below the acromion to the olecranon fossa (**FIG 5A**).

Internervous Plane

▪ There is no true internervous plane; dissection involves separating the heads of the triceps brachii muscles, all of which are supplied by the radial nerve.

▪ The medial head, which is the deepest, has a dual nerve supply (radial and ulnar nerves).

Surgical Dissection

▪ The surgeon incises the deep fascia of the arm in line with the skin incision.

▪ The triceps muscle has two layers:

▪ The outer layer consists of two heads: the lateral head arises from the lateral lip of the spiral groove, and the long head arises from the infraglenoid tubercle of the scapula (**FIG 5B**).

▪ The inner layer consists of the medial head, which arises from the whole width of the posterior aspect of the humerus

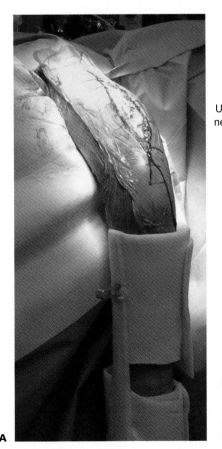

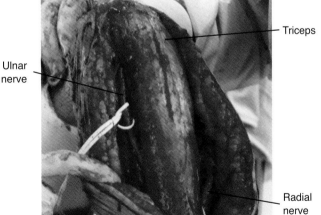

Distal

Ulnar nerve

Triceps

Radial nerve

Proximal

FIG 5 ▪ **A.** Posterior approach to the humerus, showing the longitudinal incision along the midline of the posterior aspect of the arm. **B.** Once the outer layer of the triceps is isolated, one can see the two heads, the lateral head and long head. (*continued*)

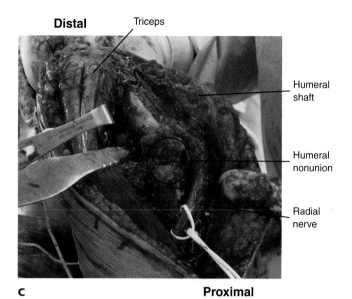

Distal Triceps

Humeral shaft

Humeral nonunion

Radial nerve

C **Proximal**

FIG 5 • (*continued*) **C.** In this humeral shaft nonunion, the triceps is reflected medially and the radial nerve can be seen passing through the spiral groove. (**A**: Courtesy of Matthew J. Garberina, MD, and Charles L. Getz, MD.)

below the spiral groove all the way down to the distal fourth of the bone.

▪ The spiral groove contains the radial nerve; the radial nerve separates the origins of the lateral and medial heads (**FIG 5C**).

▪ To avoid iatrogenic nerve injury, the surgeon should never continue dissection down to bone in the proximal two thirds of the arm until the radial nerve has been identified.

MODIFIED POSTERIOR APPROACH TO THE HUMERUS

Indications

▪ Open reduction and internal fixation of humeral shaft fractures

▪ Open reduction and internal fixation of lateral condyle fractures

▪ Treatment of humeral nonunion

▪ Exploration of the radial nerve in the spiral groove

Incision

▪ The surgeon makes a straight incision along a line between the posterolateral aspect of the acromion and the lateral edge of the olecranon.

▪ The length of the incision is dictated by the requirement for exposure.

▪ Extensile exposure is limited proximally by the axillary nerve.

Internervous Plane

▪ There is no true internervous plane, because both the medial and lateral heads of the triceps are supplied by the radial nerve.

Surgical Dissection

▪ The deep fascia is incised in line with the skin incision along the lateral aspect of the triceps.

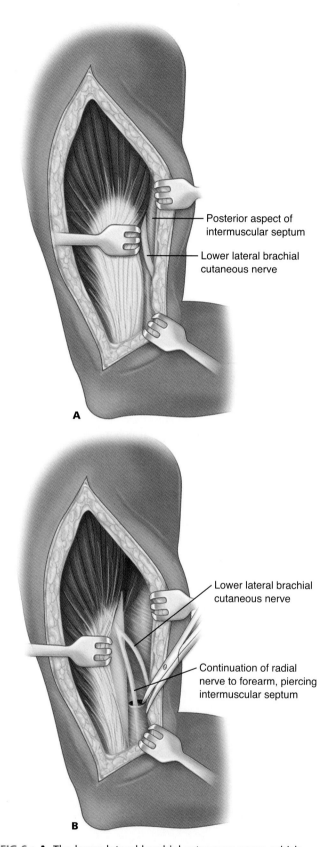

Posterior aspect of intermuscular septum

Lower lateral brachial cutaneous nerve

A

Lower lateral brachial cutaneous nerve

Continuation of radial nerve to forearm, piercing intermuscular septum

B

FIG 6 • A. The lower lateral brachial cutaneous nerve, which branches off the radial nerve, is identified along the posterior aspect of the intermuscular septum. The entire triceps here is retracted slightly medially. **B.** The intermuscular septum is divided deep to the lower lateral brachial cutaneous nerve for 3 cm to expose the radial nerve distally. (*continued*)

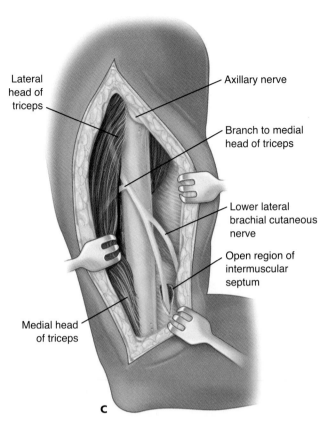

Lateral head of triceps

Axillary nerve

Branch to medial head of triceps

Lower lateral brachial cutaneous nerve

Open region of intermuscular septum

Medial head of triceps

C

FIG 6 • (*continued*) **C.** The medial and lateral heads of the triceps are retracted subperiosteally in a medial direction to expose the posterior aspect of the humeral diaphysis.

■ The triceps is retracted medially and the lower lateral brachial cutaneous nerve branch from the radial nerve is identified. This nerve is traced proximally to the main trunk of the radial nerve (**FIG 6A**).

■ The intermuscular septum is divided distally to allow the radial nerve to be mobilized (**FIG 6B**).

■ Subperiosteally, the medial and lateral heads of the triceps are reflected medially to expose the humeral shaft (**FIG 6C**).

ELBOW APPROACHES

■ The surgical exposures described for the elbow are divided into posterior, medial, and lateral approaches. These descriptions denote the deep surgical interval employed.

■ Often, these deep approaches can be performed through a direct medial or lateral skin incision or a more versatile posterior incision.

POSTERIOR APPROACH TO THE ELBOW

■ Releasing the triceps attachment to the olecranon is not advisable, owing to the difficulty of adequate repair and possible disruption during rehabilitation. Today, there are four choices of posterior exposure:
- Triceps splitting
- Triceps reflecting
- Triceps preserving
- Olecranon osteotomy

Triceps-Splitting Approaches

Posterior Triceps-Splitting Approach (Campbell)

■ Care must be exercised to maintain the medial portion of the triceps expansion over the forearm fascia in continuity with the flexor carpi ulnaris.

■ Laterally, the anconeus and triceps are more stable, with less chance of disruption.

INDICATIONS

■ Total elbow arthroplasty
■ Distal humerus fracture
■ Removal of loose bodies
■ Capsulectomies
■ Posterior exposure of the joint for ankylosis, sepsis, synovectomy, and ulnohumeral arthroplasty

APPROACH

■ Skin incision begins in the midline over the triceps, about 10 cm above the joint line, and is generally placed laterally or medially across the tip of the olecranon. It continues distally over the lateral aspect of the subcutaneous border of the proximal ulna for about 5 to 6 cm (**FIG 7A**).

■ Triceps is exposed, along with the proximal 4 cm of the ulna.

■ A midline incision is made through the triceps fascia and tendon as it is continued distally across the insertion of the triceps tendon at the tip of the olecranon and down the subcutaneous crest of the ulna (**FIG 7B**).

■ Triceps tendon and muscle are split longitudinally, exposing the distal humerus.

■ Anconeus is then reflected subperiosteally laterally, while the flexor carpi ulnaris is similarly retracted medially.

■ Insertion of the triceps is carefully released from the olecranon, leaving the extensor mechanism in continuity with the forearm fascia and muscles medially and laterally (**FIG 7C**).

■ Ulnar nerve is visualized and protected in the cubital tunnel.

■ Closure of the triceps fascia is required only proximal to the olecranon, but the insertion should be repaired to the olecranon with a suture passed through the ulna.

■ The incision is then closed in layers.

Triceps-Splitting, Tendon-Reflecting Approach (Van Gorder)

■ A variation of the technique described earlier
■ Allows lengthening of the triceps if necessary
■ Has been largely abandoned in favor of the triceps-reflecting techniques

INDICATIONS

■ Same as those for midline-splitting approach described earlier

APPROACH

■ A posterior midline incision begins 10 cm proximal to the olecranon and extends distally onto the subcutaneous border of the ulna between the anconeus and the flexor carpi ulnaris.

■ Triceps fascia and aponeurosis are exposed along the tendinous insertion into the ulna.

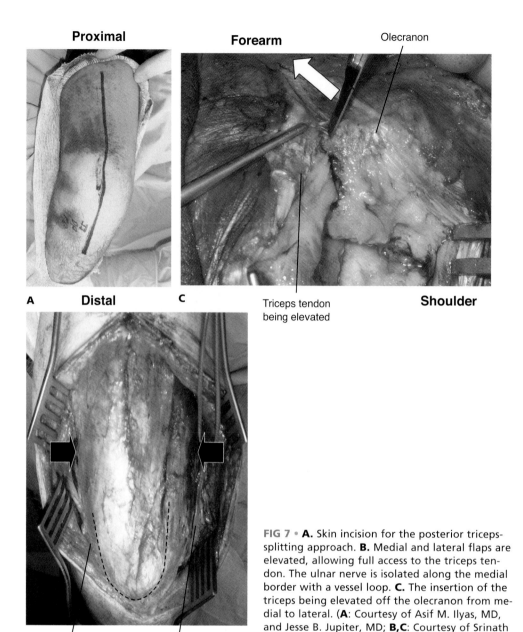

FIG 7 • A. Skin incision for the posterior triceps-splitting approach. **B.** Medial and lateral flaps are elevated, allowing full access to the triceps tendon. The ulnar nerve is isolated along the medial border with a vessel loop. **C.** The insertion of the triceps being elevated off the olecranon from medial to lateral. (**A**: Courtesy of Asif M. Ilyas, MD, and Jesse B. Jupiter, MD; **B,C**: Courtesy of Srinath Kamineni, MD.)

▪ Tendon is reflected from the muscle in a proximal to distal direction, freeing the underlying muscle fibers while preserving the tendinous attachment to the olecranon (**FIG 8**).

▪ Triceps muscle is then split in midline, and the distal humerus is exposed subperiosteally.

▪ Periosteum and triceps are elevated for a distance of about 5 cm proximal to the olecranon fossa, exposing the posterior aspect of the joint.

▪ If more extensive exposure is desired, the subperiosteal dissection is extended to the level of the joint, exposing the condyles both medially and laterally.

▪ Ulnar nerve should be identified and protected.

▪ After the procedure, if an elbow contracture has been corrected, the joint should be maximally flexed.

▪ The tendon slides distally from its initial position, and the proximal muscle and tendon are reapproximated in the lengthened relationship.

▪ The distal part of the triceps is then securely sutured to the fascia of the triceps expansion, and the remainder of the wound is closed in layers.

Triceps-Reflecting Approaches

▪ The triceps mechanism may be preserved in continuity with the anconeus and simply reflected to one side or the other.

▪ Three surgical approaches have been described that preserve the triceps muscle and tendon in continuity with the distal musculature of the forearm fascia and expose the entire joint.

Bryan-Morrey Posteromedial Triceps-Reflecting Approach

▪ Developed to preserve the continuity of the triceps with the anconeus

INDICATIONS

▪ Total elbow arthroplasty
▪ Interposition arthroplasty

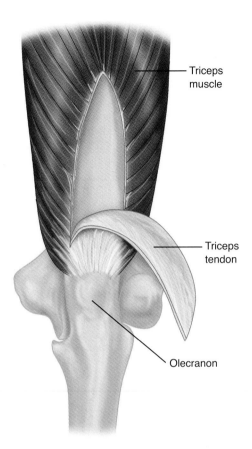

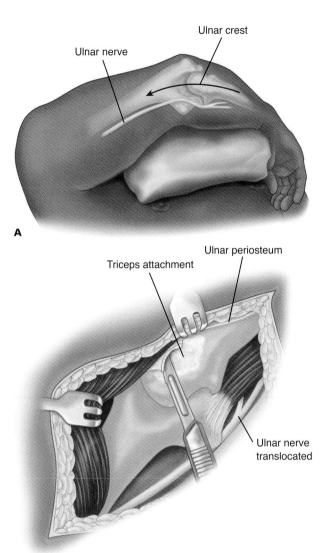

FIG 8 • Triceps-splitting, tendon-reflecting approach. The tendon is reflected from the muscle in a proximal to distal direction.

- Elbow dislocation
- Distal humerus fracture
- Synovial disease
- Infection

APPROACH

- A straight posterior incision is made medial to the midline, about 9 cm proximal and 8 cm distal to the tip of the olecranon (**FIG 9A**).
- The ulnar nerve is identified proximally at the margin of the medial head of the triceps and, depending on the procedure, is either protected or carefully dissected to its first motor branch and transposed anteriorly.
- The medial aspect of the triceps is elevated from the posterior capsule.
- The fascia of the forearm between the anconeus and the flexor carpi ulnaris is incised distally for about 6 cm.
- The triceps and the anconeus are elevated as one flap from medial to lateral, skeletonizing the olecranon and subcutaneous border of the ulna (**FIG 9B**). This should be performed at 20 to 30 degrees of flexion to relieve tension on the insertion, thereby facilitating dissection.
- The collateral ligaments may be released from the humerus for exposure as needed (**FIG 9C**).
  - If stability is important, these ligaments should be preserved or anatomically repaired at the conclusion of the surgery.
  - When performing a linked total elbow replacement, it is not necessary to preserve or repair the collateral ligaments.

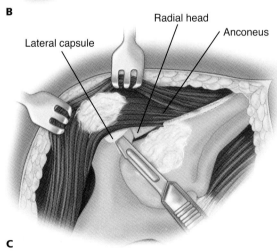

FIG 9 • The Bryan-Morrey posterior approach. **A.** Straight posterior skin incision. **B.** The ulnar nerve has been translocated anteriorly. The medial border of the triceps is identified and released and the superficial forearm fascia is sharply incised to allow reflection of the fascia and periosteum from the proximal ulna. **C.** The extensor mechanism has been reflected laterally and the collateral ligaments have been released.

- The triceps attachment can be thin at the attachment to the ulna and it is not uncommon for a buttonhole to be created when reflecting the triceps.
  - To prevent this, the flap can be raised as an osteoperiosteal flap (see osteocutaneous flap approach).
    - A small osteotome is used to elevate the fascia with the petals of bone.
    - The flap is mobilized laterally, elevating the anconeus origin from the distal humerus until it can be folded over the lateral humeral condyle.
    - At this point, the radial head can be visualized.
- The tip of the olecranon can be excised to help expose the trochlea.

Osteoanconeus Flap Approach

- This provides excellent extension and reliable healing of the osseous attachment to the olecranon.
- This approach exposes only the ulnar nerve, whereas the Mayo approach translocates the nerve.

INDICATIONS

- This is a triceps-reflecting approach similar in concept to the Bryan-Morrey triceps-reflecting approach.
- Most often used for joint replacement or distal humeral fractures

APPROACH

- A straight posterior incision is made medial to the midline, about 9 cm proximal and 8 cm distal to the tip of the olecranon.
- The ulnar nerve is identified and protected, but not translocated.
- The triceps attachment is released from the ulna by osteotomizing the attachment with a thin wafer of bone.
  - This is the essential difference from the Bryan-Morrey approach.
- The medial aspect of the triceps, in continuity with the anconeus, is elevated from the ulna (**FIG 10A,B**).
- The collateral ligaments are either maintained or released, depending on the pathology being addressed and the need for stability.
- After the surgical procedure, the wafer of bone is secured to its bed by nonabsorbable sutures placed through bone holes (**FIG 10C**).
- Interrupted sutures are used to repair the remaining distal portion of the extensor mechanism.

Extensile Kocher Posterolateral Triceps-Reflecting Approach

INDICATIONS

- Joint arthroplasty
- Ankylosis
- Distal humerus fractures
- Synovectomy
- Radial head excision
- Infection

APPROACH

- Extensile exposure from the Kocher approach
- Skin incision begins 8 cm proximal to the joint just posterior to the supracondylar ridge and continues distally over the Kocher interval between the anconeus and extensor carpi ulnaris about 6 cm distal to the tip of the olecranon

- Proximally, the triceps is identified and freed from the brachioradialis and extensor carpi radialis longus along the intramuscular septum to the level of the joint capsule.
- The interval between the extensor carpi ulnaris and the anconeus is identified distally.
- The triceps in continuity with the anconeus is subperiosteally reflected. Sharp dissection frees the bony attachment of the triceps expansion to the anconeus from the lateral epicondyle.
- The triceps remains attached to the tip of the olecranon.
- The lateral collateral ligament complex is released from the humerus.
- The joint may be dislocated with varus stress. If additional exposure is necessary, the anterior and posterior capsule can be released.
- Routine closure of layers is performed, but the radial collateral ligament should be reattached to the bone through holes placed in the lateral epicondyle.

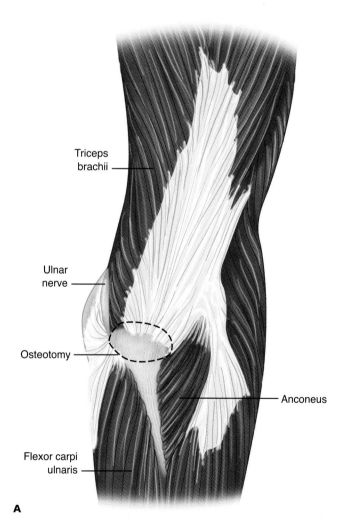

A

FIG 10 • Posterior view of the right elbow demonstrates a straight fascial incision to the lateral aspect of the tip of the olecranon. **A.** The line of release after the ulnar nerve has been identified and protected. *(continued)*

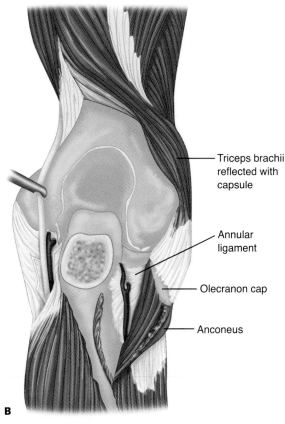

Triceps brachii
reflected with
capsule

Annular
ligament

Olecranon cap

Anconeus

B

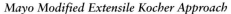

C

FIG 10 • *(continued)* **B.** The olecranon has been osteotomized and the triceps swept from medial to lateral in continuity with the anconeus and forearm fascia. **C.** Closure with sutures placed through bone and the distal extensor mechanism is done with interrupted sutures.

Mayo Modified Extensile Kocher Approach

▪ The extensile Kocher approach and the Mayo modification of the extensile Kocher approach provide sequentially greater exposure from the initial Kocher approach.

INDICATIONS

▪ Release of ankylosed joint
▪ Interposition arthroplasty
▪ Replacement arthroplasty

APPROACH

▪ A modification of the extensile Kocher approach consists of reflecting the anconeus and triceps expansion from the tip of the olecranon by sharp dissection.
▪ The extensor mechanism (triceps in continuity with the anconeus) may be reflected from lateral to medial.
▪ The ulnar nerve should be decompressed or transposed if an extensile lateral approach is used.
▪ The triceps is reattached in a fashion identical to that described for the Mayo approach.

Triceps-Preserving Approaches

Posterior Triceps-Sparing Approach

▪ Because the triceps is not elevated from the tip of the olecranon, rapid rehabilitation is possible.

INDICATIONS

▪ Tumor resection
▪ Joint reconstruction for resection of humeral nonunion
▪ Joint replacement

APPROACH

▪ A posterior incision is made medial to the tip of the olecranon.
▪ Medial and lateral subcutaneous skin flaps are elevated.
▪ The ulnar nerve is identified and transposed anteriorly.
▪ The medial and lateral aspects of the triceps are identified and developed distally to the triceps attachment on the ulna.
▪ For distal humerus fractures fixation:
  ▪ The common flexors and common extensors are partially released from the distal humerus to expose the supracondylar column for plate fixation.
▪ For total elbow arthroplasty or tumor resection:
  ▪ The common flexors and extensors are fully released from the medial and lateral epicondyle. The collateral ligaments and capsule are released and the distal humerus is excised.
  ▪ The distal humerus is exposed by bringing it through the defect along the lateral margin of the triceps.
  ▪ The ulna is exposed by supinating the forearm.
  ▪ After the implant has been inserted, the joint is articulated.

■ There is no need to close or repair the extensor mechanism with this approach.

Olecranon Osteotomy

■ Worldwide, the transosseous approach is probably the exposure most often used, especially for distal humeral fractures. The oblique osteotomy has almost been abandoned, and the transverse osteotomy has largely been replaced by the chevron.

Chevron Transolecranon Osteotomy

■ Intra-articular osteotomy, first described by MacAusland, was originally recommended for ankylosed joints.
■ It has been adapted by some for radial head excision and synovectomy and used or modified by others for T and Y condylar fractures.
■ The chevron osteotomy enhances rotational stability compared to a transverse osteotomy.

INDICATIONS

■ Ankylosed joints
■ T or Y condylar fractures

APPROACH

■ A posterior incision is made medial to the tip of the olecranon.
■ Medial and lateral subcutaneous skin flaps are elevated.
■ The ulnar nerve is identified and transposed anteriorly.
■ The medial and lateral aspects of the triceps are identified and developed distally to the triceps attachment on the ulna.
■ An apex-distal chevron or V osteotomy is performed with a thin oscillating saw but not completed through the subchondral bone. An osteotome completes the osteotomy, creating irregular surfaces that interdigitate increasing stability (**FIG 11A,B**).
■ The triceps tendon, along with the osteotomized portion of the olecranon, may then be retracted proximally, and by flexing the elbow joint, the joint can be exposed (**FIG 11C**).

■ Occasionally the medial or lateral collateral ligaments are released for better exposure.
   ■ These ligaments are then repaired at the end of the procedure.
■ At the completion of the procedure, the tip of the olecranon is secured via tension-band or plate fixation.

LATERAL APPROACH TO THE ELBOW

■ Lateral exposures to the elbow are widely used to treat a variety of elbow pathologies. The exposures differ according to the deep interval used.
■ With any of the lateral exposures to the joint or to the proximal radius, the surgeon must be constantly aware of the possibility of injury to the posterior interosseous or recurrent branch of the radial nerve.

Anterolateral Approach to the Elbow (Kaplan)

Indications

■ Anterior capsular release
■ Posterior interosseous nerve exposure
■ Capitellar/lateral column fractures

Approach

■ Deep interval for the anterolateral approach lies between the extensor digitorum communis and the extensor carpi radialis longus muscles. (Intermuscular interval is best found by observing where vessels penetrate the fascia along the anterior margin of the extensor digitorum communis aponeurosis.)
■ Fascia is split longitudinally between the extensor digitorum communis and the extensor carpi radialis longus. (As the dissection is carried deep through the extensor carpi radialis longus, the extensor carpi radialis brevis is encountered.)
■ Deep to the extensor carpi radialis brevis, the transversely oriented fibers of the supinator are encountered, along with the posterior interosseous nerve. The posterior interosseous

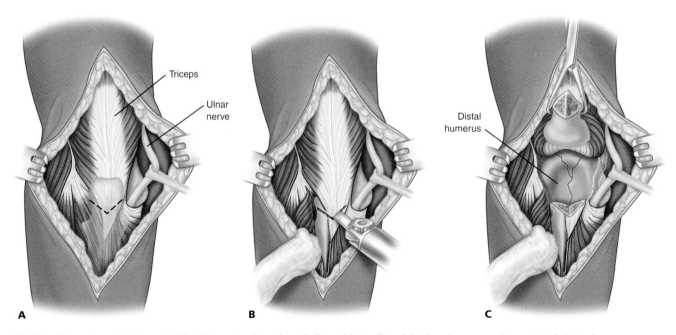

FIG 11 • Olecranon osteotomy. **A.** The triceps is released medially and laterally, while the ulnar nerve is protected. **B.** A chevron osteotomy with a distal apex is initiated with an oscillating saw. **C.** The proximal portion containing the olecranon osteotomy and triceps tendon is retracted proximally, exposing the elbow joint.

nerve defines the distal extent of the exposure. Pronation moves the radial nerve away from the surgical field.

■ If required, proximal dissection with elevation of the extensor carpi radialis longus, extensor carpi radialis brevis, and brachioradialis anteriorly from the lateral supracondylar ridge of the humerus provides exposure of the anterior joint capsule.

Modified Distal Kocher Approach

Indications

■ Reconstruction of the lateral ulnar collateral ligament

Approach

■ The skin incision begins just proximal to the lateral epicondyle of the humerus and extends obliquely for about 6 cm in line with the fascia of the anconeus and extensor carpi ulnaris muscles (**FIG 12A**).
■ The Kocher interval between the anconeus and flexor carpi ulnaris is incised (**FIG 12B**).
■ Development of the Kocher interval reveals the lateral joint capsule.

■ The anconeus is then reflected posteriorly off the joint capsule distally to expose the crista supinatoris.
■ The extensor carpi ulnaris and the common extensor tendon are released from the lateral epicondyle and reflected anteriorly, exposing the lateral capsule. The radial nerve is at a safe distance from the dissection, and it is protected by the extensor carpi ulnaris and extensor digitorum communis muscle mass (**FIG 12C**).
■ A longitudinal incision is made through the capsules to expose the radiocapitellar joint.

Boyd (Posterolateral) Approach

■ Radioulnar synostosis may occur as the proximal radius and ulna are exposed subperiosteally.

Indications

■ Monteggia fracture-dislocations
■ Radial head fractures
■ Radioulnar synostosis

Approach

■ The incision begins just posterior to the lateral epicondyle lateral to the triceps tendon and continues distally to the lat-

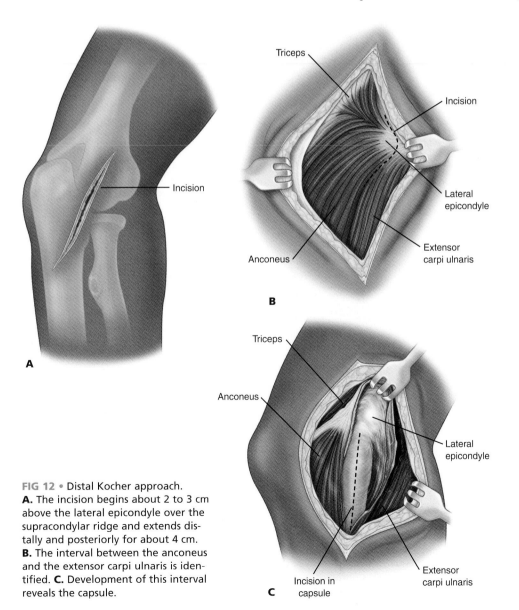

FIG 12 • Distal Kocher approach.
A. The incision begins about 2 to 3 cm above the lateral epicondyle over the supracondylar ridge and extends distally and posteriorly for about 4 cm.
B. The interval between the anconeus and the extensor carpi ulnaris is identified. **C.** Development of this interval reveals the capsule.

eral tip of the olecranon and then down to the subcutaneous border of the ulna.

■ The anconeus and supinator are subperiosteally elevated from the subcutaneous border of the ulna (anconeus and supinator) (**FIG 13A,B**).

■ Retraction of the anconeus and supinator exposes the joint capsule overlying the radial head and neck.

■ The supinator muscle protects the posterior interosseous nerve.

■ This lateral capsule contains the lateral ulnar collateral ligament, and its division can lead to posterolateral rotatory instability.

■ To expose the radial shaft, the incision may be continued along the subcutaneous ulnar border, elevating the muscles off the lateral aspect of the ulna (extensor carpi ulnaris, abductor pollicis longus, and extensor pollicis longus).

■ The posterior interosseous and recurrent interosseous arteries may need ligation.

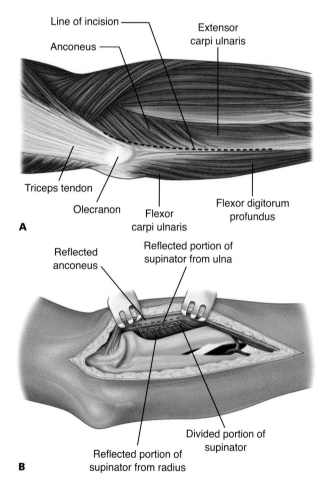

A

B

FIG 13 • The Boyd approach. **A.** The incision begins along the lateral border of the triceps about 2 to 3 cm above the epicondyle and extends distally over the lateral subcutaneous border of the ulna about 6 to 8 cm past the tip of the olecranon. The ulnar insertion of the anconeus and the origin of the supinator muscle are elevated subperiosteally. More distally, the subperiosteal reflection includes the abductor pollicis longus, the extensor carpi ulnaris, and the extensor pollicis longus muscles. The origin of the supinator at the crista supinatorus of the ulna is released, and the entire muscle flap is retracted radially, exposing the radiohumeral joint. **B.** The posterior interosseous nerve is protected in the substance of the supinator.

MEDIAL APPROACH TO THE ELBOW

■ There are relatively few indications for medial exposure of the elbow joint. This has been superseded by arthroscopic approaches.

■ The most valuable contribution to medial joint exposure is that described by Hotchkiss. This extensile exposure provides greater flexibility, particularly for exposure of the coronoid and for contracture release.

Extensile Medial Over-the-Top Approach

■ Excellent visualization of the anteromedial and posteromedial elbow

■ Not a sufficient approach for excision of heterotopic bone on the lateral side of the joint

■ Does not provide adequate access to the radial head

Indications

■ Coronoid fractures

■ Contracture release (when ulnar nerve exploration required)

■ Anterior and posterior access to the joint

■ May be converted to a triceps-reflecting exposure of Bryan-Morrey

Approach

■ Superficial dissection

  ■ Skin incision can vary between the boundaries of a pure posterior skin incision and midline medial incision (**FIG 14A**).

  ■ Subcutaneous skin is elevated.

  ■ The medial supracondylar ridge of the humerus, the medial intramuscular septum, the origin of the flexor pronator mass, and the ulnar nerve are identified.

  ■ Anterior to the septum, running just on top of the fascia (not in the subdermal tissue), the medial antebrachial cutaneous nerve is identified and protected.

  ■ The ulnar nerve is identified. If the patient previously had surgery, the ulnar nerve should be identified proximally before the surgeon proceeds distally.

    ■ If anterior transposition was performed previously, the nerve should be mobilized carefully before the operation proceeds.

  ■ The surface of the flexor pronator muscle mass origin is found by sweeping the subcutaneous tissue laterally with the medial antebrachial cutaneous nerve in this flap of subcutaneous tissue.

  ■ The medial intramuscular septum divides the anterior and posterior compartments of the elbow. The medial intramuscular septum is ultimately excised from the medial epicondyle to 5 cm proximal to it (**FIG 14B**).

  ■ The ulnar nerve is protected and the veins at the base of the septum are cauterized.

■ Deep anterior exposure

  ■ The flexor pronator mass origin is identified and totally or partially released from the medial epicondyle.

    ■ If extensile exposure is needed, the entire flexor pronator mass is elevated from the medial epicondyle (**FIG 14C,D**).

    ■ If less extensile exposure is needed, the flexor pronator mass is divided parallel to the fibers, leaving about 1.5 cm of flexor carpi ulnaris tendon attached to the epicondyle.

    ■ A small cuff of fibrous tissue of the origin can be left on the supracondylar ridge as the muscle is elevated; this facilitates reattachment when closing.

  ■ The flexor pronator origin should be dissected down to the level of bone but superficial to the joint capsule. As this plane is developed, the brachialis muscle is encountered from the underside.

▪ The brachialis muscle is identified along the supracondylar ridge and released in continuity with the flexor pronator mass.

▪ These muscles should be kept anterior and elevated from the capsule and anterior surface of the distal humerus.

▪ The median nerve and the brachial vein and artery are superficial to the brachialis muscle and protected with the subperiosteal release of the brachialis.

▪ Dissection of the capsule proceeds laterally and distally to separate it from the brachialis.

▪ In the case of contracture, the capsule, once separated from the overlying brachialis and brachioradialis, can be sharply excised (**FIG 14E**).

▪ Deep posterior capsule exposure

▪ The ulnar nerve is mobilized to permit anterior transposition with a dissection carried distally to the first motor branch to allow the nerve to rest in the anterior position without being sharply angled as it enters the flexor carpi ulnaris.

▪ With the Cobb elevator, the triceps is elevated from the posterior distal surface of the humerus.

▪ The posterior capsule can be separated from the triceps as the elevator sweeps from the proximal to distal.

▪ Closure

▪ The flexor pronator mass should be reattached to the supracondylar ridge.

▪ The ulnar nerve should be transposed and secured with a fascial sling to prevent posterior subluxation.

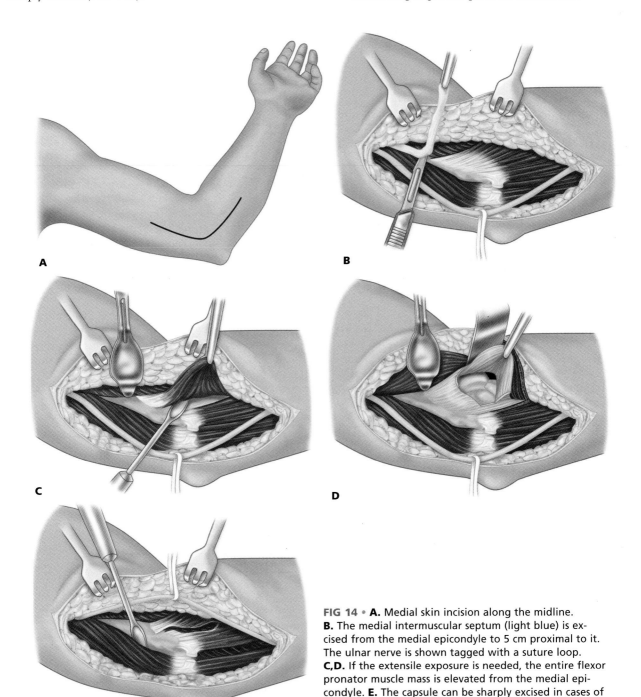

FIG 14 • **A.** Medial skin incision along the midline. **B.** The medial intermuscular septum (light blue) is excised from the medial epicondyle to 5 cm proximal to it. The ulnar nerve is shown tagged with a suture loop. **C,D.** If the extensile exposure is needed, the entire flexor pronator muscle mass is elevated from the medial epicondyle. **E.** The capsule can be sharply excised in cases of capsular contracture.

Table 1	**Indications and Recommended and Alternative Surgical Approaches**	
Indication	**Recommended Approach**	**Alternative Approach**
Total elbow arthroplasty	Bryan-Morrey, extended Kocher	Gschwend et al, Campbell, and Wadsworth
Soft tissue reconstruction	Global	Kocher, Bryan-Morrey, and Hotchkiss
T intercondylar fracture	MacAusland with chevron olecranon osteotomy	Alonso-Llames
Radial head fracture	Kocher	Kaplan
Capitellum fracture	Kaplan extended lateral approach	Kocher with or without Kaplan
Coronoid fracture	Taylor and Scham	Hotchkiss
Extra-articular distal humerus fracture	Alonso-Llames	Bryan-Morrey, Campbell
Monteggia fracture-dislocation	Gordon	Boyd
Radioulnar synostosis excision	Kocher or Gordon	Boyd or Henry

ANTERIOR APPROACH TO THE ELBOW

▪ Because of the vulnerability of the brachial artery and median nerve, the anterior medial approach to the elbow is not recommended.

▪ The extensile exposure described by Henry, and modified by Fiolle and Delmas, is best known and is the most useful for anterior exposure of the joint. Minor modifications of the Henry approach have been described, and a limited anterolateral exposure has been described by Darrach.

Modified Anterior Henry Approach

Indications

▪ Anteriorly displaced fracture fragments
▪ Excision of tumors in this region
▪ Reattachment of the biceps tendon to the radial tuberosity
▪ Exploration of nerve entrapment syndromes
▪ Anterior capsular release for contracture

Approach

▪ The skin incision begins about 5 cm proximal to the flexor crease of the elbow joint and extends distally along the anterior margin of the brachioradialis muscle to the flexion crease.
▪ At the elbow flexion crease, the incision turns medially to avoid crossing the flexor crease at a right angle. The incision continues transversely to the biceps tendon and then turns distally over the medial volar aspect of the forearm (**FIG 15A**).
▪ The fascia is released distally between the brachioradialis and pronator teres (**FIG 15B**).
▪ The interval between the brachioradialis laterally and the biceps and brachialis medially is identified. This interval is entered proximally, and gentle, blunt dissection demonstrates the radial nerve coursing on the inner surface of the brachioradialis muscle (**FIG 15C**).
▪ Care is taken to avoid injury to the superficial sensory branch of the radial nerve.

▪ Because the radial nerve gives off its branches laterally, it can safely be retracted with the brachioradialis muscle.
▪ At the level of the elbow joint, as the brachioradialis is retracted laterally and the pronator teres is gently retracted medially, the radial artery can be observed where it emerges from the medial aspect of the biceps tendon, giving off its muscular and recurrent branches in a mediolateral direction.
▪ The muscle branch is ligated, but the recurrent radial artery should be sacrificed only if the lesion warrants an extensive exposure.
▪ The posterior interosseous nerve enters the supinator and continues along the dorsum of the forearm distally.
▪ Dissection continues distally, exposing the supinator muscle, which covers the proximal aspect of the radius and the anterolateral aspect of the capsule (**FIG 15C**).
▪ Muscle attachments to the anterior aspect of the radius and those distal to the supinator include the discrete tendinous insertion of the pronator teres and the origins of the flexor digitorum sublimis and the flexor pollicis longus.
▪ The brachialis muscle is identified, elevated, and retracted medially to expose the proximal capsule.
▪ If more distal exposure is needed, the forearm is fully supinated, demonstrating the insertion of the supinator muscle along the proximal radius.
  ▪ This insertion is incised and the supinator is subperiosteally retracted laterally (**FIG 15D**).
▪ The supinator serves as a protection to the deep interosseous branch of the radial nerve, but excessive retraction of the muscle should be avoided.
▪ The proximal aspect of the radius and the capitellum are thus exposed.
▪ Additional visualization may be obtained both proximally and distally, because the radial nerve has been identified and can be avoided proximally.
▪ The posterior interosseous nerve is protected distally by the supinator muscle, and the radial artery is visualized and protected medially if a more extensile exposure is required.

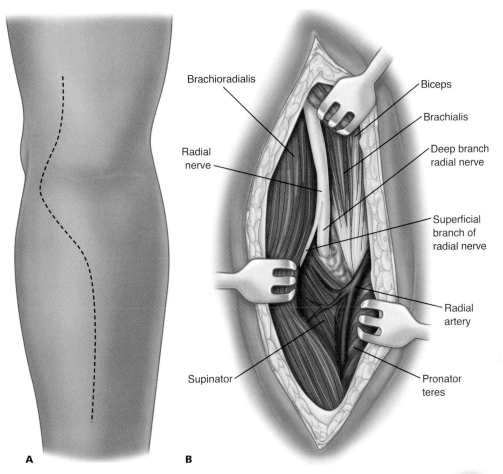

Brachioradialis

Radial nerve

Supinator

Biceps

Brachialis

Deep branch radial nerve

Superficial branch of radial nerve

Radial artery

Pronator teres

A

B

FIG 15 • The anterior Henry approach. **A.** An incision is made about 5 cm proximal to the elbow crease on the lateral margin of the biceps tendon. It extends transversely across the joint line and curves distally over the medial aspect of the forearm. The interval between the brachioradialis and brachialis proximally and the biceps tendon and pronator teres in the distal portion of the wound is identified. The radial nerve is protected and retracted along with the brachialis. **B.** The supinator muscle is released from the anterior aspect of the radius, which is fully supinated. **C.** The radial recurrent branches of the radial artery and its muscular branches are identified and sacrificed if more extensive exposure is required. The biceps tendon is retracted medially along with the brachialis muscle. **D.** This interval may now be developed to expose the anterior aspect of the elbow joint.

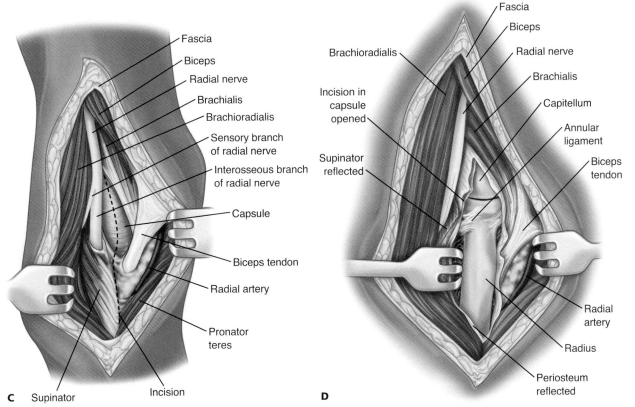

Fascia
Biceps
Radial nerve
Brachialis
Brachioradialis
Sensory branch of radial nerve
Interosseous branch of radial nerve
Capsule
Biceps tendon
Radial artery
Pronator teres

C Supinator   Incision

Fascia
Biceps
Radial nerve
Brachialis
Capitellum
Annular ligament
Biceps tendon

Brachioradialis

Incision in capsule opened

Supinator reflected

Radial artery
Radius
Periosteum reflected

D

Chapter 3

Bankart Repair and Inferior Capsular Shift

Theodore A. Blaine, Andrew Green, and Louis U. Bigliani

DEFINITION

■ Shoulder instability is caused by a disruption of the normal stabilizing anatomic structures of the shoulder, leading to recurrent dislocation or subluxation of the glenohumeral joint.

ANATOMY

■ Glenohumeral stability depends on the integrity of static and dynamic components.

■ Dynamic stabilizers include the rotator cuff muscles, which provide a concavity compression effect, the scapular stabilizers, and the biceps tendon, which contributes to anterior stability when the arm is in an abducted and externally rotated position (**FIG 1A,B**).

■ Static stabilizers consist of the bony and articular anatomy of the glenoid and humeral head, the negative intra-articular pressure supplied by the intact glenohumeral capsule, and the capsule–labral complex, which contains the glenoid labrum and anterior, middle, and superior glenohumeral ligaments (**FIG 1C**).

■ The glenoid labrum plays an important role in deepening the glenoid socket and as an attachment site for the glenohumeral ligaments (**FIG 1D**).

■ The primary restraint to anterior inferior translation of the humeral head in 90 degrees of abduction and external rotation is the inferior glenohumeral ligament (IGHL).

■ The middle glenohumeral ligament (MGHL) has a variable attachment site into the glenoid labrum, glenoid neck, and biceps tendon origin. The MGHL is important in resisting anterior subluxation of the humeral head in the middle range of shoulder abduction (45 degrees).

■ The superior glenohumeral ligament (SGHL) is located in the rotator interval capsule, and prevents inferior and posterior subluxation of the humeral head with the arm in an ad-

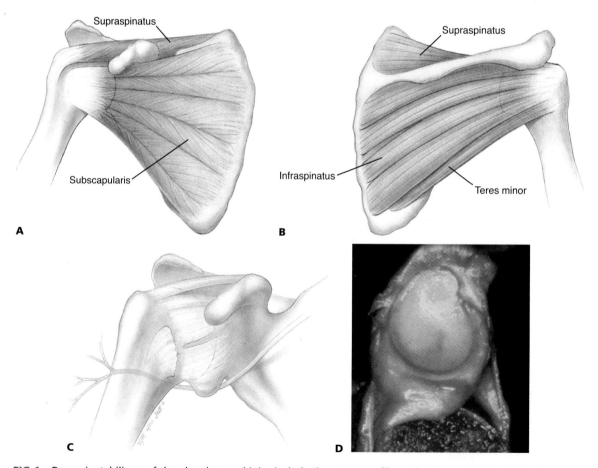

FIG 1 • Dynamic stabilizers of the glenohumeral joint include the rotator cuff muscles (supraspinatus, infraspinatus, teres minor, subscapularis; **A,B**). The static stabilizers of the glenohumeral joint include the glenohumeral ligaments of the capsule (**C**), and the glenoid labrum (**D**), which deepens the socket and serves as an attachment for the glenohumeral ligaments and biceps tendon.

ducted and neutral or internally rotated position. The SGHL is important in inferior and posterior translation of the humeral head.

PATHOGENESIS

- Glenohumeral instability (subluxation or dislocation) occurs when the static or dynamic stabilizers of the glenohumeral joint are disrupted, either from acute rupture or repetitive microtrauma.
- The "essential anatomical defect," or Bankart lesion, was first described by a British pathologist, A. Blundell Bankart, in 1923, and the operative procedure was first described in 1938 (**FIG 2A**).[3,20]
  - The Bankart lesion is present in at least 40% of shoulders undergoing anterior instability procedures.
  - The "essential" nature of the Bankart lesion has been challenged, since a simulated Bankart lesion without capsular stretching does not lead to significant increases in glenohumeral translation.
- In addition to tearing of the glenoid labrum, the labrum may also be avulsed from the glenoid rim as a sleeve of tissue (anterior labral periosteal sleeve avulsion [ALPSA]) (**FIG 2B**).[17]
- Recurrent major trauma and repetitive microtrauma creates substantial deformation to the IGHL, producing subsequent episodes of symptomatic subluxation.
  - Biomechanical studies of this ligament have demonstrated that failure typically occurs at the glenoid insertion (40%), followed by the ligament substance (35%) and the humeral attachment (25%). Significant capsular stretching can occur (23% to 34%) before failure.
- Osseous deficiency on the anterior rim (bony Bankart) may contribute to glenohumeral instability (**FIG 2C**).
  - Significant defects accounting for instability occur when 30% of the glenoid is involved, and the glenoid acquires an "inverted pear" appearance (**FIG 2D**).

NATURAL HISTORY

- The incidence of glenohumeral instability has been estimated at 8.2 to 23.9 per 100,000 person-years.[23]
- The incidence in at-risk populations is significantly higher (military population, 1.69 per 1000 person-years; NCAA athletes, 0.12 injuries/1000 athletic exposures).[19]
- Overhead athletes are prone to this repeat injury as their motions in the abducted, externally rotated position put stress on the capsulolabral structures. Contact athletes (football players and wrestlers) have the highest incidence of shoulder dislocations as compared to other sports.
- Depending on the patient's age and activity level, redislocation rates in active patients may be as high as 92% with nonoperative treatment.[13,19,24]

PATIENT HISTORY AND PHYSICAL FINDINGS

- Evaluation of the patient with suspected instability begins with a thorough history.
- Arm dominance, sport, position, and level of competition should be noted, as well as associated factors, including other sporting activities, training modalities, and past history of injuries.
- Traumatic causes of instability should be determined, as these are more likely to be associated with Bankart lesions.
- The character of the problem should be elicited.
  - Does the athlete complain of pain or instability?
  - Does the shoulder subluxate or dislocate?
  - What arm positions reproduce symptoms?
- Any prior treatments (physical therapy, training modifications, medication, and surgery) should be noted.
- Physical examination should include assessment of both shoulders.
- Inspection should be performed to identify any skin incisions, evidence of wasting in the deltoid, rotator cuff, or periscapular

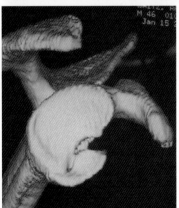
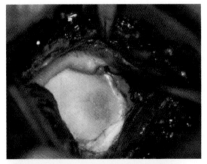
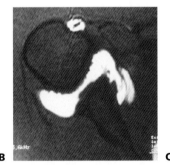
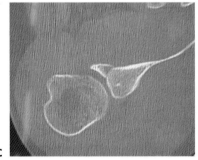

FIG 2 • **A.** The Bankart lesion: tear of the anterior inferior glenoid labrum. **B.** Axial view MRI scan showing the anterior labral periosteal sleeve avulsion (ALPSA). **C,D.** CT scan with axial view and reconstruction image, respectively, showing a large anterior inferior glenoid "bony Bankart" fracture.

musculature, and gross evidence of laxity, including sulcus signs or signs of generalized ligamentous laxity.

▪ Palpation is performed to identify point tenderness; anterior joint line tenderness may be present in acute anterior dislocations; subacromial tenderness may be present with impingement secondary to subtle instability.

▪ Active and passive motion tests are an important part of the instability examination. Significant variations in motion are encountered in throwing athletes, with increased external rotation and decreased internal rotation common in the affected shoulder.

▪ Provocative testing is perhaps the most important aspect in the clinical evaluation of shoulder instability.

▪ The sulcus sign is often elicited in patients with inferior instability.

▪ Anterior translation and posterior translation are similarly graded with the patient supine and with an anterior or posterior load and shift test, although this test is performed only in the anesthetized patient.

▪ In the awake patient, signs of instability can be more subtle. The apprehension test is routinely performed with the arm abducted, extended, and externally rotated. A sensation of impending subluxation or dislocation in the patient is diagnostic of instability. Pain is less specific and may instead indicate internal impingement of the articular surface of the rotator cuff or functional impingement of the bursal side of the rotator cuff on a prominent coracoacromial ligament.

▪ A posterior-directed force on the arm by the examiner that relieves the apprehension in this position (Jobe relocation test) suggests an unstable shoulder.

▪ Subscapularis integrity and strength should be evaluated in patients with glenohumeral instability.

▪ Inability to press the hand to the belly is a positive result of the belly press test and indicates subscapularis muscle weakness or tear.

▪ Inability to lift the hand from the back is a positive result in the lift-off test and indicates subscapularis muscle weakness or tear.

IMAGING AND OTHER DIAGNOSTIC STUDIES

▪ Radiographs include anteroposterior (AP), lateral, and axillary views (**FIG 3A,B**).

▪ The axillary view is particularly important for assessing anterior glenoid rim defects.

▪ The Hill-Sachs lesion of the posterosuperior humeral head is best seen on the AP internal rotation or Stryker notch views.

▪ CT scan is not necessary in all cases but may be helpful in patients with bony defects (see Fig 2C,D).

▪ MRI scan is not necessary in all cases but can be useful in identifying labral lesions as well as subscapularis tears (**FIG 3C**).

▪ MRI arthrogram is more sensitive in identifying labral pathology and may be necessary when superior or posterior labral pathology is suspected.

DIFFERENTIAL DIAGNOSIS

▪ External impingement, subacromial bursitis, rotator cuff tendinitis
▪ Internal impingement
▪ SLAP (superior labral tear)
▪ Voluntary instability
▪ Collagen disorder (Ehlers-Danlos syndrome, Marfan syndrome)
▪ Subscapularis insufficiency, tear

NONOPERATIVE MANAGEMENT

▪ After reduction of an acute dislocation, a sling is used for immobilization. The duration of immobilization has been controversial, but 3 to 6 weeks is recommended.[21]

▪ Some surgeons recommend immobilization in a position of abduction and external rotation to improve healing. However, many patients will not tolerate this position, and a position of adduction and internal rotation therefore is more commonly used.

▪ For treatment of acute injuries, rotational and scapular strengthening exercises of the affected shoulder are started after the initial immobilization period. The program is progressed toward normalization of strength and motion through increased resistance training.

▪ Return to sports is allowed when the patient has a full and pain-free range of motion, normal strength, and little or no apprehension.[21]

▪ For chronic and recurrent instability, strengthening is focused on the rotator cuff and scapular stabilizers, as well as core strengthening of the abdominal and trunk musculature. Resistive exercises of the rotator cuff are begun with the arm in neutral below 90 degrees and are progressed gradually. Strengthening of scapular stabilizers is particularly important.

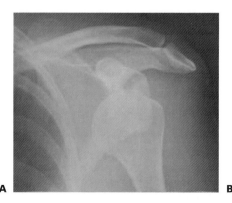
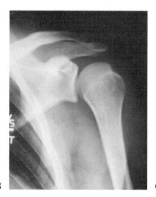
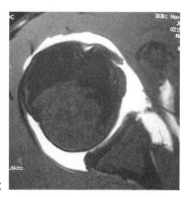

FIG 3 ▪ AP radiographs of the left shoulder showing a dislocated shoulder (**A**) and subsequent reduction (**B**). There is a Hill-Sachs fracture of the posterolateral humeral head. **C.** Axial MRI scan in a patient with deficient glenoid labrum and subscapularis tendon tear.

■ The rate of redislocation after nonoperative treatment depends on the patient's age and activity level. In young patients participating in high-risk activities (eg, military cadets), the rate of redislocation is as high as 92%.[24]

■ In a meta-analysis comparing operative to nonoperative treatment for first-time dislocators, 50% of the conservatively treated patients eventually opted for surgery.[19]

SURGICAL MANAGEMENT

■ Surgical treatment options are generally categorized into anatomic and nonanatomic procedures.

■ Nonanatomic procedures (Putti-Platt, Magnuson-Stack) are aimed at tightening the anterior structures and preventing at-risk arm positions (ie, abduction and external rotation). These procedures have largely been abandoned after it was discovered that overtightening the anterior structures could lead to posterior subluxation and glenohumeral arthritis.[11,18]

 ■ The Putti-Platt procedure consists of a vertical incision through both the subscapularis tendon and capsule followed by repair of the lateral flap to the soft tissue at the glenoid rim.[18]

 ■ The Magnuson-Stack procedure is a transfer of the subscapularis tendon lateral to the bicipital groove (**FIG 4A**).

■ Coracoid transfer procedures are other nonanatomic procedures where the coracoid process, with its attached short head of the biceps and coracobrachialis tendons, is transferred to the anterior glenoid rim and secured with screws.[1]

 ■ The Bristow procedure uses the tip of the coracoid and typically a single bicortical cancellous screw.

 ■ The Laterjet procedure lays the coracoid on its side and is typically secured with two screws (**FIG 4B**).

 ■ Although several authors have achieved excellent success with these procedures, the concern for hardware migration and late resorption of the bone block have made these procedures less popular than the anatomic procedures. They are used mainly for revision procedures and in cases where there is deficient glenoid bone stock.

■ Anatomic reconstruction procedures have been aimed at reconstructing the anterior labrum using sutures, staples, or tacks.[2,8,9,12,22] These anatomic procedures have had excellent success, with minimal (less than 5%) recurrence rates, and therefore are the procedure of choice in the surgical treatment of glenohumeral instability.

■ The Bankart repair and inferior capsular shift procedures are the most commonly used anatomic reconstruction procedures.

■ Although recurrence rates for arthroscopic Bankart repair and capsular shift were initially higher than open procedures, these rates have become comparable to open as the arthroscopic techniques have evolved.

■ Open treatment, however, is recommended over arthroscopic treatment in the following situations:
 ■ Significant bony Bankart lesions (over 30%)
 ■ Significant Hill-Sachs defects where the defect "engages" the glenoid rim with external rotation as visualized during diagnostic arthroscopy
 ■ Revision procedures
 ■ Some contact athletes (football) and extreme sports, where a slightly lower recurrence rate can be expected in comparison to the arthroscopic procedure

Preoperative Planning

■ A careful assessment of the patient's expectations of the surgery and postoperative care, including thorough discussions with the patient and family, are required as part of the preoperative plan.
 ■ Noncompliance with the postoperative restrictions will increase the risk of redislocation after surgical repair.

■ It is important to assess mental status and any secondary gain issues in patients with multidirectional instability. Patients with voluntary dislocations and malingering (Munchausen syndrome) patients have a high rate of failure and should be identified before surgery.

■ It is important to identify before surgery any glenoid bony deficiency that may require bony augmentation via coracoid transfer or allograft reconstruction. Special equipment (allograft bone and instrumentation to perform ORIF) may be required and should be arranged before surgery.

Positioning

■ Interscalene block anesthesia is preferred because of the excellent muscle relaxation and postoperative pain relief it offers. If an adequate block cannot be performed, however, general anesthesia can also be used.

■ The patient is positioned in the beach-chair position with the back elevated. The patient should be moved to the edge of the table or the shoulder cut-out removed to allow access to the anterior and posterior shoulder as required.

■ A hydraulic arm positioner (Tenet Spider) is particularly helpful and can obviate the need for an additional assistant to hold the arm (**FIG 5**).

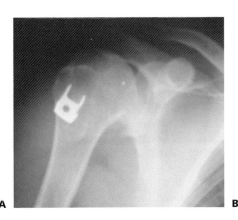
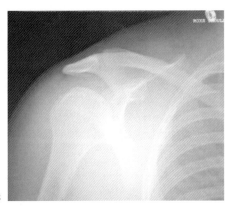

A   **B**

FIG 4 • **A.** AP radiograph of the right shoulder in a patient with previous Magnuson-Stack procedure (the subscapularis tendon has been stapled laterally to the bicipital groove). **B.** AP radiograph of the right shoulder in a patient with a Laterjet procedure. There are two screws securing the coracoid bone block to the glenoid.

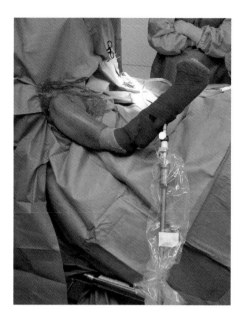

FIG 5 • Hydraulic arm positioner (Spider, Tenet Medical Engineering, Calgary, Alberta, Canada) used to position the arm during surgery.

Approach

- The bony landmarks of the shoulder are identified, including the acromion, clavicle, and coracoid process.
- Approaches to the shoulder that may be used include the deltopectoral, the concealed axillary incision, and the mini-incision approach. All of these are variations of the standard deltopectoral approach.
- Standard deltopectoral approach
  - This is the utility approach to the shoulder.
  - A 7- to 15-cm incision is made lateral to the coracoid process beginning below the clavicle and extending toward the anterior humeral shaft at the deltoid insertion. Skin flaps are elevated and the deltopectoral interval is identified.
  - The remainder of this approach is described in detail below.
- Concealed axillary incision
  - Whereas the traditional deltopectoral approach is about 15 cm in length, the concealed axillary incision begins 3 cm inferior to the coracoid and extends only 7 cm into the

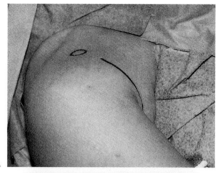

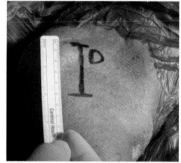

FIG 6 • **A.** The concealed axillary incision is made from below the coracoid process toward the axillary fold. **B.** The mini-incision is made in line with the deltopectoral interval and is centered one-third above and two-thirds below the coracoid process.

axillary crease (**FIG 6A**). Skin flaps are widely elevated and the deltopectoral interval is identified.
  - This incision is cosmetically appealing and is useful in patients where cosmesis is important.
- Mini-incision approach
  - A 5-cm incision just lateral to the coracoid process can be used in shoulder stabilization procedures (**FIG 6B**). Wide subcutaneous flaps are created and the deltopectoral interval is identified. The remainder of the exposure is similar to the standard deltopectoral approach.
  - The location of this incision is important to achieve direct access to the glenoid without extending the incision: one third of the incision should be above and two thirds below the coracoid process.

BANKART PROCEDURE

- The skin incision is based on surgeon preference as described above. The concealed axillary incision is the most commonly used.
- Skin flaps are elevated and the deltopectoral interval is identified (**TECH FIG 1A**).
- The cephalic vein is taken laterally with the deltoid muscle, and the clavipectoral fascia overlying the subscapularis tendon and strap muscles is exposed.
- When additional exposure is needed, it is helpful to incise and tag with a suture the upper third of the pectoralis major insertion into the humerus. Great care should be taken not to injure the biceps tendon, which lies just underneath the pectoralis major insertion.

- The clavipectoral fascia is incised lateral to the strap muscles, and a retractor is placed between them to expose the subscapularis muscle and tendon.
- A small wedge of the coracoacromial ligament can be removed to increase superior exposure (**TECH FIG 1B**).
- The branches of the anterior circumflex humeral vessels at the inferior margin of the subscapularis muscle should be cauterized at this time to control bleeding.
- The subscapularis tendon is exposed and incised vertically just medial to its insertion. The tendon can be peeled off the underlying capsule with a combination of the periosteal elevator for blunt dissection and the needle-tip Bovie cautery for sharp dissection (**TECH FIG 1C,D**).

TECHNIQUES

- The anterior capsule is then incised vertically at the level of the glenoid rim (**TECH FIG 1E,F**).
- With a curette or osteotome, the anterior glenoid rim is roughened and any soft tissue removed to allow for healing of the repair (**TECH FIG 1G**).
- Transosseous sutures are passed through holes made with pointed forceps or a drill.
    - Alternatively, suture anchors may be placed at the margin of remaining articular cartilage. Often, two and sometimes three anchors are used between the 2:30 and 6:00 positions (**TECH FIG 1H**).
- The capsule is shifted or repaired anatomically as required. Typically, an inferior capsular shift procedure is performed in combination with the Bankart procedure as described below.
- The subscapularis tendon is repaired anatomically at its insertion.

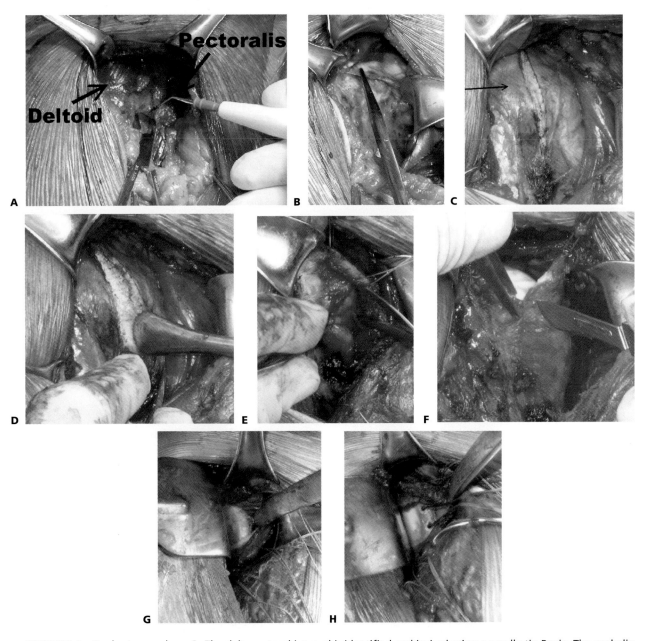

TECH FIG 1 • Bankart procedure. **A.** The deltopectoral interval is identified and incised using a needle-tip Bovie. The cephalic vein is retracted laterally with the deltoid. **B.** The anterolateral leading edge of the coracoacromial ligament (indicated by the clamp) is resected for improved superior exposure. **C.** The subscapularis is incised about 1 cm medial to its insertion, leaving a stout cuff of tissue laterally (*arrow*) for subsequent repair. **D.** Blunt dissection inferiorly, where the subscapularis muscle is not adherent to the capsule, facilitates finding the plane of separation between the subscapularis and anterior capsule. **E.** The capsule is sharply incised, taking care not to damage the humeral head cartilage below. **F.** An adequate cuff of tissue is left behind for subsequent repair. **G.** The glenoid rim is prepared using an osteotome or curette. **H.** Suture anchors are placed at the apex of the glenoid rim.

T-PLASTY MODIFICATION OF THE BANKART PROCEDURE

- To address capsular laxity in addition to the Bankart lesion, Altchek and Warren[2] described a modification of the Bankart procedure by performing a T incision in the capsule.
- The approach is the same as in the Bankart procedure described and involves dissection of the subscapularis from the anterior glenohumeral capsule.
- Unlike the inferior capsular shift procedure, the T-plasty involves a medially based capsular incision at the glenoid margin.
  - The T capsulotomy is made two thirds from the top of the capsule, with the vertical component adjacent to the glenoid rim (**TECH FIG 2**).
- The Bankart lesion is repaired using suture anchors or transosseous sutures.
- The laterally based inferior flap of capsule is advanced superiorly and medially and secured to the glenoid rim.
- The superior flap is then advanced medially and oversewn to the inferior flap.
- The subscapularis tendon is repaired anatomically at its insertion.

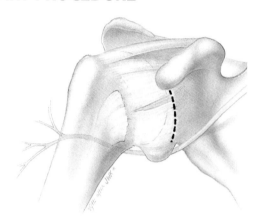

TECH FIG 2 • T-plasty modification of the Bankart procedure. The T capsulotomy is made two thirds from the top of the capsule, with the vertical component adjacent to the glenoid rim.

ANTERIOR CAPSULOLABRAL RECONSTRUCTION

- Because of the loss of strength and velocity in throwing athletes undergoing anterior stabilization procedures, Jobe[12] in 1991 proposed a subscapularis-sparing procedure in which the tendon is split in line with its fibers and its humeral attachment left intact.
- A deltopectoral approach to the shoulder is used and the strap muscles are retracted medially to expose the subscapularis tendon.

- The subscapularis is then divided horizontally in line with its fibers at the junction of the upper two thirds and lower one third (**TECH FIG 3A,B**).
- A horizontal capsulotomy is now made in the middle of the capsule extending medial to the glenoid rim. The capsule is elevated off the glenoid subperiosteally to allow for superior and inferior capsular advancement (**TECH FIG 3C**).

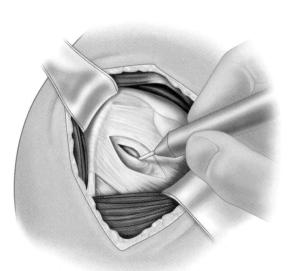
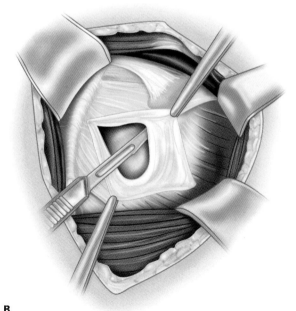

A **B**

TECH FIG 3 • The anterior capsulolabral reconstruction procedure. **A.** The subscapularis is divided horizontally in line with its fibers at the junction of the upper two thirds and lower one third. **B.** A horizontal capsulotomy is now made in the middle of the capsule extending medial to the glenoid rim. *(continued)*

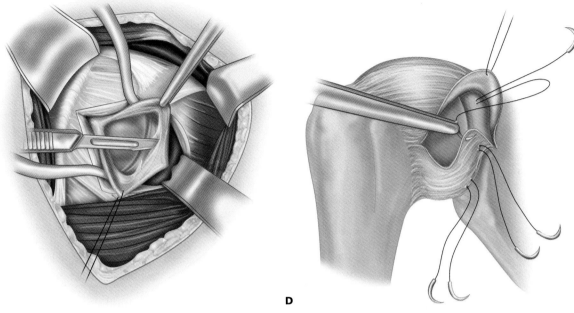

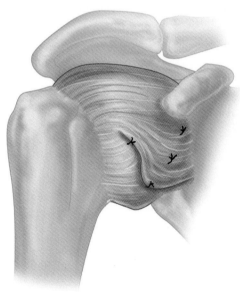

C

D

TECH FIG 3 • *(continued)* **C.** The capsule is elevated off the glenoid subperiosteally to allow for superior and inferior capsular advancement. **D.** The laterally based inferior flap is shifted superiorly and secured to the intra-articular portion of the glenoid rim using transosseous sutures to attempt to recreate the labral "bumper." **E.** The superior flap is then shifted medially and oversewn to the inferior flap.

E

- The laterally based inferior flap is then shifted superiorly and secured to the intra-articular portion of the glenoid rim using transosseous sutures to attempt to recreate the labral "bumper" (**TECH FIG 3D,E**).
- The superior flap is then shifted medially and oversewn to the inferior flap.

- Because the subscapularis tendon is not detached, active assistive rehabilitation exercises are begun immediately on postoperative day 1, and rehabilitation is progressed more rapidly.

ANTERIOR INFERIOR CAPSULAR SHIFT

- The anterior inferior capsular shift operation was first described by Charles Neer[16] in 1980.
    - The procedure was designed to treat involuntary inferior and multidirectional instability of the shoulder that could not be addressed by repair of the anterior glenoid labrum alone (the Bankart procedure).
- The skin incision may be chosen based on the desired approach.

- The subscapularis tendon is incised about 1 to 2 cm medial to its insertion at the lesser tuberosity, leaving an adequate cuff of tissue for repair.
- The subscapularis consists of both a superior tendinous portion (two thirds) and inferior muscular (one third) portion.[14]
    - To expose the inferior portion of the glenohumeral joint capsule, it is important to carefully separate the

muscle fibers' insertion from the underlying anterior capsule using a combination of sharp and blunt dissection. The arm should be in a position of adduction and external rotation during this inferior dissection, and great care is taken to protect the axillary nerve.

- A laterally based capsular shift is then performed by incising the capsule vertically about 5 to 10 mm medial to its insertion on the humeral neck (see Tech Fig 1E,F).
- The medial leaf of the capsule is tagged sequentially with nonabsorbable sutures as the capsular incision is continued inferiorly to at least the 6 o'clock position (**TECH FIG 4A**).
- By placing traction on the capsular tag sutures in a superior and lateral direction, the axillary pouch should be obliterated when an adequate amount of capsular dissection has been performed.
- It is important to release the inferior capsular attachments to the humerus, which have a broad insertion inferior to the articular surface. This is typically done with blunt subperiosteal dissection with the periosteal elevator and needle-tip Bovie cautery (**TECH FIG 4B,C**).
- The medial insertion of the glenohumeral ligaments and glenoid labrum should then be assessed for avulsion or tear. Bankart lesion and ALPSA both describe a disrup-

tion of the medial capsulolabral complex that must be repaired.
- This technique is described in the Bankart repair technique section.
- Once secure fixation to bone is achieved, the capsule is shifted superiorly and laterally and the nonabsorbable sutures are passed through the capsule from an intra-articular to extra-articular location.
- It is important to place the sutures as close to the glenoid rim as possible so that the capsule is not shortened by medial plication.
- A bimanual technique can be used in which one needle driver is used to pass the suture and a second to "catch" the needle on the extra-articular side.
- The sutures are then tied on the extra-articular side to secure the capsule to the glenoid rim.
- If excess anteromedial capsular redundancy (AMCR) exists after the Bankart repair, a "barrel stitch" technique has been described in which a nonabsorbable pursestring suture is placed to imbricate the anterior capsule.[7]
- The barrel stitch is placed vertically at the level of the glenoid rim and tied on the extra-articular side. Its size is titrated to the amount of AMCR encountered (**TECH FIG 4D,E**).

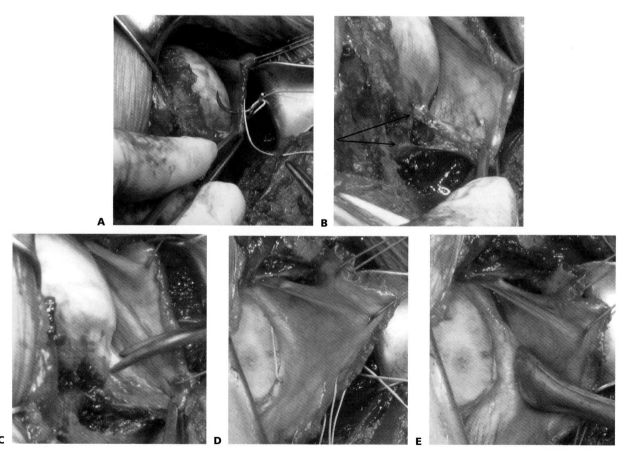

TECH FIG 4 • A. In the inferior capsule shift procedure, the laterally based capsular incision is continued inferiorly using tag stitches on the released anterior capsule to apply traction. **B.** There is a dual attachment of the inferior capsule on the humeral neck. **C.** Release of the dual inferior capsular attachment, allowing a complete shift of the capsule. **D.** An anterior crimping (barrel) stitch is used to decrease the redundancy of the anteroinferior capsule. This is a mattress stitch started on the superficial side of the capsule. **E.** Once tied, the barrel stitch reduces anterior medial capsular redundancy and an anterior inferior bolster is created. *(continued)*

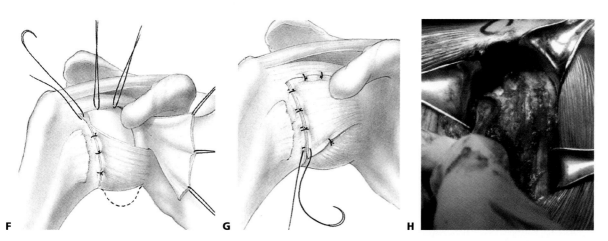

TECH FIG 4 • *(continued)* **F.** The anteroinferior capsule is advanced superiorly and reattached to the capsular sleeve preserved on the humeral neck. **G.** The superior flap is sewn to the inferior flap to reduce volume and increase strength. **H.** The rotator interval capsule is palpated between the subscapularis and supraspinatus tendons.

- Once the medial instability repair is complete, attention is directed to lateral repair of the capsule to the remaining cuff of tissue at the humeral neck.
- The capsule is shifted superiorly and laterally (**TECH FIG 4F**).
- The amount of external rotation should be titrated to the patient and should be based on the patient's age, quality of tissue, the presence of the generalized or local ligamentous laxity, sport, level of competition, arm dominance, and expected level of compliance with the prescribed rehabilitation program.
  - A good general guideline is to repair the shifted anterior capsule with the arm in 20 degrees of abduction and 30 degrees of external rotation.
- Throwers require an increased amount of external rotation in abduction and may require more laxity than a patient who is noncompliant or not involved in throwing sports.
- Excess tightening of the anterior capsule should be avoided to prevent the development of postcapsulorrhaphy arthropathy.[11]
- As the capsule is shifted superiorly and laterally, a lax capsule will have an abundance of capsular tissue remaining superiorly. In these shoulders, the capsular incision can be converted to a laterally based T capsulorrhaphy by incising the capsule between the inferior and middle glenohumeral ligaments down to the glenoid rim.
  - The inferior limb of the capsule is first repaired to its lateral insertion on the humerus.
  - The superior limb is folded down in a pants-over-vest fashion and repaired laterally to the insertion point (**TECH FIG 4G**). This will both reduce capsular volume and reinforce the anterior capsuloligamentous tissues.
- In addition to assessing residual capsular laxity, the rotator interval should also be assessed (**TECH FIG 4H**).
- If the rotator interval is widened or attenuated, it should be imbricated and closed using interrupted nonabsorbable sutures.
  - The amount of interval closure should also be titrated to the patient as mentioned previously, because excess tightening of the rotator interval can lead to restriction of external rotation.[10]
  - It may be preferable to close only the lateral portion of the rotator interval to preserve glenohumeral motion in competitive athletes.
- The subscapularis tendon is repaired anatomically at its insertion.

PEARLS AND PITFALLS

Voluntary instability	▪ Patients with voluntary instability should be carefully screened before surgery. If there are significant issues of secondary gain, surgical treatment will not be successful and should be discouraged. Preoperative psychiatric evaluation has been suggested but is seldom helpful in screening these patients.
Humeral bone defects (Hill-Sachs lesions)	▪ It is important to recognize and quantitate humeral bone defects, which are best seen on the radiograph (AP in internal rotation or Stryker notch view), CT scan, or MRI, or by diagnostic arthroscopy. With "engaging" defects, open treatment is favored over arthroscopic, and filling of the defect (autograft, allograft) may be considered.
Glenoid bone defects (bony Bankart)	▪ Glenoid defects can be assessed with preoperative imaging (radiographs, CT scan, MRI) and diagnostic arthroscopy. Significant defects (more than 30% of the glenoid) require a coracoid transfer (Bristow or Laterjet) procedure.

Posterior instability	■ The direction of instability should be assessed with preoperative examination and examination under anesthesia. If there is a significant posterior component, stability may be restored with a thorough inferior capsular shift. However, in some cases, an additional posterior approach may be required.
Associated SLAP (superior labral) tears	■ Additional labral pathology may be present in some patients with Bankart lesions. These injuries are often best managed arthroscopically, and if suspected, may require diagnostic arthroscopy to confirm and repair before an open incision.

POSTOPERATIVE CARE

■ The rehabilitation protocol must be planned individually.
■ The patient remains in a sling for 4 weeks postoperatively.
■ Passive forward elevation to 110 degrees and external rotation to 15 degrees is begun at 10 days to 2 weeks, and is gradually increased to 140 degrees forward elevation and 30 degrees external rotation by 4 weeks. During this period, isometric strengthening exercises are begun.
■ From 4 to 6 weeks, elevation is increased to about 160 degrees and external rotation to 40 degrees.
■ After 6 weeks, motion is increased to achieve a normal range.
■ Exercises should be progressed slowly to avoid apprehension and resubluxation.
■ Resistive exercises are begun with the arm in neutral below 90 degrees and progressed gradually.
■ Strengthening of scapular stabilizers is particularly important.
■ Full motion and strength should be regained before contact sports are resumed, usually between 6 and 9 months, depending on the sport and the patient.

OUTCOMES

■ The first long-term follow-up study of the Bankart procedure was reported by Carter Rowe[22] in 1978, with only a 3.5% rate of redislocation.
■ Neer[16] reported on 40 unstable shoulders that were repaired with the anterior inferior capsular shift between 1974 and 1979, 11 of which had undergone prior procedures for glenohumeral instability. Satisfactory results were achieved in all except one patient, who had postoperative subluxation of the shoulder.
■ Since Neer's initial report, multiple series have been published that have used the anterior inferior capsular shift procedure for anteroinferior instability. Although the surgical technique and the extent of capsular shift may vary with different surgeons, recurrence rates have ranged from 1.5% to 9%.[5,6,9,16,25]

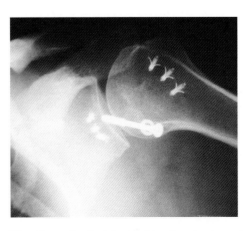

FIG 7 • AP radiograph of a left shoulder showing loose hardware after a prior coracoid transfer procedure.

■ T-plasty results: In 42 shoulders with an average of 3 years of follow-up in this initial series, 95% of the patients were satisfied and there were four recurrences (10%).[2]
■ A report on the results of anterior capsulolabral reconstruction at an average of 39 months of follow-up in 25 throwing athletes found excellent or good results in 92% of patients, and 17 (68%) returned to their prior level of competition.
  ■ A subsequent series of 22 subluxators and 9 dislocators found 97% good to excellent results and 94% return to sport.[15]
■ Return-to-sport rates of 32% to 94% have been reported for open surgical treatment of anteroinferior instability in various series.[2,5,12]

COMPLICATIONS

■ Injury to the axillary nerve can occur as it travels an average of only 2.5 mm deep to the IGHL and lies only 12 mm from the glenoid at the 6 o'clock position.
  ■ Nerve injury typically involves sensory function only, and function usually recovers spontaneously.
■ Recurrent dislocations may occur in up to 5% of patients. However, this rate may be higher when appropriate indications for surgery are not strictly followed.
■ Hardware-related complications may occur owing to loosening, bending or breakage of screws, anchors, or tacks (**FIG 7**).[26]
■ Synovitis in response to PLLA absorbable implants has also been described.
■ Misplacement of labral tacks or suture anchors, both metallic and absorbable, may lead to early arthrosis or arthritis.
■ Complications due to positioning have been described including deep venous thrombosis and compression neurapraxia. Bony prominences should be well padded and constrictive bandaging avoided during and after surgery.
■ Infection in shoulder surgery is uncommon. When it occurs, however, *Propionibacterium acnes* is a common organism, and specific cultures should be requested.

REFERENCES

1. Allain J, Goutallier D, Glorion C. Long-term results of the Latarjet procedure for the treatment of anterior instability of the shoulder. J Bone Joint Surg Am 1998;80A:841–852.
2. Altchek DW, Warren RF, Skyhar MJ, et al. T-plasty modification of the Bankart procedure for multidirectional instability of the anterior and inferior types. J Bone Joint Surg Am 1991;73A:105–112.
3. Bankart AS. The pathology and treatment of recurrent dislocation of the shoulder joint. Br J Surg 1938;26:23–29.
4. Bigliani LU, Kelkar R, Flatow EL, et al. Glenohumeral stability: biomechanical properties of passive and active stabilizers. Clin Orthop Relat Res 1996;330:13–30.
5. Bigliani LU, Kurzweil PR, Schwartzbach CC, et al. Inferior capsular shift procedure for anterior-inferior shoulder instability in athletes. Am J Sports Med 1994;22:578–584.
6. Cooper RA, Brems JJ. The inferior capsular-shift procedure for multidirectional instability of the shoulder. J Bone Joint Surg Am 1992;74A:1516–1522.

7. Flatow EL. Glenohumeral instability. In: Bigliani LU, Flatow EL, Pollock RG, et al., eds. The Shoulder: Operative Technique. Baltimore: Williams & Wilkins, 1998:183–184.

8. Gill TJ, Micheli LJ, Gebhard F, et al. Bankart repair for anterior instability of the shoulder: long-term outcome. J Bone Joint Surg Am 1997;79A:850–857.

9. Hamada K, Fukuda H, Nakajima T, et al. The inferior capsular shift operation for instability of the shoulder: long-term results in 34 shoulders. J Bone Joint Surg Br 1999;81B:218–225.

10. Harryman DT, Sidles JA, Harris SL, et al. The role of the rotator interval capsule in passive motion and stability of the shoulder. J Bone Joint Surg Am 1992;74A:53–66.

11. Hawkins RJ, Angelo RL. Glenohumeral osteoarthrosis: a late complication of the Putti-Platt repair. J Bone Joint Surg Am 1990;72A: 1193–1197.

12. Jobe FW, Giangarra CE, Kvitne RS, et al. Anterior capsulolabral reconstruction of the shoulder in athletes in overhand sports. Am J Sports Med 1991;19:428–434.

13. Kirkley A, Griffin S, Richards C, et al. Prospective randomized clinical trial comparing the effectiveness of immediate arthroscopic stabilization versus immobilization and rehabilitation in first traumatic anterior dislocations of the shoulder. Arthroscopy 1999;15:507–514.

14. Klapper RJ, Jobe FW, Matsuura P. The subscapularis muscle and its glenohumeral ligament like bands: a histomorphologic study. Am J Sports Med 1992;20:307–310.

15. Montgomery WH III, Jobe FW. Functional outcomes in athletes after modified anterior capsulolabral reconstruction. Am J Sports Med 1994;22:352–358.

16. Neer CS II, Foster CR. Inferior capsular shift for involuntary inferior and multidirectional instability of the shoulder: a preliminary report. J Bone Joint Surg Am 1980;62A:897–908.

17. Neviaser TJ. The anterior labroligamentous periosteal sleeve avulsion lesion: a cause of anterior instability of the shoulder. Arthroscopy 1993;9:17–21.

18. Osmond-Clarke H. Habitual dislocation of the shoulder: the Putti-Platt operation. J Bone Joint Surg Br 1948;30B:19–25.

19. Owens BD, Dawson L, Burks R, et al. The incidence of shoulder dislocation in the United States military: demographic considerations from a high-risk population. J Bone Joint Surg [Am] 2009;91:791-796.

20. Perthes G. Uber Operationen bei habitueller Schulterluxation. Deutsche Zeitschr Chir 1906;85:199–227.

21. Pollock RG, Bigliani LU. Glenohumeral instability: evaluation and treatment. J Acad Orthop Surg 1993;1:24–32.

22. Rowe C, Patel D, Southmayd WW. The Bankart procedure, a long-term end result study. J Bone Joint Surg Am 1978;60A:1–16.

23. Simonet WT, Melton LJ, Cofield RH, et al. Incidence of anterior shoulder dislocation in Olmstead County, Minnesota. Clin Orthop Relat Res 1984;186:186–191.

24. Wheeler JH, Ryan JB, Arciero RA, et al. Arthroscopic versus non-operative treatment of acute shoulder dislocation in young athletes. Arthroscopy 1989;5:513–517.

25. Wirth MA, Groh GI, Rockwood CA Jr. Capsulorrhaphy through an anterior approach for the treatment of atraumatic posterior glenohumeral instability with multidirectional laxity of the shoulder. J Bone Joint Surg Am 1998;80A:1570–1578.

26. Zuckerman J, Matsen F. Complications about the shoulder related to the use of screws and staples. J Bone Joint Surg Am 1984;66A:175–180.

Chapter 4

Treatment of Recurrent Posterior Shoulder Instability

Jeffrey S. Noble, Daniel D. Noble, and Robert H. Bell

DEFINITION

■ Symptomatic recurrent posterior instability represents up to 12% of all cases of shoulder instability and is subdivided into two discrete entities.[28,35]

■ The first, true posterior dislocation is acute in nature and often related to trauma. It is readily managed with shoulder reduction and carries a low recurrence rate if not associated with a large engaging humeral head defect or a primary uncontrolled seizure disorder.

■ If the primary dislocation is overlooked, this condition can manifest itself as a chronic locked posterior dislocation with its pathognomonic internally rotated position and loss of external rotation on physical examination.

■ The second entity is recurrent unidirectional posterior subluxation, which often represents the more challenging dilemma confronting the orthopaedic surgeon and will be the principal topic of this chapter.

■ Whether due to an increase in awareness by physicians or a more active athletic population, recurrent unidirectional posterior instability is being recognized, diagnosed, and treated more frequently.

■ Patients with recurrent posterior subluxation complain primarily of pain and weakness. As time progresses, symptoms of posterior subluxation become a secondary complaint. Eventually patients often learn the selected muscular contractions, scapular winging, and arm position (forward elevation, adduction, and internal rotation) needed to demonstrate their instability.

■ See Table 1 for the classification of posterior instability.

ANATOMY

■ Posterior instability may be secondary to a tear of the posteroinferior labrum or a patulous posterior capsule.

■ Rarely it can involve a posterior labrocapsular periosteal sleeve avulsion or an avulsion of the posterior glenohumeral ligaments as they insert on the humerus (posterior HAGL lesion).

■ Recently Kim described a concealed and incomplete avulsion of the posteroinferior labrum (type II marginal crack or Kim lesion).[20]

■ Pathology may also be bony in nature and secondary to posterior glenoid avulsions, erosions, increased glenoid retroversion or large engaging reverse Hill-Sachs impression defects.

PATHOGENESIS

■ A significant percentage of patients (40% to 50%) with recurrent posterior subluxation relate a history of trauma. Usually athletes, these individuals are 18 to 30 years of age and are involved in competitive contact sports.

■ Traumatic cases are often associated with the arm in a straight and locked position such as in weight lifting or during football while line blocking. A fall or collision with the individual's arm in at-risk position (forward elevation, adduction, internal rotation) can also be the cause.

■ Frequently, instead of a traumatic event, subluxation episodes with a poorly defined onset are clearly documented.

■ In many cases, especially with repetitive overhead endeavors such as swimming, gymnastics, baseball, and volleyball, the athlete recalls first the gradual onset of discomfort, with subluxation episodes occurring later. Such an onset is thought to be atraumatic and involves repetitive "microtrauma" with resultant stretching of the capsular restraints.

PATIENT HISTORY AND PHYSICAL FINDINGS

■ Whether the patient presents with a clear traumatic episode or a longer atraumatic course, he or she often has a feeling of the shoulder "coming out." Such instability episodes occur when the arm is in the at-risk position of forward elevation, adduction, and internal rotation.

■ Patients often describe a vague discomfort, pain, or weakness as their principal complaint. This actually may lead to misdiagnosis at first.

■ True apprehension or a feeling of "impending doom" when the extremity is placed in the provocative position is less common but can be present.

■ Overhead throwers may complain of a loss of velocity, fatigue, or aching over the posterior shoulder.

■ Usually there is no obvious asymmetry of the muscles on inspection.

■ Palpation may elicit some tenderness along the posterior glenohumeral joint line.

■ Crepitation or a click along the posterior joint line due to labral pathology may be noted.

■ The range of motion is full, often with a decrease in internal rotation and an excess of external rotation.

Table 1	Classification of Posterior Instability

Acute posterior dislocation
Without impression defect
With impression defect

Chronic posterior dislocation
Locked (missed) with impression defect

Recurrent posterior subluxation
Voluntary
    Habitual (willful)
    Muscular control (not willful)
Involuntary
    Positional (demonstrable)
    Nonpositional (not demonstrable)

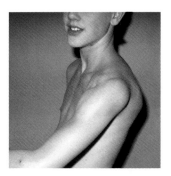

FIG 1 • Younger patient able to voluntarily demonstrate, with muscular contraction and positioning of the upper extremity, his posterior instability.

- Often patients, if voluntary subluxators, can reproduce the subluxation episode on command with arm position and selective muscular contraction (**FIG 1**).
- Physical examination should include the following:
  - Modified load shift test: documents direction and degree of instability
  - Supine load shift test (Gerber and Ganz)[13]: documents direction and degree of instability
  - Seated load shift test: documents direction and degree of instability
  - Posterior stress test: documents direction and degree of instability
  - Sulcus sign: evaluates for an inferior component of the posterior instability (bidirectional) or a more global instability (ie, multidirectional instability)
  - Scapular compression test: verifies the importance of scapular winging in the patient's ability to reproduce the instability and proves to the patient the need to strengthen the periscapular musculature to control instability
  - Jerk test: to document instability. A painful jerk test suggests a posteroinferior labral lesion and is a predictor of the success of nonoperative treatment.
  - Kim test: evaluates for the presence of a labral tear posteriorly
  - Pivot shift of the shoulder: documents direction of the instability

IMAGING AND OTHER DIAGNOSTIC STUDIES

- Radiographic evaluation includes a three-view trauma series of the shoulder, including a true anteroposterior (AP) view of the shoulder, a scapular lateral, and, more importantly, an axillary view.
  - A Velpeau axillary view can be substituted if the attempted axillary view is impossible because of painful abduction of the shoulder.
  - Axillary radiographs of patients with a voluntary component to their instability can be taken while the patient reproduces and maintains the subluxation episode to document the direction (**FIG 2A**).
  - A computed tomography (CT) scan is rarely needed but can be helpful to evaluate humeral head defects and associated fractures of the tuberosities, humeral shaft, and posterior glenoid rim. Significant posterior glenoid retroversion can also be demonstrated on CT scanning (**FIG 2B**).

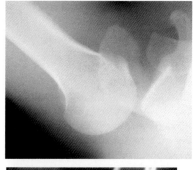

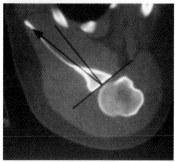

FIG 2 • **A.** Axillary radiograph of patient with voluntary posterior instability, reproducing the instability while taking the radiograph. **B.** CT scan demonstrating significant posterior glenoid retroversion in a patient with posterior instability.

- MRI is the imaging modality of choice after plain radiographs to evaluate the posterior capsule and labrum for tears and associated pathology.
- In certain situations a MRI arthrogram can help diagnose a posteroinferior labral tear.

DIFFERENTIAL DIAGNOSIS

- Superior labrum anterior from posterior tear (SLAP)
- Anterior instability
- Multidirectional instability
- Internal impingement
- Posterior Bennett lesion

NONOPERATIVE MANAGEMENT

- Nonsurgical treatment of posterior unidirectional instability is reportedly successful in up to 80% of the patients.[9,18]
  - The physical therapy program consists of concentric and eccentric resistive band exercises that strengthen the external rotators, the deltoid, and the important periscapular musculature.
    - Resistive upright and seated rows, with an emphasis on trying to pinch the medial scapular borders together during the exercise, are key, especially in patients whose scapular winging contributes to their instability.
  - A strengthening program as well as a sport-specific attempt to decrease those activities that place the arm at risk is key.
- The length of nonoperative treatment must be individualized.
  - Patients who have lower physical demands, are younger, and have an atraumatic history are treated 6 months or more.
  - Higher-level athletes or those who have a traumatic cause with an associated labral tear are more likely to respond to surgical treatment. Despite their associated labral tears, such

elite athletes are often treated with an exercise strengthening program for at least 3 months.

SURGICAL MANAGEMENT

- Although open procedures have been the mainstay and gold standard in the treatment of patients with recurrent unidirectional posterior subluxation, when nonoperative care has failed, arthroscopic treatment has become common.
- As with anterior instability 20 years ago, arthroscopic evaluation in posterior instability patients has led to the diagnosis and treatment of an increasing number of associated soft tissue and articular injuries. Obviously, arthroscopic treatment of posterior capsular avulsions or redundancy in the absence of soft tissue deficiencies or bony abnormalities can have similar success rates without the morbidity of more extensive open surgery.[2,6,20,33]
- Surgical treatment is considered only after an adequate trial of strengthening has failed and the patient remains significantly symptomatic.
- The ideal surgical candidates are those with recurrent posterior unidirectional subluxation secondary to a traumatic episode. These patients often have an associated traumatic posterior labral tear, which is optimal for arthroscopic repair.

- Patients with atraumatic subluxation due to capsular redundancy can be managed either through an open procedure or an arthroscopic capsular shift or plication procedure.
- Patients who have multifactorial causes for their instability or are revision situations are better treated with an open approach.

Preoperative Planning

- An extensive history and physical examination are key to establishing the direction and degree of the patient's instability.
- All imaging studies are reviewed. Plain films and MRI studies are reviewed for the presence of old fractures, loose bodies, and hardware from previous procedures. More importantly, the MRI establishes whether the instability is due to an associated traumatic posterior labral tear or capsular redundancy.
- Associated bony pathology (traumatic glenoid avulsions, glenoid retroversion) and soft tissue deficiencies (from previous procedures) should be addressed concurrently.
- Examination, this time under anesthesia, should be accomplished before positioning to confirm the direction and degree of the instability.

TECHNIQUES

ARTHROSCOPIC POSTERIOR RECONSTRUCTION (AUTHORS' PREFERRED TECHNIQUE)

Positioning

- The patient is positioned in a lateral decubitus position with the operative arm placed in about 40 degrees of abduction and no more than 10 pounds of longitudinal traction.
- All pressure points are carefully identified and an axillary roll is placed under the down axilla.
- The patient's body is placed close to the operating surgeon and tipped posteriorly 15 to 20 degrees.
- We do not employ a double traction set-up, as we do in anterior instability, because increased adduction tends to close down visualization of the posteroinferior joint line, and we have found optimal visualization with 40 degrees of abduction when viewing from the anterior portal.

Portal Placement

- Most posterior reconstructions are performed using only two portals.
- The first is a posterior portal established just lateral to the posterior lateral corner of the acromion.
    - This differs from the traditional posterior viewing portal, which is 1 cm medial and 2 cm inferior from the posterior lateral corner of the acromion.
    - Lateralization of this portal and moving it somewhat superiorly provides an optimal angle of attack to the posterior and inferior portion of the posterior glenoid.

- The anterior portal is established in the rotator interval under direct visualization using needle localization.
- A 6.5-mm cannula is established to allow insertion of the arthroscope and an 8-mm cannula is placed in the posterior portal to allow the passage of the Spectrum crescent suture-passing devices (ConMed Linvatec, Largo, FL).

Site Preparation

- Repair is begun by assessing the posterior labral construct for the presence of labral displacement and tearing (**TECH FIG 1A**).
- A grasper is used to capture the posterior band of the inferior glenohumeral ligament (IGHL), attempting to mobilize it superiorly to determine the amount of capsular laxity and ultimate position for repair.
- If a posterior Bankart lesion is identified, a Liberator knife (ConMed Linvatec, Largo, FL) is used to mobilize the labrum (**TECH FIG 1B**), while a shaver or burr is used to débride the posterior face of the glenoid in preparation for anchor placement (**TECH FIG 1C**).
- This is a critical step so that a freely mobile labrum can be placed up on the glenoid, thereby restoring its bumper effect. Anchor placement begins at the most inferior aspect of the glenoid, usually the 5:30 or 6:30 position, depending on the side involved (**TECH FIG 1D**).
- This position allows secure placement of an anchor while allowing optimal inferior capsular plication. Bioabsorbable anchors are employed for this reconstruction (**TECH FIG 1E**).

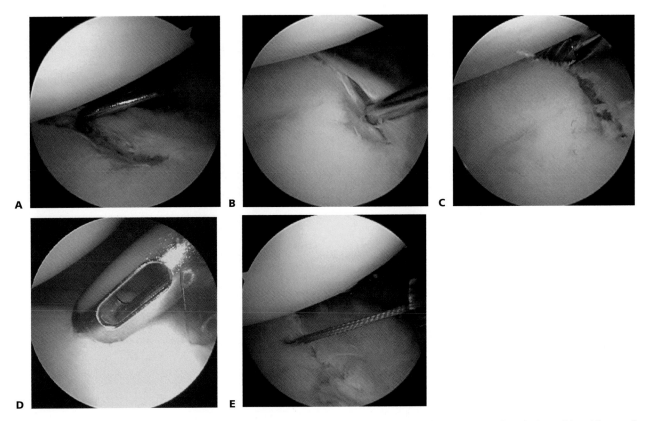

TECH FIG 1 • A. Probe entering the posterior cannula is demonstrating mobility of posterior Bankart lesion with evidence of granulation tissue in the defect. **B.** After the lesion is defined, a Liberator knife is introduced to take down the fibrous interface in the posterior Bankart lesion. **C.** After preparation using a high-speed burr, the posterior inferior aspect of the glenoid is lightly decorticated in preparation for anchor placement. **D.** Initial anchor placement begins at the inferior extent of the glenoid with the use of a guide. **E.** First anchor in place 2 mm up on the articular surface.

Suturing

- A Spectrum 45-degree-offset suture passer, preloaded with a number 0 polydioxanone (PDS) monofilament suture (Ethicon, Somerville NJ), is passed through the posterior cannula, capturing the inferior capsule in the area of the posterior band of the IGHL (**TECH FIG 2A**).
    - This tissue is brought superiorly and the second pass comes deep, exiting at the posterior labral defect.
- The PDS suture is reeled into the joint through the passer

and retrieved in the posterior cannula using a ring grasper (**TECH FIG 2B,C**).
- The deep limb of the PDS is tied to one limb of the anchor suture, and using a pulling technique, the PDS is drawn in a retrograde fashion, with the anchor suture attached, through the capsule and labral tissue, thereby creating a simple stitch (**TECH FIG 2D**).
    - This allows the inferior capsule to be drawn superiorly and medially while at the same time closing the posterior Bankart lesion.

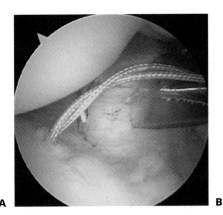

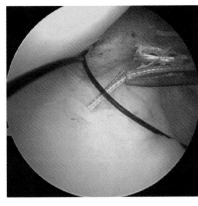

TECH FIG 2 • A. The Spectrum suture passer is used to capture inferior capsular tissue and the posterior band of the inferior glenohumeral ligament. **B.** After anchor placement, stability is assessed with gentle traction on the anchor sutures and a monofilament suture is passed through the suture passer. *(continued)*

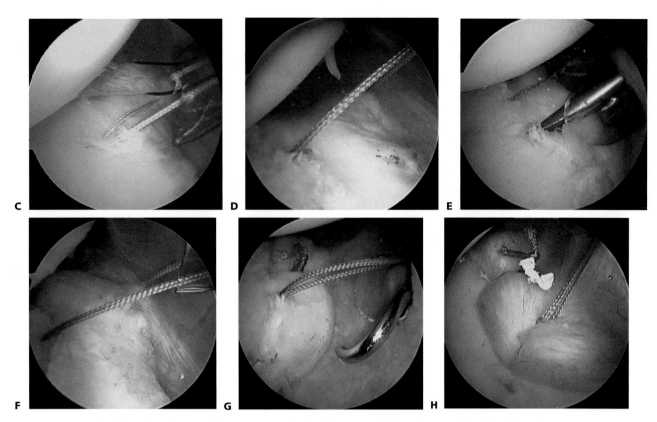

TECH FIG 2 • *(continued)* **C.** The monofilament suture, having been passed through a capsule inferiorly, is drawn up to assess capsular mobility and determine the amount of translation. **D.** One limb of the anchor suture is tied to the monofilament suture, which is then drawn back out the posterior cannula, thus creating a simple stitch. **E.** Having tied the suture on the first anchor, a drill hole is created 7 to 8 mm superiorly for the second anchor. **F.** A second anchor suture has been passed, demonstrating the purchase of additional posterior capsule. **G.** With the final superior anchor in position, the suture passer is directed superiorly to capture additional posteromedial capsule and superior labrum. **H.** Final anchor sutures are tied, demonstrating excellent reconstruction of the posterolabral defect, recreating the posterior labrum bumper effect.

- A second suture is placed after tying the first suture in a similar fashion, again incorporating the capsule as well as labrum (**TECH FIG 2E,F**).
- This process is repeated as many times as is necessary, moving superiorly at 6-mm to 8-mm increments, thereby obliterating any labral defect and capsular redundancy (**TECH FIG 2G,H**).

Capsular Plication

- Alternatively, if no labral detachment is identified and only excessive capsular redundancy exists, a posterior superior capsular shift without anchors is performed.
- The posterior capsule is lightly abraded with a synovial shaver or rasp to promote healing.
- A Spectrum suture passer is used again to pierce the capsule 1 cm lateral to the labrum at the 6:30 position on the glenoid.
- The capsule is then advanced superiorly and medially, with the suture passer re-entering the joint at the junction between the intact labrum and the glenoid rim articular cartilage.

- This is repeated at least two or three times, depending on amount of laxity.
- With each suture the capsule is advanced about one hour's position on the glenoid face (ie, 6:30 capsular stitch to the 7:30 labral position, 7:30 to 8:30, and so on).

Rotator Interval Plication

- In individuals with a significant component of ligamentous laxity, additional closure of the rotator interval is accomplished by moving the arthroscope back to the posterior portal.
- Through the anterior portal, a number 0 PDS suture is passed through the upper border of the middle glenohumeral ligament, capturing the superior glenohumeral ligament and rotator interval capsule.
  - This suture is used as a pulling stitch for a number 2 braided polyester fiber (TI•CRON) suture (Tyco, United States Surgical, Norwalk, CT).
- This is repeated again and sutures are tied just outside the capsule.

OPEN POSTERIOR HUMERAL-BASED CAPSULAR SHIFT (AUTHORS' PREFERRED TECHNIQUE)

Positioning

- Under general anesthesia the patient is positioned in the lateral decubitus position using a full-length beanbag.
- A large axillary roll is placed under the down nonsurgical axilla.
- The operative arm and shoulder are draped free.

Incision and Dissection

- A longitudinal incision in the posterior axillary fold is made beginning at a point 2 cm medial to the posterolateral corner of the acromion and extending distally, following the posterior axillary line (**TECH FIG 3**).
- The underlying deltoid muscle is split along its fibers bluntly, and a self-retaining retractor is placed.[34]
  - Caution should be exercised as to not split the deltoid distally greater than 4 to 5 cm to avoid injuring the axillary nerve.[8,34]
  - If the individual is larger and more exposure is needed, the deltoid can be detached from its scapular origin for a short distance, leaving a small tendinous attachment to repair later.
- Repair of the deltoid origin can also be accomplished by placing drill holes along the scapular spine for suture passage.

- The underlying infraspinatus is identified by its bipennate nature, a central fatty raphe dividing the muscle, and the fiber direction change compared with the teres minor inferiorly.
- The infraspinatus can be handled in three ways:
  - It can be split horizontally to expose the underlying capsule.[32] Care is taken with this technique not to extend the split farther than 1.5 to 2 cm medial to the glenoid rim, as the infraspinatus branches of the suprascapular nerve are coursing along the inferior fascia of the infraspinatus directly on the scapular surface. Extension of the split into the branches or elevation of the fascia off the scapula will injure a number of, if not all, the branches to the infraspinatus.
  - The second method is to identify the interval between the infraspinatus and teres minor. This interval is developed with the muscle being worked superiorly, thereby exposing underlying capsule.
  - Third, the infraspinatus may be completely detached, leaving a 2-cm remnant of the tendon still attached for later repair (**TECH FIG 4**). It is tagged and carefully released from the underlying thin capsule.

Capsulotomy

- A vertical capsulotomy is made on the humeral side with the arm in neutral rotation (**TECH FIG 5A**).

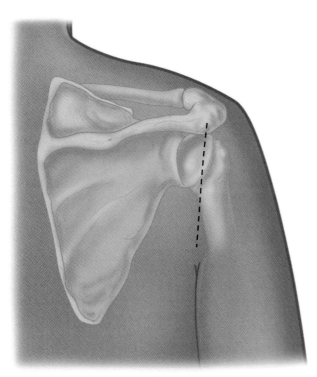

TECH FIG 3 • The posterior longitudinal incision begins about 2 cm medial to the posterolateral corner of the acromion and extends into the axillary crease.

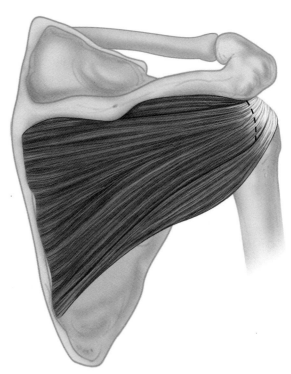

TECH FIG 4 • With the deltoid fibers bluntly split, a vertical incision is made directly through the infraspinatus while keeping a small stump of infraspinatus tendon attached laterally for reattachment later.

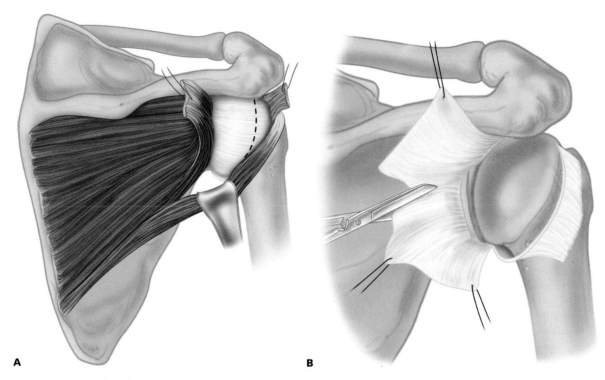

TECH FIG 5 • A. The infraspinatus is elevated as a single layer, exposing the underlying posterior capsule. A vertical capsulotomy is then made based on the humeral side from the 12 o'clock to the 6 o'clock position. **B.** Traction stitches are then placed as the medial capsule is divided horizontally, between the sutures, toward but not through the glenoid labrum.

- A small amount of capsule, 3 to 4 mm, can be left on its humeral attachment to aid in repair of the capsular flaps laterally during the shift.
- Care is taken to protect the axillary nerve inferiorly from retractors as it is traversing from anterior to posterior to exit in the quadrangular space inferiorly.
- With the vertical capsulotomy completed, two traction stitches are placed at the midposition and the capsule is horizontally divided, between the stitches, toward the middle of the glenoid rim, stopping 1 to 2 mm from the posterior glenoid labrum (**TECH FIG 5B**).

T Capsulorrhaphy

- Although both medial and lateral capsular shifts have been described, we prefer a humeral-based T capsulorrhaphy because we believe tensioning of the capsular flaps is easier to control and a larger volume reduction can be achieved, if desired.
- Those who prefer a glenoid-based T-capsular shift cite advantages of a muscle-splitting approach and ease of repair if an associated reverse Bankart lesion is encountered.
    - If a glenoid-based shift is selected, most authors position the arm in 20 degrees of abduction and neutral to 20 degrees of external rotation while doing the capsular repair.

Posterior Inferior Capsular Shift

- The posterior glenoid labrum is inspected and if there is a small detachment, it is repaired before completing the capsular shift procedure.

- The inferior flap of the capsule is carefully mobilized past the 6-o'clock position, inferiorly on the humerus.
    - This step is critical as an inadequate release of the inferior capsule will prevent correction of the posteroinferior capsular redundancy and volume.
- The nonarticular sulcus, medial to the capsular remnant left behind, is then decorticated with a high-speed burr to facilitate healing (**TECH FIG 6A**).
- The inferior capsular flap is brought superiorly and slightly laterally with the arm held in 40 to 45 degrees of abduction and 15 to 20 degrees of external rotation.
- This inferior flap is sutured in place with multiple figure eight nonabsorbable sutures.
    - If the capsular remnant to suture to is of poor quality, suture anchors are used for repair. In a similar fashion, the superior capsular flap is shifted inferiorly down over the inferior flap and sutured (**TECH FIG 6B,C**).
- The horizontal portion of the T capsulorrhaphy is then closed and reinforced with nonabsorbable sutures.
    - The degree of closure of this horizontal portion can further tighten the posterior capsule if desired.
- If the infraspinatus was released with a small remnant left attached to the humeral side, the infraspinatus is sutured back to its tendinous stump anatomically with nonabsorbable suture.
- If the infraspinatus was split, it is allowed to fall back in position and the fascia is closed with absorbable suture.
- Routine closure is performed, and the arm is placed into a shoulder orthosis or spica cast depending on patient compliance, incorporating 20 degrees of abduction and 20 degrees of external rotation.

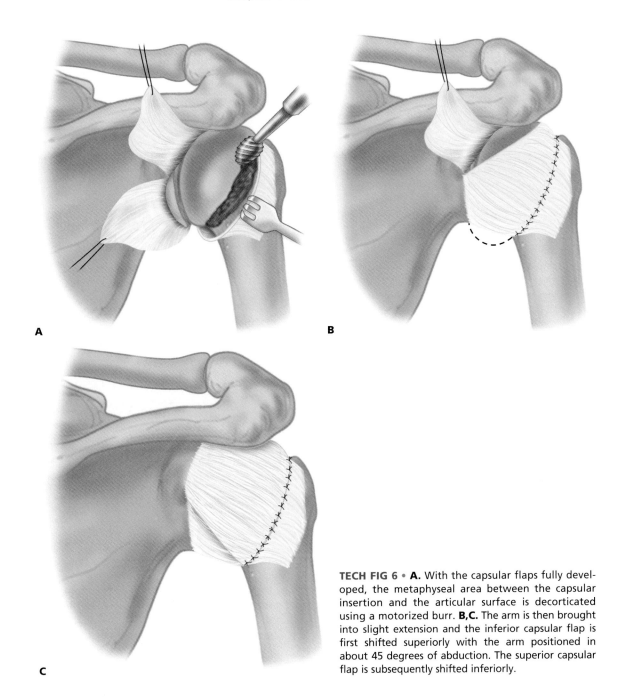

TECH FIG 6 • A. With the capsular flaps fully developed, the metaphyseal area between the capsular insertion and the articular surface is decorticated using a motorized burr. **B,C.** The arm is then brought into slight extension and the inferior capsular flap is first shifted superiorly with the arm positioned in about 45 degrees of abduction. The superior capsular flap is subsequently shifted inferiorly.

OPEN POSTERIOR LABRAL REPAIR (REVERSE BANKART REPAIR)

- The patient positioning and surgical exposure are similar down to the infraspinatus musculature.
- The infraspinatus can be split, as is our preference, or a horizontal incision can be made 2 cm lateral to the glenoid rim through both the infraspinatus and capsule as one layer.
- The posterior capsulolabral tissue is freely mobilized from the glenoid neck.
- The scapular neck is then decorticated with a motorized burr to promote healing and the labrum is reattached using the surgeon's preferred commercially available absorbable suture anchors or through transosseous tunnels.

- Again, the goal is to roll the labrum up onto the posterior glenoid rim, restoring the capsulolabral bumper effect.
- Although this procedure is usually done as a primary procedure, it may be combined with a humeral or glenoid based posterior-inferior T-capsular shift in patients with excessive laxity or instability on clinical examination.
- Care must be taken not to overtighten the repair when both procedures are used, since postoperative stiffness and loss of motion, especially internal rotation, can occur.

OPEN POSTERIOR INFRASPINATUS CAPSULAR TENODESIS

- The posterior infraspinatus and capsular tenodesis, as described by Hawkins, is reproducible and takes advantage of the thick quality of the infraspinatus tendon and underlying capsule layer.[4,16]
- It is extremely useful, in our opinion, in situations of poor-quality capsular tissue, since often the posterior capsule is only 1 to 2 mm thick, and in revision cases in which multiple posterior procedures have failed (**TECH FIG 7**).

Positioning

- This technique is performed using the same positioning and exposure as described earlier down to the infraspinatus musculature.
- Preoperatively the patient can be placed into an outrigger shoulder spica cast with a fiberglass long-arm component and a detachable spica bar or a shoulder orthosis.
- Preparation and draping are done with the involved arm free.

Incision and Approach

- The same posterior axillary incision and split of the underlying deltoid muscle described earlier are used.
- With the arm in neutral position, the glenoid rim is located under the infraspinatus using a spinal needle, starting medially and walking the needle laterally over the glenoid rim until the exact location of the joint is identified.
- This position is then marked to confirm the lateral extent of the glenoid rim.
  - This is a crucial step because if the vertical incision to be made through both the infraspinatus and capsule is made too far laterally, severe overtightening will result.

Vertical Arthrotomy

- A single vertical incision is made through the infraspinatus tendon and underlying capsule parallel to and 1.0 to

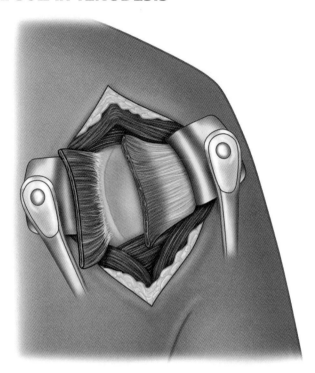

TECH FIG 8 • The arm is positioned in neutral rotation and the infraspinatus and underlying posterior capsule are incised together and parallel to the glenoid rim.

1.5 cm lateral to the joint line with the arm in neutral rotation (**TECH FIG 8**).
  - Most of the infraspinatus tendon runs on its inferior surface, with visible overlying muscle. This anatomic situation leads to a feeling of uneasiness as the surgeon begins to incise through the fleshy infraspinatus musculature portion posteriorly.
  - However, one should not worry, since the thicker tendinous portion of the infraspinatus will be encountered deeper during the vertical incision.
- With the capsulotomy complete, a Fukuda retractor is placed in the joint and the posterior labrum is inspected.

Posterior Repair

- The retractor is then removed and the arm is externally rotated 20 degrees (**TECH FIG 9A**).
- The lateral stump of the infraspinatus and capsule (one layer) is sutured to the intact posterior labrum using nonabsorbable sutures (**TECH FIG 9B**).
- The remaining medial portion of the infraspinatus and capsule is then reflected laterally overlapping the primary repair and sutured, again with nonabsorbable sutures (**TECH FIG 9C**).
- The deltoid is allowed to fall back together and the fascia is closed. Routine wound closure is performed.

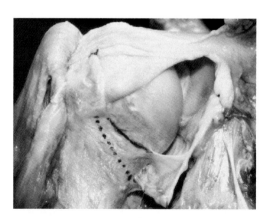

TECH FIG 7 • Anatomic dissection with the posterior rotator cuff musculature reflected, revealing the often thin posterior capsular structures.

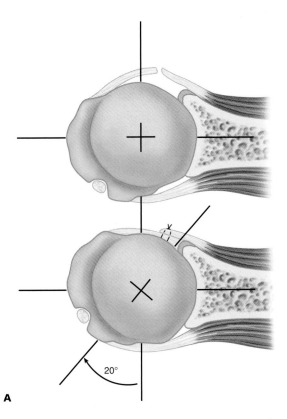

TECH FIG 9 • A. After completing the posterior capsulotomy, the arm is positioned in about 20 degrees of external rotation and the lateral tendon portion of the infraspinatus and capsule are sutured to the intact posterior labrum. **B.** The arm is then externally rotated 20 degrees and the lateral flap of infraspinatus and capsule is sutured to the posterior glenoid labrum. **C.** The medial flap of the infraspinatus is then overlapped and sutured to its lateral tendon.

20°

A

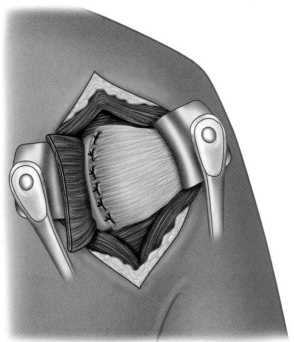

B

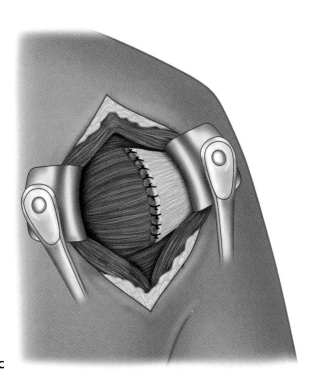

C

OPEN POSTERIOR GLENOID OSTEOTOMY

- Preoperative evaluation will rarely identify a patient who demonstrates excessive glenoid retroversion in excess of 20 degrees.[30,31]
  - In these situations, the surgeon may need to consider a posterior glenoid osteotomy as the primary procedure or in combination with a posterior capsulorrhaphy or shift.[17]
- This procedure is rarely needed, however, and is reserved for those special circumstances. This procedure is technically demanding and should be performed by a surgeon with previous exposure to the procedure.

Positioning and Approach

- The initial steps, including preoperative spica application and positioning, are repeated.
- The standard approach down to the infraspinatus is used, with the infraspinatus released from its lateral insertion.

Vertical Capsulotomy

- A vertical capsulotomy is made 1 cm lateral to the glenoid rim.
- The medial capsule is detached sharply from the posterior aspect of the glenoid, with the labrum left attached to the posterior glenoid rim.
  - Caution is again exercised because the suprascapular nerve is running superiorly around the spine of the scapula about 2 to 3 cm from the glenoid rim.
- The Fukuda retractor is placed into the joint to permit visualization of the glenoid retroversion and orientation of the plane of the glenoid.

Glenoid Osteotomy

- With the orientation determined and the line of the osteotomy marked, drill holes are made through both anterior and posterior cortices.
  - These holes should be no closer than 1 cm from the glenoid articular surface.
- The concavity of the glenohumeral joint as well as its superior to inferior and anterior to posterior orientation is kept in mind to avoid accidental intra-articular penetration and fracture.

- A depth gauge is used to measure each hole to get an idea of the depth of the glenoid neck.
- The oscillating saw blade is marked just short of this glenoid depth, thus decreasing the potential for traversing both the anterior and posterior cortices with the saw blade, which would result in creation of a free-floating glenoid (**TECH FIG 10A**).
- With the osteotomy complete, a 1-inch osteotome is gently tapped into place and the osteotomy is opened by moving the osteotome and glenoid laterally.
  - The partially intact anterior periosteum and cortex maintain the appropriate position of the glenoid fragment.
- The osteotomy is then opened with a 1-inch osteotome and a quarter-inch osteotome is placed perpendicular to the osteotomy at either the superior or inferior margin to hold the osteotomy in the open position (**TECH FIG 10B**).
- A tricortical graft harvested from the posterior acromion or iliac crest is placed into the osteotomy and its position and stability are checked.
  - Usually the humeral head against the glenoid will provide an adequate compressive force to close down the osteotomy and stabilize its position without hardware or internal fixation (**TECH FIG 10C**). If fixation is required, small fascial or hand set plates are ideal.
- This procedure can be combined, depending on how the infraspinatus is handled, with a humeral-based posteroinferior capsular shift or infraspinatus capsular tenodesis.
- The arm is placed in a shoulder spica postoperatively and held for 4 to 6 weeks to allow consolidation of the posterior bone graft.

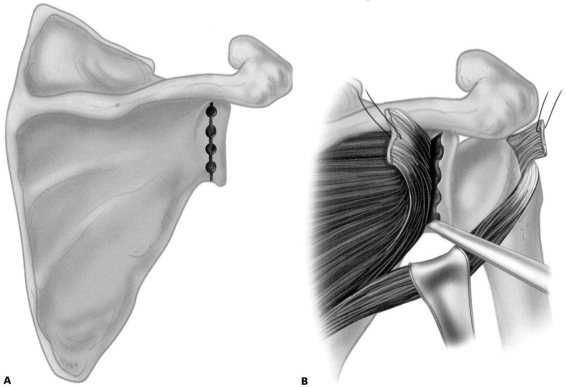

A   **B**

TECH FIG 10 • A. Bicortical drill holes are created about 1 cm medial and parallel to the posterior glenoid rim. An oscillating saw then completes the osteotomy posteriorly. **B.** A small osteotome is used to gently hinge open the osteotomy site laterally, thus preserving somewhat the integrity of the anterior cortex and its periosteal and soft tissue attachments. *(continued)*

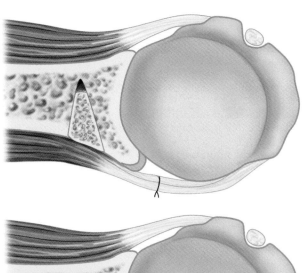

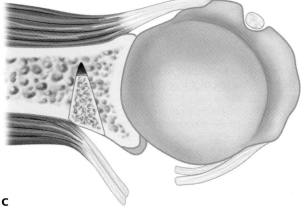

C

TECH FIG 10 • *(continued)* **C.** A tricortical graft is harvested from the posterior acromion or iliac spine and inserted into the osteotomy site. This procedure can be also combined with a posteroinferior capsular shift or also infraspinatus tenodesis.

OPEN POSTERIOR BONE BLOCK GRAFT AUGMENTATION

- A posterior-placed bone block may be selected as the primary procedure but is usually needed as an additional augmentation procedure to back up a soft tissue procedure in revision situations with inadequate capsular tissue.
  - This technique has been used only twice in 10 years as an augmentation procedure by the authors.
- We prefer a bone block placed extra-articularly in those often-difficult patients with soft tissue deficiencies, such as seen in Ehlers-Danlos syndrome.
  - Using the bone block extra-articularly allows the capsular repair anterior to the graft to act as a soft tissue interposition.
- The positioning and exposure down to the capsule are as earlier described.

- After the posterior capsule has been shifted, a 3 × 2-cm, 8- to 10-mm-thick bone graft is obtained either from the posterior acromial spine or iliac crest.
- After the glenoid neck is exposed and the glenoid neck decorticated, the cancellous side of the graft is placed posterior and inferior and fixated with two cancellous screws.
- The graft is tailored to its final desired shape using a motorized burr.
- Care must be used such that the graft is not placed excessively lateral to the glenoid rim with secondary impingement on the humeral head or too medial to the glenoid rim, rendering it ineffective. The goal is to increase the width and depth of the glenoid without contacting the humeral head.

PEARLS AND PITFALLS

Indications	■ Failure to make an accurate diagnosis of the direction or degree of instability ■ A complete history and physical examination is crucial and must be performed. If needed, an examination under anesthesia to rule out a more global instability is useful. ■ Patient selection is key for each planned procedure. ■ Failure to identify the habitual "pathologic" voluntary dislocator[29]
Soft tissue management	■ Failure to address associated ligamentous laxity ■ It is imperative to rule out a more global instability (multidirectional instability). ■ Beware of patients with previous failure from an extensive thermal capsulorrhaphy procedure.[36]

Bony deficiency management	▪ Significant glenoid rim deficiencies need to be addressed with reconstruction. Soft tissue procedures will not be sufficient. ▪ Rarely, excessive glenoid retroversion needs to be addressed.
Operative technique	▪ Proficiency in each procedure is key. A suboptimal attempt arthroscopically or open will doom the repair to failure. ▪ Capsular plication in conjunction with arthroscopic posterior labral repair may be required in patients with more ligamentous laxity. ▪ Care must be taken not to close down the rotator cuff interval too much, especially close to the glenoid, as a loss of external rotation can occur. It is important to close the interval based on the individual's clinical laxity. ▪ During arthroscopic repair it is crucial to place the suture anchors 1 to 2 mm over the glenoid rim onto the articular surface. This ensures that the capsulolabral tissue will be rolled up and onto the glenoid rim, restoring the bumper effect of the labrum. ▪ In patients with large capsular redundancy, inadequate release of the capsule past the 6 o'clock position on the humeral metaphysis, while performing a capsular shift, will lead to residual inferior symptomatic instability and failure. ▪ During the open infraspinatus tenodesis, the step of identifying the exact location of the glenoid rim is critical since a misplaced vertical incision through the infraspinatus and capsule, if done far laterally, will lead to overtightening, increased loss of internal rotation, and a risk of eventual secondary arthritis. ▪ Again, only rarely is glenoid osteotomy needed in those cases of excessive glenoid retroversion. Predrilling to the anterior cortex will decrease the risk of a free-floating glenoid or accidental intra-articular fracture. ▪ Postoperative loss of motion and stiffness, especially in open procedures, is often overlooked and most likely underreported. Although loss of internal rotation may be acceptable in revision cases to achieve stability, even insignificant losses of internal rotation and forward elevation in high-performance elite athletes, such as swimmers or overhead throwers, can be devastating. Thus, swimmers and elite overhead athletes are addressed arthroscopically if possible.

POSTOPERATIVE CARE

▪ Using these techniques, the procedure can be tailored to meet the patient's clinical instability; however, the rehabilitation is similar in all patients regardless of technique.

▪ After completion of the repair, the arm can be removed from traction and posterior translation reassessed.

▪ The patient is then placed in a 30-degree external rotation brace and held in this position for 3 to 4 weeks postoperatively (Ultra-Sling, DonJoy, Carlsbad, CA).

▪ At that point, gentle active-assisted range-of-motion exercises are begun, avoiding all internal rotation posterior to the coronal plane for the first 6 weeks.

▪ At the 6-week mark postoperatively, a gentle isometric strengthening program is started.

▪ Throwing activities are not started until the fourth month, with resumption of athletic endeavors anticipated at 6 months.

▪ While the surgical approach may vary, all posterior reconstructions are treated similarly in their postoperative regimen.

COMPLICATIONS

▪ Recurrent or residual instability
▪ Postoperative loss of motion or stiffness
▪ Neurovascular injury, especially posterior cord or axillary or suprascapular nerve
▪ Anchor pullout or hardware failure
▪ Infection
▪ Post–instability repair arthritis (capsulorrhaphy arthropathy)
▪ Chondral injury
▪ Chondrolysis secondary to thermal capsular shrinkage[36]
▪ Hematoma
▪ Postoperative rotator cuff atrophy or weakness

▪ Subcoracoid impingement (obligate anterior humeral head shift due to posterior capsular tightness or glenoid osteotomy)

OUTCOMES

▪ Posterior instability encompasses a continuum from acute and chronic posterior dislocation to the more frequently encountered recurrent posterior subluxation. Earlier reports in the literature have often involved small patient populations and isolated case reports with minimal follow-up.

▪ Past surgical treatment options included a number of nonanatomic reconstruction procedures to indirectly control posterior subluxation or dislocation.

▪ Eventually, a more anatomic approach developed, with procedures designed to openly repair the detached labrum (reverse Bankart repair)[3,27] or address the patient's excessive capsular redundancy (posteroinferior capsular shift).[5,12,15,21,26]

▪ Preliminary results, published in 1980 by Neer and Foster, described a humeral-based posterior and inferior capsular shift with early good results.[27] Since then, multiple authors have advocated the use of Neer's posteroinferior capsular shift with excellent results. Other authors have modified this concept by using a glenoid-based posterior T-capsular shift to similarly tighten the posterior capsule.[24]

▪ More recently, Misamore and Facibene[25] reported promising results in unidirectional posterior instability patients using such an open posterior glenoid-based capsular shift. Excellent results were achieved, with 12 of 14 returning to competitive sports.

▪ Fronek and colleagues,[11] using a similar capsular shift, reported on 10 of 11 patients without further episodes of instability and overall good results. However, only 3 patients were able to return to their preinjury ability level during sports. If the capsular laxity was not eliminated by this medial-based shift, then an additional lateral incision in the capsule and an H-type repair was used.

■ Osseous reconstructions, including a posterior opening wedge glenoid osteotomy[4,7,14,23,32] and posterior bone block procedures,[1,10,11,19,26] to augment or address bony deficiencies have been described and although rarely used still have a place under certain circumstances. Hernandez and Drez[17] combined glenoplasty with a capsulorrhaphy and infraspinatus advancement.

■ The posterior infraspinatus tenodesis, as illustrated, remains a valuable procedure, especially in cases of poor posterior capsular tissue or in revision cases. Hawkins and colleagues[16] reported an 85% success rate using such a tenodesis as a primary procedure. Even when including revision cases, Pollock and Bigliani[29] reported an 80% success rate using the same technique.

■ Papendick and Savoie,[28] followed by McIntyre and associates,[24] were among the first of many to describe their arthroscopic techniques in the treatment of unidirectional posterior subluxation with encouraging results.

■ Further improvements in arthroscopic suture repair techniques and instruments have led to the effective and reproducible arthroscopic treatment of recurrent posterior subluxation. The most promising arthroscopic repair techniques include posterior labral repair using suture anchor fixation, posterior capsulolabral plication, and the increasing role of rotator cuff interval plication as an augmentation to the primary repair.

  ■ Kim and colleagues[21] prospectively reported on 27 athletes with unidirectional recurrent posterior subluxation due to a distinct traumatic event. All were treated with an arthroscopic posterior Bankart repair and capsular shifting superiorly. Suture anchors were used in all cases and, if an incomplete labral lesion was encountered, it was converted to a complete detachment before repair. At a mean of 39 months postoperatively, patients had improved functional scores and only 1 patient out of 27 (4%) had a recurrence.

■ Recently, Bradley and colleagues,[6] in the largest prospective study to date, reviewed 91 athletes (100 shoulders) with unidirectional, recurrent posterior instability. Three types of capsulolabral repairs were performed based on preoperative clinical examination and arthroscopic findings: capsulolabral plication without suture anchors, capsulolabral plication with suture anchors and additional plication sutures, and capsulolabral plication with suture anchors.

  ■ The capsulolabral repair without suture anchors was used in cases of significant posterior capsular laxity even though the labrum was not detached. The labrum was advanced superiorly and medially. Patients with acute traumatic injuries with minimal capsular stretching underwent minimal capsular advancement during the repair. Patients with chronic capsular redundancy required more advancement.[6]

  ■ The mean follow-up in the study was 27 months. All were involved in athletics, and 51% were involved in contact sports. Of these, 66% had an isolated posterior labral tear. Of the eight failures due to recurrent instability, pain, or decreased function, only one had a traumatic reinjuring event. All failures had a patulous capsule and 25% had a recurrent labral tear. Twenty-five percent of the failures had a previous thermal capsulorrhaphy before being referred for treatment. Only 11% of the patients in the study group did not return to their sport, and 33% returned but were unable to perform at the same level of competition.[6]

REFERENCES

1. Ahlgren S, Hedlund T, Nistor L. Idiopathic posterior instability of the shoulder joint: results of operation with posterior bone graft. Acta Orthop Scand 1978;49:600–603.
2. Antoniou J, Duckworth DT, Harryman DT II. Capsulolabral augmentation for the management of posteroinferior instability of the shoulder. J Bone Joint Surg Am 2000;82A:1220–1230.
3. Arciero RA, Mazzocca AD. Traumatic posterior shoulder subluxation with labral injury: suture anchor technique. Tech Shoulder Elbow Surg 2004;5:13–24.
4. Bell RH, Noble JS. An appreciation of posterior instability of the shoulder. Clin Sports Med 1991;4:887–899.
5. Bigliani LU, Pollock RG, McIlveen SJ, et al. Shift of the posteroinferior aspect of the capsule for recurrent posterior glenohumeral instability. J Bone Joint Surg Am 1995;77A:1101–1120.
6. Bradley JP, Baker CL, Kline AJ, et al. Arthroscopic capsulolabral reconstruction for posterior instability of the shoulder. Am J Sports Med 2006;34:1061–1071.
7. Brewer B, Wubben RC, Carrera GF. Excessive retroversion of the glenoid cavity: a cause of non-traumatic posterior instability of the shoulder. J Bone Joint Surg Am 1986;68A:724–731.
8. Bryan WJ, Schauder K, Tullos HS. The axillary nerve and its relationship to common sports medicine shoulder procedures. Am J Sports Med 1986;14:113–116.
9. Burkhead WZ Jr, Rockwood CA Jr. Treatment of instability of the shoulder with an exercise program. J Bone Joint Surg Am 1992;74A:890–896.
10. Fried A. Habitual posterior dislocation of the shoulder joint: a case report on 5 operated cases. Acta Orthop Scand 1949;18:329.
11. Fronek J, Warren RF, Bowen M. Posterior subluxation of the glenohumeral joint. J Bone Joint Surg Am 1989;71A:205–216.
12. Fuchs B, Jose B, Gerber C. Posterior-inferior capsular shift for the treatment of recurrent, voluntary posterior subluxation of the shoulder. J Bone Joint Surg Am 2000;82:16–25.
13. Gerber C, Ganz R. Clinical assessment of instability of the shoulder; with special reference to the anterior and posterior drawer tests. J Bone Joint Surg Br 1984;66B:551–556.
14. Gerber C, Ganz R, Vinh TS. Glenoplasty for recurrent posterior shoulder instability: an anatomic reappraisal. Clin Orthop Relat Res 1987;216:70–79.
15. Goss TP, Costello G. Recurrent symptomatic posterior glenohumeral subluxation. Orthop Rev 17;1988:1024–1032.
16. Hawkins RJ, Janda DH. Posterior instability of the glenohumeral joint: a technique of repair. Am J Sports Med 1996;24:275–278.
17. Hernandez A, Drez D. Operative treatment of posterior shoulder dislocations by posterior glenoidplasty, capsulorrhaphy, and infraspinatus advancement. Am J Sports Med 1986;14:187–191.
18. Hurley JA, Anderson TE, Dear W, et al. Posterior shoulder instability: surgical versus conservative results with evaluation of glenoid version. Am J Sports Med 1992;20:396–400.
19. Jones V. Recurrent posterior dislocation of the shoulder: report of a case treated by posterior bone block. J Bone Joint Surg Br 1958;40:203–207.
20. Kim SH, Ha KI, Yoo JC, et al. Kim's lesion: an incomplete and concealed avulsion of the posteroinferior labrum in posterior or multidirectional posteroinferior instability of the shoulder. Arthroscopy 2004;20:712–720.
21. Kim SH, Ha KI, Park JH, et al. Arthroscopic posterior labral repair and capsular shift for traumatic unidirectional recurrent posterior subluxation of the shoulder. J Bone Joint Surg Am 2003;85A:1479–1487.
22. Kim SH, Kim HK, Sun JI, et al. Arthroscopic capsulolabroplasty for posteroinferior multidirectional instability of the shoulder. Am J Sports Med 2004;32:594–607.
23. Kretzler HH. Scapular osteotomy for posterior shoulder dislocation. J Bone Joint Surg Am 1974;56A:197.
24. McIntyre LF, Caspari RB, Savoie FH III. The arthroscopic treatment of posterior instability: two-year results of a multiple suture technique. Arthroscopy 1997;13:426–432.
25. Misamore GW, Facibene WA. Posterior capsulorrhaphy for the treatment of traumatic recurrent posterior subluxations of the shoulder in athletes. J Shoulder Elbow Surg 2000;9:403–408.

26. Mowery CA, Garfin SR, Booth R, et al. Recurrent posterior dislocation of the shoulder: treatment using a bone block. J Bone Joint Surg Am 1958;67:777–781.

27. Neer CS II, Foster CR. Inferior capsular shift for involuntary inferior and multidirectional instability of the shoulder. J Bone Joint Surg Am 1980;62A:897–908.

28. Papendick LW, Savoie FH III. Anatomy specific repair techniques for posterior shoulder instability. J South Orthop Assoc 1995;4: 169–176.

29. Pollock RG, Bigliani LU. Recurrent posterior shoulder instability: diagnosis and treatment. Clin Orthop Relat Res 1993;291:85–96.

30. Rowe CR, Pierce DS, Clark JG. Voluntary dislocation of the shoulder: a preliminary report on a clinical, electromyographic, and psychiatric study of 26 patients. J Bone Joint Surg Am 1973;55A:445–460.

31. Schutte JP, Lafayette LA, Hawkins RJ, et al. The use of computerized tomography in determining humeral retroversion. Orthop Trans 1988;12:727.

32. Scott DJ Jr. Treatment of recurrent posterior dislocations of the shoulder by glenoplasty. J Bone Joint Surg Am 1967;49: 471–476.

33. Shaffer BS, Conway J, Jobe FW, et al. Infraspinatus muscle-splitting incision in posterior shoulder surgery. Am J Sports Med 1994;22: 113–120.

34. Williams RJ, Strickland S, Cohen M, et al. Arthroscopic repair for traumatic posterior instability. Am J Sports Med 2003;31: 203–209.

35. Wirth MA, Butters KP, Rockwood CA. The posterior deltoid splitting approach to the shoulder. Clin Orthop Relat Res 1993;296: 92–96.

36. Wolf EM, Eakin CL. Arthroscopic capsular plication for posterior shoulder instability. Arthroscopy 1998;14:153–163.

37. Wong KL, Williams GR. Complications of thermal capsulorrhaphy of the shoulder. J Bone Joint Surg Am 2001;83:151–155.

Chapter 5

Latarjet Procedure for Instability With Bone Loss

John Lunn, Juan Castellanos-Rosas, and Gilles Walch

DEFINITION

- Glenoid bone loss after anterior dislocation is the loss of bone due to fracture, abrasion, or compression at the anteroinferior glenoid.
- This bone loss is frequently seen after anterior dislocation and varies greatly in its extent and significance.[4,6]
- The use of a coracoid bone block to prevent anterior dislocation was first proposed by Latarjet[7] in 1954.
- In 1958 Helfet[5] described the Bristow technique, in which the tip of the coracoid is sutured to the capsuloperiosteal elements of the anterior glenoid. This was later modified to screw fixation.
- Patte[9] described the effectiveness of the Latarjet procedure as being due to the "triple blocking effect":
  - The effect of the conjoint tendon when the arm is in the abducted and externally rotated position, where it acts as a sling on the inferior subscapularis and the inferior capsule (**FIG 1**).
  - The effect of the anterior bone block
  - The effect of repairing the capsule to the stump of the conjoint tendon
- The original technique described by Latarjet involved cutting the subscapularis tendon, but this has been modified to a subscapularis split, thus preserving the integrity of its fibers.

ANATOMY

- The glenoid has a pear shape, with an average height of 35 mm and an average width of 25 mm.
- The fibrous glenoid labrum provides attachment for the glenohumeral ligaments to the bony glenoid and increases the depth of the glenoid by 50%.
- The inferior glenohumeral ligament (IGHL) attaches to the glenoid between the 2 o'clock and 4 o'clock positions in a right shoulder.

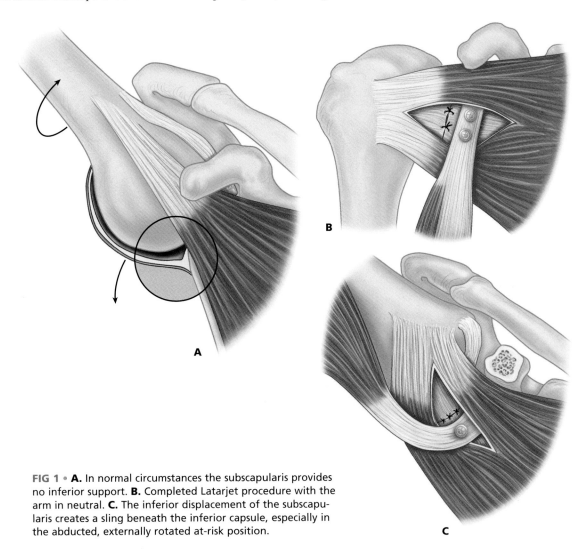

FIG 1 • **A.** In normal circumstances the subscapularis provides no inferior support. **B.** Completed Latarjet procedure with the arm in neutral. **C.** The inferior displacement of the subscapularis creates a sling beneath the inferior capsule, especially in the abducted, externally rotated at-risk position.

- The coracoid is directed anteriorly and then hooks laterally and inferiorly from its origin on the anterior scapular neck.
- The distal and lateral coracoid is the portion osteotomized for the Latarjet procedure. It is the origin for the short head of biceps and the coracobrachialis tendons (conjoint tendon) at its tip. Medially the pectoralis minor is attached, and laterally there is the insertion of the coracoacromial and the coracohumeral ligaments.
- Proximal to the "knee" of the coracoid and untouched by the osteotomy are the conoid and trapezoid ligaments.
- The musculocutaneous nerve enters the conjoint tendon from the medial aspect on its deep surface at an average of 5 cm from the tip of the coracoid (range 1.5 to 9 cm).
- The axillary nerve runs on the anterior surface of the subscapularis muscle lateral to the axillary artery before it enters the quadrilateral space at the inferior portion of the subscapularis.
- The anterior inferior glenohumeral ligament lies deep to the middle and lower portions of the subscapularis muscle.

PATHOGENESIS

- Anterior glenoid bone loss occurs because of either impaction of the humeral head on the anterior glenoid at the moment of dislocation or recurrent subluxation or dislocation.
- Acute impaction may result in anteroinferior glenoid fractures, the so-called bony Bankart lesions.
- Recurrent subluxation or dislocation may also result in erosion or impaction of the glenoid rim.
- Recurrent dislocation occurs owing to multiple factors, one of which is the presence of a bony lesion.
- Following Bankart repair, loss of external rotation is 25 degrees per centimeter of anterior glenoid defect. This is due to anterior capsular tightness.[6]
- An osseous defect with a width that is at least 21% of the glenoid length may cause instability.[6]
- The normally pear-shaped glenoid assumes the shape of an inverted pear.
- Redislocation in contact athletes after arthroscopic anterior stabilization occurs more frequently in those with anterior bone loss.[3]

NATURAL HISTORY

- Bone loss of varying degrees is seen in 90% to 95% of individuals with anterior shoulder instability.[4,10]

- This bone loss occurs more frequently with recurrent dislocation than subluxation.[4]
- A bony fragment was seen in 50% of 100 cases in a series using CT reconstruction, of which only one fragment was greater than 20% of the glenoid surface area.[10]

PATIENT HISTORY AND PHYSICAL FINDINGS

- The history should include the mechanism of dislocation (although this is often not clear), the site of the pain, maneuvers required for reduction, recurrence, and associated injuries.
- Recurrent anterior subluxation may be difficult to diagnose. A history of pain in the abducted externally rotated arm, pain resulting in a temporarily useless arm (dead arm syndrome), and more subtle variations can occur. Diagnosis is aided by a good clinical examination and imaging showing lesions of passage.
- The clinician should always assess for axillary nerve injury by checking sensation in the regimental badge area and motor power in the deltoid.
- Clinical examination should include:
  - Sulcus sign: presence suggests multidirectional hyperlaxity
  - External rotation with elbow at side: more than 90 degrees suggests multidirectional hyperlaxity
  - Anterior and posterior drawer tests: positive results suggests multidirectional hyperlaxity
  - Anterior apprehension test: apprehension anterior instability
  - Posterior apprehension test: positive apprehension suggests posterior instability
  - Gagey sign: Asymmetric difference in abduction of more than 30 degrees implies severe IGHL distention.

IMAGING AND DIAGNOSTIC STUDIES

- Plain radiographs should include anteroposterior (AP) views in neutral, internal and external rotation, and a profile view of the glenoid (ie, as per Bernageau[2]) of the normal and abnormal sides (**FIG 2A,B**).
- Radiographic accuracy and quality are improved when images are taken with fluoroscopic assistance.
- CT scanning may supplement radiographs (**FIG 2C**).

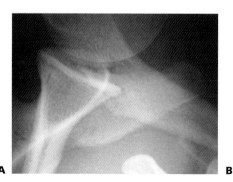
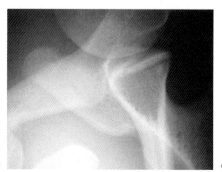
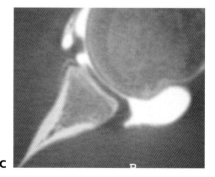

FIG 2 • A. This patient had recurrent dislocation of his shoulder; note the normal contour of the anterior glenoid on the unaffected side. **B.** The bone loss at the anterior border of the glenoid on the side with recurrent dislocation is clearly seen (Cliff sign). **C.** The CT scan also illustrates the bone loss.

DIFFERENTIAL DIAGNOSIS

- Posterior dislocation
- Posterosuperior cuff pathology in throwers
- Voluntary subluxation or dislocation
- Recurrent subluxation or dislocation

SURGICAL MANAGEMENT

Preoperative Planning

- Preoperative radiographs are analyzed to establish the presence and size of any bony glenoid defect.
- We use the Latarjet procedure for all individuals with anterior instability requiring surgery. The size of the glenoid defect does not change our operative technique.
- MRI or CT scans are not part of the standard preoperative planning but may assist in the diagnosis in cases of subtle instability.
- The presence of large Hill-Sachs lesions, SLAP lesions (superior labrum, from anterior to posterior), or other intra-articular pathology has no influence on outcome after the Latarjet procedure and hence does not influence the operative technique.

Positioning

- Under general anesthesia in association with an interscalene block for postoperative pain control, the patient is placed in the beach-chair position.
- A folded sheet is placed under the scapula to reduce scapula protraction and enable better access to the coracoid and glenoid (**FIG 3**).
- The arm is draped free to allow intraoperative abduction and external rotation.

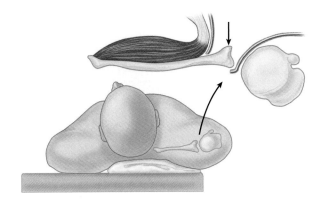

FIG 3 • Placement of the folded sheet on the medial border of the scapula reduces scapula protraction, making it easier to place your drill holes in the glenoid parallel to the articular surface.

Approach

- A deltopectoral approach is used.
- The skin incision is from the tip of the coracoid extending 4 to 5 cm toward the axillary crease.
- The cephalic vein is taken laterally and its large medial branch is ligated.
- A self-retaining retractor is used to maintain exposure between the deltoid and pectoralis major.
- The arm is placed in abduction and external rotation and a Hohmann retractor is placed over the top of the coracoid process.

CORACOID OSTEOTOMY AND PREPARATION

- Maintain the arm in abduction and external rotation to tension the coracoacromial ligament, which is incised 1 cm from its coracoid attachment.
- Partially incise at the same time the coracohumeral ligament lying deep to the coracoacromial ligament and free the upper lateral aspect of the superior conjoint tendon (**TECH FIG 1A**).
- Now adduct and internally rotate the arm to allow exposure of the medial side of the coracoid process. The pectoralis minor is released from this attachment with electrocautery, taking care not to go past the tip of the coracoid and damage its blood supply.
- A periosteal elevator is then used to remove any soft tissue from the undersurface of the coracoid. This elevator also aids visualization of the "knee" of the coracoid, which is the site of the osteotomy.
- Using a 90-degree oscillating saw, the osteotomy is made from medial to lateral.
- The arm is then placed in abduction and external rotation for the second time. The coracoid is grasped with a toothed forceps and any remnants of the coracohumeral ligament are released.

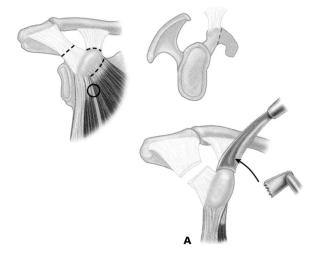

TECH FIG 1 • **A.** After release of the pectoralis minor and division of the coracoacromial ligament, the osteotomy is made distal to the coracoclavicular ligaments. *(continued)*

TECHNIQUES

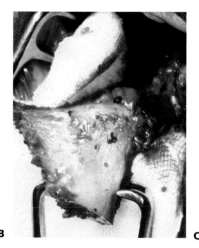
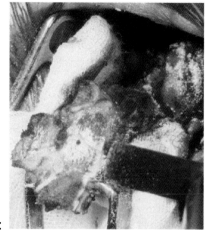
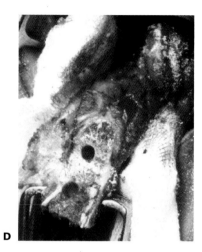

B C D

TECH FIG 1 • *(continued)* **B.** The coracoid is delivered onto a swab at the inferior part of the wound and held with a pointed grasping forceps. **C.** All cortical bone must be removed from this surface. **D.** A 3.2-mm drill is used to drill the holes.

- The arm is then returned to a neutral position and the coracoid is delivered onto a swab at the inferior aspect of the wound (**TECH FIG 1B**).
- Preparation of the bed of the coracoid is important to avoid a pseudarthrosis. Soft tissue is removed with a scalpel and then the oscillating saw is used to remove the cortical bone, exposing a cancellous bed for graft healing (**TECH FIG 1C**).
- An osteotome is placed beneath the coracoid to protect the skin and two drill holes are made using a 3.2-mm drill

(**TECH FIG 1D**). The holes are in the central axis of the coracoid and about 1 cm apart.
- The swab protecting the skin is removed, the arm is externally rotated, keeping the elbow by the side, and the lateral border of the conjoint tendon is released for about 5 cm using a Mayo scissors.
- The coracoid is then pushed beneath the pectoralis major, exposing the underlying subscapularis muscle.

GLENOID EXPOSURE

- Identify the superior and inferior margins of the subscapularis; the location for the subscapularis split is at the junction of its superior two thirds and inferior one third (**TECH FIG 2A**).
- A Mayo scissors is used to create the split. It is pushed between the fibers as far as the capsule, then opened perpendicular to the plane of the muscle fibers. Keeping the

scissors open, push a small swab into the subscapular fossa in a superomedial direction and then place a Hohmann retractor on the swab in the subscapularis fossa (**TECH FIG 2B**).
- Using a curved retractor such as a Bennett retractor on the inferior part of the subscapularis, extend the lateral part of the split with a scalpel to the lesser

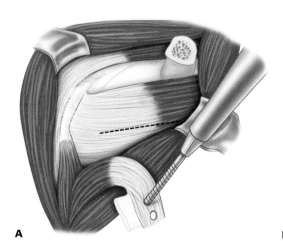
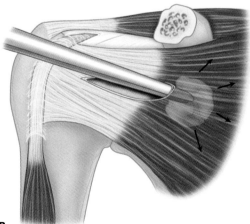

A B

TECH FIG 2 • **A.** After drilling the holes in the coracoid, the subscapularis is split at the junction between its superior two thirds and its inferior one third. **B.** A small sponge is placed superomedially between the capsule and the subscapularis muscle. *(continued)*

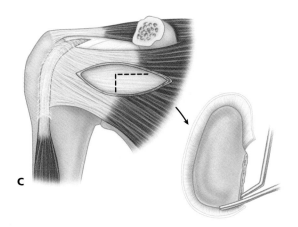

TECH FIG 2 • *(continued)* **C.** It is important to ensure the subscapularis split has been carried sufficiently laterally to allow easy visualization of the joint line.

tuberosity. The joint line is then more easily visualized and incised for about 1.5 to 2 cm, allowing a retractor to be placed in the joint (Trillat or Fukuda retractor; **TECH FIG 2C**).

- Superior exposure is created when a Steinmann pin is hammered into the superior scapular neck as high as possible.
- The medial Hohmann retractor is now exchanged for a link retractor and placed as medial as possible on the scapula neck.
- A small Hohmann retractor is placed inferiorly between the capsule on the inferior neck and the inferior part of the subscapularis.
- The anteroinferior part of the glenoid should now be easily visualized.

PREPARATION OF THE GLENOID AND CORACOID FIXATION

- The anteroinferior labrum and periosteum are incised with the electrocautery, exposing the glenoid 2 cm medially and from about 5 o'clock to 2 o'clock in a right shoulder (a vertical distance of 2 to 3 cm).
- An osteotome is then used to elevate this labral–periosteal flap from lateral to medial (**TECH FIG 3A**). The frequent presence of a Bankart lesion makes this quite simple.
- The osteotome is then used to decorticate this anteroinferior surface of the glenoid. We aim to create a flat surface on which to place our graft.
- The use of bone graft (excepting the coracoid process) is not required.
- Using the 3.2-mm drill, drill the inferior hole in the glenoid (**TECH FIG 3B**). This is at the 5 o'clock position, parallel to the plane of the glenoid and sufficiently medial that the coracoid will not overhang the glenoid (generally 7 mm, but depends on coracoid morphology). Both anterior and posterior cortices are drilled.

- The coracoid is now retrieved from its position under the pectoralis major and grasped at the cut end in a medial–lateral fashion.
- A 4.5-mm partially threaded malleolar screw is fully inserted into the inferior hole (tendinous end). The length of this screw is typically 35 mm but can be verified by adding together the depth of the coracoid and the depth of the glenoid hole (**TECH FIG 3C**).
- The screw is then placed into the already drilled inferior hole and tightened into position, ensuring that the coracoid comes to lie parallel to the anterior border of the glenoid with no overhang. A slightly medial position (2 to 3 mm) is acceptable. Rotation of the coracoid is adjusted using a heavy forceps.
- When the position of the coracoid is parallel to the glenoid, the second drill hole is made through the superior hole already drilled in the coracoid (**TECH FIG 3D**). It is important to avoid rotation of the coracoid at this stage.

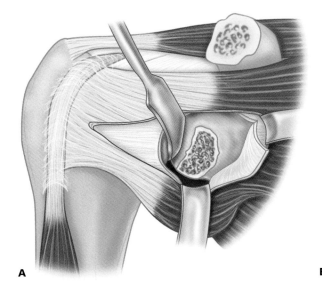

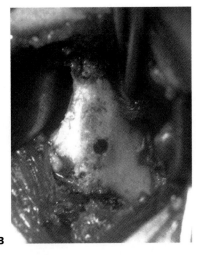

TECH FIG 3 • **A.** With an osteotome, cancellous bone is exposed on the glenoid neck. **B.** First glenoid drill hole. *(continued)*

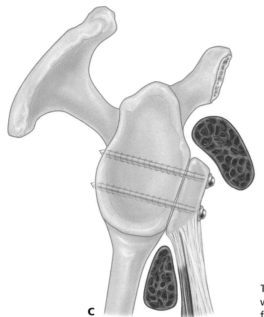

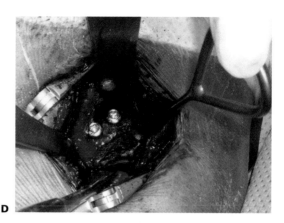

TECH FIG 3 • *(continued)* **C.** The coracoid increases the width of the anteroinferior bony glenoid. **D.** View after fixation of the coracoid to the glenoid neck.

- The hole is measured and the correct-sized malleolar screw is inserted into position.
- Repair of the capsule is then carried out by suturing the capsule to the stump of the coracoacromial ligament using a number 1 Dexon suture with the arm in external rotation, after removing the intra-articular retractor.
- The retractors are removed, as is the sponge that was on the medial scapula neck.
- There is no need to close the split in the subscapularis muscle.

PEARLS AND PITFALLS

- Dissection on the medial side of the coracoid is not necessary and risks nerve injury.
- The surgeon should not cut the subscapularis to gain access to the glenoid; the subscapularis split is used instead.
- The surgeon should decorticate the undersurface of the coracoid and the anterior glenoid to bleeding bone to avoid coracoid pseudarthrosis.
- Coracoid fracture can be avoided by using the two-fingers technique when tightening screws.
- Screws must be bicortical.
- Placing the coracoid in the "lying" position increases the coracoid–glenoid contact and decreases the risk of pseudarthrosis.
- If the coracoid fractures longitudinally, it should be turned 90 degrees. If it fractures transversely, the tip should be placed in a standing position.
- The coracoid must never overhang the glenoid, as this leads to arthritis[1] (**FIG 4**).

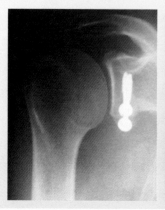

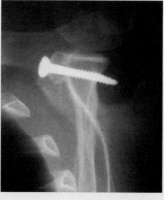

FIG 4 • Postoperative AP and lateral views showing correct placement of screws and no overhanging of the coracoid.

POSTOPERATIVE CARE

▪ A simple sling is used for 2 weeks.

▪ Rehabilitation begins on the first postoperative day with gentle active range-of-motion exercises.

▪ Full activities of daily living are allowed at 6 weeks and a return to all sports is permitted at 3 months.

OUTCOMES

▪ In a study of 160 Latarjet procedures, we had a recurrence rate of 1%. Of those who played sports, 83% returned to their preinjury level or better. Overall, 98% rated their result as excellent or good and 76% had excellent or good results using the modified Rowe score.[11]

▪ The occurrence of postoperative shoulder arthritis is related to preventable factors (ie, lateral overhang of the coracoid) and pre-existing factors (eg, increased age at the time of first dislocation, increased age at the time of surgery and the presence of arthritis before to surgery).

COMPLICATIONS

▪ Intraoperative fracture of the coracoid

▪ Infection

▪ Hematoma formation

▪ Pseudarthrosis (not associated with poor outcome)

▪ Pain related to screws (2% incidence of screw removal)

▪ Recurrence

▪ Arthritis (if graft overhangs the anterior glenoid)

REFERENCES

1. Allain J, Goutallier D, Glorion C. Long-term results of the Latarjet procedure for the treatment of anterior instability of the shoulder. J Bone Joint Surg Am 1998;80A:841–852.
2. Bernageau J, Patte D, Bebeyre J, et al. Interet du profile glenoidien dans les luxations recidivantes de l'epaule. Rev Chir Orthop 1976; 62:142–147.
3. Burkhart SS, De Beer JF. Traumatic glenohumeral bone defects and their relationship to failure of arthroscopic Bankart repairs: significance of the inverted-pear glenoid and the humeral engaging Hill-Sachs lesion. Arthroscopy 2000;16:677–694.
4. Edwards TB, Boulahia A, Walch G. Radiographic analysis of bone defects in chronic anterior shoulder instability. Arthroscopy 2003;19:732–739.
5. Helfet AJ. Coracoid transplantation for recurring dislocation of the shoulder. J Bone Joint Surg Br 1958;40B:198–202.
6. Itoi E, Lee SB, Berglund LJ, et al. The effect of a glenoid defect on anteroinferior stability of the shoulder after Bankart repair: a cadaveric study. J Bone Joint Surg Am 2000;82A:35–46.
7. Latarjet M. A propos du traitement des luxations recidivantes de l'epaule. Lyon Chir 1954;49:994–1003.
8. May VR Jr. A modified Bristow operation for anterior recurrent dislocation of the shoulder. J Bone Joint Surg Am 1970;52A: 1010–1016.
9. Patte D, Debeyre J. Luxations recidivantes de l'epaule. Encycl Med Chir. Paris-Technique chirurgicale. Orthopedie 1980;44265:4.4-02.
10. Sugaya H, Moriishi J, Dohi M, et al. Glenoid rim morphology in recurrent anterior glenohumeral instability. J Bone Joint Surg Am 200385A:878–884.
11. Walch G, Boileau P. Latarjet-Bristow procedure for recurrent anterior instability. Tech Shoulder Elbow Surg 2000;1:256–261.

Chapter 6

Glenoid Bone Graft for Instability With Bone Loss

Ryan W. Simovitch, Laurence D. Higgins, and Jon J. P. Warner

DEFINITION

▪ Anterior shoulder instability typically results from an injury to the capsule, ligaments, and labrum that stabilize the glenohumeral joint.

▪ In cases of higher-energy trauma or recurrent dislocation, however, there can be significant bone loss or erosion of the anterior glenoid rim.

▪ The key to correctly treating anterior shoulder instability is recognizing whether the lesion involves injury to only capsulolabroligamentous structures or if it also involves the anteroinferior glenoid bone.

ANATOMY

▪ Shoulder stability is provided by both dynamic and static stabilizers (**FIG 1**).

▪ Dynamic stabilizers include:
  ▪ Rotator cuff
  ▪ Biceps
  ▪ Coordinated scapulothoracic motion
  ▪ Proprioception

▪ Static stabilizers include:
  ▪ Bony anatomy of the glenoid and humeral head
  ▪ Labrum
  ▪ Glenohumeral capsule and ligaments
  ▪ Negative intra-articular pressure

▪ The inferior glenohumeral ligament (IGHL) complex limits anterior translation of the humeral head on the glenoid in abduction. It takes origin from the labrum on the glenoid inferiorly. The complex consists of an anterior band, posterior band, and intervening pouch. The anterior band is responsible for anterior restraint with the arm in high degrees of abduction with external rotation.

▪ Normal glenoid morphology is the shape of a pear. There is normally a surface area mismatch of the glenohumeral joint whereby only 20% to 30% of the humeral head contacts the glenoid surface at any point in time (Fig 1).

▪ The synchronized contraction of the rotator cuff and biceps provides a compressive force directing the convex humeral head into the concave glenoid and labrum unit. This is known as concavity compression.[7]

PATHOGENESIS

▪ Anterior shoulder instability typically follows a dislocation event that results from a fall or collision with the arm in external rotation and abduction.

▪ First-time dislocators typically require a closed reduction of their shoulder after muscle relaxation and sedation, while recurrent dislocators can often reduce their shoulders with minimal effort.

▪ An injury to the labrum in the anteroinferior quadrant of the glenoid destabilizing the IGHL complex as well as stretching or a tear of the anteroinferior capsule can result in anterior shoulder instability.

▪ A rotator cuff tear should be suspected in patients greater than 40 years old who suffer from a dislocation episode.

▪ Recurrent anterior glenohumeral instability can also occur in the setting of anterior glenoid bone loss due to glenoid fracture after a single dislocation event or erosion as a result of recurrent subluxations or dislocations.

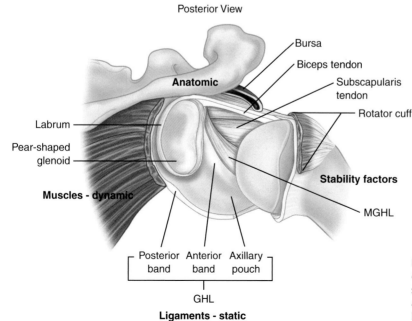

FIG 1 • Shoulder stability depends on the interaction of dynamic and static soft tissue restraints. The bony architecture of the glenoid and humerus also plays a critical role.

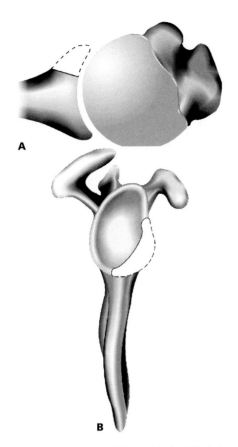

FIG 2 • Loss of anterior glenoid bone (*dashed line*) due to erosion or fracture results in loss of glenoid width (**A**) and depth (**B**). The result is an inverted-pear morphology that cannot resist displacement of the humeral head anteriorly as effectively as a normal pear-shaped glenoid.

▪ Deficiency of the anterior glenoid rim disrupts the normal mechanism of concavity–compression as a result of a decrease in width and depth of the socket (**FIG 2**).

▪ Anterior glenoid bone loss or fracture should be suspected in cases of recurrent anterior instability or acute dislocations from a high-energy mechanism.

▪ In cases of anterior glenoid bony deficiency, patients often report recurrent dislocation in their sleep and with minimal trauma.

NATURAL HISTORY

▪ In the context of anterior glenoid bone loss, both open and arthroscopic soft tissue management of anterior shoulder instability have demonstrated increased failure rates compared to the results in patients with normal bony glenoid anatomy.

▪ Burkhart and DeBeer[1] have shown that contact athletes with substantial bony glenoid defects, noted as an "inverted pear" morphology at arthroscopy, had an 87% recurrent instability rate compared to 6.5% in contact athletes with a normal bony glenoid who underwent an arthroscopic capsulolabral repair only.

▪ Given the high failure rate in patients with significant anterior glenoid bone loss, a comprehensive evaluation of the glenoid bony anatomy is imperative before treating recurrent anterior shoulder instability with a capsulolabral reconstruction alone.

PATIENT HISTORY AND PHYSICAL FINDINGS

▪ A complete examination of the shoulder should also include the evaluation of other concomitant injuries and ruling out differential diagnoses. A thorough examination includes but is not limited to the following:

▫ Apprehension test: Apprehension, not simply pain, is required for a positive apprehension test.

▫ Relocation test: Relief of apprehension with posterior pressure is necessary for a positive relocation maneuver.

▫ Load and shift test: The examiner should note the degree of displacement of the humeral head on the glenoid rim.

▫ Belly press: A positive belly press test is when the patient must flex the wrist and extend the arm to maintain the palm of the hand on the abdomen.

▫ Assessment for generalized ligamentous laxity: Specifically, hyperextension of the elbows and knees as well as the ability to oppose the thumb to the forearm should be noted.

▫ Rotator cuff: Manual strength testing of the subscapularis, supraspinatus, infraspinatus, and teres minor muscles must be done. Rotator cuff tears can contribute to instability.

▫ Subscapularis insufficiency: Weakness of internal rotation with the shoulder adducted to the side suggests a subscapularis injury but is not specific. Increased external rotation of the injured side with the shoulder adducted compared to the contralateral shoulder, pain with external rotation of the shoulder, a positive belly press sign, or positive lift-off sign should raise suspicion for subscapularis insufficiency.

▫ Axillary nerve injury: Both the deltoid motor strength and sensation in the distribution of the axillary nerve should be assessed. Atrophy of the deltoid muscle should be noted.

IMAGING AND OTHER DIAGNOSTIC STUDIES

▪ Plain radiographs are useful to detect Hill-Sachs lesion, glenoid dysplasia, and anterior glenoid fractures or erosion. Standard images should include a true anteroposterior (AP) view of the glenoid, an axillary view, and a Stryker notch view. Fractures and erosions of the glenoid as well as the position of the humerus on the glenoid should be noted.

▪ If a significant anterior bony glenoid lesion is suspected owing to plain film findings or a history of recurrent dislocations, a CT arthrogram should be obtained. This allows an evaluation of the subscapularis tendon, bony architecture of the glenoid, humeral head, and tuberosities as well the degree of capsulolabral injury and redundancy.

▪ Both Itoi[5,6] and Gerber[3] have described techniques to assess anterior glenoid bone quantitatively that serve as a guide for when bony augmentation is indicated for recurrent anterior shoulder instability. Gerber's method[3] is easily performed on oblique sagittal or 3D reconstructions of the glenoid surface (**FIG 3**). Cadaveric studies have shown that the force required for anterior dislocation is reduced by 70% from an intact glenoid if the length of the glenoid defect exceeds the maximum radius of the glenoid.

DIFFERENTIAL DIAGNOSIS

▪ Bankart lesion
▪ Multidirectional instability
▪ Hill-Sachs lesion
▪ Tuberosity fracture

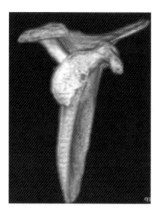

FIG 3 • A 3D CT reconstruction effectively demonstrates the degree of anterior glenoid bone loss.

- Rotator cuff tear (especially subscapularis)
- Scapular winging (especially serratus anterior dysfunction)
- Axillary nerve injury

NONOPERATIVE MANAGEMENT

- Conservative therapy for recurrent anterior shoulder dislocation includes strengthening of the rotator cuff musculature as well as the periscapular stabilizers. Deltoid muscle strengthening should be incorporated into a rotator cuff strengthening protocol. Periscapular strengthening should focus on the rhomboids, trapezius, serratus, and latissimus dorsi muscles.
- Conservative treatment of recurrent shoulder dislocation in the setting of a bony glenoid defect, however, is rarely successful.

SURGICAL MANAGEMENT

Preoperative Planning

- All imaging studies, including plain radiographs (true AP glenoid view, axillary view, Stryker notch view) and CT scan with intra-articular gadolinium, are reviewed. Additional radiographic views can be helpful. The apical oblique can demonstrate anterior glenoid lip defects as well as posterolateral impression fractures of the humeral head. Both the West Point and Bernageau views are useful to note defects of the anteroinferior glenoid rim.
- The CT arthrogram is examined for evidence of anterior glenoid bone loss:
  - The degree of bone loss is assessed on oblique sagittal reconstruction or a 3D reconstruction of the glenoid face (**FIG 4**).
  - The length of the anterior glenoid defect is measured.
  - If the length of the glenoid defect exceeds half of the maximum diameter of the glenoid, an anatomic glenoid reconstruction of the anterior glenoid with autologous iliac crest bone graft is considered.[3]
- Often, the anterior erosion is extensive, making it difficult to accurately measure the glenoid diameter. In these instances, the superoinferior axis of the glenoid should be drawn on the glenoid face image and the maximum radius determined from this line to the posterior aspect of the glenoid (Fig 4).
- Associated superior labral tears, biceps pathology, rotator cuff tears, and the presence of articular erosion and osteoarthritis should be noted preoperatively and treated appropriately at the index operation.
- An examination under anesthesia should assess passive range of motion, noting any restrictions as well as excessive motion,

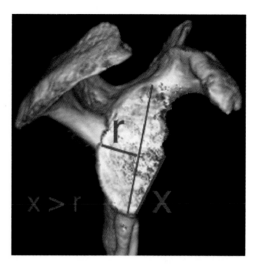

FIG 4 • Gerber's method for evaluating the degree of glenoid erosion. *x* is the length of the glenoid defect. Half of the maximum diameter of the glenoid, *r*, can be measured from a vertical line (*blue*) connecting the superior glenoid rim to the inferior glenoid rim in cases of significant erosion. If $x > r$, then the force for dislocation is decreased by 70%.

which may indicate subscapularis insufficiency. In addition, the glenohumeral joint should be assessed for laxity to ensure there is not a bidirectional or multidirectional component.

Positioning

- Although some surgeons choose to use a bean bag, we prefer to use a beach chair with an attachable hydraulic articulated arm holder (Spider Limb Positioner, Tenet Medical Engineering, Calgary, Canada) (**FIG 5**).
- The head of the beach chair is elevated 30 to 45 degrees to allow access to the ipsilateral iliac crest.

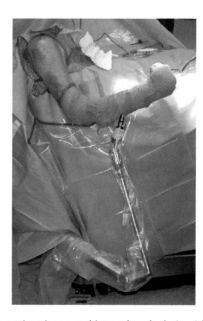

FIG 5 • The patient is secured into a beach chair with an attachable hydraulic articulated arm holder (Spider Limb Positioner, Tenet Medical Engineering, Calgary, Canada). The upper body is positioned at 30 to 45 degrees to allow access to the ipsilateral iliac crest.

■ A well-padded bump is placed behind the ipsilateral buttock and hip to ensure that the iliac crest is prominent for ease of dissection.

■ The shoulder and iliac crest are prepared and draped in the standard sterile fashion.

Approach

■ Anterior glenoid reconstruction with iliac crest bone graft requires two approaches:
  ■ Deltopectoral approach for glenoid preparation
  ■ Tricortical anterior iliac crest bone graft harvesting

EXPOSURE OF GLENOID

■ A 5- to 7-cm incision is made in the anterior axillary fold beginning at the inferior border of the pectoralis major tendon and extended superiorly to the coracoid.

■ Once the initial incision is carried through the subcutaneous tissue down to the fascia investing the pectoralis and deltoid muscles, full-thickness skin flaps are sharply developed using a no. 15 blade superiorly to the level of the coracoid as well as medially and laterally at least 1 cm to allow identification of the cephalic vein and dissection of the interval between the deltoid and pectoralis major muscles.

■ Typically, there are more crossing vessels emanating from the lateral side of the cephalic vein. Thus, the investing fascia on the medial side of the vein is incised sharply while an assistant places countertraction on the pectoralis major using a two-pronged skin hook. This allows a clean dissection and medially based crossing vessels to be coagulated in a step-by-step fashion.

■ The deep surfaces of the deltoid and pectoralis are sharply dissected using a no. 15 blade to free up adhesions and broaden the ultimate exposure.

■ A four-quadrant self-retaining retractor is positioned to retract the pectoralis major medially and the deltoid laterally (**TECH FIG 1A**).

■ There is often a leash of vessels superficial to the clavipectoral fascia at the level of the coracoid. These should be coagulated if present.

■ The clavipectoral fascia is sharply incised lateral to the conjoint tendon, making sure to stay lateral to any muscle of the short head of the biceps.

■ The musculocutaneous nerve can then be palpated on the deep surface of the conjoint tendon. The conjoint tendon is retracted medially, exposing the subscapularis tendon and muscle.

■ The coracoacromial ligament can be released if additional exposure is needed superiorly.

■ The circumflex vessels are then identified and ligated or coagulated (**TECH FIG 1B**).

■ The axillary nerve can be palpated as it passes over the inferior portion of the subscapularis and loops under the inferior capsule. A blunt retractor can be placed lateral and deep to the axillary nerve, thus retracting it gently medially away from the subscapularis musculotendinous junction.

■ The subscapularis tendon is then incised from bone off the lesser tuberosity to avoid disrupting the long head of the biceps tendon in the bicipital groove (**TECH FIG 1C**).

■ Through sharp dissection, an interval between the subscapularis tendon and capsule is developed, leaving the capsule intact. It is often easier to start inferiorly and use a blunt elevator to dissect the interval.

■ The subscapularis tendon and muscle are retracted medially using an anterior glenoid neck retractor.

■ A blunt retractor is repositioned deep to the axillary nerve to retract away from the capsule, which should be widely exposed at this point.

■ An inverted L-shaped capsulotomy is then created based on the humeral neck and extending horizontally across the rotator interval region (**TECH FIG 1D**).

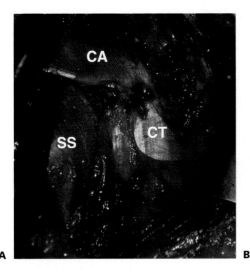

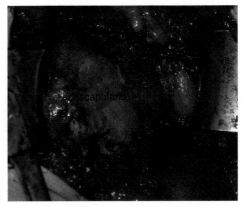

A   **B**

TECH FIG 1 • A. The pectoralis major and deltoid muscles are retracted to reveal a broad exposure of the conjoint tendon (*CT*) and muscle belly passing over the subscapularis muscle (*SS*). The coracoacromial ligament (*CA*) can be released if needed for additional exposure. **B.** A blunt curved retractor can be placed inferiorly along the subscapularis to protect the axillary nerve. *(continued)*

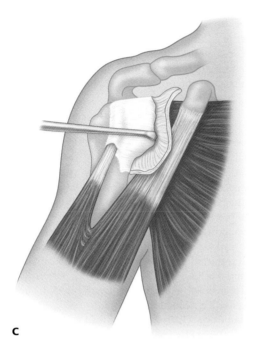

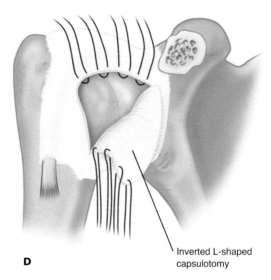

Inverted L-shaped
capsulotomy

TECH FIG 1 • *(continued)* **C.** The subscapularis is incised from its insertion on the lesser tuberosity and the layer between the deep capsule and the subscapularis muscle and tendon is developed with a blunt elevator. **D.** An inverted L-shaped capsulotomy based on the humeral neck and extending across the rotator interval region allows access to the glenohumeral joint and leaves tissue for later repair.

GLENOID PREPARATION

- The anterior glenoid and scapular neck are then exposed (**TECH FIG 2**).
- After the L-shaped capsulotomy, a periosteal elevator is used to strip the periosteal sleeve from the anterior scapular neck.
- An anterior glenoid neck retractor is positioned to retract the capsule medially.

- A Fukuda retractor or similar blunt retractor is used to retract the humeral head posteriorly, thus exposing the face of the glenoid.
- The length of the osseous defect is measured and compared to the width of the maximum AP radius of the glenoid. The measured defect length will be the basis for the size of the iliac crest bone graft harvested.
- Soft tissue and scar tissue are removed from the anterior glenoid, and this bone and the adjacent scapular neck are roughened with a high-speed burr to create punctate bleeding and a smooth surface for bone grafting.

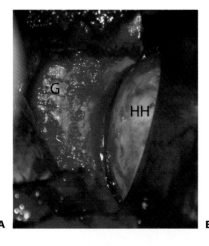

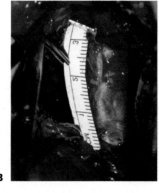

TECH FIG 2 • Glenoid preparation. **A.** The humeral head (*HH*) is retracted laterally and posteriorly using a Fukuda retractor or curved blunt retractor. The medial capsule and soft tissue are retracted medially, thus exposing the anterior scapular neck and eroded glenoid (*G*) surface. **B.** A malleable ruler is used to measure the length of the anterior glenoid defect.

HARVESTING AND PREPARING TRICORTICAL ILIAC CREST BONE GRAFT

- The iliac crest is harvested as a tricortical bone graft (**TECH FIG 3**).
- A 2- to 3-cm curved incision is made overlying the iliac crest and posterior to the anterosuperior iliac spine.

- The incision is carried sharply through subcutaneous tissue down to the periosteum, which is incised sharply and superiosteally elevated to expose the inner and outer tables. Self-retaining retractors are placed be-

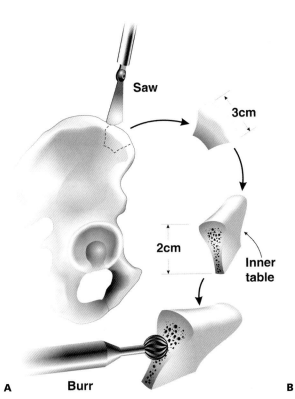

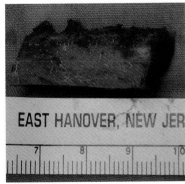

tween the crest and periosteum along the inner and outer tables.

- An oscillating saw is used to harvest a tricortical wedge-shaped graft. The graft is typically about 3 cm in length by 2 cm in width, but the size should be based on the measured defect.

- A high-speed burr and a small oscillating saw are then used to contour the graft to fit along the anterior glenoid and best re-establish concavity, depth, and length. The inner table serves as the articular portion of the graft and the cancellous surface is opposed to the anterior glenoid defect.

TECH FIG 3 • Tricortical iliac crest bone graft. **A.** Bone graft is harvested from the iliac crest using an oscillating saw and preserving both the inner and outer tables. A high-speed burr is used to contour the graft. **B.** The size of the graft is typically 3 cm in length and 2 cm in width but should be based on the measured size of the defect.

FIXATION OF TRICORTICAL GRAFT TO GLENOID

- The tricortical iliac crest graft is secured to the glenoid (**TECH FIG 4**).
- The contoured graft is then positioned onto the anterior glenoid with the inner table of the iliac crest facing laterally as the articular surface.

- Positioning of the graft is critical. Glenoid concavity should be established but impingement or articular step-off should be avoided. This can be done by avoiding too vertical or too horizontal of an angle between the graft and glenoid.

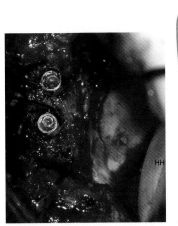

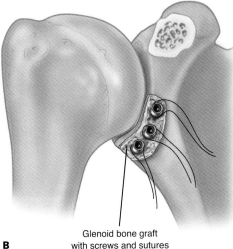

Glenoid bone graft
with screws and sutures

TECH FIG 4 • Fixation of graft to the glenoid. **A.** The graft is positioned to establish concavity to the glenoid as well as a smooth transition between the graft and native glenoid to avoid an articular step-off. **B.** A number 2 braided polyethylene suture is placed around each 4.0-mm screw before it is fully tightened to assist in later capsular repair. (*continued*)

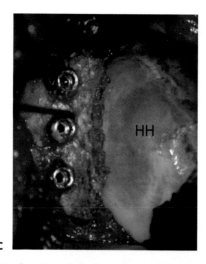

TECH FIG 4 • (continued) C. Once the graft is secured with screws, the glenohumeral retractor is removed and the position of the humeral head (*HH*) on the glenoid is noted.

- Avoid too vertical of an angle, as this may result in humeral impingement.
- Avoid too horizontal of an angle, as this may fail to re-establish glenoid concavity.
- With the graft correctly positioned, it can be temporarily secured to the anterior glenoid using two or three terminally threaded Kirschner wires from the stainless steel AO 4.0-mm cannulated screw set (AO/Synthes, Paoli, PA).
- Two or three partially threaded 4.0-mm cannulated screws are then placed over the Kirschner wires to secure the graft.
- A number 2 braided polyethylene suture is placed around the shaft of each screw before the screw is fully seated and compressing the graft. These sutures may be used for later capsular repair.
- The Fukuda retractor is gently removed and the position of the humeral head is noted. The glenohumeral joint is ranged and any incongruity or instability noted should prompt a change in graft position.

REPAIR OF CAPSULE AND SUBSCAPULARIS

- The capsulotomy and subscapularis are then repaired (**TECH FIG 5**).
- The sutures from the graft fixation screws are passed through the capsule–periosteal sleeve as horizontal mattress stitches and tied.

- The capsulotomy can be further repaired in one of two ways:
  - If the L-shaped capsulotomy can be repaired primarily, it is reapproximated using number 2 braided polyethylene suture. Often, though, the graft occupies enough space and the capsule is contracted so that a primary repair of the capsulotomy is not possible.
  - If the L-shaped capsulotomy cannot be repaired primarily to the neck of the humerus with the arm in at least 30 degrees of external rotation, then the capsule is repaired to the lateral portion of the subscapularis tendon. This will tension the anterior capsule as the subscapularis becomes more taut with external rotation.
- The lesser tuberosity is gently abraded with a high-speed burr to cause punctate bleeding.
- The subscapularis is then meticulously repaired to the lesser tuberosity with two or three suture anchors using a modified Mason-Allen stitch.
- The shoulder incision is closed in layers.

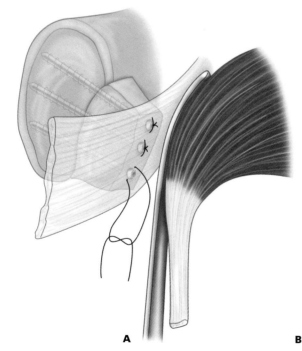

TECH FIG 5 • Repair of capsulotomy and subscapularis. **A.** The sutures around the screws are secured through the capsule with horizontal mattress stitches. **B.** If the capsule cannot be repaired back to the humeral neck without being excessively tight and restrictive of external rotation, it is secured to the deep surface of the subscapularis tendon with horizontal mattress sutures. The subscapularis is then repaired to the lesser tuberosity with suture anchors.

PEARLS AND PITFALLS

Indications	■ A complete history and physical should be performed.
	■ Associated pathology must be recognized and addressed:
	■ The glenohumeral joint must be assessed for osteoarthrosis.
	■ The humeral head must be assessed for a significant engaging Hill-Sachs lesion. It is rare for the lesion to be engaging after reconstruction of the width of the glenoid.
Tricortical graft harvest	■ Care should be exercised to avoid disrupting the anterosuperior iliac spine.
	■ The lateral femoral cutaneous and ilioinguinal nerves are at risk during dissection of the anterior ilium.
Tricortical graft placement	■ Placement of the graft in too vertical of a position may result in impingement of the humeral head and articular erosion.
	■ Placement of the graft in too horizontal of a position does not recreate concavity of the glenoid.
	■ There must be a smooth transition between the native glenoid and bone graft. This is ensured by proper positioning. A burr can be used to remove any prominences from the graft that remain after fixation.
Stiffness	■ Patients should be counseled to expect some limitation of external rotation postoperatively.
	■ The goal is to achieve a stable joint with no more than 20 degrees loss of external rotation to limit the risk of capsulorrhaphy arthropathy. This should be considered during capsular repair.

POSTOPERATIVE CARE

■ Radiographs are obtained to judge graft placement and screw position. A CT scan is helpful to estimate graft incorporation (**FIG 6**).

■ The shoulder is maintained in a sling immobilizer for 4 weeks.

■ Pendulum exercises are allowed after the first week.

■ At 4 weeks, the sling is removed to allow:

  ■ Activities of daily living

  ■ Passive range of motion, active assisted range of motion, water therapy

■ At 3 months, strengthening is initiated.

■ Participation in overhead recreational sport (golf, tennis, swimming) is allowed at 4 months.

■ Participation in contact or collision sports is allowed at 6 months.

OUTCOMES

■ With appropriate preoperative workup, diagnosis, and surgical technique, anatomic reconstruction of the glenoid with tricortical iliac crest bone graft is very effective at treating recurrent dislocations in the setting of a bony glenoid defect.

■ Hutchinson and colleagues[4] demonstrated no recurrent dislocations after tricortical iliac crest bone grafting in a population of epileptics who continued to have seizures postoperatively.

■ Warner and associates[8] reported no recurrent dislocations or subluxations after anterior glenoid bone grafting in a population of athletes with traumatic recurrent anterior instability. There was a mean loss of external rotation in abduction of 14 degrees.

COMPLICATIONS

■ Subscapularis insufficiency

■ Hardware failure and migration

■ Stiffness

■ Brachial plexus injury

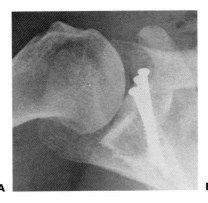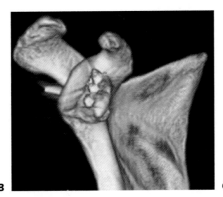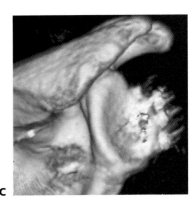

A   **B**   **C**

FIG 6 • Postoperative imaging of glenoid reconstruction with tricortical iliac crest bone graft. **A.** Axillary lateral. **B.** Anterior view of 3D CT reconstruction demonstrating position and incorporation of graft. **C.** Posterior view of 3D CT reconstruction demonstrating restored glenoid width, depth, and concavity.

REFERENCES

1. Burkhart SS, DeBeer JF. Traumatic glenohumeral bone defects and their relationship to failure of arthroscopic Bankart repairs: significance of the inverted-pear glenoid and the humeral enaging Hill-Sachs lesion. Arthroscopy 2000;16:677–694.
2. Farber AJ, Castillo R, Clough M, et al. Clinical assessment of three common tests for traumatic anterior shoulder instability. J Bone Joint Surg Am 2006;88A:1467–1474.
3. Gerber C, Nyffeler RW. Classification of glenohumeral joint instability. Clin Orthop Relat Res 2002;400:65–76.
4. Hutchinson JW, Neumann L, Wallace WA. Bone buttress operation for recurrent anterior shoulder dislocation in epilepsy. J Bone Joint Surg Br 1995;77B:928–932.
5. Itoi E, Lee SB, Berglund LJ, et al. The effect of glenoid defect on anteroinferior stability of the shoulder after Bankart repair: a cadaver study. J Bone Joint Surg Am 2000;82A:35–46.
6. Itoi E, Lee SB, Amrami KK, et al. Quantitative assessment of classic anteroinferior bony Bankart lesions by radiography and computed tomography. Am J Sports Med 2003;31:112–118.
7. Lippitt SB, Vanderhooft JE, Harris SL, et al. Glenohumeral stability from concavity-compression: a quantitative analysis. J Shoulder Elbow Surg 1993;2:27–35.
8. Warner JP, Gill TJ, O'Hollerhan JD, et al. Anatomical glenoid reconstruction for recurrent anterior glenohumeral instability with glenoid deficiency using an autogenous tricortical iliac crest bone graft. Am J Sports Med 2006;34:205–212.

Chapter 7

Management of Glenohumeral Instability With Humeral Bone Loss

Michael A. Rauh and Anthony Miniaci

DEFINITION

- The glenohumeral joint is one of the most commonly dislocated joints in the body.
- With anterior dislocations, bony defects of the anterior glenoid and posterosuperior aspect of the humeral head occur with relative frequency.
- One of the first descriptions of the lesions found on the humeral head was by Flower[4] in 1861, with many subsequent investigators reporting on these bony defects.[13]
- In 1940, two radiologists, Hill and Sachs,[6] reported that these defects were actually compression fractures produced when the posterolateral humeral head impinged against the anterior rim of the glenoid.
- Since then, Hill-Sachs lesions have been found to occur with an incidence between 32% and 51% at the time of initial anterior glenohumeral dislocation.
- In shoulders sustaining a Hill-Sachs lesion at the initial dislocation, there exists a statistically significant association with recurrent dislocation.[7,8]
- Although Hill-Sachs lesions are common after anterior glenohumeral dislocations, there are relatively few publications describing specific treatments for these humeral head defects.[14,19]
- In general, specific surgical procedures to address Hill-Sachs lesions have not been recommended in the initial surgical management of recurrent anterior dislocations because the majority of these lesions are small to moderate in size and do not routinely cause significant symptoms of instability.
- Certain subsets of patients exist with more significant bony defects and ongoing symptoms of "instability" or painful clicking, catching, or popping. This occurs even after surgical procedures directed at treating their anterior instability.

ANATOMY

- With an anterior shoulder dislocation, the humeral head is positioned anterior to the glenoid rim.
- The posterosuperior aspect of the humeral head then impacts upon the anterior aspect of the glenoid rim and creates the Hill-Sachs lesion (**FIG 1A**).
- Only after the shoulder joint is relocated can the influence of the size and shape of the Hill-Sachs lesion on overall shoulder stability be determined (**FIG 1B,C**).
- Although there is not scientific proof, our clinical experience suggests that lesions representing 25% to 30% of the articulating surface arc of the humeral head often lead to symptoms.

PATHOGENESIS

- The concept of "articular arc length mismatch" has been recently put forth by Burkhart to "explain the ongoing sensation of catching or popping" arising in the shoulder with a large Hill-Sachs lesion alone or in combination with glenoid defects."[1,2]
- Patients with these symptoms have often undergone previous anterior stabilization procedures and reconstruction of damaged glenohumeral ligaments at that time.

- This phenomenon, debatably referred to as "instability," occurs mainly in a position of abduction and external rotation of the shoulder.
  - In this position, a large "engaging" Hill-Sachs lesion encounters the anterior glenoid rim, resulting in the rim "dropping into" the Hill-Sachs lesion.
- The sudden loss of smooth articular surface on the humeral side of the joint presents an irregularly contoured area to the glenoid, causing an uneasy sensation in the patient that feels much like subluxation.
- As Burkhart and DeBeer pointed out, for every "Hill-Sachs lesion, there is a position of the shoulder at which the humeral bone defect will engage the anterior glenoid."
- Clinically, it is important to differentiate between "engaging" and "nonengaging" Hill-Sachs lesions.[1,2]
  - An *engaging* Hill-Sachs lesion is one that presents the long axis of its defect parallel to the anterior glenoid with the shoulder in a functional position of abduction and external rotation, such that the Hill-Sachs lesion encounters the rim of the glenoid.
    - Lesions can be considered engaging even in positions that are considered "nonfunctional," such as in some degree of extension, or in lesser degrees of abduction.
    - Apprehension and instability in lesser degrees of shoulder abduction often indicate a significant bony defect that is leading to the perceived instability.[14]
  - A *nonengaging* Hill-Sachs lesion is one that either fails to engage the glenoid or engages the glenoid only in a nonfunctional arm position. For example, the Hill-Sachs defect can pass diagonally across the anterior glenoid with external rotation; therefore, there is continual contact of the articulating surfaces and no engagement of the Hill-Sachs lesion by the anterior glenoid.[14]
- Hence, when a patient has symptomatic anterior instability associated with an engaging Hill-Sachs lesion with an articular arc deficit, treatment must be directed at both repairing the Bankart lesion, if present, and preventing the Hill-Sachs lesion from engaging the anterior glenoid.
- We believe that the treatment of symptomatic anterior glenohumeral instability, involving an engaging Hill-Sachs lesion with an articular arc deficit, can be accomplished satisfactorily with a technique of anatomic allograft reconstruction of the humeral head using a side- and size-matched humeral head osteoarticular allograft.
- This technique involves an anatomic reconstruction that eliminates the structural pathology while maintaining the range of motion of the glenohumeral joint.

NATURAL HISTORY

- One of the most clearly documented series of nonoperatively treated shoulder dislocations placed into immobilization is that of Hovelius and associates.[8]

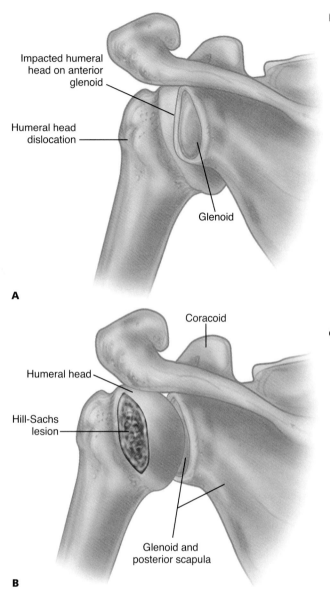

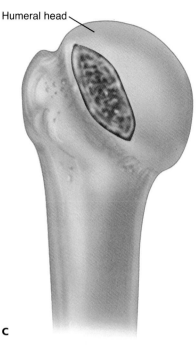

A

Impacted humeral head on anterior glenoid

Humeral head dislocation

Glenoid

B

Coracoid

Humeral head

Hill-Sachs lesion

Glenoid and posterior scapula

C

Humeral head

FIG 1 • Posterior views of an anterior glenohumeral dislocation (**A**), an "engaging" Hill-Sachs lesion after relocation of the glenohumeral joint (**B**), and a humeral head with a large Hill-Sachs lesion (**C**).

■ They determined that the "type and duration of the initial treatment had no effect on the rate of recurrence; with a higher rate of recurrence the younger the patient."

■ Overall, 52% of 247 primary anterior dislocations had no further dislocations.

■ Patients who were 12 to 22 years old had a 34% redislocation rate, while those who were 30 to 40 years had a rate of 9%.

■ Ninety-nine of 185 shoulders that were evaluated with radiographs had evidence of a Hill-Sachs lesion; and of these 99 shoulders, 60 redislocated at least once and 51 redislocated at least twice during the 10-year follow-up.

■ This compares with 38 (44%) of the 86 shoulders that did not have such a lesion documented ($P < 0.04$).

■ Acute first-time shoulder dislocations have traditionally been treated nonoperatively with reduction followed by a form of immobilization.

■ Currently recommended types of immobilization after shoulder dislocations are as follows:

■ Simple sling immobilization with the arm in internal rotation[11]

■ Immobilization in external rotation[9,10]

■ No clear evidence has quieted this discussion.

PATIENT HISTORY AND PHYSICAL FINDINGS

■ All patients are initially evaluated with complete history and physical examination.

■ Specifics of the history include questioning for the mode of onset and timing of initial symptoms, and for the details of present symptoms, including pain, frequency, instability, and level of function.

■ All previous surgical procedures performed on the shoulder should be noted.

■ Most patients will give a history of recurrent dislocations or multiple surgical attempts to correct the instability.

■ Although thought to be a procedure for failed attempts at shoulder stabilization after dislocation, there are other situations that might lead the surgeon to consider this procedure initially.

■ Significant traumatic mechanism with an extensive Hill-Sachs lesion (more than 25% to 30% of the articulating surface of the humeral head)

Patients with a history of grand mal seizures often have fairly large Hill-Sachs defects and significant apprehension about the use of their arm. Also, as a result of the violence of the dislocations, the amount of bone pathology present, and the inability to predict the onset of epileptic events, it is worth considering treating this group of patients with an allograft reconstruction of the humeral head defect at the index procedure, as soft tissue repairs alone may not be enough to prevent recurrent injury.

Physical examination should focus on inspection for previous scars, a thorough determination of active and passive range of motion, and evaluation of the integrity and strength of the rotator cuff.

The clinician should perform a detailed examination for glenohumeral laxity in the anterior, posterior, and inferior directions.

Examination for apprehension should be performed in multiple positions, as patients with large Hill-Sachs lesions usually exhibit apprehension that often occurs with the arm in significantly less than 90 degrees abduction and 90 degrees external rotation.[13,14]

A comprehensive examination should include but is not limited to:

 Anterior apprehension test: Positive apprehension can be associated with anterior labral injuries.

 Bony apprehension test: Apprehension with fewer degrees of abduction may indicate a significant and symptomatic bony contribution to the instability.

IMAGING AND OTHER DIAGNOSTIC STUDIES

Preoperative imaging includes a comprehensive plain film evaluation with anteroposterior (AP), true AP, axillary, and Stryker notch views of the involved shoulder (**FIG 2A**).

All patients require a preoperative axial imaging study (CT or MRI) to more fully define the bony architecture of the glenoid and humeral head and specifically the details of the Hill-Sachs lesion (**FIG 2B**).

One must be careful when interpreting these studies, since the plane of the Hill-Sachs defect is oblique to the plane of the axial image. Therefore, the size of these defects is often underestimated in standard axial imaging.

Three-dimensional reconstruction can be a useful tool to more clearly define the size and location of the defect and to estimate the amount of the articular surface involved.

While the volume and depth of the lesion certainly affect the stability of the shoulder, even more important may be the size of the defect in the articular arc.

DIFFERENTIAL DIAGNOSIS

Anterior shoulder dislocation with or without:

 Bankart lesion

 "Bony Bankart" or an anterior glenoid lesion

 Hill-Sachs lesion

 Combination of the above

Posterior shoulder dislocation with or without associated soft tissue and bony lesions

Inferior shoulder dislocation with or without associated soft tissue and bony lesions

NONOPERATIVE MANAGEMENT

Given a mechanism of shoulder dislocation, the presence of significant bony defects to the glenoid or the humeral head, and associated functional instability, there are not anticipated gains through nonoperative management.

SURGICAL MANAGEMENT

Several techniques have been described in the literature to address symptomatic engaging Hill-Sachs lesions.

 Open anterior procedures, such as an East–West plication to limit external rotation, designed to limit external rotation such that the humeral head defect is kept from engaging[1,2]

 Rotational proximal humeral osteotomy as described by Weber and colleagues[17]

 Transfer of the infraspinatus into the defect to render the lesion essentially extra-articular[3,18]

 Filling in of the Hill-Sachs defect so that it can no longer engage, using either a corticocancellous iliac graft or a femoral head osteoarticular allograft

If the defect is severe, prosthetic replacement using a hemiarthroplasty may become necessary.[16]

In the case of posterior glenohumeral dislocation, Gerber and coworkers[5] have reported on the successful reconstruction of the humeral head by elevation of the depressed cartilage and subchondral buttressing with cancellous bone graft, as well as femoral head osteoarticular allograft reconstruction of the humeral head defect.

The indications for anatomic allograft reconstruction of the humeral head are as follows:

 Ongoing symptomatic anterior glenohumeral instability or painful clicking, catching, or popping in a patient with a large engaging Hill-Sachs lesion in patients who have failed to respond to previous soft-tissue stabilization procedures

 A large engaging Hill-Sachs lesion is identified before undergoing initial surgical treatment. Clinical experience suggests that lesions involving more than 25% to 30% of the articular surface may be significant.[14]

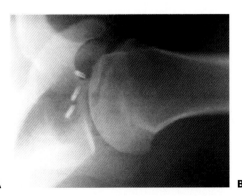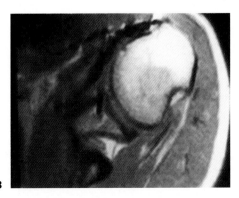

FIG 2 • A. AP radiograph of shoulder demonstrating a large Hill-Sachs lesion. **B.** Axial MRI image demonstrating large engaging Hill-Sachs lesion.

A   B

- Patients at high risk of redislocation (eg, epilepsy with recurrent anterior instability and large Hill-Sachs defects, or contact athletes with combined bony defects to the glenoid and humeral head) can consider this procedure as a primary treatment option.
- Contact athletes can be considered in this group, as time lost from an activity can be a significant issue. Thus, treatment focused on all bony and soft tissue lesions might lessen the likelihood that they would sustain a failed procedure and the associated delay in returning to full competition.
- Contraindications to this procedure include routine medical comorbidities precluding an elective surgical procedure with general anesthetic, existing infection, or presence of a nonengaging or functionally nonengaging Hill-Sachs lesion.

Preoperative Planning

- A fresh-frozen cryopreserved osteoarticular humeral head allograft is obtained from a reputable, certified tissue bank.
  - It is important to obtain a side- and size-matched graft as this allows for an optimal recreation of the radius of curvature of the humeral head.
  - The details regarding treatment, preservation, and storage then differ depending on the type of sample and the preference of the surgeon.
  - The graft serves mainly a structural function, and cartilage viability is probably not essential for success.
  - The availability of fresh-frozen tissue can be problematic, and therefore we have sometimes performed the procedure using irradiated grafts.
  - In 2 of 20 cases using irradiated grafts, however, we observed partial collapse of the grafts, which required reoperation and screw removal. Fortunately, this did not lead to recurrent instability.
  - As a result, our present protocol favors the use of fresh-frozen tissue.
- Allograft sizing of the humeral head is performed by sending copies of your patient's films to the chosen bone bank for measurement.

- Plain radiographs can be used as long as they were obtained with magnification markers. Acceptable markers include some form of recognizable currency, such as a United States quarter or dime, or a standard magnification marker obtained from your tissue bank.
- CT or MRI scan of the proximal humerus would allow for direct sizing from the scan since the magnification effect is factored into the resulting images.
- Whichever way one chooses, the tissue bank should search for a match that has a side and size match to within about ±2 mm. Clinically, we have found that this tolerance yields acceptable results for this procedure.
- Specific details should be arranged between the surgeon and the tissue bank.
- Nevertheless, availability of an allograft is sometimes a problem.
  - If waiting is not an option, one may choose to use non-matched humeral grafts or femoral head allograft.
  - The problem with this is that femoral heads often have evidence of osteoarthritis and loss of articular cartilage. This is a suboptimal situation and should be avoided.
- If different-sized grafts or femoral head grafts are used, they may not match the curvature of the native humeral head exactly and would need to be trimmed to obtain an optimal fit.
- It is important to discuss and understand the details of allograft use as it may have direct implications to your patient.

Positioning

- The patient is positioned in a modified beach chair position, inclined about 45 degrees, with the upper extremity draped free.

Approach

- An extended deltopectoral approach is used.
- The lateral border of the conjoined tendon is identified and gently retracted medially to expose the underlying subscapularis tendon.

TECHNIQUES

RELEASE OF THE SUBSCAPULARIS MUSCLE AND CAPSULOTOMY

- The entire tendon is transected vertically about 0.5 cm medial to its insertion onto the lesser tuberosity.
- Tag sutures of number 2 Control Release Ethibond Excel (#DC494, Ethicon, Somerville, NJ) are placed in the lateral aspect of the subscapularis tendon as it is released from the lesser tuberosity.
- The interval between the subscapularis and the anterior capsule is then carefully developed using sharp dissection, continuing medially to the neck of the glenoid.

- The inferior capsule is then further isolated using careful blunt dissection.
- A laterally based capsulotomy is made with the vertical limb in line with the subscapularis incision and continuing superiorly.
- The anteroinferior capsule is then released off the surgical neck of the humerus with intra-articular dissection using a periosteal elevator.

ANTERIOR LABRAL INSPECTION AND BANKART RECONSTRUCTION

- A standard humeral head retractor is placed into the glenohumeral joint, allowing inspection of the glenoid and anteroinferior capsulolabral structures for any pathology.

- If a Bankart lesion is found, it is repaired in the usual fashion using either bony drill holes or suture anchors. The sutures can be left untied until completion of the allograft reconstruction.

EXPOSURE OF THE HILL-SACHS LESION

- The humeral head retractor is withdrawn and the humerus is brought into maximal external rotation to expose the Hill-Sachs lesion.
- Unroof the synovial expansion of the supraspinatus to allow the humerus to be more fully externally rotated, allowing better visualization and access to the Hill-Sachs lesion.
- A flat narrow retractor (eg, Darach) is then placed over the reflected undersurface of the subscapularis tendon and behind the neck of the humerus on the posterior rotator cuff in order to lever out the humeral head (**TECH FIG 1**).

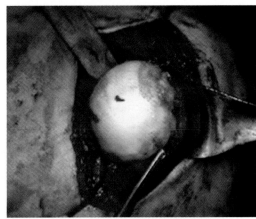

TECH FIG 1 • Intraoperative exposure of large Hill-Sachs lesion to be reconstructed.

HUMERAL HEAD OSTEOTOMY

- With the Hill-Sachs lesion adequately exposed, a micro-sagittal saw is used to smooth and reshape the defect into a chevron-type configuration.
- The piece of matching allograft humeral head to be inserted should resemble a deep-dish slice of pie (**TECH FIG 2A,B**).

- The base and side of the defect can then be further smoothed using a hand rasp to achieve precise, flat surfaces.
- The base (X), height (Y), length (Z), and rough outside partial circumference (C) of the defect are then measured to the nearest millimeter (**TECH FIG 2C**).

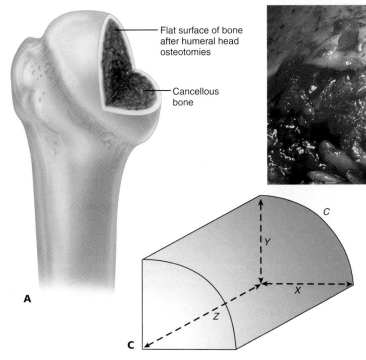

Flat surface of bone after humeral head osteotomies

Cancellous bone

TECH FIG 2 • **A.** Diagram of the humeral head after osteotomies. **B.** Reshaping of Hill-Sachs lesion to prepare to receive allograft. **C.** Schematic representation of required measurements of the defect and graft. Base (X), height (Y), length (Z), and rough outside partial circumference (C) of the defect are then measured to the nearest millimeter.

OSTEOTOMY OF THE HUMERAL HEAD ALLOGRAFT

- A corresponding piece is cut from the matched humeral head allograft that is 2 to 3 mm larger in all dimensions than the measured defect.
- The allograft segment is then provisionally placed into the Hill-Sachs defect and resized in all three planes.

- Excess graft is then carefully trimmed with the micro-sagittal saw and is reshaped in the other two planes as well.
- Fine-tuning of graft size is then continued in one plane at a time until a perfect size match is achieved in all planes, including base (X), height (Y), length (Z), and outside partial circumference (C).

FIXATION OF THE HUMERAL HEAD ALLOGRAFT

- The allograft segment is placed into the defect and aligned so as to achieve a congruent articular surface.
- It is provisionally secured in place with two or three smooth 0.045-inch Kirschner wires (**TECH FIG 3A,B**).
- The wires are then sequentially replaced with 3.5-mm fully threaded cortical or 4.0-mm cancellous screws placed in a lag fashion (**TECH FIG 3C,D**).

- Ensure that the screw heads are countersunk so that they are below the level of the articular surface.
- The joint is irrigated and taken through a range of motion to ensure that the reconstructed humeral head provides a smooth congruent articulating surface.

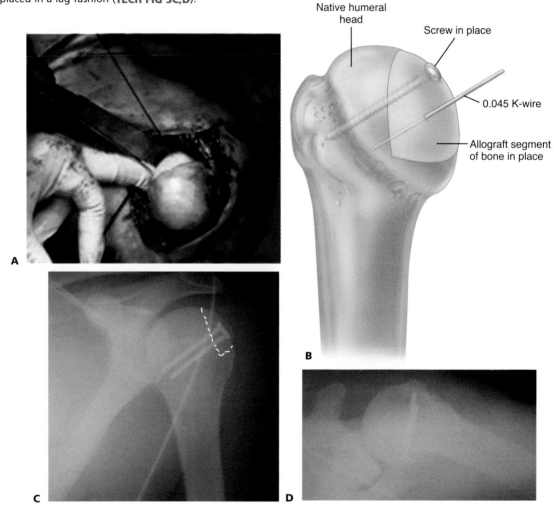

TECH FIG 3 ● A. Anatomic allograft reconstruction of Hill-Sachs defect with humeral allograft provisionally held in place with two Kirschner wires. **B.** Diagram of allograft reconstruction of Hill-Sachs defect with humeral allograft held in place with a Kirschner wire and an AO screw. **C.** AP radiograph of shoulder demonstrating anatomic allograft reconstruction of Hill-Sachs defect fixed with two countersunk cortical screws. (*Dashed line* represents the area filled by the allograft.) **D.** Axillary view of shoulder demonstrating anatomic allograft reconstruction of Hill-Sachs defect fixed with two countersunk cortical screws.

LABRAL REPAIR AND SUBSCAPULARIS REAPPROXIMATION

- The capsulotomy is closed with absorbable suture, tying any previously placed sutures used to repair the capsulolabral pathology if present.
- The subscapularis tendon is then reapproximated to its stump anatomically, without shortening, using suture anchors or a soft tissue repair with nonabsorbable suture.

- Allow the conjoined tendon, deltoid, and pectoralis major muscles to return to their normal anatomic positions.
- A routine subcutaneous and skin closure is then performed.
- Sterile dressing is applied.
- The arm is placed into a shoulder immobilizer.

PEARLS AND PITFALLS

Anterior labral injury	■ The surgeon should ensure this injury pattern is identified early after exposure of the joint. Anchors or sutures are placed in the anterior glenoid for later labral repair after reconstruction of the Hill-Sachs lesion.
Exposure of the posterior superior humeral head	■ This area of the humeral head can be accessed through external rotation and forward flexion of the upper extremity. Appropriately placed retractors assist in this exposure.
Allograft sizing	■ The surgeon should ensure the allograft obtained is larger in dimension by 2 to 3 mm than the actual defect. This allows for in situ sizing.
Screw placement	■ It is easier to initially place two 0.045-inch Kirschner wires for fixation and then replace them with two 3.5-mm stainless steel AO screws lagged into position. ■ Screw heads are countersunk beneath the surface of the allograft articular surface to prevent hardware penetration.

POSTOPERATIVE CARE

■ After surgery, patients are given a sling for comfort and allowed full passive range of motion immediately as tolerated.
■ Because of the subscapularis detachment, we protect against active and resisted internal rotation for 6 weeks.
■ After the initial 6-week period, patients are allowed terminal stretching and strengthening exercises.
■ The shoulders are imaged with repeat radiographs at 6 weeks and 6 months, and with CT scans at 6 months to assess for consolidation and incorporation of the graft.

OUTCOMES

■ Between 1995 and 2001, we performed and reviewed this procedure in 18 patients who had failed previous attempts at surgical stabilization.[13,14]
■ Fifteen patients had a history of traumatic anterior glenohumeral instability related to sports, and three patients had instability related to seizures or other trauma.
■ All had posterolateral humeral head defects (Hill-Sachs lesions) that represented greater than about 25% to 30% of the humeral head.
■ One patient had both anterior and posterior humeral head defects from bidirectional shoulder instability sustained as a result of a seizure disorder.
■ No patients had true multidirectional instability.
■ Patients in the formal review were assessed preoperatively and postoperatively with:
  ■ Detailed history
  ■ Physical examination
  ■ Radiographic evaluation (plain films and axial imaging [CT, MRI, or both])
  ■ Validated clinical evaluation measures (Constant-Murley shoulder scale, Western Ontario Shoulder Instability Index [WOSII], and SF-36)
■ Findings at the time of surgery included:
  ■ Nine patients with recurrent Bankart lesions
  ■ Nine patients with capsular redundancy only
  ■ No patients with subscapularis tears
  ■ One patient with posterior glenoid erosion
  ■ Three patients with anterior glenoid deficiency (less than 20%), which was not reconstructed
■ Mean length of follow-up was 50 months (range 24 to 96 months).
■ There were no episodes of recurrent instability. Sixteen of 18 (89%) patients returned to work.

■ The average Constant-Murley score postoperatively was 78.5. The WOSII, which is a validated quality-of-life scale specific to shoulder instability using a visual analog scale response format, decreased and patients were significantly improved.
■ Overall, this represents the first reported series of anatomic allograft reconstruction of Hill-Sachs defects for recurrent traumatic anterior instability after failed repairs.
■ This technique has been shown to be effective for a difficult problem with few available treatment options.
■ The patients demonstrated improvement in stability, loss of apprehension, and high subjective approval, allowing return to near-normal function with no further episodes of instability.
■ Although infrequently a cause for clinical concern, Hill-Sachs defects can be the source of significant disability and recurrent instability in a subset of patients.
■ One should consider anatomic allograft reconstruction of these defects as a viable treatment alternative.

COMPLICATIONS

■ Complications that occurred in our series of humeral osteoarticular allograft reconstruction of the Hill-Sachs lesions included radiographic follow-up evidence of partial graft collapse in 2 of 18 patients, early evidence of osteoarthritis in 3 patients (marginal osteophytes), and 1 mild subluxation (posterior).[12–14]
■ Hardware complications developed in two patients, who complained of pain with extreme external rotation.
  ■ The screws were removed at about 2 years postoperatively in both patients, thereby relieving their symptoms.
■ One must weigh the risks of continued shoulder dysfunction versus the risk associated with the use of fresh osteoarticular allografts.

REFERENCES

1. Burkhart SS, Danaceau SM. Articular arc length mismatch as a cause of failed Bankart repair. Arthroscopy 2000;16:740–744.
2. Burkhart SS, De Beer JF. Traumatic glenohumeral bone defects and their relationship to failure of arthroscopic Bankart repairs: significance of the inverted-pear glenoid and the humeral engaging Hill-Sachs lesion. Arthroscopy 2000;16:677–694.
3. Connolly J. Humeral head defects associated with shoulder dislocations: their diagnostic and surgical significance. AAOS Instr Course Lect 1972;1972:42–54.
4. Flower WH. On the pathological changes produced in the shoulder-joint by traumatic dislocations, as derived from an examination of all specimens illustrating this injury in the museums of London. Trans Pathol Soc London 1861;12:179.

5. Gerber C, Lambert SM. Allograft reconstruction of segmental defects of the humeral head for the treatment of chronic locked posterior dislocation of the shoulder. J Bone Joint Surg Am 1996;78A: 376–382.

6. Hill HA, Sachs MD. The groove defect of the humeral head: a frequently unrecognized complication of dislocations of the shoulder joint. Radiology 1940;35:690–700.

7. Hovelius L. Anterior dislocation of the shoulder in teen-agers and young adults: five-year prognosis. J Bone Joint Surg Am 1987;69: 393–399.

8. Hovelius L, Augustini BG, Fredin H, et al. Primary anterior dislocation of the shoulder in young patients: a ten-year prospective study. J Bone Joint Surg Am 1996;78A:1677–1684.

9. Itoi E, Hatakeyama Y, Kido T, et al. A new method of immobilization after traumatic anterior dislocation of the shoulder: a preliminary study. J Shoulder Elbow Surg 2003;12:413–415.

10. Itoi E, Sashi R, Minagawa H, et al., Position of immobilization after dislocation of the shoulder: a cadaveric study. J Bone Joint Surg Am 1999;81A:385–390.

11. Matsen FA, Thomas SC, Rockwood CA. Glenohumeral instability. In Rockwood CA, ed. The Shoulder. Philadelphia: Elsevier, 2004:655–780.

12. Miniaci A. Reconstruction of large humeral head defects in patients with failed instability surgery. In Norris TR, ed. Surgery of the Shoulder and Elbow: An International Perspective. Rosemont, IL: American Academy of Orthopaedic Surgeons, 2006.

13. Miniaci A, Gish MW. Management of anterior glenohumeral instability associated with large Hill-Sachs defects. Tech Should Elbow Surg 2004;5:170–175.

14. Miniaci A, Martineau PA. Humeral head bony deficiency (large Hill-Sachs). In El Attrache NS, ed. Surgical Techniques in Sports Medicine. Philadelphia: Lippincott Williams & Wilkins, 2006.

15. Neer CS II, Foster CR. Inferior capsular shift for involuntary inferior and multidirectional instability of the shoulder: a preliminary report. J Bone Joint Surg Am 1980;62A:897–908.

16. Pritchett JW, Clark JM. Prosthetic replacement for chronic unreduced dislocations of the shoulder. Clin Orthop Relat Res 1987;216: 89–93.

17. Weber BG, Simpson AL, Hardegger F. Rotational humeral osteotomy for recurrent anterior dislocation of the shoulder associated with a large Hill-Sachs lesion. J Bone Joint Surg Am 1984;66A:1443–1450.

18. Wolf E, Pollack ME, Smalley C. Hill-Sachs "remplissage": an arthroscopic solution for the engaging Hill-Sachs lesion. Arthroscopy Association of North America, San Francisco, CA, 2007.

19. Yagishita K, Thomas BJ. Use of allograft for large Hill-Sachs lesion associated with anterior glenohumeral dislocation: a case report. Injury 2002;33:791–794.

Chapter 8

Acromioplasty, Distal Clavicle Excision, and Posterosuperior Rotator Cuff Repair

Robert J. Neviaser and Andrew S. Neviaser

DEFINITION

■ Posterosuperior tears of the rotator cuff involve the supraspinatus, infraspinatus, and occasionally the teres minor.

■ Some of the surgical techniques to be described here are not commonly used currently, as most tears can be repaired by arthroscopic approaches, either with mini-open or all-arthroscopic techniques.

■ These approaches, however, are still useful for treating those massive tears that may need special procedures to accomplish the repair.

ANATOMY

■ The rotator cuff is a group of four musculotendinous structures arising from the scapula: the supraspinatus, the infraspinatus, the teres minor, and the subscapularis. The first three insert on the greater tuberosity of the humerus, while the subscapularis inserts on the lesser tuberosity. The cuff muscles not only rotate the humerus at the glenohumeral joint but also act to keep the humeral head centered in the glenoid fossa, providing a fixed fulcrum for the arm to be elevated, primarily by the deltoid. The subacromial bursa overlies the tendons.

■ These structures, in turn, sit under the coracoacromial arch, which consists of the acromion, the coracoacromial ligament, and the outer end of the clavicle at the acromioclavicular joint.

■ The three parts of the deltoid arise from the acromion and lateral clavicle, and this muscle lies over the cuff and bursa. It acts to elevate, abduct, and extend the humerus at the shoulder joint.

PATHOGENESIS

■ Rotator cuff tears have a multifactorial pathogenesis.

■ Among the factors are tendon insertional degeneration (enthesopathy), shear (the inferior third of the cuff tendons being more susceptible to shear failure than the superior two thirds), hypovascularity, impingement, and microtrauma.

■ Although impingement was felt to be the sole underlying cause of cuff disease for some time, it is now felt to be a secondary factor, in that it likely comes into play once the cuff is weakened and is unable to balance the upward pull of the deltoid. This then brings the cuff into contact with the undersurface of the anteroinferior acromion and the rest of the coracoacromial arch.

■ Major injury is uncommonly a factor and usually involves an already degenerative tendon. A common major injury, which can result in a rotator cuff tear, is a primary, or a first-time, anterior dislocation of the shoulder in a patient over age 40. The older the patient, the more likely there is a cuff tear.

NATURAL HISTORY

■ The natural history of rotator cuff tears is unknown. There have been several studies in cadavers and by MRI that have

confirmed that the incidence of asymptomatic cuff tears over the age of 60 is around 33%. These subjects have been pain-free and fully functional.

■ Any study that has tried to follow asymptomatic tears prospectively over time has suffered from an unacceptably high loss of patients being followed, thereby negating any conclusions.

■ Even the condition of cuff tear arthropathy does not occur regularly with known cuff tears, even massive ones.

■ It has been shown that after a traumatic tear, the outcome is influenced by the time interval to repair—in other words, those repaired within the first 3 weeks do better then those repaired between 3 and 6 weeks, and those older than 6 weeks do even worse. These outcomes apply only to the uncommon traumatic tear, not to the far more common degenerative type.

■ Therefore, treatment should be based purely on the presenting symptoms of pain and functional limitation, not on the possibility that a tear may progress in size or develop into cuff tear arthropathy, since the latter possibilities cannot be predicted.

PATIENT HISTORY AND PHYSICAL FINDINGS

■ Barring the unusual history of a significant injury, such as a primary anterior glenohumeral dislocation over the age of 40 resulting in a traumatic tear, most patients will present with a complaint of pain of indeterminate onset.

■ The pain is often worse at night and with use, especially overhead.

■ Use of nonsteroidal anti-inflammatories (NSAIDs) may provide some temporary relief, as might stretching.

■ The pain can radiate, but not to below the elbow or into the neck and occiput.

■ There rarely will be significant motion loss (ie, motion will be unaffected) nor will the patient often notice weakness.

■ The first step in the physical examination is to examine the neck to eliminate that as a source of the pain.

■ One should inspect the shoulder for atrophy of the supraspinatus and infraspinatus or rupture of the tendon of the long head of the biceps, which usually occurs with a large or massive tear. One should also palpate the region of the greater tuberosity and the bicipital groove for tenderness. In thin patients, it is possible to feel the cuff defect through the skin and deltoid.

■ Motion is assessed by having the patient elevate the arms actively and comparing this to passive motion and by placing the arms in 90 degrees of abduction and maximal external rotation, as well as maximal external rotation with the arm at the side.

　■ The inability to hold the arm in maximum active external rotation in abduction or at the side, causing the arm to drift toward internal rotation, is a positive lag sign, indicating a major defect in the musculotendinous unit.

Internal rotation is evaluated by having the patient reach up the back to the highest point possible. Further testing for this (subscapularis function) is discussed in another chapter.

Strength of the external rotators is tested with the arm at the side and in maximal external rotation, having the patient resist a force directed toward the body. Strength in elevation is assessed by resisting the patient's attempt to raise the arm.

Provocative signs for cuff and biceps disease include the following:

Impingement sign: Forcing the fully forward elevated arm against the fixed scapula helps to localize the finding to the rotator cuff when the patient experiences pain.

Palm-down abduction test: By internally rotating the arm, the supraspinatus and anterior infraspinatus tendons are placed directly under the coracoacromial arch. Elevating the arm in the scapular plane when it is in internal rotation compresses these tendons against the undersurface of the acromion.

Biceps resistance test (Speed's test): Pain during this maneuver indicates involvement of the long head of the biceps tendon.

IMAGING AND OTHER DIAGNOSTIC STUDIES

Standard radiographs, including anteroposterior (AP) views in internal and external rotation, an axillary view, and an outlet view at minimum, should always be taken to look for the type of acromion (**FIG 1A**), acromioclavicular joint changes, and narrowing of the acromial–humeral interval (**FIG 1B**) and to rule out other conditions.

Additional preoperative studies include MRI, ultrasound, and arthrography.

Ultrasound is institutional-specific and operator-dependent, so it is not widely used.

Arthrography once was the gold standard but now is used only under rare circumstances (ie, when an MRI cannot be done). It can show a full-thickness cuff tear (**FIG 1C**) but requires an intra-articular injection with fluoroscopy and radiography.

The most commonly used study is an MRI. It not only shows the integrity of the tendons but also provides a three-dimensional view of it (**FIG 1D–G**). This capacity makes the MRI a versatile preoperative planning tool.

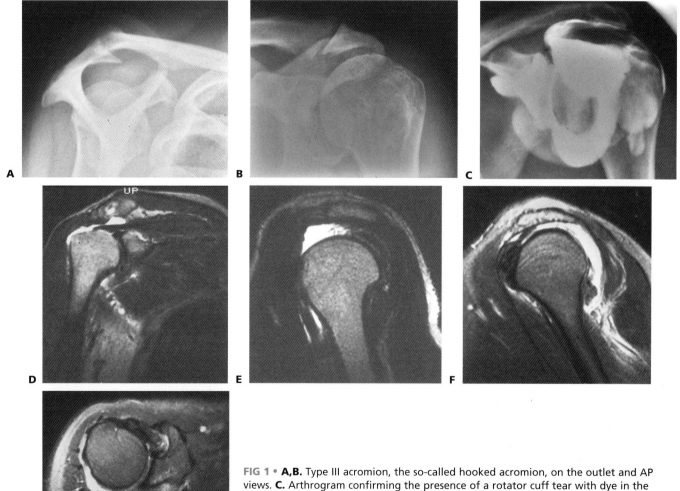

FIG 1 • A,B. Type III acromion, the so-called hooked acromion, on the outlet and AP views. **C.** Arthrogram confirming the presence of a rotator cuff tear with dye in the glenohumeral joint and the subacromial bursa simultaneously. **D.** T2-weighted coronal MRI showing cuff tear and its lateral-to-medial extent. **E.** T2-weighted sagittal oblique MRI showing the AP extent of the cuff defect. **F.** Another T2 sagittal oblique MRI showing the tear involving the teres minor but not the subscapularis. **G.** Axial T2 MRI of the same tear showing rupture of the teres minor with an intact subscapularis.

DIFFERENTIAL DIAGNOSIS

- Cuff tendinitis without tear
- Incomplete rotator cuff tear
- Bicipital tendinitis
- Calcific tendinitis
- Suprascapular neuropathy

NONOPERATIVE MANAGEMENT

- If there is a history of an acute injury with immediate inability to raise the arm, the patient can be treated symptomatically and followed every 5 to 7 days for the first 2 weeks. If the ability to raise the arm does not recover, then nonoperative treatment should be abandoned and surgery undertaken.
- The objective of treating rotator cuff disorders, in the absence of an acute injury with immediate loss of elevation, is primarily to relieve pain and secondarily to restore function or strength. Pain relief is a more predictable outcome of treatment than is restoration of function or strength. Therefore, nonoperative treatment should be directed at relieving pain.
- Although NSAIDs can help with pain, a subacromial steroid injection is often more effective and immediate in its relief.
- Once the pain is improved, physical therapy should be instituted. This involves two aspects: stretching and strengthening of the rotators and elevators.

SURGICAL MANAGEMENT

- As noted earlier, in the unusual case in which there is an acute injury resulting in an immediate loss of elevation of the arm, if symptomatic treatment fails to restore the ability to raise the arm, surgical repair should be undertaken before the 3-week mark.

- For the more common chronic attritional tear, surgery is considered if the injection, NSAIDs, and physical therapy fail to produce a level of pain relief and function that is acceptable to the patient.
- Patients make the decision to have surgery based on whether they can live with the pain and functional limitation that they have. They need to understand that the operation can help them but can also leave them unchanged or worse.

Preoperative Planning

- The radiographs and MRI should be reviewed preoperatively.
- The radiographs will help in planning the need for and extent of acromioplasty.
- The MRI will show which tendons are torn and the degree to which they are torn. It will also show the presence or absence of fatty infiltration of the muscles.

Positioning

- The patient is positioned in a sitting position, even more upright than the so-called beach chair position (**FIG 2A**). The arm is draped free to allow uninhibited mobility of the extremity (**FIG 2B**).
- This allows the surgeon to look down on the cuff from above, therefore, being able to see posterosuperiorly as well as superiorly and anteriorly. It also permits better access to the posterior part of the infraspinatus and the teres minor.

Approach

- There are basically three approaches to cuff repair:
  - The all-arthroscopic approach (discussed in another chapter)
  - Arthroscopic decompression and mini-open repair of the cuff
  - Open repair of the cuff: includes direct repair, grafting, and tendon transfers

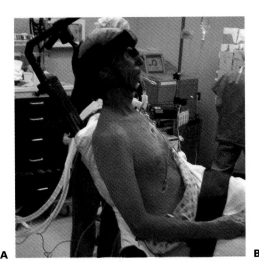
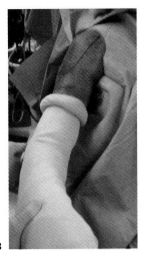

A   **B**

FIG 2 • **A.** Sitting position for surgery allows the surgeon to look down on the cuff and see posterior superior. **B.** The arm is draped free, giving extensive access to the entire shoulder.

ARTHROSCOPIC SUBACROMIAL DECOMPRESSION AND MINI-OPEN CUFF REPAIR

- The standard posterior viewing portal is established, and the glenohumeral joint is evaluated. The defect in the cuff is viewed from the articular side, and the long head of the biceps is assessed.
  - Any débridement or other intra-articular procedures deemed necessary can be carried out at this time.
- The arthroscope is then redirected into the subacromial space and enough bursa resected to allow adequate visualization of the cuff tear, the anterior inferior surface of the acromion, and the coracoacromial ligament. If deemed appropriate (as discussed later), the ligament is released and the anterior and anterolateral margins of the acromion are defined.
  - A burr is used to perform an acromioplasty to the same degree that is done in the open technique. This is an important point. Although the means of accomplishing the decompression differ, the ultimate result is the same: an adequate decompression.
- Through a small lateral portal, a suture punch is used to pass several traction sutures through the leading edge of the torn tendons. Using these sutures as handles to control and apply traction to the cuff, a small elevator is introduced through the same lateral portal and used to free the surrounding adhesions on both surfaces of the cuff. The degree of mobility achieved can be assessed by applying traction through the previously placed sutures.

- Once enough mobility of the cuff has been restored, an incision is made at the anterolateral corner of the acromion for about 1.5 to 2 cm (**TECH FIG 1**). The deltoid is split in the same line as the skin, and additional subdeltoid freeing is done. Narrow retractors are placed under the acromion and anteriorly to expose the tear.
- The procedure at this point is the same as described in the next section.

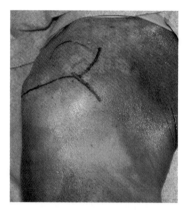

TECH FIG 1 • Skin incision for the mini-open repair technique.

OPEN REPAIR OF THE CUFF

Incision and Dissection

- With the patient in the position described above and the arm draped free, an incision is made beginning superiorly at the posterior aspect of the acromioclavicular joint, continuing over the top of the joint, and ending at a point at the lateral tip of the coracoid (**TECH FIG 2A**).
- After mobilization of the skin flaps, the deltotrapezial aponeurosis and the superior acromioclavicular ligament are incised into the acromioclavicular joint.
- The deltoid muscle is split in line with its fibers only as far distally as the tip of the coracoid.

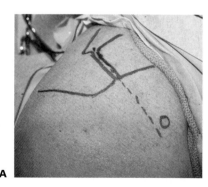

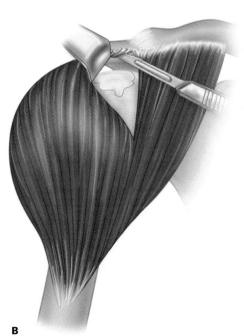

A   B

TECH FIG 2 • **A.** Skin incision for the standard anterosuperior approach. **B.** Subperiosteal dissection of deltoid origin from superior aspect of the lateral clavicle, acromioclavicular joint, and anterior acromion, without cutting across the deltoid origin. *(continued)*

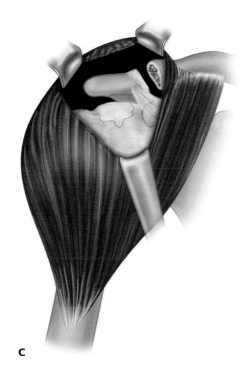

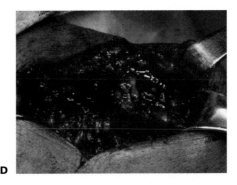

TECH FIG 2 • *(continued)* **C.** Completed elevation of the anterior deltoid origin. **D.** The completed dissection. (**A**: From Neviaser R, Neviaser AS. Open repair of massive rotator cuff tears: tissue mobilization techniques. In: Zuckerman J, ed. Advanced Reconstruction: Shoulder. Chicago, American Academy of Orthopaedic Surgery, 2007:177–184.)

- Using a sharp knife blade, the deltoid origin is dissected subperiosteally from the lateral clavicle for about 1 cm. It is also dissected from the anterior, superior, and undersurface of the acromion out to the anterolateral corner of the acromion (**TECH FIG 2B–D**).
  - No incision is made across the tendon of origin of the deltoid on the acromion; that is, the deltoid is not detached from the acromion.

Clavicular Resection and Acromioplasty

- The coracoacromial ligament is identified and isolated. If, in the judgment of the surgeon, the cuff can be securely repaired, the ligament is released from its attachment on the acromion. If the repair is tenuous, the ligament is not released, or if it is, it is dissected from the undersurface of the acromion to achieve maximal length and repaired back to the acromion through drill holes in the acromion at the end of the procedure.
  - This is necessary to prevent anterosuperior escape of the humerus, which occurs when the cuff is deficient and there is no coracoacromial arch to contain the humeral head, which is being pulled upward by the unopposed deltoid.
- Using a reciprocating saw, the lateral 7 to 8 mm of the lateral end of the clavicle are removed without damaging the periosteum or posterior capsule. The portion removed is trapezoidal in shape, with the larger base being posterior, to prevent contact of the clavicle with the acromion posteriorly.

- The clavicular resection allows the acromion and scapula to be rotated posteriorly more easily and gives greater access to the posterior cuff.
- Using the same instrument, an acromioplasty is performed by removing the anteroinferior surface of the acromion from the medial articular margin out to the anterolateral corner. The anterior edge is not recessed beyond its normal anatomy, and it is not the removal of the full thickness of the acromion, creating a type I acromion (**TECH FIG 3**). The portion removed is a triangular piece, with its base being the anterior edge.

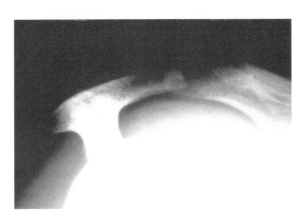

TECH FIG 3 • Type I acromion on outlet view.

- The entire subacromial space is freed bluntly of adhesions between the bursa and the undersurface of the deltoid. Retractors are placed into the subacromial space under the acromion to avoid tension on the deltoid.

Tear Repair

- The bursa is incised, undermined, and reflected. The tear in the cuff can now be seen. The friable, avascular edges are trimmed with a sharp knife. This resection is minimal—only until healthy tendon is seen (**TECH FIG 4A**), not to bleeding tendon. This usually requires the removal of only a few millimeters.
- Number 1 nonabsorbable traction sutures are placed in the edges of the freshened cuff. Applying traction through these sutures, blunt mobilization is done using an elevator, dissecting scissors, or the surgeon's finger.
  - This step of mobilization is critical, and as the musculotendinous unit becomes free, additional sutures are placed successively medially until the apex of the tear is identified (**TECH FIG 4B**).
- If the cuff edge cannot be brought sufficiently far to reach its original insertion, interval releases are done by incising between the supraspinatus and the subscapularis and between the infraspinatus and the teres minor. This restores the differential gliding between these adjacent tendons.
- When the leading edge of the cuff can be brought to its insertion on the greater tuberosity, a shallow trough is made in the anatomic neck at the greater tuberosity (**TECH FIG 4A**).
- Drill holes are made in the trough and the lateral side of the tuberosity and connected with a punch. Locking horizontal mattress sutures or modified Mason-Allen sutures are placed in the cuff and passed through the bone tunnels created by connecting the drill holes (**TECH FIG 4C**). Suture anchors can also be used in the trough and the tuberosity in a double-row fashion instead of the bone tunnels.
- With the arm in some internal rotation and slight abduction, the sutures are tied securely to bring the free edge of the cuff into the trough.
- This leaves a longitudinal split, which is sutured side to side, not only closing the split but also helping to relieve tension on the cuff advanced into the trough (**TECH FIG 4D**).

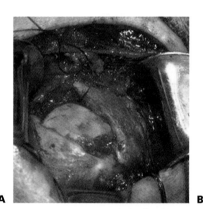
A

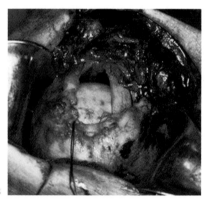
B

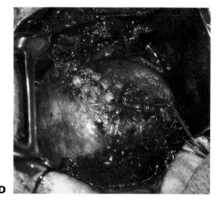
D

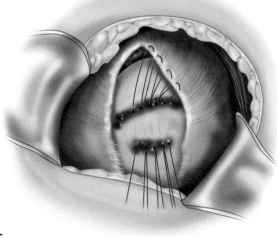
C

TECH FIG 4 • A. Intraoperative photograph showing freshened edges of tear. Healthy tendon is seen but not bleeding edges. Note cancellous trough at the anatomic neck and the greater tuberosity. **B.** Triangular tear with apex medially. **C.** Drawing of sutures passed through bone tunnels in the trough and greater tuberosity, pulling the edge of the cuff into the trough. Anchors can be used instead. **D.** Completed L-shaped repair. (**D:** From Neviaser R, Neviaser AS. Open repair of massive rotator cuff tears: tissue mobilization techniques. In: Zuckerman J, ed. Advanced Reconstruction: Shoulder. Chicago, American Academy of Orthopaedic Surgery, 2007:177–184.)

BICEPS GRAFT

- If the cuff cannot be brought to the greater tuberosity and there is a residual defect of modest size, an interpositional graft of the tendon of the long head of the biceps can be used. The critical requirement to use this or any graft is that the musculotendinous motor must be functional, not fixed and immobile. If there is no springy give when traction is applied to the tendon, no graft should be done.
- First, the tendon of the long head is tenodesed to the transverse humeral ligament in the bicipital groove using three figure 8 nonabsorbable number 1 sutures. The tendon is transected just above the most proximal suture and then released from its origin at the supraglenoid tubercle.
- This segment of tendon is filleted (TECH FIG 5A) and placed into the cuff defect. It is trimmed to fit the defect and contoured to accommodate it.
- It is sutured side to side to the cuff and to a trough in the anatomic neck at the greater tuberosity, as described above (TECH FIG 5B).

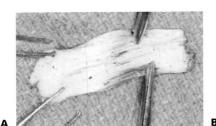
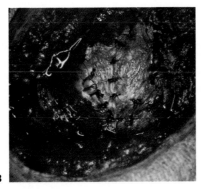

TECH FIG 5 • **A.** Filleted intra-articular portion of the tendon of the long head of the biceps. **B.** Biceps graft in place. (**A**: From Neviaser RJ. Tears of the rotator cuff. Orthop Clin North Am 1980;11:295–306. **B**: From Neviaser JS. Ruptures of the rotator cuff of the shoulder: new concepts in the diagnosis and treatment of chronic ruptures. Arch Surg 1971;102:483–485.)

FREEZE-DRIED CADAVER ROTATOR CUFF GRAFT

- If the residual defect is too large for a biceps graft to cover, a larger graft is needed. The best choice is a freeze-dried graft of human rotator cuff. As with every graft, the musculotendinous motor (ie, the native rotator cuff) must be a functional unit, as noted above.
- After the described mobilization techniques have reduced the size of the defect as much as possible, the graft is reconstituted in sterile saline for 30 minutes so that it becomes soft and pliable (TECH FIG 6A).
- It is then trimmed and contoured to accommodate the free edge of the native cuff and then sutured to it with nonabsorbable number 1 sutures.
- It is also trimmed to reach a trough in the anatomic neck adjacent to the greater tuberosity and secured in the same fashion as the direct repair through drill holes in the bone or by anchors, as previously described (TECH FIG 6B).

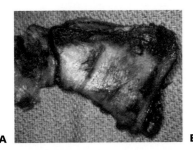
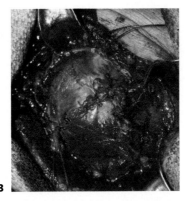

TECH FIG 6 • **A.** Reconstituted freeze-dried cadaver rotator cuff graft. **B.** Reconstituted freeze-dried cadaver rotator cuff graft sutures in place. (**A**: From Neviaser JS, Neviaser RJ, Neviaser TJ. The repair of chronic massive ruptures of the rotator cuff by use of a freeze-dried rotator cuff. J Bone Joint Surg Am 1978;60A:681–684. **B**: From Neviaser R, Neviaser AS. Open repair of massive rotator cuff tears: tissue mobilization techniques. In: Zuckerman J, ed. Advanced Reconstruction: Shoulder. Chicago, American Academy of Orthopaedic Surgery, 2007:177–184.)

LOCAL TENDON TRANSFERS

- When the cuff cannot be closed by direct repair and the proximal native cuff is not mobile, the subscapularis and teres minor can be used as local tendon transfers.
- The interval between the subscapularis and the anterior capsule is identified near the musculotendinous junction and traced laterally toward the insertion on the lesser tuberosity.
- The tendon is separated from the capsule and released from the insertion. A traction suture is placed in the tendon, and the subscapularis is mobilized so that it can be shifted superiorly.
- The subscapularis is then transferred superiorly (**TECH FIG 7A**) to close the residual defect. Its superior border is sutured to the intact portion of the cuff, its distal end to the greater tuberosity, and its inferior border to the superior edge of the undisturbed anterior capsule (**TECH FIG 7B,C**).
- If the subscapularis alone does not provide adequate closure of the tear, the teres minor can also be trans-

ferred from posterior to superior. The interval between the tendon of the teres minor and the posterior capsule is developed (**TECH FIG 7D**), starting medially at the musculotendinous junction, and freed laterally to its insertion on the greater tuberosity. It is detached from the tuberosity.
- The muscle–tendon unit is mobilized bluntly and transferred superiorly to meet the transposed subscapularis (**TECH FIG 7E**).
- The two tendons are sutured together to form a new broad tendon, which is inserted into a trough at the greater tuberosity, as described earlier.
- The inferior borders of the respective tendons are sutured to the superior edges of the undisturbed capsules (teres minor to the posterior capsule and the subscapularis to the anterior capsule) (**TECH FIG 7F,G**).
- If none of these techniques allows the cuff to be reconstructed satisfactorily, a latissimus dorsi transfer is undertaken; this is described elsewhere.

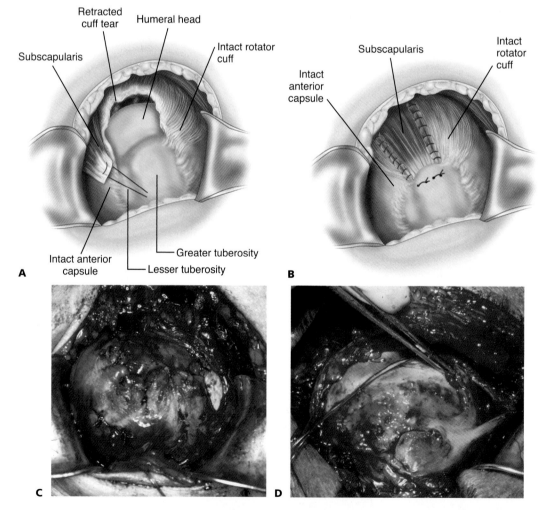

TECH FIG 7 • **A.** Detached subscapularis mobilized and moved superiorly. **B.** Subscapularis transferred and sutured to residual cuff, the greater tuberosity, and the superior border of the undisturbed anterior capsule. **C.** Subscapularis transferred and sutured. **D.** Interval between the teres minor and posterior capsule developed. (*continued*)

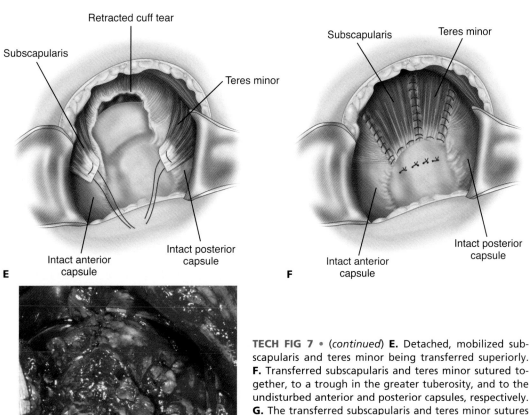

TECH FIG 7 • (*continued*) **E.** Detached, mobilized subscapularis and teres minor being transferred superiorly. **F.** Transferred subscapularis and teres minor sutured together, to a trough in the greater tuberosity, and to the undisturbed anterior and posterior capsules, respectively. **G.** The transferred subscapularis and teres minor sutures in place. (**D** and **G**: From Neviaser RJ, Neviaser TJ. Transfer of the subscapularis and teres minor for massive defects of the rotator cuff. In Bayley I, Kessel L, eds. Shoulder Surgery. Heidelberg: Springer-Verlag, 1982:60–69.)

CLOSURE

- The closure is the same for all procedures.
- Since the deltoid has not been detached from its origin, it is allowed to fall back to its normal anatomic position or brought back by the surgeon. Simple sutures with the knots buried under the deltoid are placed to repair the side-to-side split, being sure to pass the suture through the external muscle fascia, the muscle itself, and the internal muscle fascia.
- If the deltotrapezial aponeurosis and superior acromioclavicular ligament have been incised, they are repaired side to side with figure 8 sutures.
- The skin is closed with a subcuticular 3-0 nylon suture and Steri-Strips. A sterile dressing is applied, and the extremity is immobilized in an immobilizer with the elbow forward of the midline of the body and the shoulder in internal rotation.

PEARLS AND PITFALLS

Postoperative deltoid detachment	▪ This can be avoided by subperiosteally elevating the origin and not incising across it.
Axillary nerve injury with deltoid split	▪ This can be avoided by not splitting the deltoid beyond the tip of the coracoid. Exposure is achieved by superior access, not distally.
Excessive tendon resection	▪ Friable, poor-quality tendon should be trimmed only to healthy fibers, not to bleeding tendon.
Postoperative repair failure	▪ Tendons should be repaired to bone under only normal resting tension. If this is not possible, the described grafts or tendon transfers should be used. ▪ The early postoperative rehabilitation program is used to regain motion; strengthening is avoided until at least 3 weeks.

POSTOPERATIVE CARE

- Within 24 to 72 hours of the surgery, the dressing is changed. The patient is instructed in passive-only forward elevation and external rotation at the side while lying supine. The operative arm must be completely relaxed with no muscle activity at all, and the arm is elevated to at least 90 degrees forward and external rotation to neutral only.
- Over the next 4 to 6 weeks the amount of passive forward elevation is slowly increased, as is the external rotation at the side, but the latter should not go beyond 10 to 15 degrees of external rotation at most.
- The extremity is kept in the immobilizer at all other times during this period. At 4 to 6 weeks postoperatively, depending on the security of the repair and the technique used, formal active and assisted exercises are permitted, along with continued passive stretching. Strengthening, weights, or resistive exercises are avoided until at least 3 months.

OUTCOMES

- Repairs of small and medium-sized tears have a high rate of success in relieving pain and recovering motion and function while remaining structurally intact, regardless of whether repaired by arthroscopic, mini-open, or open techniques.
- Repairs of large and massive tears also have resulted in good pain relief and functional recovery but have a much lower incidence of remaining intact structurally.

COMPLICATIONS

- Deltoid origin detachment
- Cuff repair dehiscence
- Anterosuperior instability or escape
- Infection
- Loss of motion
- Cuff tear arthropathy

REFERENCES

1. Cofield RH. Subscapularis muscle transposition for repair of chronic rotator cuff tears. Surg Gynecol Obstet 1982;154:667–672.
2. Karas SE, Giacello TL. Subscapularis transfer for reconstruction of massive tears of the rotator cuff. J Bone Joint Surg Am 1996;78A: 239–245.
3. Neviaser JS. Ruptures of the rotator cuff: new concepts in the diagnosis and operative treatment for chronic tears. Arch Surg 1971; 102:483–485.
4. Neviaser JS, Neviaser RJ, Neviaser TJ. The repair of chronic massive ruptures of the rotator cuff by use of a freeze-dried rotator cuff graft. J Bone Joint Surg Am 1978;60A:681–684.
5. Neviaser RJ, Neviaser TJ. Transfer of the subscapularis and teres minor for massive defects of the rotator cuff. In Bayley I, Kessel L, eds. Shoulder Surgery. Heidelberg: Springer-Verlag, 1982:60–69.
6. Neviaser RJ, Neviaser TJ. Major ruptures of the rotator cuff. In Watson M, ed. Practical Shoulder Surgery. London: Grune & Stratton, 1985:171–224.

Chapter 9

Subscapularis Repair, Coracoid Recession, and Biceps Tenodesis

Steven Milos and Allen Deutsch

DEFINITION

▪ Subscapularis tears are less common than supraspinatus or infraspinatus tears. They occur in 2% to 8% of rotator cuff tears and are often missed.[5,12]

▪ Subscapularis tears can be:
  ▪ Isolated tears (partial or complete)
  ▪ Partial-thickness tears
  ▪ Anterosuperior (involving the supraspinatus)
  ▪ Rotator interval lesions (with associated biceps tendon injury)

▪ There is a high association of concomitant biceps tendon pathology.[12,18]

ANATOMY

▪ The subscapularis is innervated by the upper and lower subscapular nerves (C5–C8). Its origin is at the subscapularis fossa, and the upper two thirds inserts onto the lesser tuberosity, while the inferior third inserts onto the humeral metaphysis.

▪ The subscapularis is the strongest of the rotator cuff muscles. It acts to internally rotate the humerus along with the teres major, latissimus dorsi, and pectoralis major muscles. It resists anterior and inferior translation of the humeral head.[10,17]

▪ The upper fibers of the subscapularis and the anterior fibers of the supraspinatus contribute to the rotator interval as well as the transverse humeral ligament.

▪ The coracohumeral ligament is the roof of the rotator interval and blends with the supraspinatus and subscapularis. The coracohumeral ligament and the superior glenohumeral ligament are the primary stabilizers of the biceps.[2]

▪ The biceps muscle is innervated by the musculocutaneous nerve (C5–C6). It is composed of a long head, which originates from the supraglenoid tubercle, and a short head, which originates from the coracoid process. Both heads insert onto the bicipital tuberosity of the radius and the ulnar fascia of the forearm.

▪ The long head of the biceps tendon provides superior shoulder stability when the arm is abducted. It also provides posterior shoulder stability when the arm is in midranges of elevation.[14,21]

▪ The coracoid is located just anterior to the superior border of the subscapularis. It projects laterally, anteriorly, and inferiorly toward the glenoid.
  ▪ The subcoracoid bursa does not communicate with the glenohumeral joint but can communicate with the subacromial bursa.

PATHOGENESIS

▪ In the young patient, subscapularis tears occur as a result of trauma. The typical mechanisms include hyperextension of an externally rotated arm or forced external rotation of an adducted arm.[5,8]

▪ In older patients a tear is typically degenerative in nature, although it may be the result of a glenohumeral dislocation or other trauma.[13,15,16]

▪ Frequently, there is associated long head of the biceps pathology. This may include tenosynovitis, subluxation, dislocation, degeneration, or complete rupture.[12,19]

▪ Subcoracoid impingement may also be a cause of subscapularis tendon tears.

NATURAL HISTORY

▪ Isolated subscapularis tendon ruptures are relatively rare. Subscapularis tears are often associated with tears of the supraspinatus and infraspinatus.

▪ One study found that subscapularis tears occur in 8% of rotator cuff tears.[7]

▪ An MRI study was performed on 2167 patients with rotator cuff tears.[12]
  ▪ 2% of the patients had subscapularis tendon tears.
  ▪ 27% of those tears were partial-thickness tears and 73% were full-thickness tears.

▪ One study found a high correlation between subscapularis tendon tears and medial biceps subluxation, biceps tendinopathy, superior labral pathology, and fluid within the subscapular recess or the subcoracoid space.[12,18]

▪ The above-listed MRI study found that 25 of the 45 patients with subscapularis tendon tears had associated biceps pathology.

PHYSICAL FINDINGS

▪ Patients with complete tears of the subscapularis have increased passive external rotation compared with the unaffected shoulder.

▪ Several muscles contribute to internal rotation of the shoulder, including the pectoralis major, latissimus dorsi, and teres major, and can compensate for loss of the subscapularis.
  ▪ Passive external rotation: Increased passive external rotation may indicate a complete rupture of the subscapularis.
  ▪ Passive forward flexion, external rotation, and internal rotation: Limited passive range of motion is indicative of adhesive capsulitis.
  ▪ Active forward flexion: Limited active forward flexion is indicative of a possible large rotator cuff tear.

▪ The lift-off test isolates the subscapularis muscle. Inability to lift the hand off the back is a positive test.

▪ Internal rotation lag sign[11]: The examiner measures the lag between maximal internal rotation and the amount the patient can maintain. A positive sign shows increased sensitivity over the classic lift-off test.

▪ Belly press (Napoleon test)[8]: A positive test is the inability to bring the elbow forward. An intermediate test is the ability to bring the elbow forward partially. A positive test indicates a complete rupture, while an intermediate test indicates a partial tear of the subscapularis.

▪ The bear hug test[1]: If the examiner is able to lift the hand off the shoulder, then the patient likely has a partial or complete tear of the upper subscapularis tendon. This is perhaps the most sensitive test for a subscapularis tear.

■ Coracoid impingement[6]: Reproduction of pain or a painful click indicates a positive test. A positive test indicates impingement of the coracoid onto the subscapularis.

■ Speed's test[4]: If the maneuver produces pain or tenderness, the test is positive, which may indicate bicipital pathology, although the test is not specific.

■ Yerguson test[22]: The patient will experience pain as the biceps tendon subluxes out of the groove with a positive test; this indicates biceps instability.

■ Pain may inhibit a patient from maneuvering the arm behind the body into the lift-off position, thereby preventing assessment.

■ A complete rupture of the long head of the biceps tendon will result in an obvious cosmetic deformity in the anterior arm as the muscle retracts distally.

■ Tests used to diagnose superior labral lesions will be discussed in a separate section.

IMAGING AND DIAGNOSTIC STUDIES

■ Anteroposterior (AP), outlet, and axillary view radiographs should be obtained to rule out any fractures or associated injuries.

■ In chronic cases of subscapularis tears, anterior subluxation of the humeral head may be noted on the axillary view.[18]

■ MRI is the modality of choice for diagnosing subscapularis tears (**FIG 1**).

■ MR arthrography improves the study accuracy to detect partial-thickness tears.

■ Fatty degeneration of the subscapularis correlates with poor tendon quality.[20]

■ Although not sensitive, these signs are highly specific for subscapularis tears[15]:

■ Leakage of contrast material onto the lesser tuberosity

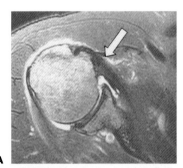
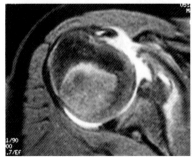

FIG 1 • Axial T2-weighted MR images of right shoulders with an intact subscapularis tendon (**A**; *arrow*) and a complete rupture of the subscapularis tendon.

■ Fatty degeneration of the subscapularis muscle
■ Abnormalities in the course of the long biceps tendon
■ Biceps dislocation deep to the subscapularis tendon is pathognomonic for a subscapularis tear.

■ Ultrasound is a noninvasive method for assessing the subscapularis and can be performed in the office. It is less expensive than MRI, but results are operator-dependent.

DIFFERENTIAL DIAGNOSIS

■ Impingement syndrome
■ Subscapularis tendinitis
■ Bicipital tendinitis
■ Posterosuperior rotator cuff tear (supraspinatus, infraspinatus, teres minor)
■ Biceps pathology
■ Coracoid impingement
■ Labral tear
■ Glenoid fracture
■ Glenohumeral instability
■ Glenohumeral arthritis
■ Pectoralis major injury
■ Contusion
■ Cervical radiculopathy

NONOPERATIVE MANAGEMENT

■ For subscapularis tears, nonoperative management is reserved for some chronic and atraumatic, degenerative, and asymptomatic tears.

■ Treatment includes activity modification, anti-inflammatory medications, and physical therapy.

■ Corticosteroid injections may be performed in the bicipital groove or subcoracoid bursa to treat biceps tendinitis and coracoid impingement.

■ It is likely that some degenerative subscapularis tendon tears are successfully treated nonsurgically without ever being diagnosed.

■ In most cases, an acute symptomatic subscapularis tear should be managed operatively and whenever possible within the first 6 to 8 weeks, when retraction and scarring are minimal, to reduce the risks of dissection in the axillary recess.

■ In young, active patients, attempts are made to repair acute biceps ruptures.

■ In older, less active patients and in cases of chronic biceps ruptures more than 8 weeks old, biceps repair is discouraged.

SURGICAL MANAGEMENT

Preoperative Planning

■ Physical therapy or a home exercise program emphasizing range of motion may be used to prevent stiffness and improve range of motion before surgery.

■ All imaging studies are reviewed.

■ An examination under anesthesia is performed before beginning surgery to evaluate for instability, increased external rotation, or decreased range of motion.

Positioning

■ The patient is placed in a low beach chair position with the arm draped free.

■ A McConnell arm holder (McConnell Orthopedic Manufacturing Co., Greenville, TX) is useful for maintaining arm positions throughout the case (**FIG 2**).

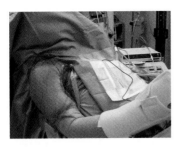

FIG 2 • Positioning for a subscapularis repair. The patient is placed in a beach chair position with the arm stabilized in a McConnell holder.

Approach

- Both the deltopectoral and anterolateral deltoid-splitting approaches have been described.[20]
- The anterolateral deltoid-splitting approach is useful for partial tears of the upper subscapularis and tears associated with supraspinatus tears. It is not recommended for large retracted full-thickness subscapularis tears.
- The deltopectoral approach provides greater visualization and access to the inferior portion of the subscapularis. It also allows for concomitant biceps tenodesis and coracoplasty.

INCISION AND DISSECTION

- The deltopectoral approach is started just proximal to the coracoid process and extended distally 8 to 10 cm.
- Adducting the arm identifies the major axillary crease.
- The cephalic vein and deltoid muscle are carefully retracted laterally and the pectoralis muscle is retracted medially to facilitate exposure (**TECH FIG 1A**).
- Once the deltopectoral interval is developed, the clavipectoral fascia is identified.
- The clavipectoral fascia is divided at the lateral aspect of the conjoined tendon.
- Avoid excessive retraction on the conjoined tendon to avoid injuring the musculocutaneous nerve.
- The tendon of the subscapularis is often retracted inferiorly and medially and requires mobilization.
- A layer of scar tissue may be seen overlying the lesser tuberosity, which can mimic the subscapularis tendon.

- If the subscapularis tendon cannot be brought back to the lesser tuberosity easily, then the subscapularis requires systematic release from the glenohumeral ligaments.
- Begin by releasing the superior aspect of the tendon from the coracohumeral ligament. The rotator interval is opened from the glenoid to the bicipital groove to facilitate the release.
- Next release the inferior portion of the tendon from the capsular attachments. Care must be taken to identify and protect the axillary nerve and vascular supply inferiorly.
- Finally, release the remaining capsular attachments on the undersurface of the subscapularis (**TECH FIG 1B**).

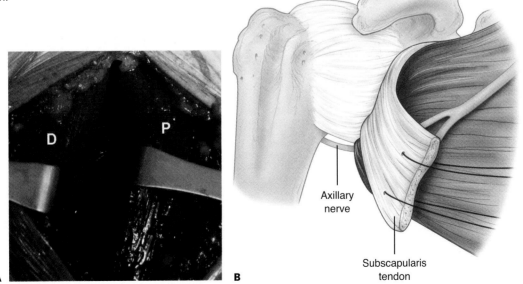

Axillary nerve

Subscapularis tendon

TECH FIG 1 • **A.** Deltopectoral interval in a right shoulder. The deltoid muscle (*D*) and cephalic vein are retracted laterally and the pectoralis muscle (*P*) is retracted medially. **B.** The subscapularis is released from the capsule to facilitate mobilization of the tendon. Note the proximity of the axillary nerve inferiorly.

BICEPS TENODESIS

- If a biceps tenotomy is performed, it is important to warn the patient of the resultant cosmetic deformity when the biceps retracts distally.
- Indications for biceps tenodesis include the following:
  - Tears involving more than 50% of the biceps tendon
  - Medial subluxation of the biceps tendon
- Open the bicipital groove from the medial side to expose the biceps tendon.

- The biceps tendon is released from the superior glenoid with curved scissors.
- The tendon is retracted distally from the bicipital groove.
- To ensure proper tensioning of the biceps tendon, the proximal portion of the tendon is resected to leave about 20 to 25 mm of tendon proximal to the musculotendinous junction.
- Running locking Krakow or whipstitches are placed up and down the proximal 15 mm of the biceps tendon.
- Abrade the bicipital groove to develop a bleeding surface.
- A burr hole the size of the biceps tendon is made in the bicipital groove about 15 mm from the articular surface. Two smaller 3.2-mm holes are made 15 mm distal to the burr hole in a triangular configuration.
- The tendon end is passed into the proximal hole by pulling the sutures out the distal holes. The sutures are then passed through and tied over the overlying biceps tendon (**TECH FIG 2A,B**).
- Another fixation option is to use a biotenodesis screw for the biceps tendon.
  - The tendon is prepared as above.
  - An 8-mm reamer is used to make a 25-mm-deep bone tunnel about 15 mm from the articular surface.
  - An 8 × 23-mm Arthrex Bio-Tenodesis screw is used for fixation.
  - One end of the suture is passed through the biotenodesis screw while the other suture passes outside of the screw. This ensures that the tendon will be pulled into the hole as the screw is advanced.
  - When the screw is flush with the bone tunnel, the sutures are tied over the screw (**TECH FIG 2C**). This provides both an interference fit and suture anchor stability.

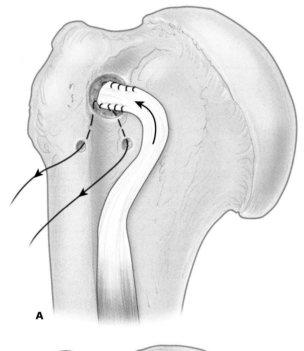

A

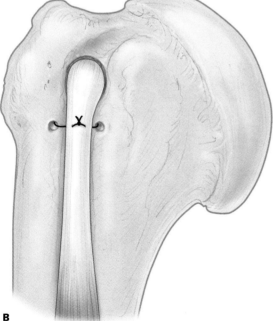

B

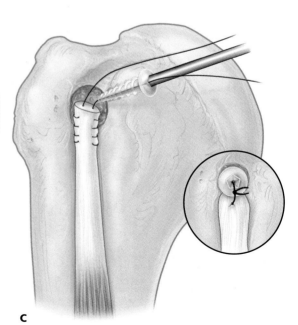

C

TECH FIG 2 • A,B. The tunnel technique uses bone tunnels to fix the biceps tendon upon itself. **C.** A biceps tenodesis with interference screw fixation.

CORACOPLASTY

- The conjoined tendons are identified.
- Care is taken not to retract vigorously on the conjoined tendons to avoid injury to the musculocutaneous nerve.
- The coracoacromial ligament is released from the coracoid.
- The posterior aspect of the coracoid is exposed by removing the overlying soft tissue. The posterolateral portion is then resected in line with the subscapularis muscle with an osteotome (**TECH FIG 3**). Alternatively, a burr may be used to accomplish the same resection. Protect the neurovascular structures by placing a retractor on the posterior aspect of the coracoid.
- A rasp is then used to smooth out the bony surface.
- The goal is a 7- to 10-mm clearance between the coracoid and subscapularis.

- Confirmation of adequate decompression can be determined by manipulating the arm into the impingement position and confirming that there is adequate clearance for the subscapularis.

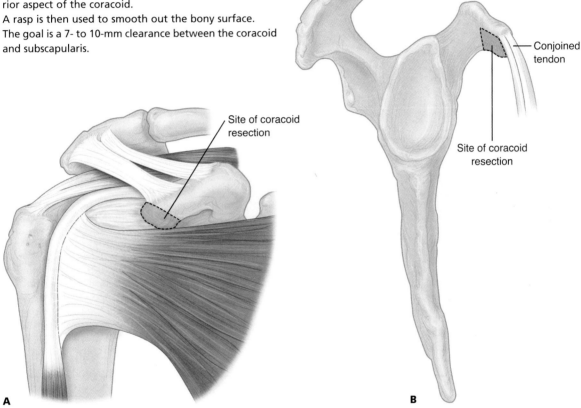

TECH FIG 3 • The posterolateral portion of the coracoid is resected, leaving the conjoined tendon attached. The goal is a 7- to 10-mm clearance space for the subscapularis.

SUBSCAPULARIS REPAIR

- The residual soft tissue is cleaned from the lesser tuberosity. A burr is then used to expose bleeding bone for the tendon to heal to.
- To recreate the anatomic footprint of the subscapularis insertion, four suture anchors are used for the repair.
- Two anchors are placed at 1-cm intervals along the medial aspect of the lesser tuberosity and two are placed at the lateral aspect of the lesser tuberosity (**TECH FIG 4A**).
- The sutures from the medial anchors are passed in a mattress fashion near the musculotendinous junction of the subscapularis (**TECH FIG 4B**).

- The sutures from the lateral anchor are passed through the lateral edge of the tendon in a simple fashion and tied down to the lesser tuberosity.
- After repair of the subscapularis tendon, the shoulder is taken through a gentle range of motion to determine the safe arcs for postoperative rehabilitation.
- The lateral aspect of the rotator interval is closed while maintaining about 30 degrees of external rotation of the arm to prevent overtightening of the subscapularis repair.

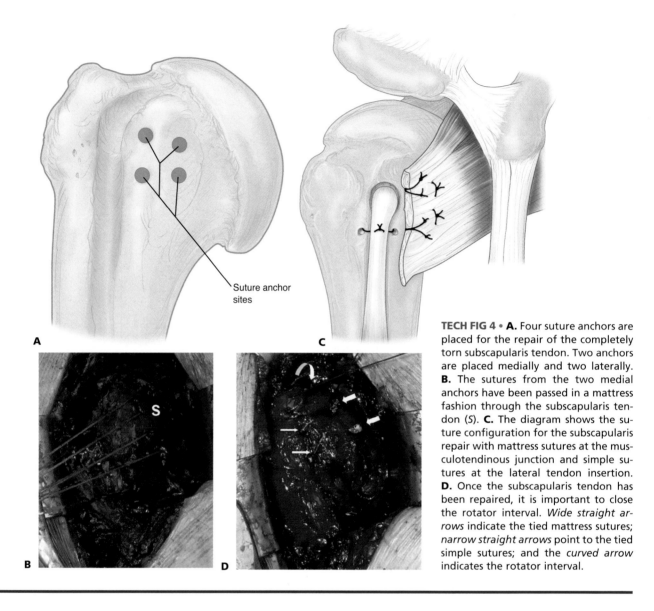

Suture anchor
sites

A

C

B

D

TECH FIG 4 • A. Four suture anchors are placed for the repair of the completely torn subscapularis tendon. Two anchors are placed medially and two laterally. **B.** The sutures from the two medial anchors have been passed in a mattress fashion through the subscapularis tendon (*S*). **C.** The diagram shows the suture configuration for the subscapularis repair with mattress sutures at the musculotendinous junction and simple sutures at the lateral tendon insertion. **D.** Once the subscapularis tendon has been repaired, it is important to close the rotator interval. *Wide straight arrows* indicate the tied mattress sutures; *narrow straight arrows* point to the tied simple sutures; and the *curved arrow* indicates the rotator interval.

PEARLS AND PITFALLS

Indications	■ A complete history and physical examination should be performed. ■ The surgeon should identify and address all associated pathology. ■ Any limitations of motion should be addressed before surgery.
Coracoplasty	■ The surgeon should take care to protect the musculocutaneous nerve. ■ A 7- to 10-mm clearance should be achieved for the subscapularis.
Biceps tenodesis	■ Tears in the biceps tendon of over 50% and subluxing tendons should be tenodesed. ■ The surgeon should maintain proper tension of the biceps muscle; typically, 20 to 25 mm of tendon should be maintained proximal to the musculotendinous junction. ■ A "hidden lesion" describes the presence of a partial undersurface subscapularis tear with a medially dislocated or subluxed biceps. This injury can be missed at the time of open surgery because the bursal surface of the subscapularis remains intact. Diagnostic arthroscopy or proper imaging will prevent missing this lesion.
Subscapularis repair	■ In chronic cases, a scar layer covers the lesser tuberosity and is usually attached at its medial extent to the retracted and scarred subscapularis tendon. The presence of this scar layer may lead to the misdiagnosis of an intact subscapularis. ■ The surgeon should prepare a bleeding bony surface for the tendon to heal to. ■ The rotator interval is closed in external rotation to avoid loss of motion. ■ External rotation is limited for 6 weeks postoperatively to protect the repair.

POSTOPERATIVE CARE

▪ The most important postoperative management for subscapularis tears is limitation of external rotation for 6 weeks to avoid stressing the repair.
 ▪ Complete tears are not allowed to externally rotate past 0 degrees.
 ▪ Partial tears are allowed to externally rotate 20 to 30 degrees.
▪ At 6 weeks the patient may begin active and active-assisted external rotation exercises, as well as overhead stretching.
▪ At 12 weeks strengthening exercises are initiated for partial tears. At 16 weeks strengthening exercises are initiated for complete tears.

OUTCOMES

▪ Isolated subscapularis tears have favorable surgical outcomes.
 ▪ At 2 years of follow-up, good or excellent results were reported in 13 of 14 isolated subscapularis tears.[4]
 ▪ Another study demonstrated good or excellent results in 13 of 16 patients with acute traumatic subscapularis tears at 43 months of follow-up. The Constant scores were 82% of age-matched controls.[8]
▪ Poor prognostic factors include chronic tears (symptoms for more than 6 months), fatty degeneration of the subscapularis muscle, and anterosuperior tears (combination of subscapularis and supraspinatus tears).[19]
▪ Comparative outcomes between open and arthroscopic techniques remain to be determined.

COMPLICATIONS

▪ Repair failure
▪ Infection
▪ Loss of motion
▪ Axillary nerve injury
▪ Vascular injury

REFERENCES

 1. Barth JRH, Burkhart SS, DeBeer JF. The bear hug test: the most sensitive test for diagnosing a subscapularis tear. Arthroscopy 2006;22:1076–1084.
 2. Burkhead WZ Jr, Arcand MA, Zeman C, et al. The biceps tendon. In: Rockwood CA Jr, Matsen FA III, Wirth MA, Lippitt SB, eds. The Shoulder, 3rd ed. Philadelphia: Saunders, 2004;1059–1119.
 3. Constant CR, Murley AH. A clinical method of functional assessment of the shoulder. Clin Orthop Relat Res 1987;214:160–164.
 4. Crenshaw AH, Kilgore WE. Surgical treatment of bicipital tenosynovitis. J Bone Joint Surg Am 1966;48A:1496–1502.
 5. Deutsch A, Altchek DW, Veltri DM, et al. Traumatic tears of the subscapularis tendon: clinical diagnosis, magnetic resonance imaging findings, and operative treatment. Am J Sports Med 1997;25:13–22.
 6. Dines DM, Warren RF, Inglis AE, et al. The coracoid impingement syndrome. J Bone Joint Surg Br 1990;72B:314–316.
 7. Frankle MA, Cofield RH. Rotator cuff tears including the subscapularis [abstract]. Fifth International Conference of Surgery of the Shoulder, Paris, France, 1992:52.
 8. Gerber C, Krushell RJ. Isolated rupture of the tendon of the subscapularis muscle: clinical features in 16 cases. J Bone Joint Surg Br 1991;73B:389–394.
 9. Gerber C, Rippstein R. Combined lesions of the subscapularis and supraspinatous tendons: a multi-center analysis of 56 cases [abstract]. Fifth International Congress of Surgery of the Shoulder, Paris, France, 1992:51.
10. Halder AM, Itoi E, An KN. Anatomy and biomechanics of the shoulder. Orthop Clin North Am 2000;31:159–176.
11. Hertel R, Ballmer F, Lombert SM, et al. Lag signs in the diagnosis of rotator cuff rupture. J Shoulder Elbow Surg 1996;5:307–313.
12. Li XX, Schweitzer ME, Bifano JA, et al. MR evaluation of subscapularis tears. J Comput Assist Tomogr 1999;23:713–717.
13. Neviaser RJ, Neviaser TJ. Recurrent instability of the shoulder after age 40. J Shoulder Elbow Surg 1995;4:416–418.
14. Pagnani MJ, Deng XH, Warren RF, et al. Role of the long head of the biceps brachii in glenohumeral stability: a biomechanical study in cadavers. J Shoulder Elbow Surg 1996;5:255–262.
15. Pfirrmann CW, Zanetti M, Weishaupt D, et al. Subscapularis tendon tears: detection and grading at MR arthrography. Radiology 1999;213:709–714.
16. Symeonides PP. The significance of the subscapularis muscle in the pathogenesis of recurrent anterior dislocations of the shoulder. J Bone Joint Surg Br 1972;54B:276–283.
17. Tillett F, Smith M, Fulcher M, et al. Anatomic determination of humeral head retroversion: the relationship of the central axis of the humeral head to the bicipital groove. J Shoulder Elbow Surg 1993;2:255–256.
18. Travis RD, Burkhead WZ, Doane R. Technique for repair of the subscapularis tendon. Orthop Clin North Am 2001;32:495–500.
19. Tung GA, Yoo DC, Levine SM, et al. Subscapularis tendon tear: primary and associated signs on MRI. J Comput Assist Tomogr 2001;25:417–424.
20. Warner JJ, Higgins L, Parsons IM, et al. Diagnosis and treatment of anterosuperior rotator cuff tears. J Shoulder Elbow Surg 2001;10:37–46.
21. Warner JJ, McMahon PJ. The role of the long head of the biceps brachii in superior stability of the glenohumeral joint. J Bone Joint Surg Am 1995;77A:366–372.
22. Yergason RM. Supination sign. J Bone Joint Surg Am 1931;13A:60.

Chapter 10

Latissimus Transfer for Irreparable Posterosuperior Rotator Cuff Tear

Jesse A. McCarron, Michael J. Codsi, and Joseph P. Iannotti

DEFINITION

- Irreparable posterosuperior rotator cuff tears are tears that involve the supraspinatus and infraspinatus tendons, where there is an inability to repair the tendons back to the anatomic footprint of the greater tuberosity with the arm at the side.
- Some tears can be determined to be irreparable preoperatively, if the MRI or CT scans demonstrate severe muscle atrophy of the supraspinatus or infraspinatus muscles.
  - This may help indicate that a patient has an irreparable tear and may be a candidate for muscle transfer, but the final determination of whether a tear is reparable is made at the time of surgery.

ANATOMY

- The latissimus dorsi is normally an adductor and internal rotator of the humerus however, after transfer it is expected to act as an abductor and external rotator of the humerus.
  - The ability of the patient to retrain his or her neural pathways to achieve this active in-phase function varies dramatically.
  - In some cases, the latissimus dorsi transfer has only a tenodesis effect.
- Originating from the supraspinatus and infraspinatus fossa respectively, the supraspinatus and infraspinatus muscle–tendon units become confluent and insert as a common tendon on the greater tuberosity of the humerus immediately lateral to the humeral head articular margin.
  - Their combined footprint area averages 4.02 cm^2.
  - The insertion of the supraspinatus averages 1.27 cm from medial to lateral and 1.63 cm from anterior to posterior.
  - The infraspinatus insertion averages 1.34 cm medial to lateral and 1.64 cm anterior to posterior.[6]
- Over the superior aspect of the glenohumeral joint, the deepest fibers of the supraspinatus and infraspinatus tendons are intimately interwoven with the joint capsule such that the rotator cuff tendons and joint capsule function as a single unit. As a result, rotator cuff tears involving the supraspinatus or infraspinatus tendons result in direct communication between the glenohumeral and subacromial spaces.
- The latissimus dorsi muscle has a broad origin from the aponeurosis of spinous processes T7 through L5, the sacrum, the iliac wing, ribs 9 through 12, and the inferior border of the scapula.
- The latissimus dorsi tendon averages 3.1 cm wide and 8.4 cm long at its insertion between the pectoralis major and teres major tendons on the proximal, medial humerus.[13]
- The fibers of the latissimus dorsi twist 180 degrees from origin to insertion, allowing the latissimus dorsi muscle to originate posterior to the teres major muscle on the posterior chest wall but insert immediately anterior to the teres major tendon on the proximal humerus.

- The latissimus dorsi humeral insertion never extends more distal along the shaft than that of the teres major.
- In most patients, the latissimus dorsi and teres major tendons insert separately onto the proximal humerus; however, 30% of patients have conjoined latissimus dorsi and teres major tendons that cannot be separated without sharp dissection.[13]
- The neurovascular pedicle to the latissimus dorsi is the thoracodorsal artery and nerve (posterior cord, C6 and C7). The thoracodorsal artery and nerve enter the anterior, inferior surface of the latissimus dorsi, about 13 cm from the humeral insertion site.
  - Anatomic studies have shown that this neurovascular pedicle is of adequate length to allow transfer and excursion of the latissimus dorsi without risk of undue tension, once any adhesions and fibrous bands have been released from the anterior surface of the muscle belly.[14]
- Several important neurovascular structures lie close to the latissimus dorsi insertion, and careful attention to these structures must be given at the time of its release from the humerus to avoid injury.
  - Anterior to the latissimus, the radial nerve passes an average of 2.4 cm medial to the humeral shaft at the superior border of the tendon.
    - This distance increases with external rotation and abduction and decreases with internal rotation and adduction[2] (**FIG 1A,B**).

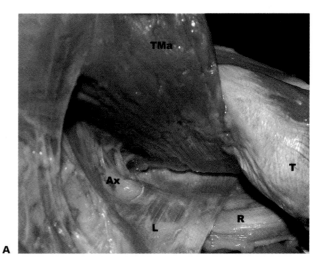

A

FIG 1 • **A.** Cadaveric dissection of the interval between the teres major (*TMa*) and latissimus dorsi (*L*) tendons running deep to the long head of the triceps (*T*) near their humeral insertion. The view is from a posterior approach to the right shoulder. Note the proximity of the radial nerve (*R*) lying deep to the latissimus tendon, and the axillary nerve (*Ax*) running with the posterior humeral circumflex artery over the superior border of the latissimus and teres major as it passes through the quadrilateral space. *(continued)*

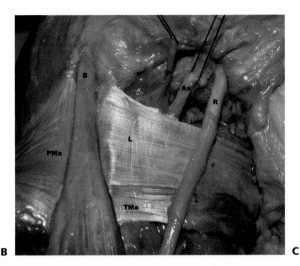

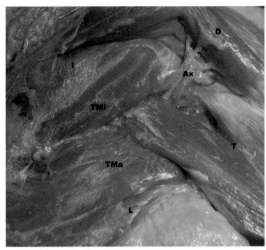

FIG 1 • *(continued)* **B.** Cadaveric dissection demonstrating the insertion of the latissimus dorsi (*L*) and teres major (*TMa*) tendons viewed from an anterior exposure. The pectoralis major (*PMa*) tendon has been reflected laterally and the long head of the biceps (*B*) tendon remains in the bicipital groove. Note the more distal insertion of the teres major relative to the latissimus dorsi. *Ax*, axillary nerve; *P*, posterior humeral circumflex vessel; *R*, radial nerve. **C.** Cadaveric dissection of the superficial muscular anatomy of the posterior shoulder. The axillary nerve (*Ax*) and posterior humeral circumflex artery are seen exiting the quadrilateral space before entering the posterior deltoid (*D*). *L*, latissimus dorsi; *TMa*, teres major; *TMi*, teres minor; *I*, infraspinatus; *T*, triceps.

■ The axillary nerve runs superior to the latissimus dorsi tendon before exiting the quadrangular space (**FIG 1C**). In neural rotation and adduction, the average distance between the nerve and the superior border of the tendon is 1.9 cm.

  ■ This distance increases with external rotation and abduction and decreases with internal rotation.[2]

■ The anterior humeral circumflex artery runs along the superior border of the latissimus dorsi tendon.

PATHOGENESIS

■ Multiple causes have been proposed for the development of rotator cuff tears, including decreased vascular supply, mechanical compression between the humeral head and the coracoacromial ligament or the undersurface of the acromion, and traumatic causes such as humeral head dislocation, or rapid or repetitive eccentric loading of the rotator cuff muscle–tendon units.

■ Isolated, acute traumatic events may cause massive rotator cuff tears, the majority of which can be repaired open or arthroscopically if diagnosis and surgical intervention are timely.

■ Alternatively, most degenerative tendon tears start small and progressively get larger until the muscle retraction, muscle atrophy, and tendon loss prevent primary repair.

■ Tear size may not predict reparability at the time of surgery, but it does influence healing postoperatively, with larger tears having a lower incidence of healing.

■ Tissue quality and tendon retraction are the major determinants intraoperatively of whether a repair is possible. These factors also influence healing of a primary repair.

■ Increased size and duration of a tear lead to retraction of the rotator cuff and fatty infiltration of the muscle belly within weeks to months of developing a tear. These changes result in decreased tendon excursion and tissue compliance that is often irreversible (**FIG 2**).

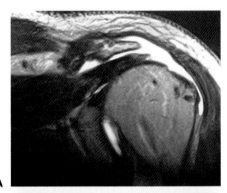

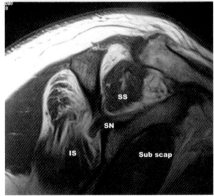

FIG 2 • **A.** Coronal MRI of a massive cuff tear showing tendon retraction to the midhumeral head. **B.** Sagittal MRI through lateral supraspinatus and infraspinatus fossae showing fatty degeneration and muscle wasting consistent with decreased muscle compliance and increased risk of repair failure at the time of surgery. The suprascapular nerve (*SN*) can be seen crossing through the spinoglenoid notch. *SS*, supraspinatus; *IS*, infraspinatus; *Sub scap*, subscapularis.

■ As a result, the longer these massive tears go untreated, the higher the likelihood that the tear will be irreparable at the time of surgery.

■ Presentation of the patient with a massive irreparable cuff tear is often precipitated by a minor traumatic event such as a fall onto an outstretched hand, resulting in an acute-on-chronic tear and functional decompensation of the shoulder. Others present with a history of longstanding, worsening symptoms that finally reach a point that is no longer tolerable to the patient.

NATURAL HISTORY

■ Massive posterosuperior rotator cuff tears are uncommon, representing less than one third of all rotator cuff tears even in practices limited to the treatment of shoulder pathology.[15]

■ Not all patients with large posterosuperior cuff tears experience enough loss of function or pain to require surgery or even seek treatment.

■ It can be difficult to predict who will have significant shoulder dysfunction based on radiographic or MRI findings or direct inspection of a torn rotator cuff.

■ Some patients with large tears can still use their arm for many activities, and some even retain the ability to perform overhead activities.

■ Others with smaller tears may have significant difficulty or an inability to use their arm for anything above chest level.

■ Regardless of tear size, it is loss of the rotator cuff muscles' ability to perform their role as humeral head stabilizers that eventually leads to functional decompensation.

■ As the tear progresses in size, behavioral and biomechanical compensation will allow maintenance of function to a point. However, once the rotator cuff can no longer stabilize the humeral head to create a fulcrum around which the deltoid can act to forward flex and abduct the arm, rapid decompensation, loss of function, and increased pain ensue.

PATIENT HISTORY AND PHYSICAL FINDINGS

■ The patient history should elicit the mechanism and duration of the current symptoms with the intent of determining if there was a specific traumatic event leading to the rotator cuff tear and whether symptoms of rotator cuff pathology were present before any such event.

■ Determining if the tear is a result of an acute injury as opposed to an acute-on-chronic process will help in estimating the quality of the tissues and whether they will be amenable to repair at the time of surgery.

■ The duration of dysfunction is also important in determining the likelihood of being able to repair any rotator cuff tear, since fatty degeneration of the supraspinatus and infraspinatus muscle bellies may start within weeks of the injury and will greatly decrease tissue compliance and increase tension placed on a potential repair.[9,16]

■ A careful neurologic examination, starting with the neck, must be performed to rule out neurologic causes of shoulder symptoms.

■ An understanding of the patient's current functional limitations as well as expectations for postoperative function is necessary to elicit whether the patient's disability is significant enough to benefit from the procedure.

■ A focused examination for the rotator cuff-deficient shoulder includes but is not limited to:

■ Active forward flexion examination: Patients with function at or above shoulder level are more likely to have improved active forward flexion postoperatively.

■ Active external rotation examination: Decreased external rotation on the affected side indicates partial or complete loss of infraspinatus function due to tear involvement or muscle dysfunction.

■ External rotation lag sign: Inability to maintain maximal external rotation (greater than or equal to a 20-degree lag sign) suggests tear extension well into the infraspinatus.

■ Passive range of motion should be compared to the contralateral limb. Decreased range of motion suggests joint contracture, which requires treatment before consideration for muscle transfer.

■ Modified belly press test: Inability to perform this action demonstrates a dysfunctional or torn subscapularis tendon, and these patients will have a higher rate of clinical failure with muscle transfer.

■ Abduction strength testing: This tests deltoid muscle strength. A weak deltoid suggests less postoperative active range of motion secondary to inadequate strength.

■ External rotation strength testing: Full strength suggests no infraspinatus tear involvement, whereas weakness suggests progressive infraspinatus involvement or dysfunction.

■ Evaluation for superior escape: Superior escape suggests an incompetent coracoacromial arch and a high likelihood of failure to improve with muscle transfer.

IMAGING AND OTHER DIAGNOSTIC STUDIES

■ A true anteroposterior (AP) radiographic view of the shoulder in the plane of the scapula and axillary view is obtained (**FIG 3A,B**).

■ This allows evaluation of glenohumeral arthritis, superior migration of the humeral head, and identification of any abnormal bony anatomy (**FIG 3C,D**).

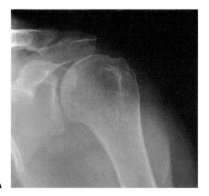

FIG 3 • A. True AP radiographic view of the glenohumeral joint showing minimal superior migration of the humeral head and preservation of the joint space. *(continued)*

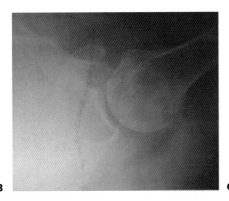
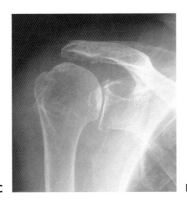
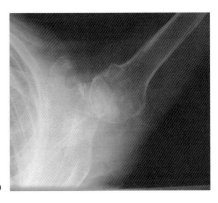

B **C** **D**

FIG 3 • *(continued)* **B.** Axillary lateral view of the glenohumeral joint demonstrating joint space preservation and the absence of osteophytes with a centered humeral head. **C,D.** Radiographic findings of degenerative arthritis, suggestive of a poor surgical candidate for a latissimus dorsi transfer. **C.** True AP radiographic view of the glenohumeral joint showing osteoarthritic changes, osteophyte formation, and superior migration of the humeral head. **D.** Axillary lateral view of the glenohumeral joint showing osteoarthritis with early posterior glenoid wear.

■ MRI allows evaluation of the rotator cuff, biceps tendon, and labral and capsular pathology (see Fig 2):
■ The size of the rotator cuff tear, especially the extent of subscapularis and infraspinatus involvement
■ Distance of tendon retraction from the greater tuberosity
■ Extent of fatty degeneration seen in involved muscle bellies
■ Electromyography is used to evaluate nerve function around the shoulder girdle.
■ It is necessary when nerve pathology is suspected as a cause of shoulder dysfunction.

DIFFERENTIAL DIAGNOSIS

■ Frozen shoulder
■ Adhesive capsulitis
■ Massive rotator cuff tear that can be repaired
■ Cervical nerve root compression
■ Suprascapular nerve palsy
■ Deltoid dysfunction

NONOPERATIVE MANAGEMENT

■ Nonoperative management is directed toward optimizing the patient's current function, managing pain, and modifying activities and expectations.
■ Treatment of irreparable cuff tears begins with physical therapy focused on maintaining motion and strengthening the deltoid and scapular stabilizers.
■ Physical therapy includes strengthening of the periscapular muscles and internal and external rotators, and stretching to prevent stiffness and further loss of motion.
■ Cortisone injection: Forty to 80 mg triamcinolone with 5 to 10 mL 1% Xylocaine is placed in the subacromial–glenohumeral space to decrease synovitis and bursitis, improve pain, and facilitate physical therapy.
■ Activity and expectation modification: The physician should explain avoidance of inciting activities that increase pain and discuss realistic functional goals for patients with irreparable cuff tears.
■ Most patients with irreparable cuff tears who fail to gain adequate improvement from physical therapy and activity modification are still not good candidates for latissimus dorsi muscle transfers. For these patients, alternative surgical inter-

ventions such as limited-goals arthroscopic débridement or reverse total shoulder arthroplasty in low-demand patients, versus shoulder fusion in young, high-demand manual laborers, may be options.
■ Limited-goals arthroscopy: If nonoperative management has failed but the patient is not a good candidate for latissimus transfer, an arthroscopic glenohumeral and subacromial débridement may be an option.
■ The ideal patient is over the age of 65 and retired, has low functional demands, and has an irreparable tear, and the primary indication for surgery is pain (not weakness).
■ These patients should have at least shoulder-level active elevation with an improvement in active elevation after having a positive injection test (10 cc lidocaine into the glenohumeral joint) and without shoulder arthritis.
■ This débridement can include synovial débridement, bursectomy, abrasion chondroplasty, acromioplasty–greater tuberosity-plasty, and biceps tenotomy or tenodesis to decrease mechanical symptoms and remove inflamed and painful tissues.
■ Successful results are characterized by a decrease in pain followed by a fairly aggressive postoperative strengthening program.

SURGICAL MANAGEMENT

■ The treatment decisions regarding management of massive irreparable rotator cuff tears must be made in the context of the patient's current functional deficits, level of pain and its suspected cause, and physical examination findings.
■ What the patient should expect in terms of postoperative pain relief and functional improvement must be clearly delineated before surgery, since return of full (normal) strength, active range of motion, and complete resolution of pain are not realistic goals for even the best latissimus transfer candidates.
■ Only a carefully selected subset of patients with irreparable rotator cuff tears are good candidates for latissimus dorsi transfers.
■ Ideal patients are younger and have good deltoid and subscapularis muscle strength, limited glenohumeral arthritis, and the ability to get shoulder-level active forward flexion preoperatively.
■ Table 1 lists specific prognostic factors.

Table 1	Prognostic Factors for Latissimus Dorsi Transfers	
Parameter	Better Prognosis	Worse Prognosis
Age	<60 years	>60 years
Gender	Male	Female
Function	Chest level or better	Below chest level
Subscapularis condition	Intact, functional	Torn, dysfunctional
Deltoid condition	Intact	Detached, dysfunctional
Previous surgery	No	Yes

Preoperative Planning

▪ Before surgery, plain radiographs and MRI must be reviewed to rule out other sources of pathology.

▪ Glenohumeral osteoarthritis should be ruled out as a predominant cause of the patient's current pain.

▪ An estimate should be made of the likelihood of successful primary repair based on the degree of cuff retraction and tissue quality.

▪ The equipment needed for both an attempted cuff repair and for muscle transfer should be available at the time of surgery.

▪ The possibility of needing to use autograft or allograft tendon to augment the length of the latissimus dorsi transfer should be discussed with the patient and the site for autograft harvest must be draped appropriately at the time of surgery, or allograft tissue must be available.

Positioning

▪ The patient is placed in the lateral decubitus position and secured with a bean-bag or hip positioner posts (**FIG 4A**).

▪ The patient is draped to keep the affected arm free during the case and allow access to the back, the superior aspect of the shoulder, and the arm down to the elbow (**FIG 4B,C**).

▪ An arm holder attached to the opposite side of the table will allow abduction, flexion, and rotation for positioning of the arm during the case.

Approach

▪ The surgical approach must allow wide access to the rotator cuff and to the muscle belly of the latissimus dorsi and its insertion.

▪ Although a single-incision technique has been described,[11] most authors prefer a two-incision technique—one incision for exposure and preparation of the rotator cuff and a second for dissection and release of the latissimus dorsi.[3,5,8,12,15]

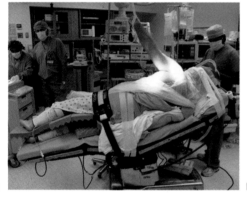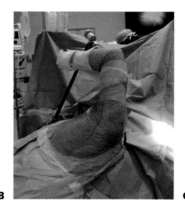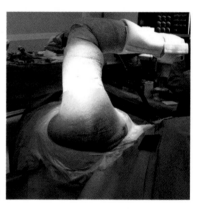

FIG 4 • Lateral decubitus positioning of the patient with a bean-bag, viewed from the back (**A**) and from the foot of the bed (**B**). Slight reverse Trendelenburg positioning of the table facilitates superior exposure of the subacromial space. **C.** Lateral decubitus positioning of the patient with a bean-bag after draping with the arm placed in an arm holder, viewed from the head of the table.

TECHNIQUES

SUPERIOR APPROACH TO THE ROTATOR CUFF

▪ An incision is made at the lateral edge of the acromion parallel to the acromion's lateral border (**TECH FIG 1A**).

▪ Subcutaneous flaps are raised just superficial to the deltoid fascia.

▪ The anterior deltoid is taken off the acromion from the acromioclavicular joint to the midpoint between the anterior and posterior borders of the acromion.

  ▪ This dissection is done in the subperiosteal plane to ensure strong fascial and periosteal tissue for later closure.

▪ The deltoid is split distally in line with its muscle fibers at the mid-lateral or posterolateral corner of the acromion (depending on the amount of deltoid released), and a stay suture is placed in the deltoid about 5 cm distal to the lateral edge of the acromion to prevent propagation of the split distally, which may result in injury to the axillary nerve (**TECH FIG 1B**).

▪ This exposure removes at least half and in some cases all of the middle deltoid origin. This extensive exposure helps in repair of the cuff as well as for transfer and repair of the latissimus dorsi tendon.

▪ A complete bursectomy is performed, the size and pattern of the rotator cuff tear are delineated, and the leading edge of the cuff tear is débrided (**TECH FIG 1C**).

▪ Inspection of the subscapularis tendon should be performed at this stage and partial detachments should be repaired.

  ▪ Irreparable subscapularis tears should be considered for concomitant pectoralis major transfers.

  ▪ Double muscle transfers are rarely performed and have a worse prognosis than single muscle transfers.

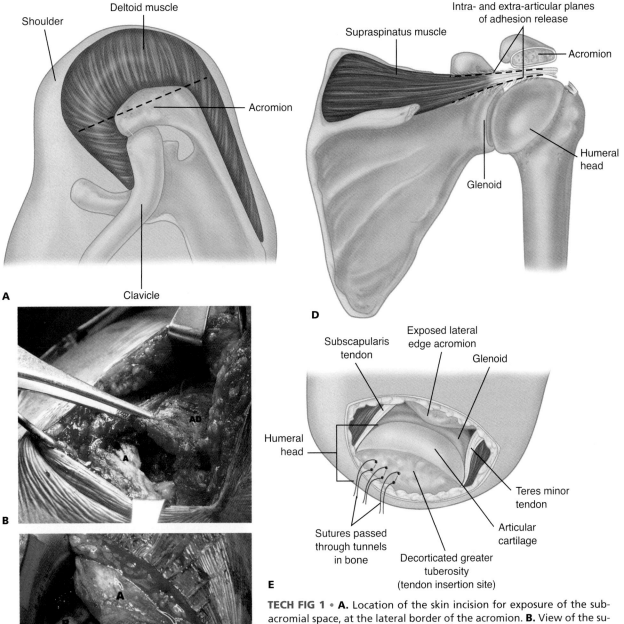

TECH FIG 1 • A. Location of the skin incision for exposure of the subacromial space, at the lateral border of the acromion. **B.** View of the superior approach to the shoulder with the patient in a lateral decubitus position. A subperiosteal release of the anterior deltoid (*AD*) from the acromioclavicular joint to the midpoint of the lateral border of the acromion (*A*) ensures strong tissue for later deltoid reattachment. A stay suture is placed in the deltoid split 5 cm distal to the lateral acromial edge to prevent traction injury to the axillary nerve. *PD,* posterior deltoid. **C.** The subacromial space after complete bursectomy and débridement of the irreparable rotator cuff tear. *A,* acromion; *B,* biceps tendon; *H,* humeral head; *TMi,* teres minor. **D.** A Cobb or periosteal elevator is used to perform a capsulotomy and release of adhesions around the superior glenoid rim. Articular and subacromial-sided release of adhesions from the retracted rotator cuff allows full mobilization of the torn tendons for an attempted primary repair. **E.** The prepared greater tuberosity, lightly decorticated, with sutures in place to allow tendon fixation.

- An acromioplasty is performed as needed.
    - Remove only that portion of the acromion that extends inferior to the plane of the posterior acromion.
    - Avoid decreasing the anteroposterior dimension of the acromion, which can increase the risk of superior escape of the humeral head.

- Keep the coracoacromial ligament at its maximum length and attached to the deep surface of the deltoid.
- At wound closure, place sutures in the acromial end of the coracoacromial ligament and suture this back to the anterior acromion to reconstruct the coracoacromial arch.

■ Reconstruction of the coracoacromial arch also helps minimize the risk of postoperative superior subluxation of the humeral head.

■ If degenerative changes are seen in the biceps tendon, it can be tenodesed in the bicipital groove and the intra-articular portion excised to remove it as a potential pain generator.

■ Complete mobilization of the retracted rotator cuff should be performed on both the intra-articular and extra-articular sides of the tendon.

■ This is best performed with a scalpel, Cobb or periosteal elevator, and use of electrocautery where necessary on the intra-articular side of the tendons.

■ Do not exceed 1.5 to 2.0 cm of medial dissection of the rotator cuff muscles within the fossa. Excessive medial dissection could injure the suprascapular nerve (**TECH FIG 1D**).

■ Débridement of remaining tissue and light decortication of the greater tuberosity with a rongeur or burr is per-

formed to prepare the site for rotator cuff reattachment or muscle transfer.

■ Any portion of the cuff that is reparable to the tuberosity should be attached with number 2 or larger nonabsorbable suture to bone.

■ Bone tunnels or suture anchors are placed in the lateral edge of the greater tuberosity (**TECH FIG 1E**).

■ If full mobilization of the rotator cuff will not allow solid repair of the tendon back to the greater tuberosity with the arm at the side, then the decision is made to proceed with the latissimus dorsi transfer.

■ If a full repair is achieved but the quality of the repair or the tissue quality is fair or poor, we still prefer to perform the latissimus transfer when the likelihood for healing of the primary repair is low and the need for postoperative strength is high and of primary importance to the patient.

SURGICAL APPROACH TO THE LATISSIMUS DORSI

■ A 15-cm incision is made along the posterolateral border of the latissimus dorsi, extending proximally to the posterior axillary fold (**TECH FIG 2A**).

■ The incision can be extended proximally as needed for exposure, being careful to change directions when crossing skin creases in the axilla to avoid webbing and excessive scarring in the skin of the posterior axillary crease.

■ Skin flaps are raised just superficial to the muscular fascia of the latissimus dorsi, and the upper and lower borders of the muscle are defined (**TECH FIG 2B,C**).

■ Identification of the inferior (lateral) border of the latissimus is the most reliable method for correctly identifying the muscle belly, as there is no large muscle inferior (lateral) to the latissimus on the posterior chest wall.

■ Blunt dissection is used to define and trace the tendon proximally toward its insertion on the proximal humerus (**TECH FIG 2D**).

■ Abduction and internal rotation of the arm provides the best visualization of the tendon at its insertion.[13]

■ Careful attention to neurovascular structures is critical at this stage, as the axillary and radial nerves, brachial plexus, and humeral circumflex vessels are all in proximity to the surgical field during this phase of the procedure.

■ Internal rotation of the arm in abduction is necessary for adequate exposure but also brings the radial nerve closer to the latissimus dorsi tendon along its anterior, medial surface.[2]

■ The axillary nerve and posterior humeral circumflex artery run along the superior border of the teres

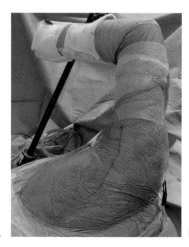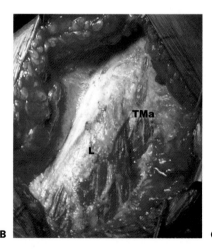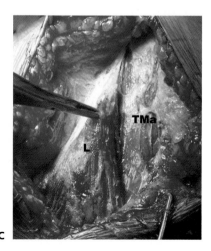

A **B** **C**

TECH FIG 2 • A. The posterior incision for harvest of the latissimus dorsi runs along the posterolateral border of the latissimus muscle belly, extending to the posterior axillary fold. It may be extended proximally to improve exposure, crossing skin creases at an angle to avoid postoperative contracture. **B.** Subcutaneous flaps are raised superficial to the muscular fascia of the latissimus dorsi (*L*) and teres major (*TMa*). **C.** The latissimus dorsi is the most inferior muscle belly running along the posterior and lateral chest wall. *(continued)*

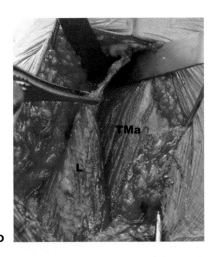

TECH FIG 2 • *(continued)* **D.** Exposure of the tendinous insertion of the latissimus dorsi (*L*) and teres major (*TMa*) on the proximal, medial humerus is facilitated by abduction and internal rotation of the arm.

major just proximal to the latissimus dorsi before exiting the quadrangular space.

- The anterior humeral circumflex vessels run along the superior border of the latissimus dorsi tendon and can be a source of significant bleeding if inadvertently cut.
- Dissection and release of the tendon should be carried out by working from the posterior surface of the tendon, as this keeps all important neurovascular structures anterior (deep) to the tendon.

■ A significant number of patients will have latissimus dorsi and teres major tendons that fuse into one tendon along their superior border where they insert on the humerus, a condition that requires sharp dissection to separate the two.

■ Once the humeral insertion of the latissimus dorsi has been identified, it should be released directly off the bone on the humeral shaft to ensure adequate tendon length for transfer.

TRANSFER AND FIXATION OF THE LATISSIMUS DORSI TO THE HUMERAL HEAD

■ Once released from its insertion, the latissimus dorsi tendon is prepared by weaving number 2 fiberwire (Arthrex, Naples FL) through the tendon with a locking Krackow technique along both its superior and inferior borders (**TECH FIG 3A,B**).

■ These locking sutures should be placed as soon as the tendon is released to minimize extensive handling of the tendon itself, which is easily frayed because it has few crossing fibers.

■ These sutures can now be used as traction stitches, and the latissimus is freed from any adhesions on its anterior surface.
- Be sure to pull the sutures in line with the long axis of the tendon.
- Do not pull the locking sutures in divergent directions as it will separate the parallel fibers of the tendon.

■ The neurovascular pedicle is identified and freed as well to prevent traction and damage to these structures during the transfer.
- The pedicle is located on the deep surface of the muscle about 13 cm from the musculotendinous junction.
- It is best seen and dissected after the tendon is released from its insertion and the muscle is flipped posteriorly, thereby exposing the undersurface of the muscle.

■ Mobilization of the latissimus dorsi for transfer requires dissection of the deep fascial investments of the muscle from surrounding tissues into the chest wall.
- If this is not performed, maximum excursion of the transfer will not be achieved and the tendon will not be long enough to reach the top of the humeral head.

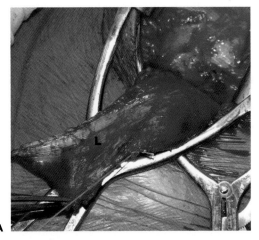

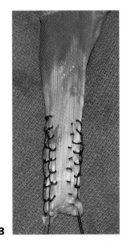

TECH FIG 3 • A single-strand (**A**) or double-strand (**B**) locking Krackow stitch is run along the upper and lower borders of the released latissimus tendon (*L*). This minimizes the risk of damage to the tendon fibers and facilitates passage of the latissimus into the subacromial space. *(continued)*

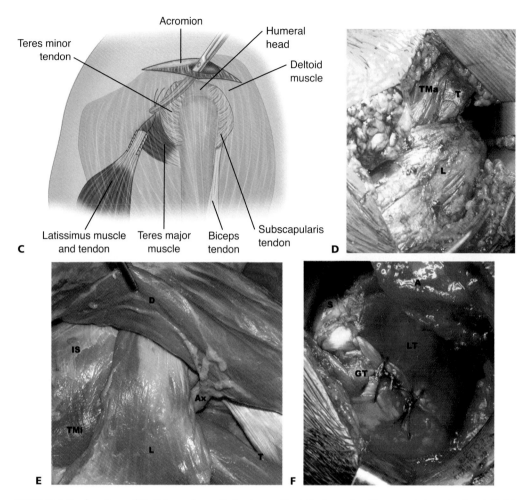

TECH FIG 3 • *(continued)* **C.** Using a large Kelly clamp, the latissimus dorsi is passed deep to the deltoid over the posterior surface of the rotator cuff muscles into the subacromial space. **D.** Intraoperative photo showing the transferred latissimus dorsi (*L*) viewed from the posterior chest wall incision on the left shoulder. **E.** Cadaveric dissection showing the subdeltoid passage of the released latissimus tendon in the right shoulder. Note the proximity of the axillary nerve (*Ax*) to the latissimus during this stage of the procedure. *D*, deltoid; *T*, triceps; *TMa*, teres major; *TMi*, teres minor; *IS*, infraspinatus. **F.** The latissimus dorsi tendon (*LT*) is anchored to the greater tuberosity (*GT*) laterally and sutured to the upper border of the subscapularis (*S*) anteriorly and to the leading edge of the torn, retracted rotator cuff tendons medially.

- Using sharp and scissor dissection and some blunt dissection, the plane underneath the deltoid and superficial to the rotator cuff muscles across the back of the shoulder is developed (about 4 to 6 cm wide) to connect the superior (rotator cuff exposure) and the posterior (latissimus exposure) wounds.
  - A large Kelly clamp is passed in this plane from the superior to the posterior wounds.
- Attention must be paid to enlarging this plane (4 to 6 cm) to prevent binding of the latissimus muscle belly within the tunnel, compromising its excursion.
- Grasping the previously placed traction sutures with the large curved Kelly clamp, the surgeon then passes the latissimus dorsi deep to the deltoid and into the subacromial space with the arm in adduction and neutral rotation (**TECH FIG 3C**).
- The effectiveness of this transfer depends on achieving a tenodesis effect of the transfer, thereby creating a passive humeral head depressor effect.

- To accomplish this, the arm is positioned in 45 degrees of abduction and at least 30 degrees of external rotation.
- In this position the transferred tendon is pulled to its maximum length over the top of the humeral head, and the traction sutures placed along the sides of the tendon are passed through the leading edge of the subscapularis tendon and tied. This step establishes the tendon transfer tension and places the tendon over the top of the humeral head (**TECH FIG 3D,E**).
- When the arm is brought to the patient's side and in internal rotation, the transfer is tensioned further, bringing the humeral head lower within the glenoid fossa.
- We believe that this is one of the most important steps in the surgery to achieve proper transfer function.
- The lateral border of the latissimus dorsi tendon is now fixed to the greater tuberosity with three number 2 fiberwires passed through bone tunnels or with 5.5-mm biocorkscrew suture anchors (**TECH FIG 3F**).

- The medial edge of the latissimus tendon is sutured to the retracted edge of the supraspinatus and infraspinatus tendons with several nonabsorbable sutures.
- Although some authors believe that the latissimus tendon should be attached only to the greater tuberosity to act as an external rotator of the humerus, we believe that repair of the leading edge to the upper border of

the subscapularis allows the transfer to act as a humeral head depressor (either passively by a tenodesis effect or actively if the patient can learn how to fire the muscle actively [isotonically] in phase with external rotation or forward elevation).

- This suturing of the latissimus to the subscapularis can be done with two heavy, nonabsorbable sutures.

WOUND CLOSURE

- The anterior deltoid and middle deltoid are reattached to the acromion with nonabsorbable sutures placed through bone tunnels in the acromion as well as to the intact fascia (**TECH FIG 4A**).
- A drain is placed in the latissimus dorsi harvest site as

needed, and both skin incisions are closed without closure of any deep fascial layers.

- Before emergence from general anesthesia, the patient is placed in a brace with 20 degrees of abduction and neutral rotation (**TECH FIG 4B**).

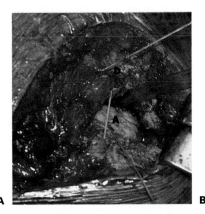 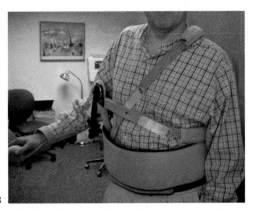

A   **B**

TECH FIG 4 • A. The deltoid (*D*) is reattached to the anterior and lateral edges of the acromion (*A*) with heavy, nonabsorbable sutures placed through bone tunnels. **B.** Patients are placed into an abduction brace in 20 degrees abduction and neutral rotation before extubation.

PEARLS AND PITFALLS

Indications and patient selection	■ Ideal candidates: physiologically young, thin, male gender, minimal muscle wasting, shoulder level function, minimal glenohumeral arthritis ■ Poor candidates: older, obese (big heavy arm), female gender, deltoid weakness, moderate arthritis, poorly compliant patient, subscapularis involvement, more limited preoperative function (less than shoulder-level active elevation), superior humeral head escape
Preoperative assessment of whether cuff can be repaired	■ Duration: Within weeks to months, rotator cuff muscle–tendon units demonstrate decreased compliance and inferior mechanical properties. ■ Cuff retraction: Retraction of torn tendons medial to the midpoint of the humeral head on MRI suggests the need for significant mobilization at the time of surgery to attempt a primary repair. ■ Muscle degeneration: MRI or CT imaging showing fatty degeneration of the rotator cuff muscle bellies suggests tendons will have limited excursion and inferior mechanical properties at the time of attempted repair.
Surgical	■ The surgeon should internally rotate the arm to fully visualize the latissimus insertion on the humerus. Inadequate exposure limits the ability to harvest the entire length of tendon, necessitating additional tendon graft. ■ The released latissimus tendon should be handled carefully to prevent fraying. ■ Release and mobilization of the latissimus dorsi muscle belly along the chest wall ■ The surgeon should ensure that the tunnel for the latissimus rerouting is large enough to prevent constriction of the latissimus muscle belly in the subdeltoid space.
Postoperative	■ Retraining of the latissimus to work in phase with forward flexion and external rotation of the arm

POSTOPERATIVE CARE

- The patient is placed into a brace postoperatively for 4 to 6 weeks to prevent internal rotation.
- During this time the brace can be removed for dressing and bathing, keeping the arm in neutral rotation.
- Passive forward flexion and external rotation is performed during the first 4 weeks to prevent shoulder stiffness.
- At 4 weeks, bracing is discontinued and passive range of motion in all planes is performed.
- At 7 to 9 weeks, active range of motion is started and physical therapy is begun, focused on retraining the latissimus dorsi to function as an abductor and external rotator of the arm.
  - External rotation training: A pillow is placed between the arm and chest wall holding the arm abducted 30 degrees. The patient is told to actively externally rotate the arm while adducting the arm against the pillow.
  - Forward elevation training: The patient squeezes a large rubber ball between the palms of the hands while raising both arms forward over the head.
  - Biofeedback can also be used to show the patient when he or she is actively contracting the latissimus during external rotation and forward elevation.

OUTCOMES

- Significant improvement in pain scores postoperatively is a consistent finding (80% to 100% of patients) across outcome studies, even for patients less satisfied with their final results.[7,11]
- Sixty-six to 81% of patients report satisfaction postoperatively. Patient satisfaction tends to be associated more with improved active shoulder function than pain relief.[7,11]
- Patients with better preoperative function tend to have greater postoperative improvements in range of motion and strength compared to patients starting with greater shoulder dysfunction.
- Based on our experience and that reported in the literature, postoperative range of motion improves by an average of 35 to 50 degrees in forward flexion and 9 to 40 degrees of external rotation.[1,7,11,16]
- Patients undergoing latissimus transfer as the first procedure to treat their rotator cuff pathology can expect better outcomes with regard to satisfaction, pain relief, and active range of motion compared to patients undergoing latissimus transfer who have had prior failed surgery for treatment of their rotator cuff.[16]
- Electromyographic studies show that about 40% to 50% of patients can be retrained to use in-phase latissimus dorsi contraction with active forward flexion or external rotation.[7,11]
- Female gender and advanced age are associated with worse outcomes.
- Subscapularis tendon tears and superior escape of the humeral head are associated with a higher failure rate.
- Patients with multiple negative preoperative prognostic factors should not undergo isolated latissimus muscle transfer, and other options should be considered either alone or in conjunction with a latissimus transfer.

COMPLICATIONS

- Deltoid detachment
- Wound infection
- Rupture of the transferred tendon
- Decreased active forward flexion

REFERENCES

1. Aoki M, Okamura K, Fukushima S, et al. Transfer of latissimus dorsi for irreparable rotator-cuff tears. J Bone Joint Surg Br 1996;78B:761–766.
2. Cleeman E, Hazrati Y, Auerbach JD, et al. Latissimus dorsi transfers for massive rotator cuff tears: a cadaveric study. J Shoulder Elbow Surg 2003;12:539–543.
3. Codsi MJ, Hennigan S, Herzog R, et al. Latissimus dorsi tendon transfer for irreparable posterosuperior rotator cuff tears: factors affecting outcomes. J Bone Joint Surg Am 2007;89A(Suppl 2):1–9.
4. Cofield RH. Rotator cuff disease of the shoulder. J Bone Joint Surg Am 1985;67A:974–979.
5. Costouros JG, Gerber C, Warner JP. Management of irreparable rotator cuff tears: the role of tendon transfer. In: Iannotti JP, Williams GR, ed. Disorders of the Shoulder: Diagnosis and Management, 2nd ed. Philadelphia: Lippincott-Raven, 1999.
6. Dugas JR, Campbell DA, Warren RF, et al. Anatomy and dimensions of rotator cuff insertions. J Shoulder Elbow Surg 2002;11:498–503.
7. Gerber C. Latissimus dorsi transfer for the treatment of irreparable tears of the rotator cuff. Clin Orthop Relat Res 1992;275:152–160.
8. Gerber C, Vinh TS, Hertel R, et al. Latissimus dorsi transfer for the treatment of massive tears of the rotator cuff: a preliminary report. Clin Orthop Relat Res 1988;232:51–60.
9. Goutallier D, Postel JM, Bernageau J, et al. Fatty muscle degeneration in cuff ruptures: pre- and postoperative evaluation by CT scan. Clin Orthop Relat Res 1994;304:78–83.
10. Habermeyer P, Magosch P, Rudolph T, et al. Transfer of the tendon of latissimus dorsi for the treatment of massive tears of the rotator cuff: a new single incision technique. J Bone Joint Surg Br 2006;88B:208–212.
11. Iannotti JP, Hennigan S, Herzog R, et al. Latissimus dorsi tendon transfer for irreparable posterosuperior rotator cuff tears. J Bone Joint Surg Am 2006;88A:342–348.
12. Miniaci A, MacLeod M. Transfer of the latissimus dorsi muscle after failed repair of a massive tear of the rotator cuff: a two- to five-year review. J Bone Joint Surg Am 1999;81A:1120–1127.
13. Pearle AD, Kelly BT, Voos JE, et al. Surgical techniques and anatomic study of latissimus dorsi and teres major transfers. J Bone Joint Surg Am 2006;88A:1524–1531.
14. Schoierer O, Herzberg G, Berthonnaud E, et al. Anatomical basis of latissimus dorsi and teres major transfers on rotator cuff tear surgery with particular reference to the neurovascular pedicles. Surg Radiol Anat 2001;23:75–80.
15. Warner JP. Management of massive irreparable rotator cuff tears: the role of tendon transfers. AAOS Instr Course Lect 2001;50:63–71.
16. Warner PJ, Parsons IM. Latissimus dorsi tendon transfer: a comparative analysis of primary and salvage reconstruction of massive, irreparable rotator cuff tears. J Shoulder Elbow Surg 2001;10:514–521.

Chapter 11

Pectoralis Major Transfer for Irreparable Subscapularis Tears

Leesa M. Galatz

DEFINITION

▪ The subscapularis is one of four muscles making up the rotator cuff. Tears can result from chronic attenuation secondary to age or overuse, but more commonly they result from trauma.

▪ Subscapularis tears commonly occur after a fall on the outstretched arm, traction injuries resulting in a strong external rotation force applied to the arm, or an anterior shoulder dislocation.

▪ Many tears affect only the upper tendinous portion of the insertion. Other tears result in a complete tear of the tendinous and muscular portions of the insertion.

▪ Subscapularis tears are often missed early in the course of treatment. Tears older than about 6 months are usually not reparable because of atrophy and degeneration of the muscle, necessitating a pectoralis major muscle transfer.

ANATOMY

▪ The subscapularis muscle (**FIG 1A**) arises from the deep, volar surface of the scapular body (the subscapular fossa) and inserts on the lesser tuberosity. The upper two thirds of the insertion is tendinous and the lower third is a muscular insertion.

▪ The anterior humeral circumflex artery courses laterally along the demarcation between the tendinous and muscular portions of the muscle.

▪ Tears of the subscapularis differ from tears of the other rotator cuff muscles in that there is often an intact soft tissue sleeve across the front of the shoulder with the torn tendon retracted medially within this "sheath." In contrast, the supraspinatus and infraspinatus tear leaving exposed humeral head. The remaining soft tissue over the anterior humeral head after a subscapularis tear can be mistaken for an intact or partially torn tendon.

▪ The pectoralis major muscle is composed of two major heads (**FIG 1B**).

▪ The clavicular head originates from the medial third of the clavicle. The sternal head originates from the manubrium, the upper two thirds of the sternum, and ribs 2 to 4. The muscle courses laterally to insert on the lateral lip of the biceps groove.

▪ The sternal head lies deep to the clavicular head, forming the posterior lamina, and inserts slightly superior to the clavicular head. The clavicular head forms the anterior lamina. The laminae are usually continuous inferiorly.

▪ Some of the deep muscular fibers from the inferior aspect of the pectoralis major muscle course toward and insert on the more proximal or superior aspect of the muscle insertion. These inferior-to-superior–directed fibers tend to make the muscle "flip" when it is released. The superior corner should be tagged to assist with orientation if used for the transfer.

▪ The mean width of the pectoralis major insertion is 5.7 cm (range, 4.8 to 6.5 cm).[6] The undersurface of the insertion has a broad tendinous insertion, whereas the anterior surface is primarily muscular; only the most distal insertion is tendinous.

▪ The pectoralis major muscle is innervated by the medial and lateral pectoral nerves, which arise from the medial and lateral cords of the brachial plexus, respectively.

▪ The medial pectoral nerve enters the pectoralis major muscle about 11.9 cm (range, 9.0 to 14.5 cm) from the

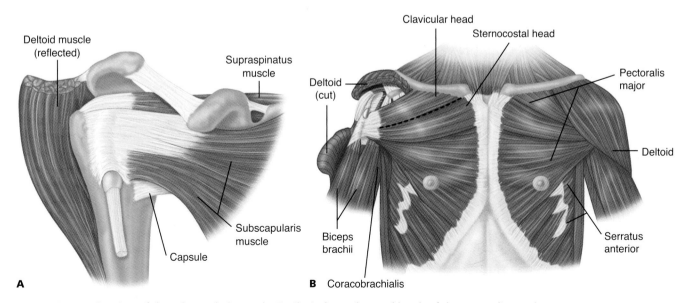

FIG 1 • **A.** Anterior view of the subscapularis muscle. **B.** Clavicular and sternal heads of the pectoralis muscle.

humeral insertion and 2.0 cm from the inferior edge of the muscle.[6]

◾ The lateral pectoral nerve enters the pectoralis major muscle at a mean of 12.5 cm (range, 10.0 to 14.9 cm) from the insertion.[6]

◾ The musculocutaneous nerve arises from the lateral cord of the brachial plexus and enters the conjoint tendon an average of 6.1 cm (range, 3.5 to 10 cm) from the coracoid (95% confidence interval, 3.1 to 9.1 cm).[6]

◾ In some patients, a proximal branch enters the conjoint tendon proximal to the main branch of the musculocutaneous nerve. The function of this proximal branch is not known. It is likely innervation to the coracobrachialis, and its release has little clinical effect.

PATHOGENESIS

◾ Subscapularis tears result from:
◾ Anterior shoulder dislocations
◾ Traction injuries to the arm with extension and external rotation forces to the arm
◾ Rarely, chronic attenuation from age and overuse
◾ Possible relationship to coracoid impingement
◾ The subscapularis muscle is particularly prone to atrophy and degeneration after a tear. With complete, retracted tears of the muscle, there is a window of opportunity for about 6 months when a primary repair can be performed. Beyond that time point, the muscle is increasingly difficult to mobilize and repair is under substantial tension, leading to early failure.

NATURAL HISTORY

◾ Subscapularis tears can result in pain, loss of motion, and loss of strength in the affected shoulder.
◾ Failure to recognize the injury can result in a delay in treatment and possibly an irreparable tear.
◾ An untreated rotator cuff tear can lead to progressive loss of function, stiffness, and possibly arthritis. Loss of the subscapularis may result in dynamic proximal migration of the humeral head with arm elevation that can eventually become static elevation.

PATIENT HISTORY AND PHYSICAL FINDINGS

◾ Lift-off test: The patient will not be able to lift the hand off the back if the subscapularis is deficient.
◾ Abdominal compression test: With a tear, the patient will not be able to maintain this position and will flex wrist or hand will release from the belly if positive.
◾ Range-of-motion testing: A subscapularis tear will result in increased external rotation at the side, with a "softer" endpoint.

IMAGING AND OTHER DIAGNOSTIC STUDIES

◾ A standard shoulder series of radiographs comprising a shoulder anteroposterior (AP) view, a true scapular AP view, an axillary view, and a scapular Y view is obtained to rule out fractures, arthritis, or other injury.
◾ A subscapularis tear may result in proximal migration of the humeral head relative to the glenoid, depending on the degree of tear and involvement of other rotator cuff muscles.

◾ In the absence of a subscapularis tear, slight anterior subluxation of the humeral head may be noted on the axillary view.
◾ An MRI will reveal the tear and also is helpful in assessing the degree of retraction, atrophy, and fatty degeneration of the subscapularis muscle. The proximal portion of the long head of the biceps tendon becomes unstable from the intertubercular groove when the subscapularis tears. An MRI can demonstrate a dislocated or subluxed biceps tendon.
◾ A CT arthrogram is an alternative to an MRI.
◾ Subscapularis tears can be diagnosed with ultrasound if performed by a competent, experienced ultrasonographer. Ultrasound is very sensitive for biceps tendon subluxation or dislocation from the groove.[1]

DIFFERENTIAL DIAGNOSIS

◾ Supraspinatus tears
◾ Infraspinatus tears
◾ Biceps tendon pathology
◾ Anterior instability
◾ Rotator cuff insufficiency secondary to neurologic etiology

NONOPERATIVE MANAGEMENT

◾ Physical therapy focusing on strengthening the intact rotator cuff muscles can be beneficial to maximize the function of remaining musculature.
◾ Range-of-motion exercises focus on any areas of loss of motion or capsular contracture.
◾ Rotator cuff strengthening with the use of light-resistance Therabands at waist level is an effective initial exercise. Progression to higher-resistance exercises is as tolerated.
◾ Cortisone injections may give some temporary pain relief but are unlikely to result in permanent resolution of symptoms.
◾ Nonsteroidal anti-inflammatory medication may be helpful for pain relief of mild to moderate pain.

SURGICAL MANAGEMENT

◾ An attempt is made at the time of surgery to repair the native subscapularis. Within reasonable limits, the subscapularis is mobilized by releasing surrounding soft tissues. Even a partial repair is recommended in conjunction with a pectoralis major transfer.
◾ Surrounding soft tissues include the rotator interval and coracohumeral ligament, the anterior capsule of the shoulder (middle and inferior glenohumeral ligaments), and superficial soft tissue adhesions deep to the coracoid and conjoint tendon.
◾ The subscapularis differs from the other rotator cuff muscles in that it has a fascial sleeve that remains attached to the lesser tuberosity and covers the anterior humeral head. This is in contrast to the other rotator cuff muscles, which leave exposed greater tuberosity and cartilage without soft tissue coverage. This material is easily mistaken for an intact subscapularis, emphasizing the significance of preoperative evaluation.

Preoperative Planning

◾ Patient history, physical examination, and all imaging studies are reviewed. A soft tissue imaging study such as MRI or ultrasound of the rotator cuff is a necessity.

▪ Plain films should be assessed for proximal migration, anterior subluxation, and deformity secondary to trauma and arthritis. An MRI is useful for assessing the condition of the subscapularis. A high degree of retraction and degeneration of the muscle is highly suggestive of a chronic, irreparable tear that will necessitate a pectoralis major muscle transfer.

▪ Subscapularis tears result in instability of the long head of the biceps tendon with medial subluxation into the joint. The surgeon should be prepared to perform a biceps tenotomy or tenodesis of the tendon if it has not already ruptured from chronic, attritional changes.

▪ Associated tears of the other rotator cuff muscles are addressed concurrently. Isolated arthritic lesions are débrided, as is degenerative labral fraying or tear.

Positioning

▪ The pectoralis major transfer is most easily performed with the patient in the beach chair position. The head of the bed or positioning device is elevated about 60 degrees. The head is secured to avoid cervical injury. The arm is prepared and draped free and held in a commercially available arm holder that allows flexible arm positioning.[5]

Approach

▪ Several different variations of the pectoralis major transfer have been described.

▪ Wirth and Rockwood[8] described a split pectoralis major muscle transfer superficial to the coracoid.

▪ Resch and colleagues[7] described a split pectoralis major transfer deep to the coracoid.

▪ Jost and colleagues[4] and Gerber and associates[3] recommended transfer of the whole pectoralis major muscle superficial to the coracoid.

▪ Gerber and associates[3] described transfer of the sternal head of the pectoralis major with or without the teres major tendon.

▪ The procedure can be performed through a deltopectoral or anterior axillary incision.

▪ The deltopectoral incision allows a more extensile approach and is recommended in revision cases.

▪ The anterior axillary incision from the coracoid to the anterior axillary crease is useful in primary cases in smaller patients.

▪ Both incisions use the deltopectoral interval for deep exposure.

SPLIT PECTORALIS MAJOR MUSCLE TRANSFER

▪ The deltopectoral interval is identified. The cephalic vein is usually retracted laterally with the deltoid. The subdeltoid and subacromial spaces are released of adhesions.

▪ Regardless of technique, the native subscapularis is examined and mobilized to its full extent. If repair is not possible, a muscle transfer is performed.

▪ The superior 2.5 to 3 cm of the pectoralis major insertion is identified along the lateral edge of the biceps groove. This contains portions of both the anterior and posterior laminae. The identified portion of the pectoralis major in-

sertion is released sharply from its insertion. Care is taken to avoid injury to the long head of the biceps tendon, which lies directly under the insertion in this case. The distal tendon is tagged with three or four stay sutures.

▪ Tension is applied to the stay sutures to facilitate the muscle split of the pectoralis major muscle. Muscle dissection is performed bluntly in a medial direction at the inferior portion of the split to mobilize the superior muscle for transfer. Dissection should be limited to 6 to 8 cm to preserve the medial pectoral nerve (**TECH FIG 1A**).

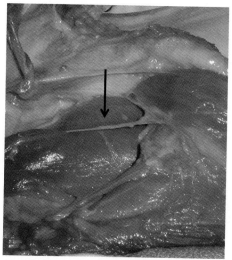

A

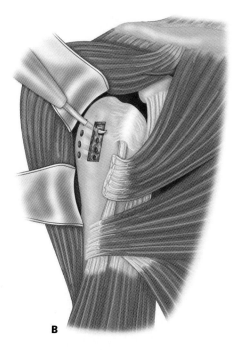

B

TECH FIG 1 • A. The medial pectoral nerve (*arrow*) arises from the medial cord of the brachial plexus and enters the pectoralis major muscle 6 to 8 cm medial to the muscle insertion. Thus, medial dissection and mobilization is limited to 6 to 8 cm to avoid denervating the muscle. **B.** The superior half of the pectoralis major insertion is freed from the humerus and mobilized. This half is transferred to the humeral head and secured in a small bone trough with drill holes for the sutures.

TECHNIQUES

- The humerus is rotated internally to expose the greater tuberosity and humeral shaft lateral to the biceps groove. An osteotome or burr is used to make a bone trough measuring 5 × 25 mm oriented in a vertical position for reinsertion of the transferred pectoralis muscle.
- Three or four holes are drilled just lateral to the edge of the trough and a curved awl is used to connect the drill holes to the trough (**TECH FIG 1B**).

- The sutures in the tendon are passed into the trough and out through the drill holes. Tension is placed on the sutures, bringing the tendon into the trough. The sutures are then tied over the bone bridges between the holes, securing the tendon.
- A biceps tenotomy or tenodesis is performed as needed.

SUBCORACOID MUSCLE TRANSFER OF THE CLAVICULAR HEAD

- A deltopectoral incision and approach are used (**TECH FIG 2A**).
- The tendon of the pectoralis major insertion is exposed along its full length (**TECH FIG 2B**).
- The superior half to two thirds of the clavicular head is detached from the humerus. The muscle fibers corresponding to the detached section of the tendon are split or separated from the remaining muscle using blunt dissection in a medial direction. The blunt dissection is performed between the sternal and clavicular heads so that only the clavicular head muscle is released and preserved

for the transfer (**TECH FIG 2C**). The muscle fibers of the sternal portion that course into the proximal portion of the muscle are transected.
- The space between the medial border of the conjoint tendon and the pectoralis minor is gently dissected bluntly. The musculocutaneous nerve and its entry into the conjoint tendon are identified. The space deep to the conjoint tendon and superficial to the musculocutaneous nerve is developed for the muscle transfer (**TECH FIG 2D**).
- Stay sutures are attached to the distal pectoralis major tendon. The sutures are grasped with a curved forceps

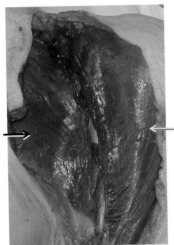

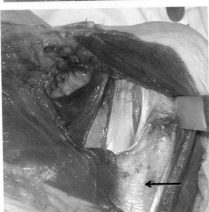

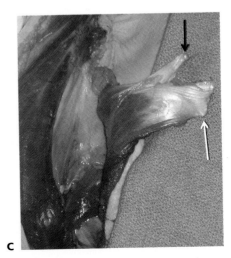

TECH FIG 2 • A. This cadaveric dissection illustrates the deltopectoral approach (*black arrow,* pectoralis major; *white arrow,* deltoid). The incision should be long enough to allow adequate exposure of the pectoralis major and the proximal humerus for reattachment. **B.** Cadaveric dissection illustrating the pectoralis major and its insertion (*arrow*). **C.** The pectoralis major has two heads, the superficial clavicular head (*white arrow*) and the deeper sternal head (*black arrow*). In this photo, the insertion has been released and is reflected medially. *(continued)*

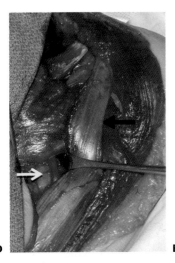
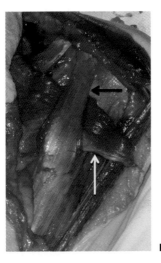
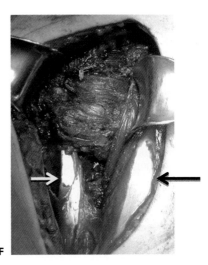

TECH FIG 2 • *(continued)* **D.** To avoid injury to the musculocutaneous nerve, it should be identified as part of the surgical procedure for a subcoracoid transfer. The muscle should be transferred deep to the conjoint tendon (*black arrow*) and superficial to the nerve (*white arrow*). **E.** The pectoralis major muscle (*white arrow*) is transferred deep to the conjoint tendon (*black arrow*), laterally to the greater tuberosity. **F.** Intraoperative photo of a right shoulder with a pectoralis major transfer secured to the greater tuberosity. *White arrow*, biceps; *black arrow*, conjoint tendon.

and passed deep to the conjoint tendon and superficial to the musculocutaneous nerve, advancing the muscle to the greater tuberosity (**TECH FIG 2E**).

■ The tendon is attached to the lesser tuberosity with transosseous nonabsorbable sutures. In very large individuals with substantial muscle mass, the muscle may need to be debulked to facilitate tension-free passage deep to the coracoid (**TECH FIG 2F**).

■ The transferred muscle is reattached using anchors or transosseous sutures.

WHOLE PECTORALIS MUSCLE TRANSFER

■ The deltopectoral approach is identical to that described above.

■ An attempt is made to mobilize and repair the subscapularis. Releases are performed at the rotator interval, the base of the coracoid, the brachial plexus, and the subscapularis fossa. A partial repair is performed if possible.

■ The entire tendon of the pectoralis major tendon is exposed and released from its insertion of the humerus.

■ Three nonabsorbable sutures are passed through the tendon using a modified Mason-Allen technique.

■ The muscle and tendon is mobilized and brought over (superficial) the coracoid to the medial aspect of the greater tuberosity, where it is secured using anchor fixation or to a bone trough (**TECH FIG 3**).

  ■ If a bone trough is used, the sutures are routed through the trough and the knots are tied over a small titanium plate to prevent suture pullout. The uppermost corner of the tendon is sutured to the anterolateral supraspinatus. Care is taken not to overtighten the rotator interval.

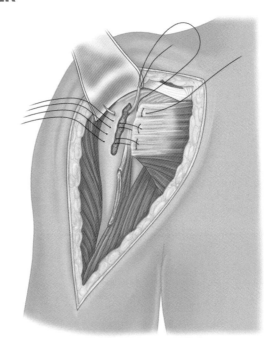

TECH FIG 3 • The whole pectoralis major muscle is released from its insertion on the humerus and transferred and secured to the humeral head using anchor fixation or a bone trough with tunnels.

SPLIT PECTORALIS MAJOR AND TERES MAJOR TENDON TRANSFER

- Setup and exposure are as described above.
- The plane between the sternal and clavicular heads is located and developed. The sternal head is sharply released from the humerus. Nonabsorbable sutures (no. 2) are placed in the tendon in Mason-Allen fashion.
- The sternal head is mobilized and pulled underneath the clavicular head to the lesser tuberosity, where it is secured (**TECH FIG 4A**). The transfer is superficial to the coracoid process and should be tight but allow 30 degrees of external rotation.
- If the subscapularis tear is completely irreparable, the authors recommend combining this transfer with the teres major muscle.
- To expose the teres major, the arm is externally rotated.

- The latissimus dorsi insertion is located and the superior and inferior aspects are demarcated. The latissimus is released, leaving a cuff of tissue laterally for repair.
- The teres major insertion is deep to the latissimus. The teres major is tagged and released. Often, the muscle must be released from confluence with the latissimus.
  - The axillary nerve and posterior humeral circumflex artery lie at the superior border of the teres major muscle. The radial nerve and brachial artery are in close approximation to the inferior border of the teres major.
- Finally, the teres major is transferred to the inferior portion of the lesser tuberosity, where it is secured with nonabsorbable sutures (**TECH FIG 4B**).

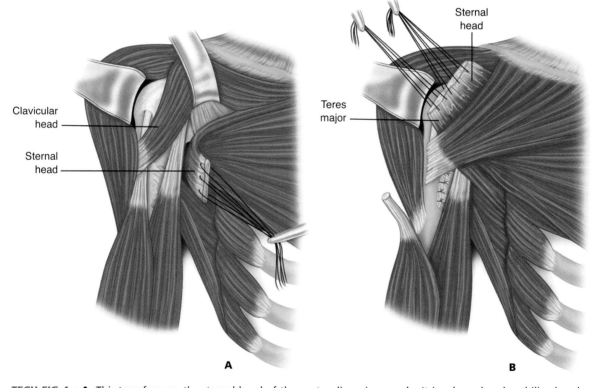

A   B

TECH FIG 4 • **A.** This transfer uses the sternal head of the pectoralis major muscle. It is released and mobilized underneath the clavicular head to the lesser tuberosity. **B.** The teres major muscle is released from its insertion on the humerus and transferred along with the sternal head of the pectoralis major to the lesser tuberosity. The teres major inserts deep to the latissimus dorsi, which is reattached in its anatomic position.

PEARLS AND PITFALLS

Indications	■ Subscapularis tears are often missed, resulting in a delayed diagnosis. ■ Elderly patients with generalized atrophy should be considered for a whole muscle transfer, whereas more muscular individuals are better candidates for split or sternal head transfers.
Pectoralis major muscle detachment and mobilization	■ Mobilization of the muscle should not proceed greater than 8 cm from the insertion in order to protect the pectoral nerves. ■ In whole muscle transfers, the medial pectoral nerve can enter the muscle within 1.2 cm of the inferior edge. ■ Muscle split is performed bluntly.

Subcoracoid transfer of the pectoralis major muscle	■ The musculocutaneous nerve and its proximal branches are at risk. ■ The musculocutaneous nerve is identified. ■ Transferred muscle should course deep to the conjoint tendon and superficial to the nerve to avoid excessive traction and neurapraxia. ■ Scar in revision cases can make this dissection difficult; an intraoperative nerve stimulator may help identify structures of the brachial plexus if necessary.
Fixation problems	■ Mason-Allen or Krackow sutures are used to grasp the tendon securely.
Orientation	■ Before release of the muscle, the superior corner is tagged to keep muscle in its anatomic orientation (some inferior muscle fibers course to the superior insertion, so the muscle tends to flip after release).

POSTOPERATIVE CARE

■ A drain should always be used because release and transfer of the pectoralis major muscle[5] results in dead space, and hematoma formation is common.

■ The operative arm is placed in a sling postoperatively. Passive exercises are started on postoperative day 1.

　■ The surgeon should evaluate tension on the transfer intraoperatively before closure to determine the limits of external rotation during early rehabilitation.

　■ Forward elevation is performed in internal rotation or neutral rotation to minimize tension on the transfer.

　■ Active internal rotation and extension are avoided for 6 weeks.

■ Active assisted and active range-of-motion exercises are started 6 weeks after surgery. Resistance exercises commence as tolerated thereafter. No internal rotation resistance exercises are recommended until 12 weeks postoperatively.

OUTCOMES

■ Jost and associates[4] reported a series of 30 transfers in 28 patients. Twelve had isolated subscapularis tears and 18 had concomitant supraspinatus–infraspinatus tears. The mean relative Constant score improved from 47% to 70% at an average of 32 months of follow-up. Thirteen patients were very satisfied, 10 patients were satisfied, 2 patients were disappointed, and 3 patients were dissatisfied.

■ Resch and colleagues[7] reported on a series of 12 patients with a subcoracoid transfer. The Constant score increased from 26.9% to 67.1%. Nine assessed their final result as good or excellent, three as fair, and none as poor. Four unstable shoulders were stable at the average of 28 months of follow-up.

■ Rockwood[8] reported a series of 13 patients. Seven had a pectoralis major transfer and six had a pectoralis minor transfer. Ten of the 13 were satisfied, but the results were not separated between the patients with the pectoralis major and minor transfers.

■ Galatz and associates[2] reported on the subcoracoid pectoralis major transfer in 14 patients as a salvage procedure for iatrogenic anterior superior instability. Nine of the 14 had satisfactory results in terms of pain relief, but the functional results are not as predictable for this particular indication.

■ Gerber and colleagues[3] reported a combination of sternal head and sternal head plus teres major transfers. In the sternal head patients, 9 of 11 had pain relief. Two had a rupture that required revision. In the sternal head plus teres major group, seven of nine patients had pain relief. One had a rupture discovered at the time of revision surgery (fusion). Final ASES scores were 61 in the sternal group and 55 in the sternal plus teres group.

■ In all series, most of the patients had had surgery before the transfer, and in most cases a pectoralis major transfer was performed for revision purposes. This has dramatic implications on outcome.

COMPLICATIONS

■ Musculocutaneous nerve injury
■ Pectoral nerve injury
■ Fixation failure
■ Mechanical impingement with the coracoid, either deep or superficial to the conjoint tendon

REFERENCES

1. Armstrong A, Teefey SA, Wu T, et al. The efficacy of ultrasound in the diagnosis of long head of the biceps tendon pathology. J Shoulder Elbow Surg 2006;15:7–11.
2. Galatz LM, Connor PM, Calfee RP, et al. Pectoralis major transfer for anterior-superior subluxation in massive rotator cuff insufficiency. J Shoulder Elbow Surg 2003;12:1–5.
3. Gerber A, Clavert P, Millett PJ, et al. Split pectoralis major and teres major tendon transfers for reconstruction of irreparable tears of the subscapularis. Tech Shoulder Elbow Surg 2004;5:5–12.
4. Jost B, Puskas GJ, Lustenberger A, et al. Outcome of pectoralis major transfer for the treatment of irreparable subscapularis tears. J Bone Joint Surg Am 2003;85A:1944–1951.
5. Klepps S, Galatz LM, Yamaguchi K. Subcoracoid pectoralis major transfer: a salvage procedure for irreparable subscapularis deficiency. Tech Shoulder Elbow Surg 2001;2:92–99.
6. Klepps SJ, Goldfarb C, Flatow E, et al. Anatomic evaluation of the subcoracoid pectoralis major transfer in human cadavers. J Shoulder Elbow Surg 2001;10:453–459.
7. Resch H, Povacz P, Ritter E, et al. Transfer of the pectoralis major muscle for the treatment of irreparable rupture of the subscapularis tendon. J Bone Joint Surg Am 2000;82:372–382.
8. Wirth MA, Rockwood CA Jr. Operative treatment of irreparable rupture of the subscapularis. J Bone Joint Surg Am 1997;79A:722–731.

Chapter 12

Acute Repair and Reconstruction of Sternoclavicular Dislocation

Steven P. Kalandiak, Edwin E. Spencer, Jr., Michael A. Wirth, and Charles A. Rockwood

DEFINITION

▪ Sternoclavicular dislocation is one of the rarest dislocations, but one most shoulder surgeons will encounter several times during a career (more in a practice with significant exposure to high-energy trauma).

▪ Sternoclavicular dislocations represented 3% of a series of 1603 injuries of the shoulder girdle reported by Cave et al.[6]

▪ The true ratio of anterior to posterior dislocations is unknown, since most reports focus on the rarer posterior type. Estimates range from a ratio of 20 anterior dislocations to each posterior by Nettles and Linscheid,[19] in a series of 60 patients (57 anterior and 3 posterior), to a ratio of approximately three to one (135 anterior and 50 posterior) in our series[23] of 185 traumatic sternoclavicular injuries.

▪ Not all sternoclavicular dislocations require surgery. Avoiding inappropriate patient selection, preventing hardware-related complications, and repairing or reconstructing the capsule and the rhomboid ligament if the medial clavicle has been resected require special emphasis.

▪ Although this region can be an intimidating one because of the surrounding anatomic structures, a knowledgeable and careful surgeon can treat this joint safely and reliably produce good results.

ANATOMY

▪ The epiphysis of the medial clavicle is the last epiphysis of the long bones to appear and the last to close. It does not ossify until the 18th to 20th year, and it generally fuses with the shaft of the clavicle around age 23 to 25.[14,15] For this reason, many sternoclavicular "dislocations" in young adults are in fact physeal fractures.

▪ The articular surface of the medial clavicle is much larger than that of the sternum. It is bulbous and concave front to back and convex vertically, creating a saddle-type joint with the curved clavicular notch of the sternum.[14,15]

▪ A small facet on the inferior aspect of the medial clavicle articulates with the superior aspect of the first rib in 2.5% of subjects.[5]

▪ There is little congruence and the least bony stability of any major joint in the body. Almost all of its integrity comes from the surrounding ligaments.

Ligaments

▪ The intra-articular disc ligament is dense and fibrous, arises from the synchondral junction of the first rib to the sternum, passes through the sternoclavicular joint, and divides it into two separate spaces[14,15] (**FIG 1**). It attaches on the superior and posterior medial clavicle and acts as a checkrein against medial displacement of the inner clavicle.

▪ The costoclavicular (rhomboid) ligament attaches the upper surface of the medial first rib to the rhomboid fossa on the inferior surface of the medial end of the clavicle.[14,15] It averages 1.3 cm long, 1.9 cm wide, and 1.3 cm thick.[5]

▪ The anterior fasciculus arises anteromedially, runs upward and laterally, and resists lateral displacement and upward rotation of the clavicle.

▪ The posterior fasciculus is shorter, arises laterally, runs upward and medially, and resists medial displacement and excessive downward rotation[1,5,15] (**FIGS 1 AND 2**).

▪ The interclavicular ligament (see Fig 1) connects the superomedial aspects of each clavicle with the capsular ligaments and the upper sternum. Comparable to the wishbone of birds, it helps the capsular ligaments to produce "shoulder poise"; that is, to hold up the lateral aspect of the clavicle.[14]

▪ The capsular ligaments cover the anterosuperior and posterior aspects of the joint and represent thickenings of the joint capsule (Figs 1 and 2). The clavicular attachment of the ligament is primarily onto the epiphysis of the medial clavicle, with some blending of the fibers into the metaphysis.[3,8]

▪ In sectioning studies, the capsular ligaments are the most important structures in preventing upward displacement of the medial clavicle caused by a downward force on the distal end of the shoulder.[1]

▪ This lateral poise of the shoulder (ie, the force that holds the shoulder up) is attributed to a locking mechanism of the ligaments of the sternoclavicular joint.

▪ Other single ligament sectioning studies[26] have shown that the posterior capsule is the most important primary stabilizer to anterior and posterior translation. The anterior capsule is an important restraint to anterior translation. The costoclavicular ligament is unimportant if the capsule remains intact,[26] although it may be an important secondary restraint if the capsular ligaments are torn, much like the coracoclavicular ligament laterally.

Applied Surgical Anatomy

▪ A "curtain" of muscles—the sternohyoid, sternothyroid, and scaleni—lies posterior to the sternoclavicular joint and the inner third of the clavicle and blocks the view of vital structures—the innominate artery, innominate vein, vagus nerve, phrenic nerve, internal jugular vein, trachea, and esophagus.

▪ The anterior jugular vein lies between the clavicle and the curtain of muscles. Variable in size and as large as 1.5 cm in diameter, it has no valves and bleeds like someone has opened a floodgate when nicked.

▪ The surgeon who is considering stabilizing the sternoclavicular joint by running a pin down from the clavicle into the sternum should not do it and should remember that the arch of the aorta, the superior vena cava, and the right pulmonary artery are also very close at hand.

PATHOGENESIS

▪ Most sternoclavicular joint dislocations result from high-energy trauma, usually a motor vehicle accident. They occasionally result from contact sports.

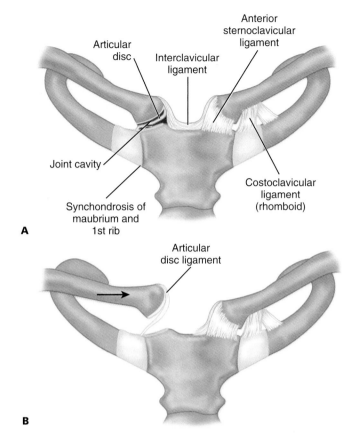

FIG 1 • **A.** Normal anatomy around the sternoclavicular joint. The articular disc ligament divides the sternoclavicular joint cavity into two separate spaces and inserts onto the superior and posterior aspects of the medial clavicle. **B.** The articular disc ligament acts as a checkrein for medial displacement of the proximal clavicle.

- A force applied directly to the anteromedial aspect of the clavicle can push the medial clavicle back behind the sternum and into the mediastinum.
- More commonly, a force is applied indirectly, from the lateral aspect of the shoulder. If the shoulder is compressed and rolled forward, a posterior dislocation results; if the shoulder is compressed and rolled backward, an anterior dislocation results.
- As noted above, many injuries of the sternoclavicular joint in patients under 25 years of age are, in fact, fractures through the medial physis of the clavicle.

NATURAL HISTORY

- Mild or moderate sprain
  - The mildly sprained sternoclavicular joint is stable but painful.
  - The moderately sprained joint may be slightly subluxated anteriorly or posteriorly, and may often be reduced by drawing the shoulders backward as if reducing and holding a fracture of the clavicle.
- Anterior dislocation
  - Although most anterior dislocations are unstable after closed reduction, we still recommend an attempt to reduce the dislocation closed.
  - Occasionally the clavicle remains reduced, but typically the clavicle remains unstable after closed reduction. We usually accept the deformity, because an anteriorly dislocated sternoclavicular joint typically becomes asymptomatic, and

we believe that the deformity is less of a problem than the potential complications of operative fixation.

- When the entire medial clavicle is stripped out of the delto-trapezial fascia, the deformity can be so severe that it may be poorly tolerated, so we consider primary fixation. In those rare cases when a chronic anterior dislocation is symptomatic, one may perform a capsular reconstruction or a medial clavicle resection and costoclavicular ligament reconstruction.
- Posterior dislocation
  - In contrast to anterior dislocations, the complications of an unreduced posterior dislocation are numerous: thoracic outlet syndrome, vascular compromise, and erosion of the medial clavicle into any of the vital structures that lie posterior to the sternoclavicular joint.
  - Closed reduction for acute posterior sternoclavicular dislocation can usually be obtained, and the reduction is generally stable. Often, general anesthesia is necessary. However, when a posterior dislocation is irreducible or the reduction is unstable, an open reduction should be performed.
  - When chronic posterior dislocation is present, late complications may arise from mediastinal impingement, so we recommend medial clavicle resection and ligament reconstruction.
- Physeal injuries
  - The typical history for physeal injuries is the same as for other traumatic dislocations. The difference between these injuries and pure dislocations is that most of these injuries will heal with time, without surgical intervention.
  - In very young patients, the remodeling process can eliminate deformity because of the osteogenic potential of an intact periosteal tube. Zaslav,[31] Rockwood,[23] and Hsu et al[16] have all reported successful treatment of displaced medial clavicle physeal injury in adolescents and provided radiographic evidence of remodeling.
  - Anterior physeal injuries may be reduced, but if reduction cannot be obtained, they can be left alone without problem. Posterior physeal injuries should likewise undergo an attempt at reduction. If a posterior dislocation cannot be reduced closed and the patient is having no significant symptoms, the displacement can be observed while remod-

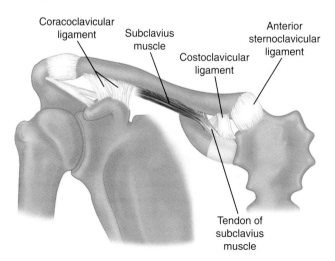

FIG 2 • Normal anatomy around the sternoclavicular and acromioclavicular joints. The tendon of the subclavius muscle arises in the vicinity of the costoclavicular ligament from the first rib and has a long tendon structure.

eling occurs. Even in older individuals, a posteriorly displaced fracture with moderate displacement and no mediastinal symptoms may be observed, as it usually becomes asymptomatic with fracture healing.

■ However, as with severely displaced dislocations, one may wish to consider operative repair for severely displaced physeal fractures. Suture repair through the medial shaft and the epiphysis and Balser plate fixation have both been successfully used in this situation.[13,27,28]

PATIENT HISTORY AND PHYSICAL FINDINGS

■ A history of high-energy trauma is almost a requirement for the diagnosis. Most cases will be due to a motor vehicle accident, a fall from a significant height, or a sports injury.

■ The absence of such a history suggests either an atraumatic instability or some other atraumatic condition of the joint.

■ Posterior displacement may be obvious, but anterior fullness can represent either anterior displacement or swelling overlying posterior displacement.

■ Careful examination is extremely important. Mediastinal injuries may occur when a traumatic dislocation is posterior, and the physician should seek evidence of damage to the pulmonary and vascular systems, such as hoarseness, venous congestion, and difficulty breathing or swallowing.

■ Evaluation should also include the remainder of the thorax, shoulder girdle, and upper extremity, as well as the contralateral sternoclavicular joint.

IMAGING AND OTHER DIAGNOSTIC STUDIES

■ Plain radiographs

■ Occasionally, routine anteroposterior chest radiographs suggest displacement compared with the normal side. However, these are difficult to interpret.

■ Serendipity view: A 45-degree cephalic tilt view is the most useful and reproducible plain radiograph for the sternoclavicular joint. The tube is centered directly on the sternum and a nongrid 11 × 14 cassette is placed on the table under the patient's upper shoulders and neck, so the beam will project the

medial half of both clavicles onto the film (**FIG 3**). The technique is the same as a posteroanterior view of the chest.

■ An anteriorly dislocated medial clavicle will appear to ride higher compared to the normal side. The reverse is true if the sternoclavicular joint is dislocated posteriorly (**FIG 4**).

■ In the past, tomograms were useful in distinguishing a sternoclavicular dislocation from a fracture of the medial clavicle and defining questionable anterior and posterior injuries of the sternoclavicular joint. Although they provide more information than plain films, at present they have been replaced with CT scans.

■ Without question, CT scanning is the best technique to study the sternoclavicular joint. It distinguishes dislocations of the joint from fractures of the medial clavicle and clearly defines minor subluxations (**FIG 5**).

■ The patient should lie supine. The scan should include both sternoclavicular joints and the medial halves of both clavicles so that the injured side can be compared with the normal.

■ If symptoms of mediastinal compression are present or displacement of the medial clavicle is severe, the use of intravenous contrast will aid in the imaging of the vascular structures in the mediastinum.

DIFFERENTIAL DIAGNOSIS

■ Arthritic conditions: sternocostoclavicular hyperostosis, osteitis condensans, Friedrich disease, Tietze syndrome, and osteoarthritis

■ Atraumatic (spontaneous) subluxation or dislocation: One or both of the sternoclavicular joints may spontaneously subluxate or dislocate during abduction or flexion during overhead motion. Typically seen in ligamentously lax females in their late teens or early 20s, it is not painful, it is almost always anterior, and it should almost always be managed nonoperatively.[22]

■ Congenital or developmental or acquired subluxation or dislocation: Birth trauma, congenital defects with loss of bone substance on either side of the joint, or neuromuscular or other developmental disorders can predispose the patient to subluxation or dislocation.

■ Iatrogenic instability may be due to failure to reconstruct the ligaments of the sternoclavicular joint adequately or to an excessive medial clavicle resection. History is significant for a prior procedure on the sternoclavicular joint.

NONOPERATIVE MANAGEMENT

■ A mild sprain is stable but painful. We treat mild sprains with a sling, cold packs, and resumption of activity as comfort dictates.

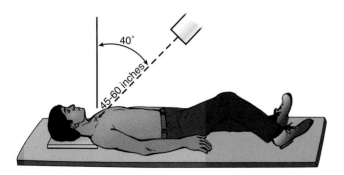

FIG 3 • Serendipity view. Positioning of the patient to take the serendipity view of the sternoclavicular joints. The x-ray tube is tilted 40 degrees from the vertical position and aimed directly at the manubrium. The nongrid cassette should be large enough to receive the projected images of the medial halves of both clavicles. In children the tube distance from the patient should be 45 inches; in thicker-chested adults the distance should be 60 inches.

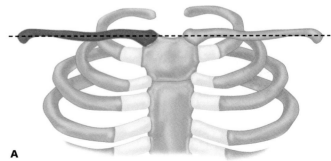

A

FIG 4 • Interpretation of the cephalic tilt films of the sternoclavicular joints. **A.** In a normal person, both clavicles appear on the same imaginary line drawn horizontally across the film. *(continued)*

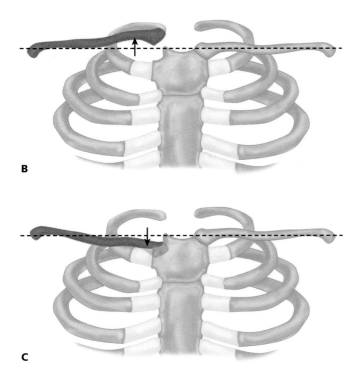

B

C

FIG 4 • (*continued*) **B.** In a patient with anterior dislocation of the right sternoclavicular joint, the medial half of the right clavicle is projected above the imaginary line drawn through the level of the normal left clavicle. **C.** If the patient has a posterior dislocation of the right sternoclavicular joint, the medial half of the right clavicle is displaced below the imaginary line drawn through the normal left clavicle.

▪ A moderate sprain may be slightly subluxated anteriorly or posteriorly. Moderate sprains may be reduced by drawing the shoulders backward as if reducing a fracture of the clavicle. This is followed by cold packs and immobilization in a padded figure 8 strap for 4 to 6 weeks, then gradual resumption of activity as comfort dictates.

▪ Anterior dislocations may undergo closed reduction with either local or general anesthesia, narcotics, or muscle relaxants.

   ▪ The patient is supine on the table, with a 3- to 4-inch-thick pad between the shoulders. Direct gentle pressure over the anteriorly displaced clavicle or traction on the outstretched

arm combined with pressure on the medial clavicle will generally reduce the dislocation.

▪ Posterior dislocation in a stoic patient may possibly be reducible under intravenous narcotics and muscle relaxation. However, general anesthesia is usually required for reduction of a posterior dislocation, because of pain and muscle spasm.

   ▪ Our preferred method is the abduction traction technique.

      ▪ The patient is placed supine, with the dislocated side near the edge of the table. A 3- to 4-inch-thick sandbag is placed between the scapulae (**FIG 6**). Lateral traction is applied to the abducted arm, which is then gradually brought back into extension. The clavicle usually reduces with an audible snap or pop, and it is almost always stable. Too much extension can bind the anterior surface of the dislocated medial clavicle on the back of the manubrium.

      ▪ Occasionally it is necessary to grasp the medial clavicle with one's fingers to dislodge it from behind the sternum. If this fails, the skin is prepared, and a sterile towel clip is used to grasp the medial clavicle to apply lateral and anterior traction (see Fig 6C). If the joint is stable after reduction, the shoulders should be held back for 4 to 6 weeks with a figure 8 dressing to allow ligament healing.

   ▪ Many investigators have reported that closed reduction usually cannot be accomplished after 48 hours. However, others have reported closed reductions as late as 4 and 5 days after the injury.[4]

▪ Physeal fractures are reduced in the same manner as dislocations, with immobilization in a figure 8 strap for 4 weeks to protect stable reductions. Fractures that cannot be reduced and are being managed nonoperatively are treated with a figure 8 strap or a sling for comfort and mobilized as symptoms permit.

SURGICAL MANAGEMENT

▪ A posterior displacement of the medial clavicle that is irreducible or redislocates after closed reduction is a well-accepted surgical indication.

▪ More controversial is anterior displacement that fails to maintain a stable reduction.

   ▪ Although the traditional treatment for persistent anterior displacement is nonoperative, extreme displacement can result in abundant heterotopic bone formation with accompanying pain, limited motion, and extraordinary deformity.

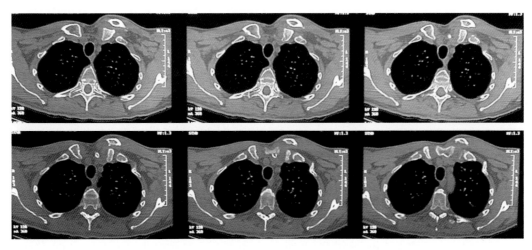

FIG 5 • CT scans of a 6-month-old medial clavicle fracture demonstrate anterior displacement without significant healing.

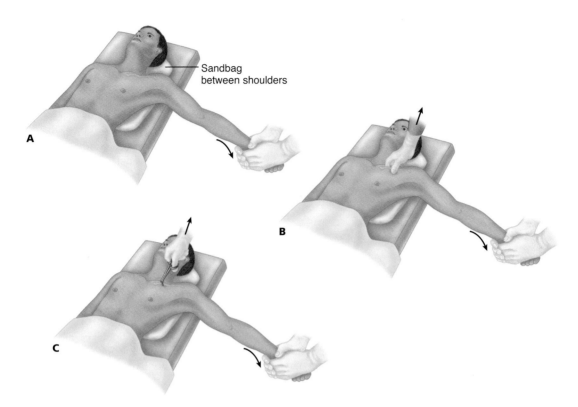

FIG 6 • Technique for closed reduction of the sternoclavicular joint. **A.** The patient is positioned supine with a sandbag placed between the two shoulders. Traction is then applied to the arm against countertraction in an abducted and slightly extended position. In anterior dislocations, direct pressure over the medial end of the clavicle may reduce the joint. **B.** In posterior dislocations, in addition to the traction it may be necessary to manipulate the medial end of the clavicle with the fingers to dislodge the clavicle from behind the manubrium. **C.** In stubborn posterior dislocations, it may be necessary to prepare the medial end of the clavicle sterilely and use a towel clip to grasp around the medial clavicle to lift it back into position.

■ We now consider operative treatment when the entire medial clavicle is torn out of the deltotrapezial sleeve.

Preoperative Planning

■ Careful review of the history and examination for symptoms of mediastinal compression is crucial.

■ Review of the CT scan for the direction and degree of displacement and determination of a very medial fracture versus pure dislocation follows.

■ If history or radiographic evidence of mediastinal compromise or potential compromise is present, a cardiothoracic surgeon should be either present or readily available.

■ Very medial fractures can occasionally be repaired with independent small-fragment lag screws or orthogonal minifragment plates. For pure dislocations, heavy nonabsorbable suture will sometimes suffice. Suture anchors are useful for augmenting ligament repairs. Allograft tendons may be used if the capsule is irreparable and must be reconstructed.

■ Closed reduction under anesthesia is then attempted and the stability of the joint is evaluated after reduction.

Positioning

■ To begin, the patient is positioned supine on the table, and three or four towels or a sandbag placed between the scapulae.

■ The upper extremity should be draped free so that lateral traction can be applied during the open reduction.

■ A folded sheet may be left in place around the patient's thorax so that it can be used for countertraction.

■ If there is concern regarding the mediastinum, the entire sternum should be draped into the field.

Approach

■ An anterior incision that parallels the superior border of the medial 3 to 4 inches of the clavicle and then extends downward over the sternum just medial to the involved sternoclavicular joint is used (**FIG 7A**).

■ As an alternative, a necklace-type incision may be created in Langer's lines, beginning at the midline and sweeping lateral and up along the clavicle.

■ Careful subperiosteal dissection around the medial clavicle and onto the surface of the manubrium allows exposure of the articular surfaces.

■ If the medial clavicle is resting posteriorly, it is safer to identify the shaft more laterally and then trace it back medially along the subperiosteal plane (**FIG 7B**).

■ Traction and blunt retractors can then be used to lever the medial clavicle back up into its anatomic location (**FIG 7C**). These retractors may be used behind the medial clavicle and manubrium to protect the posterior structures.

■ If one has chosen to operate on an anterior medial clavicle because of extreme displacement, it may generally be simply pushed back into place.

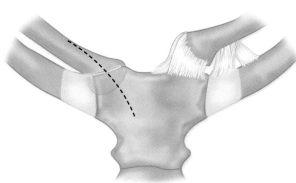

FIG 7 • **A.** Proposed skin incision for open reduction of a posterior dislocation. **B.** Subperiosteal exposure of the medial clavicle shows a posteriorly displaced medial clavicular shaft (*left*) resting posterior to the medial clavicular physis (*arrow, right*). **C.** The medial shaft of the clavicle has been lifted anteriorly with a clamp and now rests adjacent to the medial physis (*arrow, right*).

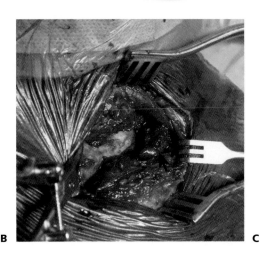

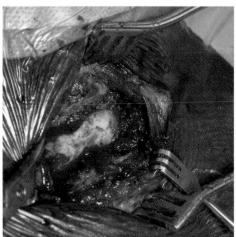

PRIMARY REPAIR: MEDIAL FRACTURE

- In children and in young adults, the dislocation of the medial clavicle may occur through the medial physis or as a fracture, leaving a small amount of bone articulating with the manubrium.
- Because much of the capsule remains intact to this medial fragment, it can serve as an anchor for internal fixation of the medial clavicle shaft. Depending on the amount of bone, the type of fixation will vary.

- The smallest fragments will permit only osseous suture fixation, but the medial clavicle is cancellous bone and heals very quickly (**TECH FIG 1A**).
- As the fragment gets larger, independent lag screw fixation may be possible (**TECH FIG 1B,C**).
- For very medial shaft fractures, it may even be possible to use two orthogonal miniframe plates.

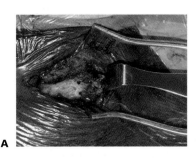

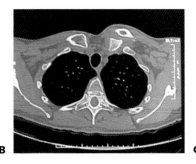

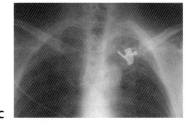

TECH FIG 1 • A. Heavy nonabsorbable suture has been placed through drill holes in the medial clavicle and through the physis to secure the fracture shown in Figure 7B,C. **B,C.** A symptomatic medial clavicle nonunion had a medial fragment large enough to allow fixation with three cortical lag screws.

TECHNIQUES

PRIMARY REPAIR: CAPSULAR LIGAMENTS AND SUTURE AUGMENTATION

- After reduction, the ligaments may be repaired primarily with heavy nonabsorbable suture. This usually allows repair of the anterior and superior capsule, but, for obvious reasons, does not allow repair of the important posterior capsule.
- The reduction is often reinforced with either simple osseous sutures through drill holes in the medial clavicle and manubrium[27,28] or with suture anchors[18] (**TECH FIG 2**). The costoclavicular ligament may also occasionally be repaired primarily.
- This technique has generally been employed in children but may also be used in adults.

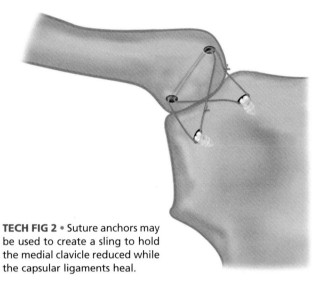

TECH FIG 2 • Suture anchors may be used to create a sling to hold the medial clavicle reduced while the capsular ligaments heal.

IMMEDIATE RECONSTRUCTION: CAPSULAR LIGAMENTS

- At times the joint may be reducible but the ligaments are damaged to the point where primary repair is not feasible. In this circumstance, the ligaments may be immediately reconstructed using tendon graft.
- This may be done by passing a tendon from the front of the sternum, through the articular surfaces and intra-articular disc, and out the front of the medial clavicle and tying the tendon to itself anteriorly.[20] Autograft or allograft tendon may be used.
- The capsule may also be reconstructed in the manner described by Spencer and Kuhn[25] (**TECH FIG 3**).
  - Drill holes 4 mm in diameter are created from anterior to posterior through the medial clavicle and the adjacent manubrium.
  - A free semitendinosus tendon graft is woven through the drill holes so the tendon strands are parallel to each other posterior to the joint and cross each other anterior to it.
  - The tendon is tied in a square knot and secured with no. 2 Ethibond suture.
  - This technique has the advantage of reconstructing both the anterior and the posterior ligament in a very strong and secure manner.

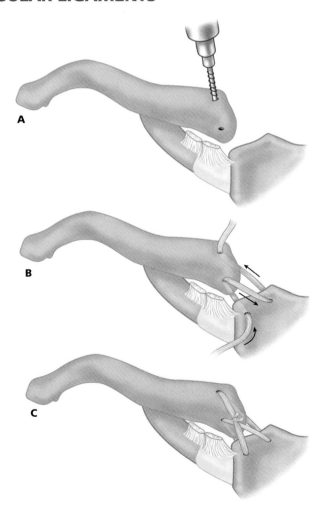

TECH FIG 3 • **A.** Semitendinosus may be used to reconstruct the capsular ligaments. **B,C.** The allograft tendon is pulled through the medial clavicle (*left*) and manubrium (*right*) and tied. *(continued)*

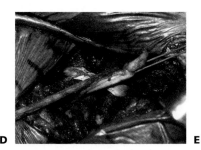 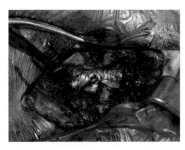

TECH FIG 3 • *(continued)* **D,E.** Intraoperative images showing the technique illustrated in **B** and **C.** (**A–C,** After Spencer EE Jr, Kuhn JE. Biomechanical analysis of reconstructions for sternoclavicular joint instability. J Bone Joint Surg Am 2004;86A:98–105.)

MEDIAL CLAVICLE RESECTION AND LIGAMENT RECONSTRUCTION

- If there is concern about the stability of a reconstruction or repair, if the dislocation is subacute and posterior, or if there is a question of impingement on the mediastinal structures, one may elect to resect the medial clavicle entirely. In this situation, it is important to repair or reconstruct the costoclavicular ligament (akin to a modified Weaver-Dunn procedure).
- The medullary canal can also be used to create an attachment point for an additional medial tether. We prefer to use the patient's own tissue, such as the sternoclavicular ligament, whenever possible (**TECH FIG 4**).

- The medial clavicle is resected and the canal curetted and prepared with drill holes on the superior surface.
- Grasping suture is woven through the remaining ligament, pulled through the superior drill holes, and tied over bone.
- Heavy nonabsorbable sutures are then passed through the remaining costoclavicular ligament and around the clavicle, and the periosteal tube is closed.
- If adequate local tissue is not present, an allograft such as Achilles tendon may also be used.[2]

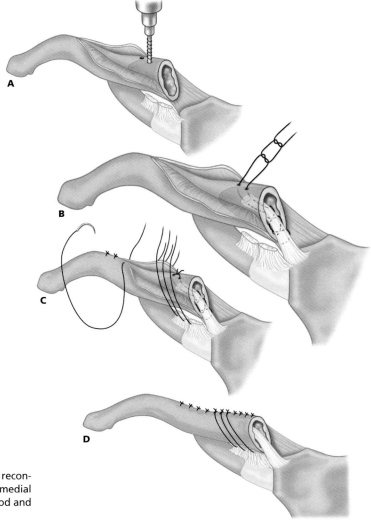

TECH FIG 4 • The residual capsule may be used to reconstruct a medial clavicular restraint, akin to a medial Weaver-Dunn procedure, as described by Rockwood and Wirth.[23]

REDUCTION AND BALSER PLATE FIXATION

- The use of K-wires around the sternoclavicular joint has been routinely condemned, and they should not be used.
  - There are reports, however, of temporary plate fixation from the medial clavicle to the sternum to maintain a reduced joint while the soft tissues heal.
- The Balser plate is a hook plate used in Europe for treatment of acromioclavicular joint separations and distal clavicle fractures. It has been used for sternoclavicular dislocations by placing the hook into the sternum and using screws to fix the plate onto the medial clavicle (**TECH FIG 5**).
  - Franck et al[12] published good results for 10 patients treated with Balser plates. They thought that the stability of this construct allowed a more rapid rehabilitation. The implant is quite bulky and removal is generally required.

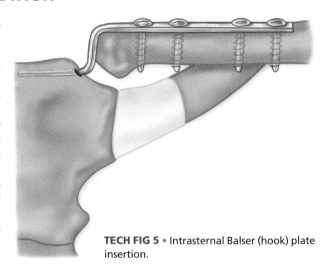

TECH FIG 5 • Intrasternal Balser (hook) plate insertion.

PEARLS AND PITFALLS

Diagnosis	▪ Conventional studies are unreliable. A high index of suspicion, a thorough examination, and a prompt CT scan will ensure correct diagnosis.
Individualize treatment when necessary	▪ Although anterior dislocations are generally treated nonoperatively, a severely anteriorly displaced medial clavicle may be reduced and fixed acutely, with a low risk of complications, in a reliable patient. ▪ Posterior dislocations generally mandate surgery because delayed impingement on mediastinal contents may occur. However, there may be situations where displacement is mild and chronic and the risks of surgery may outweigh the benefits.
Prepare for complications	▪ Although complications are uncommon, they are spectacular, and not in a good way. The surgeon needs to be ready for both pneumothorax and the unlikely possibility of a vascular injury. A cardiothoracic surgeon should be immediately available.
Use the medial clavicle	▪ Even a medial epiphysis or a tiny piece of medial clavicle in its anatomic location provides an excellent anchor for heavy suture or lag screws for primary fracture repair.
Be flexible intraoperatively	▪ Preserving the native joint is an admirable goal, but poor ligament and bone quality sometimes precludes primary repair, especially in the subacute dislocation. If the stability of the joint cannot be ensured, medial clavicle resection and costoclavicular reconstruction should be strongly considered.

POSTOPERATIVE CARE

- For sternoclavicular strains and anteriorly dislocated medial clavicles accepted in this position, a sling or figure 8 strap is prescribed and the patient is allowed to mobilize the extremity as function permits.
- Medial clavicle fractures that are stable after reduction are immobilized in a figure 8 strap for 4 to 6 weeks and then mobilized as comfort allows.
- Acute dislocations that have been reduced and are stable or have been surgically repaired receive a sling or figure 8 strap for 6 weeks to protect the reduction and allow ligament healing.
- Patients in the figure 8 strap are allowed use of the elbow and hand with the arm at the side for light activities of daily living, but the strap is conscientiously maintained.
- At 4 to 6 weeks they move to a sling and perform their own mobilization. Because the glenohumeral joint is unaffected, motion usually returns quickly to near full range.

- When full range of motion has been obtained, gentle progressive strengthening and resumption of normal activities commence.
- In general, patients treated with joint preservation can return to all activities, including heavy labor, but we have seen traumatic failure of costoclavicular reconstructions and do ask patients who have undergone medial clavicle resection and ligament reconstruction to avoid heavy overhead labor for their lifetimes.

OUTCOMES

- A recent Medline search for "sternoclavicular" and "dislocation" yielded 320 citations, most dealing with sternoclavicular instability and its sequelae. Most were case reports, a series of three or four patients, or a discussion of the complications of the injury or its treatment. There are very few large series, which makes discussing outcomes difficult. However, several themes do emerge.

- The need for proper patient selection becomes evident when one considers that some forms of sternoclavicular instability generally do well when treated without surgery.
  - Sadr and Swann[24] and Rockwood and Odor[22] have both documented the good long-term results obtained with nonoperative treatment of atraumatic sternoclavicular instability.
  - De Jong[7] has documented good long-term results in 13 patients with anterior dislocations treated nonoperatively.
- Several larger series[9,11,29] have reported on about a dozen patients treated with open reduction, ligament repair or reconstruction, and fixation with pins or sternoclavicular wiring. Good results were obtained when the medial clavicle was successfully stabilized.
  - Eskola,[10] however, noted a high failure rate if the remaining medial clavicle was not successfully stabilized to the first rib.
  - In a separate study, Rockwood et al[21] reported on seven patients who had previously undergone medial clavicle resection without ligament reconstruction. Six of the seven had worse symptoms than before their index procedure.

COMPLICATIONS

- Complications of injury
  - Anterior dislocation: cosmetic "bump" (which may occasionally be pronounced) and late degenerative changes
  - Posterior dislocation: Great vessel injuries, including laceration, compression, and occlusion, pneumothorax, rupture of the esophagus with abscess and osteomyelitis of the clavicle, fatal tracheoesophageal fistula, brachial plexus compression, stridor and dysphagia, hoarseness of the voice, onset of snoring, and voice changes from normal to falsetto with movement of the arm have all been reported. These all may occur acutely or in a delayed fashion.
  - Worman and Leagus[30] reported that 16 of 60 patients with posterior dislocations had suffered complications of the trachea, esophagus, or great vessels.
- Errors of patient selection
  - Operating in unindicated circumstances introduces another set of complications. Rockwood and Odor[22] reviewed 37 patients with spontaneous atraumatic subluxation.
  - Twenty-nine managed without surgery had no limitations of activity or lifestyle at over 8 years average follow-up. Eight treated (elsewhere) with surgical reconstruction had increased pain, limitation of activity, alteration of lifestyle, persistent instability, and significant scars.
  - Before surgery, most of these patients had minimal discomfort and excellent motion and complained only of a "bump" that slipped in and out of place with certain motions.
- Intraoperative complications
  - Little has been written about these, but a veritable jungle of vitally important structures lurks immediately behind the sternoclavicular joint. We always perform these operations with an available, in-house cardiothoracic surgeon on notice and request his or her presence in the operating suite for all but the most routine cases.
- Postoperative complications
  - Hardware migration: Because of the motion at the sternoclavicular joint, tremendous leverage is applied to pins that cross it; fatigue breakage of the pins is common. Numerous authors have reported deaths and many near-deaths from K-wires and Steinmann pins migrating into the heart, pulmonary artery, innominate artery, aorta, and elsewhere in the mediastinum. Despite numerous admonitions in the literature regarding the use of sternoclavicular pins, there have been continued reports of intrathoracic K-wire migration, most recently in 2005.[17]
  - For this reason, we do not recommend the use of any transfixing pins—large or small, smooth or threaded, bent or straight—across the sternoclavicular joint.
  - Iatrogenic instability: Failure to preserve the costoclavicular ligament when it is intact and failure to reconstruct it when it is deficient both severely compromise the surgical result. As noted above, both Rockwood[21] and Eskola[10] noted vastly inferior results when the residual medial clavicle was not stabilized to the first rib, and an inability to obtain equivalent results when the costoclavicular ligament was reconstructed in a delayed fashion.
  - Iatrogenic instability: An excessive resection that removes bone to a point lateral to the costoclavicular ligament is an extremely difficult problem that is best avoided because there is no reconstructive option. In these difficult cases, we have occasionally performed a subtotal claviculectomy to a point just medial to the coracoclavicular ligaments. This leaves the extremity without a "strut" connecting it to the thorax but can produce substantial relief of pain and improvement in motion and activity.

REFERENCES

1. Bearn JG. Direct observations on the function of the capsule of the sternoclavicular joint in the clavicular support. J Anat 1967;101: 159–170.
2. Battaglia TC, Pannunzio ME, Chhabra AB, et al. Interposition arthroplasty with bone-tendon allograft: a technique for treatment of the unstable sternoclavicular joint. J Orthop Trauma 2005;19:124–129.
3. Brooks AL, Henning CD. Injury to the proximal clavicular epiphysis [abstract]. J Bone Joint Surg Am 1972;54A:1347–1348.
4. Buckerfield CT, Castle ME. Acute traumatic retrosternal dislocation of the clavicle. J Bone Joint Surg Am 1984;66A:379–385.
5. Cave AJE. The nature and morphology of the costoclavicular ligament. J Anat 1961;95:170–179.
6. Cave EF. Fractures and Other Injuries. Chicago: Year Book Medical Publishers, 1958.
7. De Jong KP, Sukul DM. Anterior sternoclavicular dislocation: a long-term follow-up study. J Orthop Trauma 1990;4:420–423.
8. Denham RH Jr, Dingley AF Jr. Epiphyseal separation of the medial end of the clavicle. J Bone Joint Surg Am 1967;49A:1179–1183.
9. Eskola A, Vainionpaa S, Vastamki M, et al. Operation of old sternoclavicular dislocation: results in 12 cases. J Bone Joint Surg Br 1989; 71B:63–65.
10. Eskola A. Sternoclavicular dislocations: a plea for open treatment. Acta Orthop Scand 1986;57:227–228.
11. Ferrandez L, Yubero J, Usabiaga J, et al. Sternoclavicular dislocation, treatment and complications. Ital J Orthop Traumatol 1988;14: 349–355.
12. Franck WM, Jannasch O, Siassi M, et al. Balser plate stabilization: an alternate therapy for traumatic sternoclavicular instability. J Shoulder Elbow Surg 2003;12:276–281.
13. Franck WM, Siassi RM, Hennig FF. Treatment of posterior epiphyseal disruption of the medial clavicle with a modified Balser plate. J Trauma 2003;55:966–968.
14. Gray H. Osteology. In: Goss CM, ed. Anatomy of the Human Body, ed 28. Philadelphia: Lea & Febiger, 1966:324–326.
15. Grant JCB. Method of Anatomy, ed 7. Baltimore: Williams & Wilkins, 1965.
16. Hsu HC, Wu JJ, Lo WH, et al. Epiphyseal fracture–retrosternal dislocation of the medial end of the clavicle: a case report. Chinese Med J 1993;52:198–202.
17. Kamiyoshihara M, Kakegawa S, Otani Y, et al. Video-assisted thoracoscopic surgery for migration of an orthopedic fixation wire in the

mediastinum: report of a case [in Japanese]. Kyobu Geka 2005; 58:403–405.

18. Mirza AH, Alam K, Ali A. Posterior sternoclavicular dislocation in a rugby player as a cause of silent vascular compromise: a case report. Br J Sports Med 2005;39:e28.

19. Nettles JL, Linscheid R. Sternoclavicular dislocations. J Trauma 1968;8:158–164.

20. Qureshi SA, Shah AK, Pruzansky ME. Using the semitendinosus tendon to stabilize sternoclavicular joints in a patient with Ehlers-Danlos syndrome: a case report. Am J Orthop 2005;34:315–318.

21. Rockwood CA Jr, Groh GI, Wirth MA, et al. Resection-arthroplasty of the sternoclavicular joint. J Bone Joint Surg Am 1997;79A:387.

22. Rockwood CA Jr, Odor JM. Spontaneous atraumatic anterior subluxation of the sternoclavicular joint. J Bone Joint Surg Am 1989; 71A:1280–1288.

23. Rockwood CA, Wirth MA. Disorders of the sternoclavicular joint. In: Rockwood CA, Matsen FA, eds. The Shoulder, ed 2. Philadelphia: WB Saunders, 1998:555–609.

24. Sadr B, Swann M. Spontaneous dislocation of the sternoclavicular joint. Acta Orthop Scand 1979;50:269–274.

25. Spencer EE Jr, Kuhn JE. Biomechanical analysis of reconstructions for sternoclavicular joint instability. J Bone Joint Surg Am 2004; 86A:98–105.

26. Spencer EE, Kuhn JE, Huston LJ, Carpenter JE, et al. Ligamentous restraints to anterior and posterior translation of the sternoclavicular joint. J Shoulder Elbow Surg 2002;11:43–47.

27. Thacker MM, Patankar JV, Goregaonkar AB. A safe technique for sternoclavicular stabilization. Am J Orthop 2006;35:64–66.

28. Waters PM, Bae DS, Kadiyala RK. Short-term outcomes after surgical treatment of traumatic posterior sternoclavicular fracture-dislocations in children and adolescents. J Pediatr Orthop 2003;23: 464–469.

29. Witvoet J, Martinez B. Treatment of anterior sternoclavicular dislocations: apropos of 18 cases. Rev Chir Orthop Reparatrice Appar Mot 1982;68:311–316.

30. Worman LW, Leagus C. Intrathoracic injury following retrosternal dislocation of the clavicle. J Trauma 1967;7:416–423.

31. Zaslav KR, Ray S, Neer CS. Conservative management of a displaced medial clavicular physeal injury in an adolescent athlete. Am J Sports Med 1989;17:833–836.

Chapter 13

Medial Clavicle Excision and Sternoclavicular Joint Reconstruction

John E. Kuhn

DEFINITION

- Many pathologic disorders affect the medial clavicle, the most common of which is osteoarthritis.
  - Other conditions include rheumatoid arthritis, seronegative spondyloarthropathies, crystal deposition disease, sternoclavicular hyperostosis, condensing osteitis, and avascular necrosis.[6]
- Infection, while rare, must be considered. When suspected, the sternoclavicular joint should be aspirated for culture, Gram stain, and cell counts and then treated with irrigation and débridement.
- Instability of the sternoclavicular joint is rare but potentially fatal.
- Traumatic instability is defined by the direction of displacement of the clavicular head and is superior, anterior, or posterior.
- Posterior instability has been associated with a variety of potentially fatal comorbidities.
- Atraumatic instability is usually anterior and is often seen in people with generalized ligamentous laxity.
- Symptomatic traumatic instability is best treated with closed reduction and possible reconstruction of the joint, not resection of the clavicle head.

ANATOMY

- The sternoclavicular joint is a saddle-shaped joint that is the most unconstrained joint in the human body.
- Important ligamentous restraints to motion include the anterior capsule (restrains anterior and posterior translation), the posterior capsule (restrains posterior translation),[10] and the costoclavicular ligament (which is the pivot point for motion in the axial plane).[2]
  - The interclavicular ligament seems to provide little function (**FIG 1**).

PATHOGENESIS

- Osteoarthritis is the most common disorder affecting the medial clavicle that may require surgical excision.
- Osteoarthritis is most commonly seen in male laborers, in women in the perimenopausal years, and after radical neck dissection.
- Rheumatologic disorders can affect the sternoclavicular joint as part of the systemic disease. Involvement of the sternoclavicular joint is usually late.
- Other atraumatic conditions are less common and the pathogenesis is largely unknown.
- Traumatic instability typically develops from a blow to the shoulder girdle.
  - If the force impacts the anterior shoulder, it will push the shoulder girdle posteriorly. The clavicle pivots over the first rib, forcing the head of the clavicle anteriorly.

- If the force impacts the posterior shoulder, it will push the shoulder girdle anteriorly. The clavicle pivots over the first rib, dislocating the head of the clavicle posteriorly.
- Direct blows to the sternoclavicular joint can also dislocate the clavicle head posteriorly.
- Atraumatic instability develops insidiously without a history of trauma.

NATURAL HISTORY

- Many people have asymptomatic sternoclavicular joint arthritis.
- Patients with symptoms may find relief with activity modification and time. This is particularly true with the pain and swelling seen in perimenopausal women.
- Infection may present with a relatively benign clinical picture but will progress and may become serious.
- It is rare for the sternoclavicular joint to be the primary joint involved in rheumatologic conditions or crystal deposition disease.

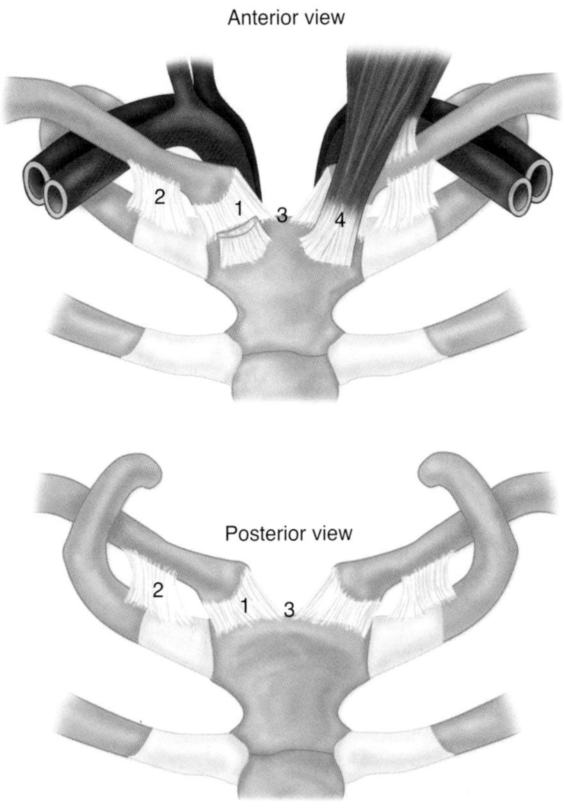

FIG 1 • Anterior and posterior anatomy of sternoclavicular joint. *1*, capsule; *2*, costoclavicular ligament; *3*, interclavicular ligament; *4*, sternocleidomastoid tendon.

Table 1	Clinical Features of Atraumatic Disorders of the Sternoclavicular Joint					
Disorder	**Age (yr)**	**Gender**	**Side**	**Pain**	**Erythema**	**Associated Conditions and Risk Factors**
Osteoarthritis	>40	M=F	B	+	Rare	Manual labor, radical neck dissection, postmenopausal women
Rheumatoid arthritis	Any	F>M	B	+	+	Symmetric polyarthritis
Seronegative spondyloarthropathies	<40	M>F	B	Occasional	−	Urethritis, uveitis, nail pitting
Septic arthritis	Any	M=F	U	+++	+++	HIV, IVDA, DM
Crystal deposition disease	>40	M>F	U	+++ during flare	++	Other joint involvement
Sternoclavicular hyperostosis	30–60	M>F	B	+	−	Synovitis, acne, pustulosis, hyperostosis, osteitis
Condensing osteitis	25–40	F>M	U	+	−	None
Friedreich's disease	Any	F>M	U	+	−	None
Atraumatic subluxation	10–30	F>M	U	Infrequent	−	Generalized ligamentous laxity

DM, diabetes mellitus; F, female; IVDA, intravenous drug abuse; M, male.

- Traumatic instability may result from high-energy injuries (eg, motor vehicle collision) or may be related to contact in athletics.
- Posterior instability may be life-threatening as the clavicular head may compress vascular structures, the trachea, or the esophagus.
- Atraumatic instability may have an insidious onset and is often associated with other signs of generalized ligamentous laxity (eg, patellar subluxation, glenohumeral subluxation).

PATIENT HISTORY AND PHYSICAL FINDINGS

- Atraumatic disorders
  - Pain at the sternoclavicular joint is localized to the joint and may be referred up the sternocleidomastoid and trapezius.[5]
  - Infection typically is unilateral and has significant pain and erythema (Table 1).
  - Osteoarthritis, rheumatoid arthritis, seronegative spondyloarthropathies, and sternoclavicular hyperostosis are typically bilateral, with mild pain, and rare erythema.
  - Crystal deposition diseases, condensing osteitis, and Friedreich's disease are typically unilateral, and mildly painful.
- Traumatic disorders
  - With acute traumatic injuries, patients will have significant pain and will be unwilling to raise the arm. They may describe difficulty with swallowing or breathing in posterior dislocations.
  - The sternoclavicular joint is often swollen and tender.
  - The affected arm may demonstrate circulatory changes with arm swelling.
  - Physical examination may not be helpful in determining if the instability is anterior or posterior.

IMAGING AND OTHER DIAGNOSTIC STUDIES

- Special radiographic projections include the Rockwood (serendipity), Hobbs, Heinig, and Kattan views but are somewhat difficult to interpret (Table 2).[4]
- Computed tomography is particularly useful in trauma as it demonstrates displacement of the joint and bony anatomy.[4]

It very useful to determine whether a dislocation is anterior or posterior.
- Arteriography should be considered in posterior dislocations if vascular injury is suspected.
- MRI is helpful in atraumatic disorders to evaluate the soft tissues and can delineate marrow abnormalities, joint effusions, and disc and cartilage injury.[4]
- Laboratory findings in atraumatic disorders of the sternoclavicular joint are covered in Table 3.

DIFFERENTIAL DIAGNOSIS

- Atraumatic disorders
  - Osteoarthritis
  - Rheumatoid or other serologic arthritis
  - Seronegative spondyloarthropathies
  - Crystal deposition disease
  - Sternoclavicular hyperostosis
  - Condensing osteitis
  - Avascular necrosis
  - Septic arthritis
  - Instability

Table 2	Radiographic Features of Atraumatic Disorders of the Sternoclavicular Joint
Disorder	**Radiographic Findings**
Osteoarthritis	Sclerosis, osteophytes
Rheumatoid arthritis	Minimal change
Seronegative spondyloarthropathies	Marginal erosions, cysts
Septic arthritis	Sclerotic, lytic, or mixed lesions
Crystal deposition disease	Calcification of soft tissue
Sternoclavicular hyperostosis	Hyperostosis, ossification of intercostal ligaments
Condensing osteitis	Medial clavicle enlargement, preserved joint space, marrow obliteration
Friedreich's disease	Irregular end of medial clavicle
Atraumatic subluxation	Normal

Table 3	Laboratory Features of Atraumatic Disorders of the Sternoclavicular Joint	
Disorder	**Laboratory Findings**	
Osteoarthritis	Normal	
Rheumatoid arthritis	May have +RF, +ANA,	
Seronegative sponyloarthropathies	+HLA-B27	
Septic arthritis	WBC, ESR, CRP elevated	
Crystal deposition disease	+BRFC, -BRFC	
Sternoclavicular Hyperostosis	ESR elevated, other markers of rheumatologic disease normal	
Condensing osteitis	Normal	
Friedrich's disease	Normal	
Atraumatic subluxation	Normal	

ANA, antinuclear antibodies; BRFC, birefringement crystals; CRP, C-reactive protein; ESR, sedimentation rate; RF, rheumatoid factor; WBC, white blood cell count.

- Traumatic disorders
  - Medial-third clavicle fracture
  - Sternal fracture
  - First rib fracture

NONOPERATIVE MANAGEMENT

- Most atraumatic conditions can be managed nonoperatively.
- Nonoperative management includes nonsteroidal anti-inflammatories (NSAIDs) and rest. Sometimes topical lidocaine patches can help with pain.
- Acute dislocations should undergo closed reduction.
- In posterior dislocations, open reduction and possible reconstruction of the joint is indicated if closed reduction fails.

SURGICAL MANAGEMENT

- Surgery is indicated for atraumatic disorders of the sternoclavicular joint in every case of septic arthritis and when nonoperative management fails for the other conditions listed in the differential diagnosis.
- When infection is suspected, surgeons should perform incision and drainage quickly to prevent late osteomyelitis.
- Contraindications for resection of the medial clavicle include atraumatic instability of the joint.
- Acute dislocations should undergo closed reduction.
- In posterior dislocations, open reduction and possible reconstruction of the joint is indicated if closed reduction fails.

Preoperative Planning

- Due to the vital structures that lie behind the sternoclavicular joint, it is important to have a thoracic surgeon available should complications develop.

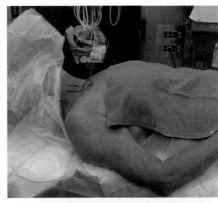

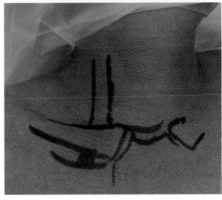

FIG 2 • **A.** Patient positioning. **B.** Anatomy is identified and marked.

Positioning

- The patient is positioned supine on the operating room table with a small rolled towel behind the middle of the back (**FIG 2A**).
- The entire chest is exposed for treatment of complications should they occur.
- Important structures, including the clavicle, manubrium, sternocleidomastoid, and costoclavicular ligament, are marked (**FIG 2B**).
- The ipsilateral hand is prepared and draped as well if the surgeon desires to use palmaris as an interposition graft.
- For reconstructions of the sternoclavicular joint, an ipsilateral hamstring may be used; as such, the knee should be prepared and draped.

Approach

- The approach is anterior. Care is taken to protect important structures during dissection, particularly the origin of the sternocleidomastoid muscle and the costoclavicular ligament.

INCISION AND DISSECTION

- The incision is made in the lines of Langer, which follow a necklace pattern over the head of the clavicle and manubrium (**TECH FIG 1A**).
- After undermining in the subcutaneous plane, the platysma is incised in line with the skin incision, exposing the joint capsule and sternocleidomastoid origin (**TECH FIG 1B**).
- The capsule of the joint is marked. Care must be taken to avoid incising the entire sternal head of the sternocleidomastoid tendon (**TECH FIG 1C**).

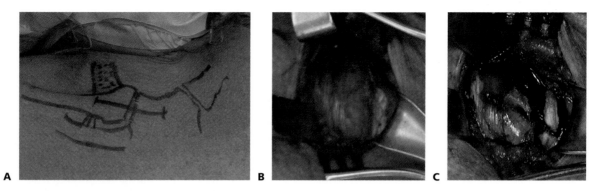

TECH FIG 1 • **A.** Location of incision. **B.** Incision of platysma. **C.** Incision in joint capsule.

ATRAUMATIC DISORDERS: REMOVING THE BONE

- Electrocautery can be used to carefully elevate the capsule from the clavicular head. It is important to avoid straying too far laterally to avoid detaching the capsule and injuring the costoclavicular ligament (**TECH FIG 2A**).
- The intra-articular disc is removed and the capsule is carefully dissected around the cartilaginous margin of the head of the clavicle (**TECH FIG 2B**).
- A self-retaining retractor is placed on the capsule, a blunt retractor is placed next to the articular surface, and

a small oscillating saw is used to remove between 0.5 and 1.0 cm of the medial clavicle (**TECH FIG 2C**).
- An osteotome may be used to lever the medial clavicle head out of the joint (**TECH FIG 2D**).
- Electrocautery is used to carefully dissect the posterior capsule from the back of the clavicular head (**TECH FIG 2E**).
- The resected head should be between 0.5 and 1.0 cm in size to preserve the costoclavicular ligaments (**TECH FIG 2F**).[3]

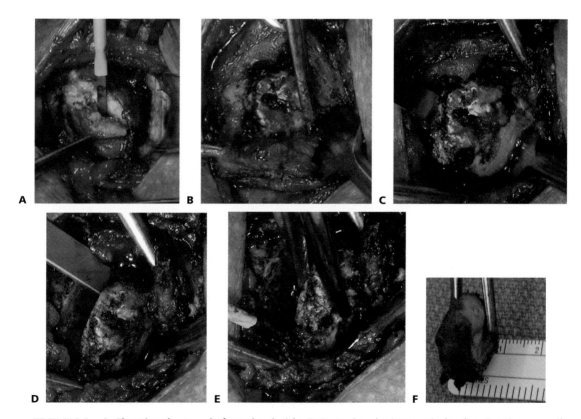

TECH FIG 2 • **A.** Elevating the capsule from the clavicle. **B.** Removing the intra-articular disc. **C.** Using an oscillating saw to remove the medial clavicle. **D.** Levering the medial clavicle from the joint. **E.** Removing the posterior soft tissue attachments. **F.** The excised medial clavicle.

TECHNIQUES

HARVESTING THE TENDON

- The palmaris tendon is isolated with a small incision in the wrist crease (**TECH FIG 3A**).
- After sutures are passed in the end of the palmaris, the tendon is removed percutaneously with a tendon stripper (**TECH FIG 3B**).
- The harvested tendon is rolled over a small spool and sutured to itself to create a rolled tendon (**TECH FIG 3C,D**).

- When resecting the clavicular head for atraumatic disorders, the rolled palmaris tendon is inserted into the defect to create a soft tissue interposition between the cut surface of the clavicle and the manubrial joint surface (**TECH FIG 3E**).
- Alternatively, the palmaris can be used to augment a reconstruction of an unstable sternoclavicular joint by passing it around the clavicle and first rib (see below).

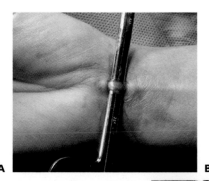
A

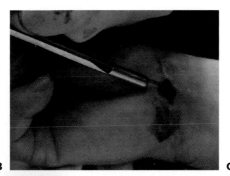
B

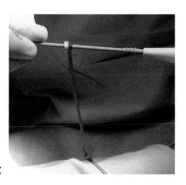
C

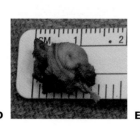
D

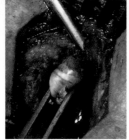
E

TECH FIG 3 • A. Palmaris tendon is identified. **B.** Percutaneous harvesting of palmaris longus tendon. **C.** Rolling the palmaris tendon graft. **D.** The rolled palmaris is sutured to itself. **E.** Insertion of the palmaris as interposition graft.

RECONSTRUCTION OF THE STERNOCLAVICULAR JOINT IN INSTABILITY

- A variety of techniques have been described. A figure 8 reconstruction has the best biomechanical properties.[11]
- With the assistance of a thoracic surgeon, the plane behind the manubrium is developed by dissecting above the sternal notch (**TECH FIG 4A**).
- With a ribbon retractor behind the manubrium, two drill holes are made in the manubrium and sutures are passed (**TECH FIG 4B**).

- Two drill holes are placed in the medial clavicle from anterior to posterior (**TECH FIG 4C**).
- The semitendinosus autograft is passed in figure 8 fashion and secured to itself (**TECH FIG 4D–F**).
- Additionally, the palmaris tendon may be passed around the first rib. This dissection behind the first rib should be performed by the thoracic surgeon to avoid injury to the internal mammary artery (**TECH FIG 4G**).

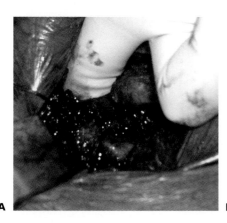
A

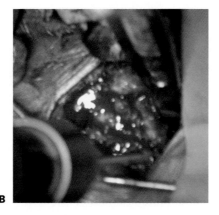
B

TECH FIG 4 • A. Development of the surgical plane behind manubrium. **B.** Drill holes are in manubrium with protection of mediastinal structures with an Army-Navy retractor. *(continued)*

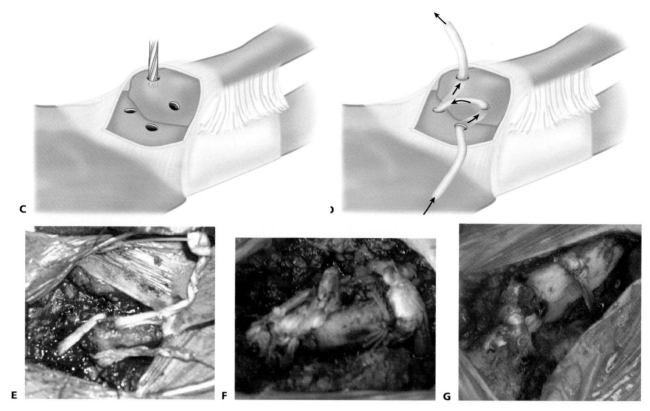

C

)

E F G

:CH FIG 4 • *(continued)* **C.** Drill holes in clavicle. **D–F.** Semitendinosus graft is passed in figure 8 fashion. **G.** Palmaris is passed ound clavicle and first rib for augmentation. (**C** and **D**, Adapted from Kuhn JE. Sternoclavicular joint reconstruction for an-rior and posterior sternoclavicular joint instability. In Zuckerman J, ed. Advanced Reconstruction of the Shoulder. Rosemont, : American Academy of Orthopaedic Surgeons, 2007:255–264.)

WOUND CLOSURE

- The capsule is closed with figure 8 interrupted perma-nent number 2 suture, and the sternal head of the stern-ocleidomastoid falls into place (**TECH FIG 5A**).

- The wound is closed in layers with 0 Vicryl in the platysma (**TECH FIG 5B**), 2-0 Vicryl in the subcutaneous layer, and 3-0 Monocryl in the skin (**TECH FIG 5C**).

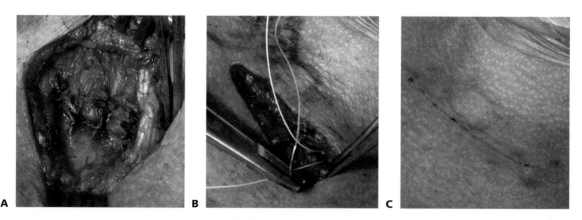

A B C

TECH FIG 5 • A. Repair of the joint capsule. **B.** Repair of the platysma. **C.** Surgical wound is closed.

PEARLS AND PITFALLS

Diagnosis	▪ CT and MRI imaging will help differentiate arthritis from other less common conditions.
	▪ The surgeon must always be diligent for infection, which may have a relatively benign appearance.
	▪ If it is unclear whether the sternoclavicular joint is the source of pain, a diagnostic injection with lidocaine can be helpful.
	▪ CT is extremely helpful to determine if a dislocation is anterior or posterior.
Removing bone	▪ Great care must be taken to avoid perforating the posterior capsule and entering the mediastinum. It is better to do a partial resection and remove residual bone with a burr.
	▪ Preserving the clavicular head is important for reconstructions of unstable sternoclavicular joints.
Preserving capsule	▪ Maintaining the integrity of the joint capsule is of critical importance. If the capsule is stripped completely off the clavicle, suture anchors in the clavicle can help restore stability.
Costoclavicular ligament	▪ If the costoclavicular ligament is sacrificed, the intra-articular disc and disc ligament can be passed into the intramedullary canal.
General surgery	▪ It is wise to have a thoracic surgeon available should complications develop in the mediastinum.

POSTOPERATIVE CARE

▪ Patients are typically admitted overnight for observation.

▪ Patients wear a sling with pillow support to support the arm when upright for 6 weeks.

▪ Patients are instructed to avoid moving the arm for 6 weeks to allow for capsular healing and preventing instability.

▪ After 6 weeks, patients gradually increase range of motion.

▪ After 12 weeks, patients can begin strengthening activities.

▪ After 16 weeks, patients have unrestricted activity.

OUTCOMES

▪ There is little reported on the outcomes after this procedure. All reports are level 4 case series.

▪ Rockwood and colleagues[9] reported that outcomes were improved if the costoclavicular ligament remained intact (eight of eight excellent with complete satisfaction). If the costoclavicular ligament was disrupted, however, the results were less predictable (three of five excellent).

▪ Arcus and associates[1] reported on 15 patients with a variety of pathologies. Sixty percent were graded as good to excellent, and 93% had significant pain relief and would have the procedure again.

▪ Pingsmann and colleagues[8] found seven of eight women with sternoclavicular joint arthritis had good to excellent results with medial clavicle excision after 31 months of follow-up.

▪ Meis and coworkers[7] modified the technique by interposing the sternal head of the sternocleidomastoid into the defect. Ten of 14 patients reported good to excellent outcomes; however, two patients reported incisional pain with head turning, and three patients had cosmesis concerns.

▪ A variety of case reports exist for other sternoclavicular joint reconstructions. To date, no reports are in the peer-reviewed literature for the figure 8 reconstruction.

COMPLICATIONS

▪ Rockwood and colleagues[9] report that patients may have severe discomfort if instability persists or develops. Consequently,

it is imperative to preserve the costoclavicular ligament. If the costoclavicular ligament is disrupted, the intra-articular disc and ligament can be transferred into the intramedullary canal of the resected clavicle. In addition, reconstructing the costoclavicular ligament with a tendon graft around the first rib should be considered.

▪ Heterotopic ossification has been reported in about half of the patients but seems to be asymptomatic.[1]

▪ Although not reported to date, complications involving the great vessels, trachea, and other mediastinal contents are possible. A thoracic surgeon should be available for assistance if required.

REFERENCES

1. Acus RW III, Bell RH, Fisher DL. Proximal clavicle excision: an analysis of results. J Shoulder Elbow Surg 1995;4:182–187.
2. Bearn JG. Direct observations on the function of the capsule of the sternoclavicular joint in clavicular support. J Anat 1967;101:159–170.
3. Bisson LJ, Dauphin N, Marzo JM. A safe zone for resection of the medial end of the clavicle. J Shoulder Elbow Surg 2003;12:592–594.
4. Ernberg LA, Potter HG. Radiographic evaluation of the acromioclavicular and sternoclavicular joints. Clin Sports Med 2003;22:255–275.
5. Hassett G, Barnsley L. Pain referral from the sternoclavicular joint: a study in normal volunteers. Rheumatology 2001;40:859–862.
6. Higgenbotham TO, Kuhn JE. Atraumatic disorders of the sternoclavicular joint. J Am Acad Orthop Surg 2005;13:138–145.
7. Meis RC, Love RB, Keene JS, et al. Operative treatment of the painful sternoclavicular joint: a new technique using interpositional arthroplasty. J Shoulder Elbow Surg 2006;15:60–66.
8. Pingsmann A, Patsalis T, Michiels I. Resection arthroplasty of the sternoclavicular joint for the treatment of primary degenerative sternoclavicular arthritis. J Bone Joint Surg Br 2002;84B:513–517.
9. Rockwood CA Jr, Groh GI, Wirth MA, et al. Resection arthroplasty of the sternoclavicular joint. J Bone Joint Surg Am 1997;79A:387–393.
10. Spencer EE, Kuhn JE, Huston LJ, et al. Ligamentous restraints to anterior and posterior translation of the sternoclavicular joint. J Shoulder Elbow Surg 2002;11:43–47.
11. Spencer EE, Kuhn JE. Biomechanical analysis of reconstructions for sternoclavicular joint instability. J Bone Joint Surg Am 2004;86A:98–108.

Chapter 14

Plate Fixation of Clavicle Fractures

David Ring and Jesse B. Jupiter

DEFINITION

- Displaced, comminuted fractures of the clavicle are at risk for nonunion and malunion[3–5,7–9] and can be considered for open reduction and internal fixation with a plate and screws.

ANATOMY

- The clavicle and scapula are tightly linked through the strong coracoclavicular and acromioclavicular ligaments and link the axial skeleton to the upper extremity.
- Clavicles are present only in brachiating animals and apparently serve to help hold the upper limb away from the trunk to enhance more global positioning and use of the limb.
- The clavicle is named for its S-shaped curvature, with an apex anteromedially and an apex posterolaterally, similar to the musical symbol clavicula. The larger medial curvature widens the space for passage of neurovascular structures from the neck into the upper extremity through the costoclavicular interval.
- The clavicle is made up of very dense trabecular bone lacking a well-defined medullary canal. In cross section, the clavicle changes gradually between a flat lateral aspect, a tubular midportion, and an expanded prismatic medial end.
- The clavicle is subcutaneous throughout its length and makes a prominent aesthetic contribution to the contour of the neck and upper part of the chest.
- The supraclavicular nerves run obliquely across the clavicle just superior to the platysma muscle and should be identified and protected during operative exposure to offset the development of hyperesthesia or dysesthesia over the chest wall.

PATHOGENESIS

- Clavicle fractures usually result from a direct blow to the point of the shoulder.
- This is usually a moderate- to high-energy injury in younger adults but can result from a low-energy fall from a standing height in an older individual.

NATURAL HISTORY

- The overall nonunion rate for diaphyseal clavicle fractures is 4.5%.[7]
- The risk of nonunion increases with age, female gender, displacement, and comminution.[7]
- The risk of nonunion for completely displaced (no apposition) and comminuted fractures is between 10% and 20% (**FIG 1**).[9]
- Malunion of the clavicle can result in shoulder girdle deformity and weakness.[3–5,9]
- Malunion and nonunion of the clavicle can result in brachial plexus compression.

PATIENT HISTORY AND PHYSICAL FINDINGS

- The mechanism and date of injury should be elicited.
- A careful neurologic examination should be performed.

- In contrast to late dysfunction of the brachial plexus after clavicular fracture, a situation in which medial cord structures are typically involved, acute injury to the brachial plexus at the time of clavicular fracture usually takes the form of a traction injury to the upper cervical roots. Such root traction injuries generally occur in the setting of high-energy trauma and have a relatively poor prognosis.
- "Tenting" of the skin by a fracture fragment is dangerous only in patients who cannot protect their skin (eg, patients who are comatose).

IMAGING AND OTHER DIAGNOSTIC STUDIES

- An anteroposterior (AP) radiograph can be supplemented by a 20- to 60-degree cephalad-tilted view.
- The so-called apical oblique view (tilted 45 degrees anterior and 20 degrees cephalad) may facilitate the diagnosis of minimally displaced fractures (eg, birth fractures, fractures in children).
- The abduction lordotic view taken with the shoulder abducted above 135 degrees and the central ray angled 25 degrees cephalad is useful in evaluating the clavicle after internal fixation. Abduction of the shoulder results in rotation of the clavicle on its longitudinal axis, which causes the plate to rotate superiorly and thereby expose the shaft of the clavicle and the fracture site under the plate.
- Computed tomography with 3D reconstructions can help understand 3D deformity.

DIFFERENTIAL DIAGNOSIS

- Lateral or medial clavicle fracture
- Acromioclavicular or sternoclavicular dislocation

NONOPERATIVE MANAGEMENT

- Closed reduction of clavicular fractures is rarely attempted because the reduction is usually unstable and no reliable means of providing external support is available.
- A simple sling provides comfort and limits activity during healing. A figure 8 bandage leaves the arm free, but it cannot improve alignment.

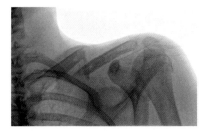

FIG 1 • An AP radiograph shows greater than 100% displacement and comminution with a vertical fracture fragment. The clavicle is shortened. (Copyright David Ring, MD.)

- There is no need to be concerned about shoulder stiffness, and patients should be encouraged keep the arm at the side and limit activity for the first 4 to 6 weeks.

SURGICAL MANAGEMENT

- Intramedullary fixation is an option when comminution is limited, but otherwise plate-and-screw fixation is preferred.
- The plate can be placed on either the superior or the anterior[1,2] aspect of the clavicle.

Preoperative Planning

- Planning of the surgery using tracings of radiographs helps limit intraoperative decision making and helps the surgeon anticipate problems and contingencies.

Positioning

- The patient is supine with a variable amount of flexion of the trunk according to surgeon preference (**FIG 2**).

Approach

- A longitudinal incision is made in line with the clavicle.

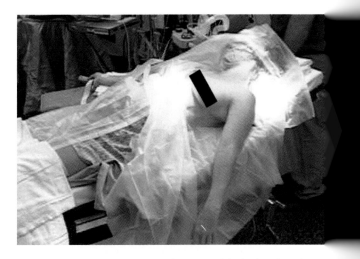

FIG 2 • The patient is positioned supine with the head and trunk elevated slightly. (Copyright David Ring, MD.)

SUPERIOR PLATE-AND-SCREW FIXATION

- An incision is made parallel and just inferior to the long axis of the clavicle (**TECH FIG 1A**). Infiltration with dilute epinephrine can help limit bleeding.
- The crossing supraclavicular nerves are identified under loupe magnification and preserved (**TECH FIG 1B**).
- Muscle attachments and periosteum are preserved as much as possible.
- Realignment and provisional fixation may be facilitated by the use of a small distractor or temporary external fixator (**TECH FIG 1C**).

- A 3.5-mm limited-contact dynamic compression plate (LCDC plate, Synthes) or a precontoured plate is applied to the superior aspect of the clavicle (**TECH FIG 1D**). A minimum of three screws should be placed in each major fragment. If the fracture pattern is amenable, placement of an interfragmentary screw greatly enhances the stability of the construct.
- When the vascularity of the fragments has been preserved, no bone graft is needed (**TECH FIG 1E**). When extensive stripping or gaps have occurred in the cortex

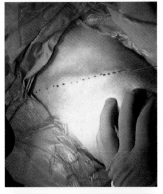
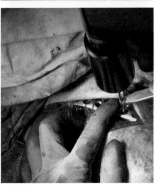
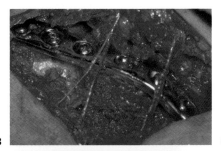
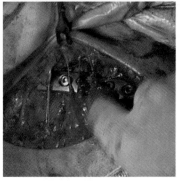
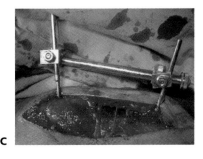

TECH FIG 1 • A. A straight incision in line with the clavicle and just inferior to it is infiltrated with dilute epinephrine. **B.** The supraclavicular nerves cross the clavicle at the level of the platysma, and an effort should be made to protect them. **C.** A small distractor or temporary external fixator can be used to facilitate realignment and provide provisional fixation. **D.** In this patient, a superior 3.5-mm LC-DCP is applied. An oscillating drill is used to limit the risk to nerves. **E.** Final plate placement. *(continued)*

TECHNIQUES

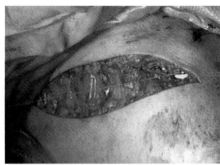

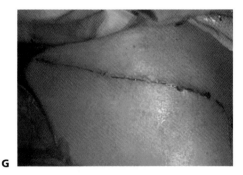

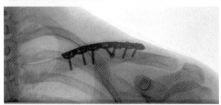

TECH FIG 1 • *(continued)* **F.** The platysma is sutured closed. **G.** A subcuticular skin closure is used. **H.** Final AP radiograph demonstrates superior plate placement with lag screw fixation of an oblique fracture line. (Copyright David Ring, MD.)

opposite the plate, one might consider adding a small amount of autogenous iliac crest cancellous bone graft.
- Close the platysma (**TECH FIG 1F**).

- If the skin condition is suitable, wound closure is accomplished in atraumatic fashion with a subcuticular suture (**TECH FIG 1G,H**).

ANTERIOR PLATE-AND-SCREW FIXATION

- The technique is identical for an anterior plate placement with the exception that the origins of the pectoralis major and deltoid are partially extraperiosteally elevated off the anterior clavicle (**TECH FIG 2**).
- The anterior plate placement may help to decrease hardware prominence, and the drill and screws are directed posterior rather than directly inferior to the clavicle, which may increase the margin of safety.

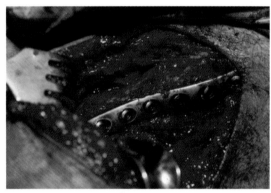

TECH FIG 2 • An alternative is to place the plate on the anterior surface of the clavicle. This limits plate prominence but requires greater stripping and muscle elevation. (Copyright David Ring, MD.)

PEARLS AND PITFALLS

Supraclavicular nerve neuroma	▪ Attempts to identify and protect these nerves are worthwhile.
Brachial plexus stretch injury	▪ Realignment should be done gradually and can be facilitated by temporary external fixation. Pulling fragments out of the wound should be limited.
Loosening of fixation	▪ At least three good bicortical screws should be placed on each side of the fracture.
Axial pull-out of locked screws	▪ Locking screws may be troublesome when used on the lateral fragment with the plate in a superior position.
Plate prominence	▪ Anterior plate placement may diminish plate prominence.

POSTOPERATIVE CARE

- Confident use of the hand at the side is encouraged immediately.
- Shoulder abduction and handling of more than 15 pounds is delayed until early healing is established.
- Shoulder stiffness is unusual and usually responds quickly to exercises. Shoulder exercises can therefore be delayed until healing is established.

OUTCOMES

- Plate loosening and nonunion occur in 3% to 5% of cases.[6]
- Healing leads to good function.

COMPLICATIONS

- Infection and wound complications occur but are uncommon.
- Neurovascular injury is very uncommon and pneumothorax has not been described.

REFERENCES

1. Collinge C, Devinney S, Herscovici D, et al. Anterior-inferior plate fixation of middle-third fractures and nonunions of the clavicle. J Orthop Trauma 2006;20:680–686.
2. Kloen P, Sorkin AT, Rubel IF, et al. Anteroinferior plating of midshaft clavicular nonunions. J Orthop Trauma 2002;16:425–430.
3. McKee MD, Pedersen EM, Jones C, et al. Deficits following nonoperative treatment of displaced midshaft clavicular fractures. J Bone Joint Surg Am 2006;88A:35–40.
4. McKee MD, Wild LM, Schemitsch EH. Midshaft malunions of the clavicle. J Bone Joint Surg Am 2003;85A:790–797.
5. Nowak J, Holgersson M, Larsson S. Can we predict long-term sequelae after fractures of the clavicle based on initial findings? A prospective study with nine to ten years of follow-up. J Shoulder Elbow Surg 2004;13:479–486.
6. Poigenfurst J, Rappold G, Fischer W. Plating of fresh clavicular fractures: results of 122 operations. Injury 1992;23:237–241.
7. Robinson CM, Court-Brown CM, McQueen MM, et al. Estimating the risk of nonunion following nonoperative treatment of a clavicular fracture. J Bone Joint Surg Am 2004;86A:1359–1365.
8. Robinson CM. Fractures of the clavicle in the adult: epidemiology and classification. J Bone Joint Surg Br 1998;80B:476–484.
9. Zlowodzki M, Zelle BA, Cole PA, et al. Treatment of acute midshaft clavicle fractures: systematic review of 2144 fractures: on behalf of the Evidence-Based Orthopaedic Trauma Working Group. J Orthop Trauma 2005;19:504–507.

Chapter 15

Intramedullary Fixation of Clavicle Fractures

Bradford S. Tucker, Carl Basamania, and Matthew D. Pepe

DEFINITION

- The clavicle is one of the most commonly fractured bones.
- The site on the clavicle most often fractured is the middle third.[9]
  - The midclavicular region is the thinnest and narrowest portion of the bone.
  - It is the only area not supported by ligament or muscle attachments.
  - It represents a transitional region of both cross-sectional anatomy and curvature.
    - It is the transition point between the lateral part, with a flatter cross section, and the more tubular medial.
- Because of the clavicle's S shape, an axial load creates a very high tensile force along the anterior midcortex. (Axial load makes a virtual right angle at midclavicle.)

ANATOMY

- The clavicle is the only long bone to ossify by a combination of intramembranous and endochondral ossification.[6]
- Its configuration is S-shaped, a double curve; the medial curve is apex anterior and the lateral curve is apex posterior (**FIG 1A**).
- The larger medial curvature widens the space for the neurovascular structures, providing bony protection.
- The clavicle is made up of very dense trabecular bone, lacking a well-defined medullary canal.

- The cross-sectional anatomy gradually changes from flat laterally, to tubular in the midportion, to expanded prismatic medially.
- The clavicle is subcutaneous throughout, covered by the thin platysma muscle.
- The supraclavicular nerves that provide sensation to the overlying skin of the clavicle are found deep to the platysma muscle.
- Very strong capsular and extracapsular ligaments attach the medial end to the sternum and first rib and the lateral end to the acromion and coracoid.
- Proximal muscle attachments include the sternocleidomastoid, pectoralis major, and subclavius. Distal muscle attachments include the deltoid and trapezius (**FIG 1B**).
- The clavicle functions by providing a fixed-length strut through which the muscles attached to the shoulder girdle can generate and transmit large forces to the upper extremity.

PATHOGENESIS

- The mechanism of clavicle fractures in the vast majority is a direct injury to the shoulder.[10] Stanley and associates studied 106 injured patients; 87% had fallen onto the shoulder, 7% were injured by a direct blow on the point of the shoulder, and only 6% reported falling onto an outstretched hand.
- Stanley suggests that in the patients who described hitting the ground with an outstretched hand, the shoulder became the next contact point with the ground, causing the fracture. Stanley

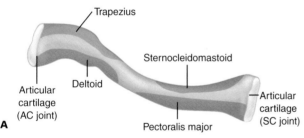

FIG 1 • **A.** The clavicle is S-shaped and has a double curve. The medial curve is apex anterior and the lateral curve is apex posterior. **B.** Proximal muscle attachments to the clavicle include the sternocleidomastoid, pectoralis major, and subclavius. Distal muscle attachments to the clavicle include the deltoid and trapezius.

stated that a compressive force equivalent to body weight would exceed the critical buckling load to cause the clavicle fracture.

NATURAL HISTORY

- In the 1960s, both Neer[7] and Rowe[9] published large series of midclavicle fractures, showing very low nonunion rate (0.1% and 0.8%) with closed treatment and a higher nonunion rate (4.6% and 3.7%) with operative treatment.
- More recent studies have shown that nonunion is more common then previously recognized and that a significant percentage of patients with nonunion are symptomatic.
- Malunion with shortening greater than 15 to 20 mm has also been shown to be associated with significant shoulder dysfunction.
- McKee and colleagues[5] identified 15 patients with malunion of the midclavicle after closed treatment. All patients had shortening of more than 15 mm, all were symptomatic and unsatisfied, and all underwent corrective osteotomy. Postoperatively all 15 patients improved in terms of function and satisfaction.
- Hill and associates[4] reviewed 52 completely displaced midshaft clavicle fractures and found that shortening of more than 20 mm had a significant association with nonunion and unsatisfactory results.
- Eskola and coworkers[3] reported on 89 malunions of the midclavicle, showing that shortening of more than 15 mm was associated with shoulder discomfort and dysfunction.

PATIENT HISTORY AND PHYSICAL FINDINGS

- The diagnosis is usually straightforward and is based on obtaining the mechanism of injury from a good history.
- On visual inspection the examiner will frequently see notable swelling or ecchymosis at the fracture site and possibly deformity of the clavicle, with drooping of the shoulder downward and forward if the fracture is significantly displaced. The skin is inspected for tenting at the fracture site and characteristic bruising and abrasions that might suggest a direct blow or seatbelt shoulder strap injury (**FIG 2A,B**).
- Palpation over the fracture site will reveal tenderness, and gentle manipulation of the upper extremity or clavicle itself may reveal crepitus and motion at the fracture site.
- The amount of shortening is identified by clinically measuring the distance of a straight line (in centimeters) from both acromioclavicular joints to the sternal notch and noting the difference (**FIG 2C**).
- It is important to perform a complete musculoskeletal and neurovascular examination of the upper extremity and auscul-

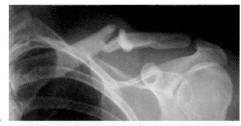
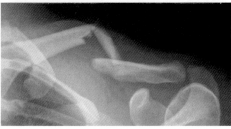

FIG 3 • Radiographs of the same displaced left clavicle fracture viewed from a standard AP projection (**A**) and a 45-degree cephalic tilt projection (**B**).

tation of the chest to identify the rare associated injuries; these are more closely related to high-energy injuries.
- Rib and scapula fracture
- Brachial plexus injury (usually traction to upper cervical root)
- Vascular injury (subclavian artery or vein injury associated with scapulothoracic dissociation)
- Pneumothorax and hemothorax

IMAGING AND OTHER DIAGNOSTIC STUDIES

- Two orthogonal radiographic projections are necessary to determine the fracture pattern and displacement, ideally 45-degree cephalic tilt and 45-degree caudad tilt views.
- Usually a standard anteroposterior (AP) view and a 45-degree cephalic tilt (**FIG 3**) view are adequate.
  - In practice, a 20- to 60-degree cephalic tilt view will minimize interference of thoracic structures.
- The film should be large enough to include the acromioclavicular and sternoclavicular joints, the scapula, and the upper lung fields to evaluate for associated injuries.
- An AP view of bilateral clavicles on a wide cassette to include the acromioclavicular joints and sternum is fairly helpful in determining the amount of shortening; however, this is a multiplanar deformity and a CT scan would have greater accuracy, although it is rarely required.

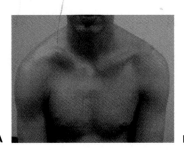
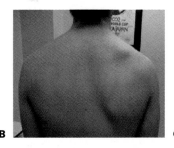
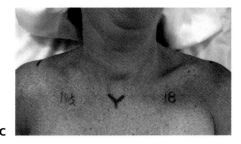

FIG 2 • **A,B.** Anterior and posterior photographs of a displaced right clavicle fracture showing deformity of the clavicle and drooping of the shoulder girdle downward and forward. **C.** Clinical picture of a displaced right clavicle fracture, showing 3.5 cm of shortening, measured from the sternal notch to the acromioclavicular joint.

DIFFERENTIAL DIAGNOSIS

▪ Sprain of acromioclavicular joint
▪ Sprain of sternoclavicular joint
▪ Rib fracture
▪ Muscle injury
▪ Contusion
▪ Hematoma
▪ Kehr sign: referred pain to the left shoulder from irritation of the diaphragm, signaled by the phrenic nerve. Irritation may be caused by diaphragmatic or peridiaphragmatic lesions, renal calculi, splenic injury, or ectopic pregnancy.

NONOPERATIVE MANAGEMENT

▪ If the clavicle fracture alignment is acceptable, generally a simple configuration with less than 15 mm of shortening, then any of a number of methods of supporting the upper extremity are adequate, including a figure 8 bandage, sling, sling and swathe, Sayre bandage, Velpeau dressing, and benign neglect, just to name a few.
▪ Nordqvist and colleagues[8] reported on 35 clavicle fracture malunions with shortening of less than 15 mm. They were all treated nonoperatively in a sling. All 35 had normal mobility, strength, and function compared to the normal shoulder.
▪ A prospective, randomized study[2] comparing sling versus figure 8 bandage showed that a greater percentage of patients were dissatisfied with the figure 8 bandage, and there was no difference in overall healing and alignment. The study concluded that the figure 8 bandage does little to obtain reduction.

SURGICAL MANAGEMENT

▪ Indications for operative treatment of acute midshaft clavicle fractures are as follows:
  ▪ Open fractures
  ▪ Fractures with neurovascular injury
  ▪ Fractures with severe associated chest injury or multiple trauma: patients who require their upper extremity for transfer and ambulation
  ▪ "Floating shoulder"
  ▪ Impending skin necrosis
  ▪ Severe displacement: possibly 15 to 20 mm of shortening

▪ In a multicenter, randomized, prospective clinical trial of displaced midshaft clavicle fractures, Altamimi and McKee[1] showed that operative fixation compared to nonoperative treatment improved functional outcome and had a lower rate of both malunion and nonunion.
▪ Potential advantages of intramedullary fixation of the clavicle are as follows:
  ▪ Less soft tissue stripping and therefore potentially better healing
  ▪ Smaller incision
  ▪ Better cosmesis
  ▪ Easier hardware removal
  ▪ Less weakness of bone after hardware removal
▪ Potential disadvantages of intramedullary fixation of the clavicle are as follows:
  ▪ Less ability to resist torsional forces
  ▪ Skin breakdown from prominence distally
  ▪ Pin breakage
  ▪ Pin migration
▪ Newer designs and techniques prevent pin migration by placing a locking nut on the lateral end and technically avoiding penetration of the medial fragment cortex.

Preoperative Planning

▪ After the decision has been made to fix a clavicle fracture, one must evaluate whether the fracture pattern is amenable to intramedullary pin fixation.
▪ A simple fracture pattern in the middle third of the bone is ideal.
▪ The fracture should not extend past the middle third of the bone.
▪ Comminution and butterfly fragments (usually anterior) are common and do not preclude intramedullary fixation as long as the medial and distal main fragments have cortical contact.

Positioning

▪ There are two good options for patient positioning that facilitate use of an image intensifier or C-arm device, which will aid you during pin placement.
▪ The patient can be placed supine on a Jackson radiolucent surgical table so the C-arm can be brought in perpendicular from the opposite side of the table, which is out of the way of the surgeon (**FIG 4A,B**).

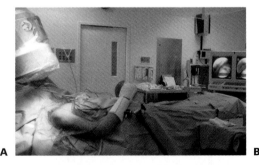
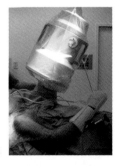
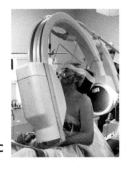
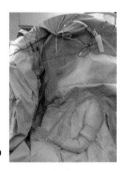

A   B   C   D

FIG 4 • **A,B.** The patient is placed supine on a Jackson radiolucent surgical table. A 1-L bag is placed under the affected shoulder, medial to the scapula, and the arm is prepared free and placed in an arm holder to aid in fracture reduction. The C-arm can be brought in perpendicular from the opposite side of the table, which is out of the way of the surgeon and facilitates getting orthogonal radiographic views of the fracture: 45-degree caudad tilt view (**A**) and 45-degree cephalic tilt view (**B**). **C,D.** Alternatively, the patient is placed in the beach chair position on the OR table, using a radiolucent shoulder-positioning device. **C.** The arm is prepared free and placed in an arm holder to facilitate fracture reduction. The C-arm is brought in from the head of the bed with the gantry rotated upside down and slightly away from the operative shoulder and oriented with a cephalic tilt. **D.** The same beach chair positioning shown sterilely draped.

■ A 1-L bag is placed under the affected shoulder, medial to the scapula, to aid in fracture reduction.

■ The arm is also prepared free and placed in an arm holder to facilitate fracture reduction.

■ This is our preferred method due to the ease and speed of the set-up and the ease of getting orthogonal radiographic views of the fracture (45-degree cephalic and caudad tilt views).

■ The other option is placing the patient in the beach chair position on the OR table, using a radiolucent shoulder-positioning device (**FIG 4C,D**).

■ The C-arm is brought in from the head of the bed with the gantry rotated upside down and slightly away from the operative shoulder and oriented with a cephalic tilt.

■ The arm is also prepared free and placed in an arm holder to facilitate fracture reduction.

INCISION AND DISSECTION

■ Mark out the clavicle, fracture site, and surrounding anatomy (**TECH FIG 1A**).

■ Use the C-arm to identify the appropriate position for the incision, which should be over the distal end of the medial fragment, in the Langer lines of the normal skin crease around the neck (**TECH FIG 1B**).

■ Make an incision of about 2 to 3 cm over the fracture site.

■ Divide the subcutaneous fat down to the platysma muscle using electrocautery (**TECH FIG 1C**).

■ Although there is usually very little subcutaneous fat, gently make full-thickness flaps to include skin and subcutaneous tissue around the entire incision to facilitate exposure.

■ Bluntly split the platysma muscle in line of its fibers to identify, protect, and retract the underlying supraclavic-

ular nerves; its middle branches are frequently found near the midclavicle (**TECH FIG 1D,E**).

■ The fracture site is then usually easily identifiable in acute injuries because the periosteum is disrupted and usually requires no further division.

■ Remove any debris, hematoma, or interposed muscle from the fracture site.

■ If there are butterfly fragments, be careful to keep any soft tissue attachments.

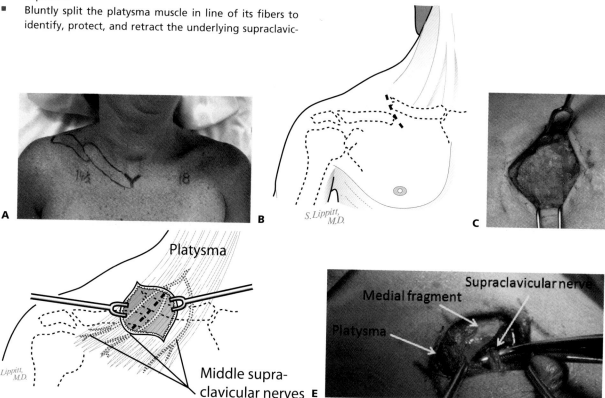

TECH FIG 1 ● **A.** Displaced right clavicle fracture, showing the clavicle and fracture site marked out. **B.** A skin incision of about 2 to 3 cm is made over the distal end of the medial clavicular fragment, in the Langer lines of normal skin creases around the neck. **C.** Incision over a clavicle fracture site, showing full-thickness flaps to include skin and subcutaneous tissue around the entire incision. This exposes the fascia that covers the platysma muscle. **D.** Skin incision over a displaced clavicle fracture, with underlying platysma muscle and the middle supraclavicular nerves. **E.** Intraoperative photo showing the platysma muscle bluntly split in the line of its fibers to identify an underlying supraclavicular nerve, which is under the clamp. The fracture site is usually easily identifiable in acute injuries because the periosteum is disrupted and usually requires no further division; as shown here, the medial clavicular fragment is easily seen. (**B,D:** Courtesy of Steven B. Lippitt, MD.)

CLAVICLE PREPARATION

- The following technique uses a modified Hagie pin called the Rockwood Clavicle Pin (DePuy Orthopaedics, Warsaw, IN) (**TECH FIG 2A**).
- Use a bone-reducing clamp or towel clip to grab and elevate the medial clavicular fragment through the incision (**TECH FIG 2B**).
- Size the diameter of the canal with the appropriate-size drill bit; the C-arm can be useful to judge canal fill and orientation of the drill.
  - The fit should be snug to maximize fixation, but not too tight, to prevent splitting the bone.
- Attach the chosen drill to the T-handle and ream out the intramedullary canal without penetrating the anterior cortex (**TECH FIG 2C–E**).
- Next, attach the appropriate-sized tap (that corresponds to the drill size) to the T-handle and tap the intramedullary canal to the anterior cortex (**TECH FIG 2F,G**).
- Elevate the lateral clavicular fragment through the incision; this can be facilitated by externally rotating the arm.
- Use the same drill bit attached to the T-handle to ream out the lateral fragment, but this time, under C-arm guidance, penetrate the posterolateral cortex of the clavicle (**TECH FIG 2H,I**).
  - The drill should exit posterior and medial to the acromioclavicular joint capsule (**TECH FIG 2J**).
  - To prevent the pin nuts from being too prominent, make sure the drill does not exit in the upper half of the posterolateral clavicle.
- Attach the appropriate-sized tap to the T-handle and tap the intramedullary canal of the lateral fragment (**TECH FIG 2K**).

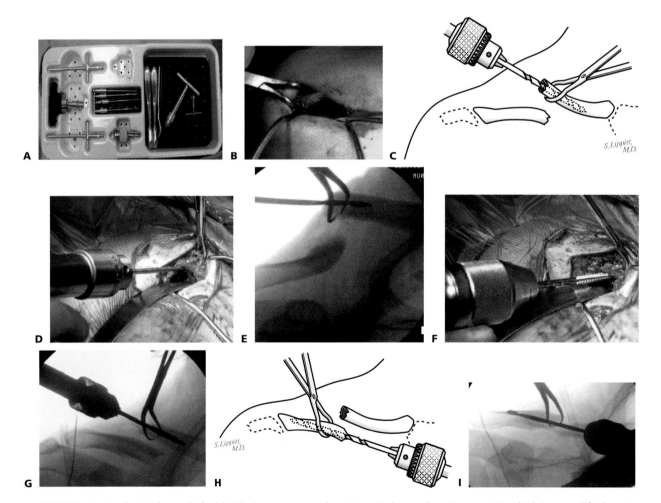

TECH FIG 2 • A. The Rockwood Clavicle Pin instrument set by DePuy Orthopaedics, Warsaw, IN, which is a modified Hagie pin. **B.** A bone-reducing clamp is used to elevate the medial clavicular fragment through the incision. **C–E.** The chosen drill is attached to a T-handle and the intramedullary canal of the medial clavicular fragment is reamed without penetrating the anterior cortex. **F,G.** An appropriate-sized tap is attached to a T-handle and the intramedullary canal of the medial clavicular fragment is tapped to the anterior cortex. **H,I.** The chosen drill is attached to a T-handle and the intramedullary canal of the lateral clavicular fragment is reamed out, penetrating the posterolateral cortex under direct C-arm guidance. *(continued)*

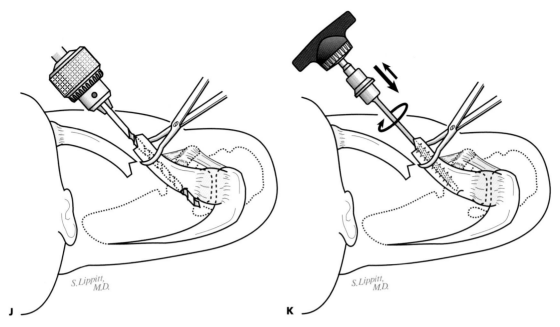

TECH FIG 2 • *(continued)* **J.** When drilling out the posterolateral cortex of the lateral clavicular fragment, the drill should exit posterior and medial to the acromioclavicular joint capsule. To prevent the pin nuts from being too prominent, the drill should not exit in the upper half of the posterolateral clavicle. **K.** The appropriate-sized tap is attached to the T-handle and the intramedullary canal of the lateral fragment is tapped. (**C,H,J,K:** Courtesy of Steven B. Lippitt, MD.)

PIN INSERTION AND FRACTURE REDUCTION

- Remove the nuts from the pin assembly and attach the T-handle using a Jacobs chuck to the medial end of the clavicle pin.
  - This is the end with the large threads.
  - Never tighten the chuck over the machined threads at either end.
- Continue firmly holding the lateral fragment while passing the trocar end (lateral end) of the clavicle pin into the intramedullary canal, out the previously drilled hole in the posterolateral cortex (**TECH FIG 3A**).
- Once you are just through the cortex, make a small incision over the palpable tip.
- Bluntly dissect the subcutaneous tissue with a hemostat until the tip of the pin can be felt, and then place the

hemostat or a small elevator under the tip of the pin to facilitate the pin's passage through the incision (**TECH FIG 3B**).
  - Drill the pin out laterally until the large medial threads engage the lateral fragment.
- Now switch the T-handle to the lateral end of the pin and retract the pin into the lateral fragment (**TECH FIG 3C,D**).
- Reduce the fracture by lifting the arm, and pass the pin into the medial fragment.
  - Use the C-arm to ensure that the pin advances correctly down the line of the medial fragment and that all the medial threads cross the fracture site.

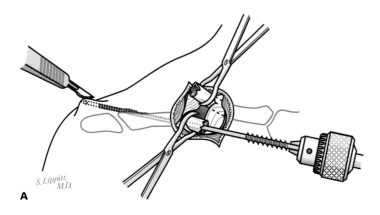

TECH FIG 3 • **A.** The surgeon continues firmly holding the lateral fragment while passing the trocar end (lateral end) of the clavicle pin into the intramedullary canal, out the previously drilled hole in the posterolateral cortex. Once just through the cortex, the surgeon makes a small incision over the palpable tip. *(continued)*

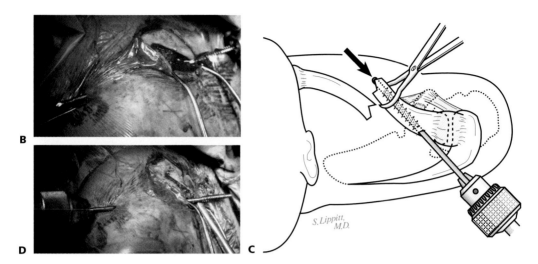

TECH FIG 3 • *(continued)* **B.** The subcutaneous tissue is bluntly dissected with a hemostat until the tip of the pin can be felt, and then the hemostat or a small elevator is placed under the tip of the pin to facilitate the pin's passage through the incision. **C,D.** The T-handle is switched to the lateral end of the pin and the pin is retracted into the lateral fragment. (**A,C:** Courtesy of Steven B. Lippitt, MD.)

FINAL POSITIONING OF PIN AND FRACTURE COMPRESSION

- Cold-weld the two nuts onto the lateral end of the pin.
  - First place the medial nut onto the pin, followed by the smaller lateral nut.
  - Grasp the medial nut with a needle-nose pliers and then tighten the lateral nut against the medial nut using the lateral nut wrench (**TECH FIG 4A,B**).
- Using the lateral nut wrench and C-arm guidance, now advance the pin assembly into the medial fragment until it contacts the anterior cortex (**TECH FIG 4C**).
- Break the cold weld by grasping the medial nut with needle-nose pliers and then loosen the lateral nut by turning it counterclockwise using the lateral nut wrench.

- Advance the medial nut against the posterolateral cortex of the clavicle to get desired compression across the fracture site.
- Cold-weld the lateral nut back onto the medial nut again.
- Use the medial nut wrench to back the pin assembly out of the soft tissues far enough to expose the nuts, usually about 1 cm. This will enable the pin to be cut flush to the lateral nut (**TECH FIG 4D,E**).
- Finally, use the lateral nut wrench to advance the pin assembly back into the medial fragment with the same desired fracture site compression (**TECH FIG 4F,G**).

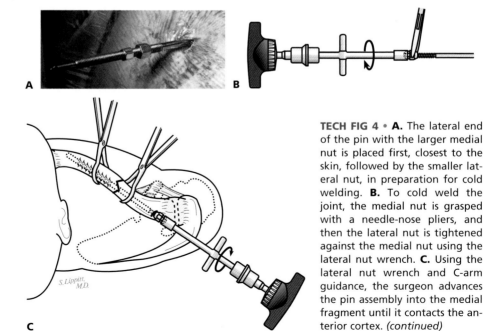

TECH FIG 4 • **A.** The lateral end of the pin with the larger medial nut is placed first, closest to the skin, followed by the smaller lateral nut, in preparation for cold welding. **B.** To cold weld the joint, the medial nut is grasped with a needle-nose pliers, and then the lateral nut is tightened against the medial nut using the lateral nut wrench. **C.** Using the lateral nut wrench and C-arm guidance, the surgeon advances the pin assembly into the medial fragment until it contacts the anterior cortex. *(continued)*

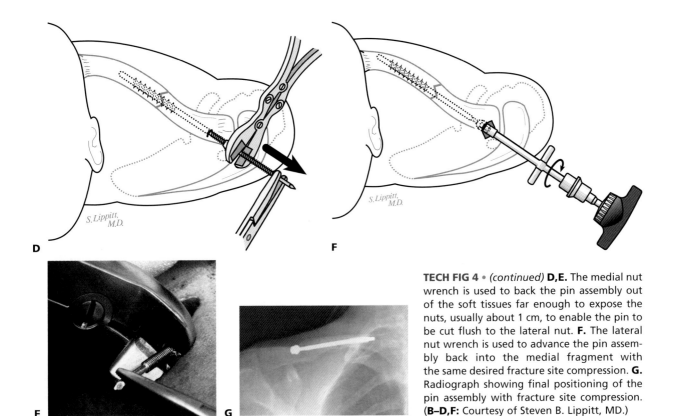

TECH FIG 4 • *(continued)* **D,E.** The medial nut wrench is used to back the pin assembly out of the soft tissues far enough to expose the nuts, usually about 1 cm, to enable the pin to be cut flush to the lateral nut. **F.** The lateral nut wrench is used to advance the pin assembly back into the medial fragment with the same desired fracture site compression. **G.** Radiograph showing final positioning of the pin assembly with fracture site compression. (**B–D,F:** Courtesy of Steven B. Lippitt, MD.)

BUTTERFLY FRAGMENT MANAGEMENT AND WOUND CLOSURE

- If an anterior butterfly fragment exists, cerclage is done using no. 0 or no. 1 absorbable suture.
  - Pass an elevator under the clavicle to deflect the sutures (**TECH FIG 5A**).

- Then pass the suture in a figure 8 manner through the periosteum of the butterfly fragment and around the fragment and the clavicle (**TECH FIG 5B**).
- Close the periosteum overlying the fracture site with no. 0 absorbable suture in an interrupted figure 8 manner.
- Reapproximate the fascia of the platysma muscle using 2-0 absorbable suture in an interrupted figure 8 manner.
- Close the subcutaneous tissue and skin of both incisions.

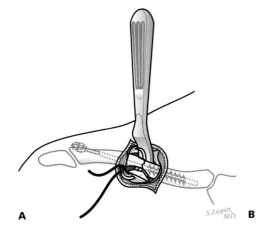

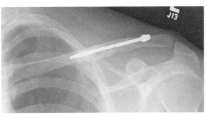

TECH FIG 5 • A. Cerclage of an anterior butterfly fragment is accomplished by first passing an elevator under the clavicle to deflect the sutures and then passing the suture, in a figure 8 manner, through the periosteum of the butterfly fragment and around the fragment and the clavicle. **B.** Radiograph showing an adequate reduction of a butterfly fragment. (**A:** Courtesy of Steven B. Lippitt, MD.)

TECHNIQUES

PIN REMOVAL

- The pin is removed at 10 to 12 weeks if the fracture has healed.
- The patient is positioned on his or her side and a local anesthetic is delivered (**TECH FIG 6A**).

- An incision is made over the same previous lateral incision and the subcutaneous tissue is dissected using the hemostat until the medial nut is identified.
- The medial nut wrench is used to extract the pin assembly (**TECH FIG 6B,C**).
- If the nut is stripped, the T-handle and chuck can be used to extract the pin assembly.

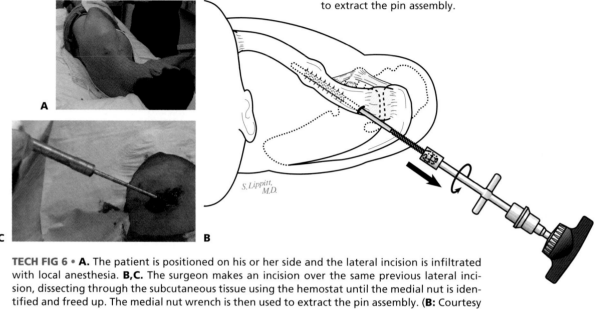

S. Lippitt, M.D.

TECH FIG 6 • A. The patient is positioned on his or her side and the lateral incision is infiltrated with local anesthesia. **B,C.** The surgeon makes an incision over the same previous lateral incision, dissecting through the subcutaneous tissue using the hemostat until the medial nut is identified and freed up. The medial nut wrench is then used to extract the pin assembly. (**B:** Courtesy of Steven B. Lippitt, MD.)

PEARLS AND PITFALLS

Avoid splitting the clavicular fragments and aid in pin insertion	▪ If tapping the medial or lateral clavicular fragments is too tight, the surgeon should redrill with the next larger drill size.
Achieve a more anatomic fracture reduction	▪ When advancing the pin into the medial clavicular fragment, the surgeon should avoid starting too superior and anterior, which can lead to malreduction. Instead, the pin should be inserted more inferior and posterior to achieve a more anatomic reduction.

POSTOPERATIVE CARE

- A sling is worn for 4 weeks. During this time the sling is removed at least five times a day for active range of motion of the elbow and active assisted range of motion of the shoulder to 90 degrees of forward flexion.
- The sling is discontinued and full active range of motion of the shoulder is started at 4 weeks.
- Progressive resistance exercises are started at 6 weeks if the patient achieved full range of motion and there is clinical and radiographic evidence of healing.
- Once the clavicle fracture has healed, the pin is removed at 10 to 12 weeks, as described in the Techniques section (**FIG 5**).

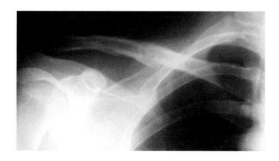

FIG 5 • Radiograph showing a healed clavicle fracture after pin assembly removal.

OUTCOMES

■ One of the authors (C.B.) has performed intramedullary fixation of some 300 acute fractures; there have been 60 malunions and 30 nonunions of the clavicle, with a nonunion rate of 1.2%.
■ Most of the nonunions occurred in older, sick patients with polytrauma.

COMPLICATIONS

■ Pin migration is rare with this technique because of the locking nut on the lateral end of the pin, the blunt tip on the medial end of the pin, and technically avoiding penetration of the medial fragment cortex.
■ The risk of skin breakdown from pin prominence laterally can be minimized by making sure the drill exits the posterolateral clavicle in the lower half.
■ Neurovascular complications are rare.
   ■ There is no drilling toward the neurovascular structures with this technique.
   ■ When exposing the fracture site, the surgeon should stay on bone at all times.
■ Nonunion rates are low as long as general fracture principles are maintained, soft tissue stripping of the fracture site is minimized, the technique is followed to get adequate fracture site compression and alignment, and the patient is compliant with the postoperative protocol.
■ Malunion can rarely occur, especially in fractures with large butterfly fragments. Good imaging with the C-arm allows the surgeon to start inserting the pin more inferior and posterior down the line of the medial clavicular fragment to achieve a more anatomic reduction.
■ Infection is rare, especially with this technique, which has a relatively short surgical time and small exposure. Preoperative antibiotics, meticulous handling of the soft tissues, and adequate irrigation should be part of any surgical technique.

REFERENCES

1. Altamimi S, McKee M. Nonoperative treatment compared with plate fixation of displaced midshaft clavicle fractures. J Bone Joint Surg Am 2008;90A:1–8.
2. Andersen K, Jensen PO, Lauritzen J. Treatment of clavicular fractures: figure-of-eight versus a simple sling. Acta Orthop Scand 1987;58:71–74.
3. Eskola A, Vainionpaa S, Myllynen P, et al. Outcome of clavicular fractures in 89 patients. Arch Orthop Trauma Surg 1986;105:337–338.
4. Hill J, McGuire M, Crosby L. Closed treatment of displaced middle-third fractures of the clavicle gives poor results. J Bone Joint Surg Br 1997;79B:537–539.
5. McKee M, Wild L, Schemitsch E. Midshaft malunions of the clavicle. J Bone Joint Surg Am 2003;85A:790–797.
6. Moseley HF. The clavicle: its anatomy and function. Clin Orthop Relat Res 1968;58:17–27.
7. Neer C. Nonunion of the clavicle. JAMA 1960;172:96–101.
8. Nordqvist A, Redlund-Johnell I, Von Scheele A, et al. Shortening of clavicle after fracture, incidence and clinical significance, a 5-year follow-up of 85 patients. Acta Orthop Scand 1997;68:349–351.
9. Rowe C. An atlas of anatomy and treatment of midclavicular fractures. Clin Orthop Relat Res 1968;58:29–42.
10. Stanley D, Trowbridge EA, Norris SH. The mechanism of clavicle fracture: a clinical and biomechanical analysis. J Bone Joint Surg Br 1988;70B:461–464.

Chapter 16

Percutaneous Pinning for Proximal Humerus Fractures

Leesa M. Galatz

DEFINITION

- *Proximal humerus fractures* are defined as those of the proximal portion of the humerus involving the shoulder joint.
- *Fracture lines* divide the proximal humerus into parts defined by anatomic structures that arise from early centers of ossification.
    - These "parts" first were described by Codman, and led to development of the Neer classification,[6] which is commonly used today.
    - The parts refer to the head of the humerus, the greater tuberosity, the lesser tuberosity, and the shaft (**FIG 1**).
    - Proximal humerus fractures are classified as two-, three-, or four-part fractures according to the Neer classfication.[6]
- Displacement of a "part" is classically defined as 1 cm of displacement or 45 degrees of angulation. Importantly, displacement is not necessarily an indication for surgery, but only a criterion for classification.
    - The type of fracture and degree of displacement, as well as patient considerations, all factor into surgical decision-making.

ANATOMY

- The proximal humerus arises from four distinct centers of ossification: the humeral head, the greater tuberosity, the lesser tuberosity, and the shaft.
    - The greater tuberosity has three distinct facets for the insertion of the supraspinatus, the infraspinatus, and the teres minor muscles of the rotator cuff.
- The lesser tuberosity is the insertion site for the subscapularis muscle.
- The rotator interval lies between the upper subscapularis and the anterior border of the supraspinatus.
    - The long head of the biceps tendon lies in a shallow groove on the anterior proximal humerus and enters the glenohumeral joint at the rotator interval.
    - The proximal 3 cm of the long head of the biceps tendon lies deep to the interval tissue intra-articularly.
- The anterior humeral circumflex artery (**FIG 2**) courses laterally along the inferior subscapularis.
    - The anterolateral branch of the anterior humeral circumflex artery travels superiorly along the lateral aspect of the biceps groove and enters the humeral head at the proximal-most aspect of the groove, providing about 85% of the blood supply to the humeral head.[1]
- The posterior humeral circumflex artery gives off several small branches that run adjacent to the inferior capsule of the shoulder, providing most of the remaining blood supply.
- The pectoralis major muscle inserts on the proximal shaft of the humerus lateral to the long head of the biceps tendon. The latissimus dorsi muscle inserts onto the proximal shaft medial to the biceps groove.

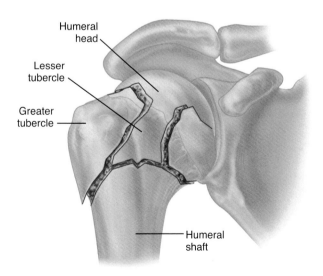

Humeral head

Lesser tubercle

Greater tubercle

Humeral shaft

FIG 1 • Fractures of the proximal humerus are classified as two-, three-, or four-part fractures based on fracture and degree of displacement of the greater tuberosity, the lesser tuberosity, the humeral head, and the humeral shaft.

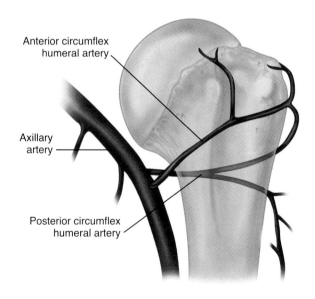

Anterior circumflex humeral artery

Axillary artery

Posterior circumflex humeral artery

FIG 2 • The rotator interval lies between the upper border of the subscapularis and the anterior border of the supraspinatus. The biceps tendon runs deep to the rotator interval tissue. Importantly, the fracture line between the greater and lesser tuberosities lies just posterior to the biceps groove. The ascending branch of the anterior humeral circumflex artery provides 85% of the blood supply to the humeral head.

PATHOGENESIS

- Proximal humerus fractures occur in a bimodal distribution.
  - Most proximal humerus fractures are "fractures of senescence" in older individuals with age-related osteopenia. They commonly result from low-energy injures such as tripping and falling.
  - They also occur in younger individuals as the result of high-energy injuries such as motorcycle or automobile accidents.
- Associated nerve injuries can occur and usually resolve spontaneously. Axillary nerve neurapraxia is the most common.

NATURAL HISTORY

- Eighty-five percent of proximal humerus fractures can be treated nonoperatively.[6]
- Displacement at the surgical neck is better tolerated than displacement at the greater tuberosity.
  - Because of the vast range of motion (ROM) of the shoulder in multiple planes, the arm can compensate for translational displacement or angulation at the surgical neck.
  - Displacement of the tuberosities, however, affects the mechanics of the rotator cuff and is very poorly tolerated.
- Four-part fractures have an extremely high incidence of avascular necrosis—45% in Neer's classic series—with the exception of valgus impacted four-part fractures, in which the incidence is only 11%.[7]
  - In most four-part fractures, the blood supply from the anterior humeral circumflex artery is disrupted, contributing to the high incidence of avascular necrosis.
  - The blood supply is maintained in most valgus impacted fractures by the branches from the posterior humeral circumflex artery along the intact medial periosteal hinge (**FIG 3**), making this particular fracture configuration very amenable to fixation.

PATIENT HISTORY AND PHYSICAL FINDINGS

- A complete history of injury is important to determine the mechanism of injury. It is helpful to differentiate low-energy from high-energy injuries.
  - Elderly individuals often sustain proximal humerus fractures as the result of low-energy injuries such as slipping and falling. These injuries often are very amenable to minimally invasive fixation techniques, because the displacement is manageable and the periosteal sleeve between fracture fragments often is intact. The rotator cuff often is intact as

a sleeve. All these qualities facilitate minimally invasive reduction and fixation techniques.
  - In younger individuals, proximal humerus fractures often result from higher-energy injuries. These fractures commonly have greater fracture fragment displacement, rotator cuff tears between the tuberosities, and disruption of the periosteal sleeve. These factors do not necessarily preclude percutaneous pinning, but make it more challenging and should be considered in preoperative planning.
- Other important aspects of the history include:
  - Previous history of injury to the affected shoulder
  - Previous shoulder function
  - History of numbness or tingling in the affected extremity
- Rule out elbow and wrist fractures, especially in osteoporotic patients with injuries resulting from a fall on an outstretched arm.
- Patients often hold the shoulder inferior on the affected side.
- Examination should include skin integrity, presence of ecchymosis, downward carriage of shoulder girdle, and deformity consistent with shoulder dislocation or acromioclavicular joint separation.
- Examine for possible associated nerve injury (usually neurapraxia) by testing sensation to light touch in individual nerve distribution, two-point discrimination, and muscle strength (testing is limited to isometric at shoulder because of limited ROM and pain).
- Possible associated vascular injury can be determined by testing radial pulse and capillary refill.

IMAGING AND OTHER DIAGNOSTIC STUDIES

- A trauma series of radiographs of the shoulder should be obtained (**FIG 4**).
  - The series includes an AP view of the shoulder, a scapular AP view, a scapular Y view, and an axillary view.
  - A complete series with these views allows the fracture configuration to be determined in sufficient detail.
- A CT scan is helpful in many cases and should be obtained if there is any question regarding the extent of fracture involvement or the level of displacement of the fragments. It also is helpful if there is any question of joint dislocation or glenoid fracture.
- Radiographs are used to determine whether the fracture is a two-, three-, or four-part fracture and to assess the degree of displacement.

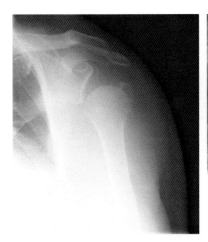
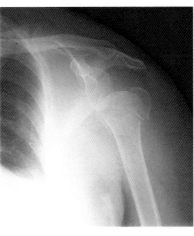

FIG 3 • Valgus impacted fractures maintain blood supply to the articular surface via ascending branches off the posterior humeral circumflex artery along the intact medial periosteal hinge.

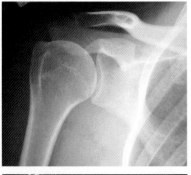
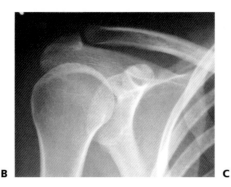
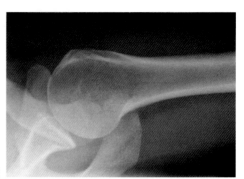
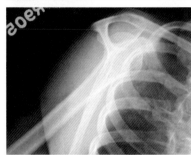

FIG 4 • A normal trauma series includes a scapular AP radiograph, an AP radiograph of the shoulder, an axillary view, and a Y lateral view. **A.** The scapular AP view is taken, by convention, with the arm in neutral rotation. **B.** The AP view of the shoulder is taken with the arm in internal rotation. **C.** The axillary lateral view is taken with the arm abducted and in neutral rotation. **D.** The Y lateral view often allows the examiner to detect any posterior displacement of subtle greater tuberosity fractures.

■ Three-dimensional reconstructions of the CT scan can be helpful in fracture evaluation, but are not routinely required.

DIFFERENTIAL DIAGNOSIS

■ Acromioclavicular joint separation
■ Glenohumeral joint dislocation
■ Humeral shaft fracture
■ Scapulothoracic dissociation
■ Elbow and wrist fractures (may coexist)

NONOPERATIVE MANAGEMENT

■ Minimally displaced fractures can be treated nonoperatively.
■ Displacement at the surgical neck is well tolerated.
    ■ An AP view of the shoulder can be misleading in the case of a surgical neck fracture.
        ■ The pectoralis major muscle exerts an anterior force on the shaft, resulting in anterior displacement of the shaft relative to the humeral head.
    ■ A scapular Y or axillary view can exhibit this angular deformity.
■ Displacement of the greater tuberosity is less well tolerated.
    ■ Historically, 1 cm of displacement has been used as the criterion for clinically significant tuberosity displacement.
    ■ Recently, however, even 5 mm of displacement has been considered an operative indication.
■ Patients wear a sling for 2 to 3 weeks or until the proximal humerus feels stable with gentle internal or external rotation of the arm.
    ■ Patients should be instructed to remove the sling for elbow and hand ROM to avoid stiffness of these joints.
    ■ Early signs of healing (eg, callus formation) also are helpful indicators of when it is safe to commence ROM exercises.
■ In borderline instances, it is better to err toward a longer period of immobilization to ensure healing, because shoulder stiffness is easier to address than a nonunion.
■ Therapy begins with passive stretching until 6 weeks when active ROM and strengthening can be started, progressing as tolerated.

SURGICAL MANAGEMENT

Preoperative Planning

■ All imaging studies should be reviewed carefully to determine the type of fracture, the degree of displacement, fracture configuration, and bone quality.
■ Certain radiographic findings that can suggest that minimally invasive fracture fixation is not appropriate for a given fracture are as follows:
    ■ *Poor bone quality.* The bone may not hold the pins and screws well and may be better treated with a more stable construct.
    ■ *Comminution of the greater tuberosity.* A comminuted bone fragment is not amenable to fixation with screws. Fractures with a comminuted greater tuberosity require suture fixation through the tendon–bone junction (required open approach).
    ■ *Comminution of the medial calcar region* leads to unstable reduction of the head onto the shaft.
■ Fractures amenable to minimally invasive fixation are two-part, three-part, and valgus impacted four-part fractures with:
    ■ Good bone quality
    ■ Substantial fracture fragments with minimal comminution of the tuberosities
    ■ Minimal or no comminution at the medial calcar region
■ Minimally invasive fixation is not appropriate for noncompliant or unreliable patients. This procedure should be performed only in patients committed to consistent follow-up in the postoperative period.
    ■ The pins require close surveillance in the early postoperative period.
    ■ Pin migration is possible and must be caught early in order to avoid potential injury to thoracic structures.

Positioning

■ Percutaneous pinning is performed with the patient in the straight supine or 10- to 15-degree beach chair position (**FIG 5**).
    ■ This allows easy intraoperative evaluation with C-arm fluoroscopy.

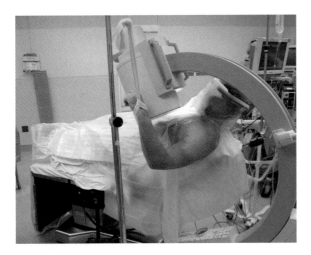

FIG 5 • The patient is placed in the supine or gently upright position. The C-arm is brought in parallel to the patient, leaving the lateral aspect of the arm free for instrumentation. The patient should be positioned laterally on the table such that an adequate fluoroscopic view can be obtained.

- The C-arm fluoroscope is placed parallel to the patient, extending over the shoulder from the cephalad direction.
  - This position leaves the lateral shoulder completely accessible for instrumentation and pin fixation.
- The patient must be positioned far lateral on the table or on a specialized shoulder surgery positioning device such that the shoulder can be imaged in the anteroposterior plane without the table obstructing the view.
  - This image should be checked before prepping and draping to confirm adequate visualization.
- The entire upper extremity is draped free.

Approach

- Closed fracture reductions are performed with the aid of a "reduction portal" (**FIG 6**).[2]
  - The reduction portal is a portal (analogous to that of an arthroscopic portal) or small incision used to access the fracture fragments.
  - Instruments can be introduced through this portal to lever fracture fragments or pull fragments into reduced position.
  - The surgeon also can insert a finger through this portal to palpate fragments.
    - Medially, the biceps tendon can be palpated.
    - The surgical neck fracture is located just deep to the portal.
    - By sweeping posterior and superior, the greater tuberosity and its extent of displacement can be palpated.
- The location of the reduction portal is critical (**FIG 6B**).
  - In three- and four-part fractures, the fracture line of the greater tuberosity is reliably 0.5 to 1 cm posterior and lateral to the biceps groove.
  - Therefore, the reduction portal is located at the level of the surgical neck and 1 cm posterior to the biceps groove.

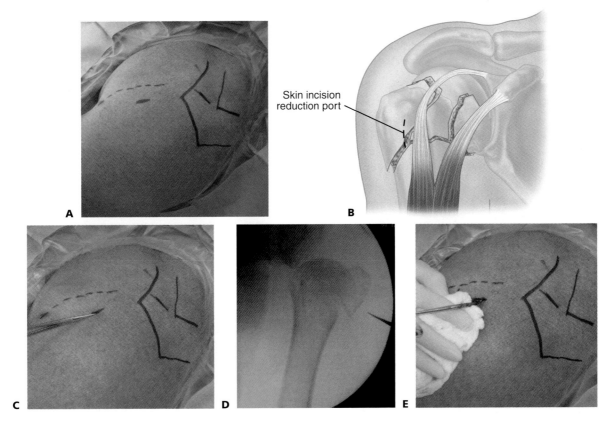

Skin incision reduction port

FIG 6 • **A.** The reduction portal is established off the anterolateral corner of the acromion. Instruments can be introduced through this portal to help reduce the fracture. **B.** The reduction portal is located at the level of the surgical neck fracture approximately 0.5 to 1 cm posterior to the biceps groove. The reduction portal is definitively localized using C-arm imagery. A hemostat is applied to the skin (**C**) and then imaged (**D**) to confirm that this portal will be directly at the level of the surgical neck fracture. **E.** A small incision is made in the skin, and the deltoid is spread bluntly to avoid injury to the underlying axillary nerve.

- The arm is held in neutral rotation.
  - The level of the surgical neck is located using fluoroscopic imagery (**FIG 6C,D**).
  - The location of the biceps tendon is estimated based on surface anatomic landmarks.

- A 2-cm incision is made in the skin (**FIG 6E**).
  - Subcutaneous tissues and the deltoid muscle are spread bluntly using a straight hemostat to avoid injury to the axillary nerve on the deep surface of the deltoid. Subdeltoid adhesions are gently released by sweeping finger if necessary.

SURGICAL NECK FRACTURE

Reduction

- The pectoralis major muscle provides the major deforming force resulting in displacement of surgical neck fractures. The shaft usually is displaced anteriorly and medially with respect to the head.
  - An axillary or scapular Y radiograph is necessary to evaluate the extent of this displacement.
- The reduction maneuver involves flexion, adduction, and possibly some slight internal rotation to relax the pull of the pectoralis major muscle[3] (**TECH FIG 1**).
  - Longitudinal traction is applied to the arm, and a posteriorly directed force is applied to the proximal shaft of the humerus.
- A blunt instrument can be inserted into the fracture at the surgical neck to lever the head back onto the shaft. This maneuver can be a powerful reduction tool, but care should be used to avoid further damage or fracture to the humeral head during this maneuver, especially on osteopenic patients.
  - The long head of the biceps tendon can become interposed between the fracture fragments, precluding reduction. Therefore, if reduction is not achieved, check the biceps tendon through the reduction portal (or consider open reduction).

Fixation

- Two or three retrograde pins are placed from the shaft into the humeral head (**TECH FIG 2**).
  - The starting point for the pins is approximately 5 to 6 cm distal to the surgical neck fracture line.

- The pins must angle steeply to enter the head fragment and not cut out posteriorly (**TECH FIG 2B,C**).
- Pins should be smooth to avoid injury to soft tissue upon insertion, and terminally threaded to avoid backing out.
- 2.5- or 2.7-mm smooth, terminally threaded pins commonly are found in external fixation or 7.3-mm cannulated screw sets of instruments.
- The pins should enter at different directions to enhance stability of fixation construct.
  - One pin should enter lateral to the biceps in a primarily anterior-to-posterior direction.
  - Another pin should enter further laterally in a primarily lateral-to-medial direction.
- Stability should be checked under fluoroscopic imaging with live, gentle internal and external rotation.

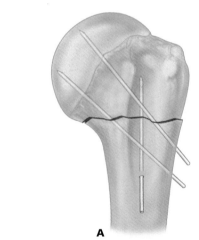

A

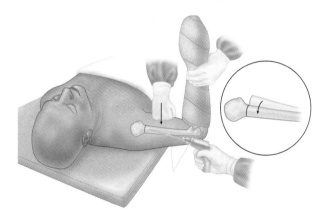

TECH FIG 1 • The reduction maneuver for surgical neck fractures involves flexion and internal rotation of the arm to negate the effect of the pectoralis major fragment on the proximal aspect of the shaft. Often a posterior vector must be applied to the shaft or an instrument can be introduced through the reduction portal to lever the head back onto the shaft.

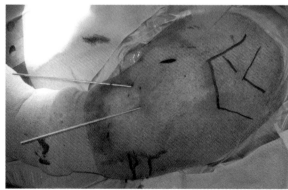

B

TECH FIG 2 • **A.** Retrograde pins are introduced several centimeters below the level of the surgical neck fracture into the head. The pins should be placed in different directions to provide stability to the construct. **B.** Placement of two pins. *(continued)*

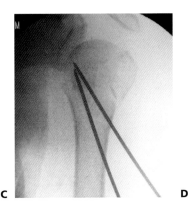

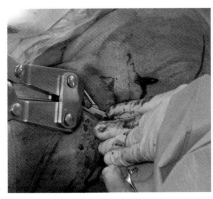

TECH FIG 2 • *(continued)* **C.** Fluoroscopic view of two retrograde pins in place. **D.** The pins should be cut below the skin after insertion to prevent pin site infection. They are easily removed a couple of weeks later with a small procedure in the office or operating room.

- Any suggestion of instability or motion at the fracture is an indication for open reduction and plate fixation at that point.
- Pins are cut below the skin to prevent pin site infection (**TECH FIG 2D**).

- The reduction portal is closed with interrupted nylon sutures.
- A soft dressing and sling are applied.

THREE-PART GREATER TUBEROSITY FRACTURES

Reduction

- Deforming forces influencing displacement of three-part fractures include the pectoralis major, as described earlier, and the rotator cuff muscles. The rotator cuff pulls the tuberosity medially (to a certain extent) and posteriorly. Posterior displacement and rotation often are underappreciated and must be considered.
- The surgical neck component is addressed first. (See Surgical Neck Fractures earlier in this section).
- The greater tuberosity fracture is reduced using the "reduction portal." A dental pick or small hooked instrument is inserted through the portal to engage the tuberosity and pull it inferior and anterior into a reduced position.

Fixation

- 4.5-mm cannulated screws are used to fix the tuberosity fragment.
  - The screw is placed through the tuberosity fragment distal to the cuff insertion through bone on the lateral cortex (**TECH FIG 3A**).
  - The proper location is confirmed with fluoroscopic imaging.
- The guidewire is first passed through a small incision in the skin just large enough to pass the drill guide and screw through the deltoid (**TECH FIG 3B,C**).
  - The guidewire is passed through the tuberosity, across the surgical neck fracture, and engages the medial cortex of the proximal humeral shaft.

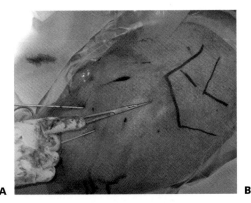

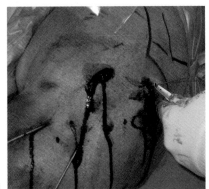

TECH FIG 3 • A. The greater tuberosity is localized under fluoroscopy using a hemostat. **B.** A small incision is made over the greater tuberosity, and a cannulated screw is used for fixation. This photograph demonstrates the drill guide used for soft tissue protection. *(continued)*

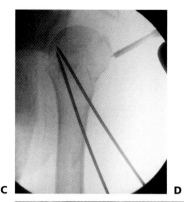

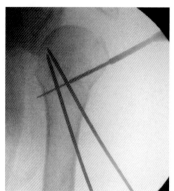

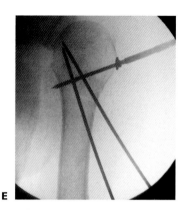

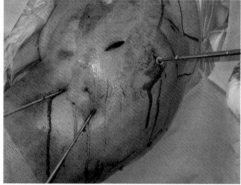

TECH FIG 3 • *(continued)* **C.** The guidewire is aimed to engage the greater tuberosity fragment as well as the medial cortex to provide compression. **D.** This fluoroscopic view demonstrates the screw being inserted over the guidewire. **E.** A washer is used to provide some compression. Over-tightening should be avoided to prevent fracture of the greater tuberosity fragment. **F.** Screw and washer insertion.

- After the guidewire is overdrilled, the screw is passed over the guidewire. We use a partially threaded screw with a washer (**TECH FIG 3D–F**).
- If the greater tuberosity fragment is large enough, a second cancellous screw is directed through the tuberosity fragment, engaging cancellous bone of the humeral head.
- Pins are cut beneath the skin.
- Incisions are closed with nylon interrupted sutures.
- A dressing and sling are applied.

VALGUS IMPACTED FOUR-PART PROXIMAL HUMERUS FRACTURES

- Valgus impacted fractures are recognized by the 90-degree angle between the long axis of the humeral shaft and the articular surface of the humeral head with loss of the normal neck shaft angle.[4] The tuberosities are displaced laterally from the head of the humerus and slightly proximally.
  - This fracture configuration results in a low incidence of avascular necrosis compared to that of other four-part fractures, because the medial periosteal hinge of soft tissues is intact along the medial and posterior anatomic neck, preserving the blood supply provided by the posterior humeral circumflex artery and its ascending vessels.
- The reduction maneuver for this fracture requires raising the humeral head back into its anatomic position.
  - The reduction portal described previously is created, and an instrument such as a blunt elevator or small bone tamp is inserted beneath the humeral head (**TECH FIG 4A,B**).
  - The instrument passes through the surgical neck fracture and through the fracture line between the tuberosities, which reliably exists 0.5 to 1 cm posterior and lateral to the biceps groove.

- The instrument is tapped with a mallet in a distal-to-proximal direction, lifting the head fragment into anatomic position (**TECH FIG 4C**).
- The surgical neck fractures and tuberosity fractures are then fixed using the techniques described earlier.

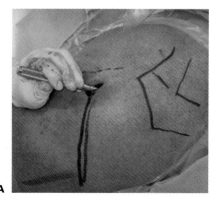

TECH FIG 4 • **A.** Valgus impacted proximal humerus fractures are reduced using a small bone tamp or other blunt-tipped instrument. *(continued)*

TECHNIQUES

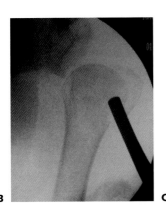
B

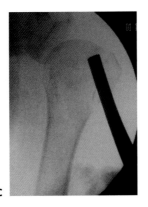
C

TECH FIG 4 • *(continued)* **B.** The instrument is inserted through the fracture line between the greater tuberosity and the lesser tuberosity, which lies posterior to the biceps groove. Position is confirmed with fluoroscopic imaging. **C.** The bone tamp is impacted in a superior direction, bringing the humeral head into a reduced position. The greater and lesser tuberosities fall naturally into a reduced position after this reduction maneuver.

- In some cases, there may be significant medial displacement of the lesser tuberosity. In these cases, the lesser tuberosity is reduced using the hook through the reduction portal and fixed with a screw placed in the anterior-to-posterior direction through the tuberosity into the head.

- In most cases, minimal medial displacement of the lesser tuberosity is well tolerated and no fixation is required.
- Pins are cut beneath the skin.
- Incisions are closed with nylon sutures.
- A dressing and sling are applied.

PEARLS AND PITFALLS

Indications	▪ Successful percutaneous pinning depends on appropriate patient selection. Criteria include good bone stock, minimal to no comminution at the greater tuberosity fragment, minimal to no comminution at the medial calcar and proximal shaft, and patient compliance. ▪ Contraindications include poor bone stock that will not hold pins, comminution of greater tuberosity or proximal shaft fragments, and a noncompliant patient with poor follow-up potential.
Positioning	▪ The patient must be lateral enough on the table to obtain unencumbered access to the shoulder and clear fluoroscopic images.
Reduction technique	▪ The location of the reduction portal is critical for maximizing its usefulness during the procedure. ▪ The surgeon must have a thorough understanding of three-dimensional anatomy, as well as interpretation and application of two-dimensional fluoroscopic images.
Pin placement	▪ Pins should engage the humerus distal to the axillary nerve, but proximal to the deltoid insertion to avoid nerve injury. ▪ The angle of insertion is steep to enter the humeral head and avoid cutting out posteriorly. ▪ At least two fluoroscopic images in different planes are necessary to confirm successful pin placement. ▪ A drill guide can be used to protect the soft tissues during pin insertion.
Screw placement	▪ The deltoid should be spread bluntly and a drill guide used to prevent injury to the axillary nerve in this location. In most cases, insertion will be proximal to the nerve, but precautionary measures should be taken. ▪ Overtightening the screw with a washer may result in fracture of the greater tuberosity. ▪ Engaging medial cortex of the proximal shaft gives stability to the screw construct.
Intraoperative assessment of stability	▪ The arm should be internally and externally rotated gently under continuous fluoroscopic imagery after completion of hardware placement. Any motion or suggestion of instability is an indication for open reduction and fixation.

POSTOPERATIVE CARE

- The operative arm is immobilized in a sling.
- The patient is instructed to begin active elbow, wrist, and hand ROM exercises.
- Radiographs are checked weekly to monitor for pin migration or loss of fixation.
  - Pins are removed as a short procedure in the office or operating room about 3 to 4 weeks postoperatively or when early signs of healing are evident radiographically.
- Pendulum exercises are initiated 2 to 3 weeks postoperatively, and passive stretching (forward elevation in scapular plane), external rotation, and internal rotation (all in supine position) is initiated when pins are removed.
  - Ideally, pins should be out and motion started no later than 4 weeks postoperatively.
- Active ROM progressing as tolerated to resistance exercises commences at 6 weeks postoperatively.

OUTCOMES

- Jaberg et al[3] reported good to excellent results in 38 of 48 fractures. There were 29 surgical neck, 3 anatomic neck, 8 three-part, and 5 four-part fractures.

- Resch et al[8] reported results of 9 three-part fractures and 18 four-part fractures. In the four-part fractures, the incidence of avascular necrosis was 11%. Good results correlated with anatomic reconstruction.
- Keener et al[5] reported a multicenter study of 35 patients— 7 two-part, 8 three-part, and 12 valgus impacted fractures. Average duration of follow-up was 35 months. All fractures healed. American Shoulder and Elbow Surgeons and Constant scores were 83.4 and 73.9, respectively. Four patients had some residual malunion, and four developed posttraumatic arthritis. Neither of these affected outcome at this early follow-up period, however.
- Most studies report very satisfactory results with this procedure. Patient selection is critical. In published studies, patients are not randomized to percutaneous pinning, but, rather, careful patient selection is left to the treating surgeon. Therefore, it can be concluded that this is an appropriate technique in certain patients who meet the outlined criteria.

COMPLICATIONS

- Nerve injury[9]
- Pin migration
- Loss of fixation
- Malunion
- Nonunion
- Infection
- Glenohumeral joint stiffness

REFERENCES

1. Gerber C, Schneeberger AG, Vinh TS. The arterial vascularization of the humeral head. An anatomical study. J Bone Joint Surg Am 1990; 72A:1486–1494.
2. Hsu J, Galatz LM. Mini-incision fixation of proximal humeral four-part fractures. In Scuderi GR, Tria A, Berger RA, eds. MIS Techniques in Orthopedics. New York: Springer, 2006:32–44.
3. Jaberg H, Warner JJ, Jakob RP. Percutaneous stabilization of unstable fractures of the humerus. J Bone Joint Surg Am 1992;74A: 508–515.
4. Jakob RP, Miniaci A, Anson PS, et al. Four-part valgus impacted fractures of the proximal humerus. J Bone Joint Surg Br 1991;73B: 295–298.
5. Keener J, Parsons BO, Flatow EL, et al. Outcomes after percutaneous reduction and fixation of proximal humeral fractures. J Shoulder Elbow Surg 2007;16:330–338. Epub 2007 Feb 22.
6. Neer CS II. Displaced proximal humerus fractures. I. Classification and evaluation. J Bone Joint Surg Am 1970;52A:1077–1089.
7. Resch H, Beck A, Bayley I. Reconstruction of the valgus impacted humeral head fracture. J Shoulder Elbow Surg 1995;4:73–80.
8. Resch H, Povacz P, Frohlich R, et al. Percutaneous fixation of three- and four-part fractures of the proximal humerus. J Bone Joint Surg Br 1997;79B:295–300.
9. Rowles DJ, McGrory JE. Percutaneous pinning of the proximal humerus: An anatomic study. J Bone Joint Surg Am 2001;83A: 1695–1699.

Chapter 17

Open Reduction and Internal Fixation of Proximal Humerus Fractures

Mark T. Dillon and David L. Glaser

DEFINITION

▪ Proximal humerus fractures may involve the surgical neck, the greater tuberosity, or the lesser tuberosity.

▪ The Neer classification, which is most commonly used, categorizes fractures based on the number of displaced parts (**FIG 1**). This classification system involves four segments: the articular surface, the greater tuberosity, the lesser tuberosity, and the humeral shaft. Fracture fragments displaced 1 cm or angulated 45 degrees are considered displaced.[17,18]

▪ The AO/ASIF (Arbeitsgemeinschaft fuer Osteosynthesefragen–Association for the Study of Internal Fixation) broadly classifies fractures into three types: type 1, unifocal extra-articular; type 2, bifocal extra-articular, and type 3, intra-articular.

  ▪ Each type is then further divided into groups and subgroups.[16]

  ▪ This system places more emphasis on the vascular supply to the humerus, with intra-articular fracture patterns having the highest risk of avascular necrosis.[26]

▪ Studies have demonstrated that interobserver reliability for both classification systems is not high.[1,23,24]

▪ Although not included in Neer's original classification, valgus impacted fractures are a unique entity that is important to recognize:

  ▪ Four-part fractures in which the humeral articular surface is impacted upon the shaft segment

  ▪ Often minimally displaced owing to an intact rotator cuff[5]

  ▪ Have a lower incidence of avascular necrosis, because the blood supply to the head is less likely to be disrupted

ANATOMY

▪ The osseous anatomy of the proximal humerus consists of the greater tuberosity, the lesser tuberosity, and the articular surface.

  ▪ The subscapularis inserts onto the lesser tuberosity, whereas the supraspinatus, infraspinatus, and teres minor insert onto the greater tuberosity.

▪ Knowledge of deforming forces associated with humerus fracture allows the surgeon to better treat proximal humerus fractures by both operative and nonoperative means.

  ▪ In a two-part surgical neck fracture, the pectoralis major pulls the humeral shaft anteromedial.

  ▪ In a two-part greater tuberosity fracture, the pull of the supraspinatus, infraspinatus, and teres minor tendons displaces the greater tuberosity superiorly and/or posteriorly.

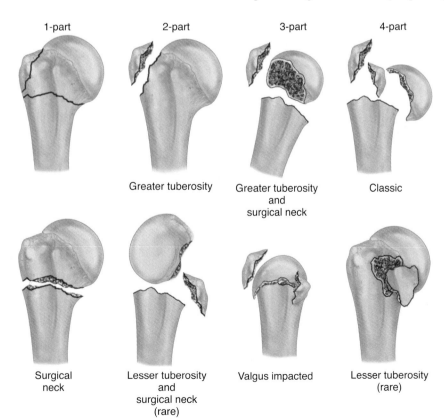

1-part	2-part	3-part	4-part
	Greater tuberosity	Greater tuberosity and surgical neck	Classic
Surgical neck	Lesser tuberosity and surgical neck (rare)	Valgus impacted	Lesser tuberosity (rare)

FIG 1 • Simplified Neer classification for fractures of the proximal humerus.

- With a three-part fracture involving the lesser tuberosity, the attachment site of these tendons into the greater tuberosity is intact, and the articular surface of the humeral head rotates externally to face anteriorly.
- Three-part fractures involving the greater tuberosity result in unopposed subscapularis function, and the humeral articular surface rotates posteriorly.
- Four-part fractures result in displacement of the shaft and both tuberosities, leaving a free head fragment with little soft tissue attachment.
- An understanding of the vascular anatomy is crucial to treat fractures of the proximal humerus effectively.
  - The main blood supply to the humeral head is the anterolateral ascending branch of the anterior circumflex artery.
  - This branch of the axillary artery runs just lateral to the bicipital groove, entering the humeral head at the proximal portion of the transition from bicipital groove to greater tuberosity.[9]
  - The intraosseous portion of this vessel, known as the *arcuate artery,* has been shown to supply the entire epiphyseal portion of the proximal humerus except for a small portion of the greater tuberosity and the posteroinferior humeral head, which is supplied by the posterior humeral circumflex artery.[9]

PATHOGENESIS

- In older patients, proximal humerus fractures usually result from a ground-level fall. Younger patients may sustain such an injury from a higher-energy mechanism such as an automobile collision or from sports.
- The presence of an associated glenohumeral dislocation also must be determined.

PATIENT HISTORY AND PHYSICAL FINDINGS

- On presentation, patients with proximal humerus fractures complain of pain in the shoulder that is made worse with attempted movement. Palpation of the proximal humerus results in diffuse pain.
- Visual inspection reveals ecchymosis and swelling of the arm.
- It is necessary to determine the stability of the fracture. If the shaft and the proximal portion move as a unit when taken through internal and external rotation, the fracture usually is stable. Unstable fractures will not move as a unit, and crepitus often is appreciated.
- If there is an associated dislocation, it may be possible to palpate the humeral head as an anterior fullness.
- It is crucial to perform a thorough neurovascular examination to determine the presence of associated injuries.
  - Patients over 50 years of age are more prone to nerve injuries. One study demonstrated nerve injury, usually of the axillary nerve, in nearly 40% of patients in this age group who sustained shoulder dislocations or surgical neck fractures.[2]

IMAGING AND OTHER DIAGNOSTIC STUDIES

- Initial imaging studies consist of anteroposterior, scapular Y, and axillary views.
  - Additional views also may include internal and external rotation views if the fracture pattern is stable. Internal rotation views help to visualize the lesser tuberosity, whereas external rotation shows the greater tuberosity.

- Traction views also may prove helpful if tolerated by the patient.
- A CT scan may be helpful if radiographs do not demonstrate the fracture pattern adequately.
  - Studies have shown that the addition of a CT scan improves intraobserver reproducibility only minimally and does not affect interobserver reliability.[1]
  - However, CT scanning may prove valuable in determining the method of fixation as well as identifying associated injuries such as Hill-Sachs fractures and bony Bankart lesions.
- Indications for MRI are limited, although it may prove useful if there is any concern regarding soft tissue injuries, including the glenoid labrum and rotator cuff.

DIFFERENTIAL DIAGNOSIS

- Glenohumeral dislocation
- Scapula fracture
- Head-splitting fracture
- Clavicle fracture
- Humeral shaft fracture
- Neurovascular injury
- Neuropathic arthropathy

NONOPERATIVE MANAGEMENT

- Historically, conservative treatment usually is recommended for fractures with less than 1 cm of displacement and 45 degrees of angulation.[17] About 85% of proximal humerus fractures can be treated nonoperatively.[15] With newer fixation devices, however, indications for surgical management have been expanded. Whether a more aggressive approach leads to improved outcomes remains to be seen.
- There is less tolerance for displacement in isolated greater tuberosity fractures. It has been suggested that more than 5 mm of displacement leads to poor functional results.[14]
- For proximal humerus fractures not involving the humeral shaft, patients initially are immobilized in a simple sling.
  - When pain improves and the fracture moves as a unit, passive range of motion (ROM) is started. Patients begin with pendulum exercises, usually 2 to 3 weeks after injury, then progress to ROM in all planes.
  - Between 6 and 10 weeks, the fracture usually has healed enough that strengthening exercises may be started.[13]
- Physical therapy is very important when treating proximal humerus fractures conservatively. Koval et al[11] showed significant improvement with one-part fractures when physical therapy was initiated before 2 weeks.
- Several studies have shown that nonoperative management can lead to acceptable results with proximal humerus fractures.[22,25,28]
- Studies comparing patients treated surgically and nonsurgically have shown no difference in outcome with two-part surgical neck fractures[4] and displaced three- and four-part fractures,[27] although these studies were done before the advent of anatomic proximal humeral plating.

SURGICAL MANAGEMENT

- It is imperative that patients have reasonable expectations of their outcome following surgery. Patients also must be aware of the importance of physical therapy postoperatively.

Preoperative Planning

▪ Acceptable imaging studies, either plain radiographs or a CT scan, are necessary before proceeding to surgery.

▪ Each proximal humerus fracture is unique, and in most cases a planned method of fixation is chosen before entering the operating room. However, the definitive choice of fixation is not made until the fracture is visualized at surgery. Consequently, the surgeon should be prepared with an arsenal of different fixation techniques.

  ▪ If the fracture is not deemed suitable for internal fixation intraoperatively, the surgeon must be prepared to perform a hemiarthoplasty.

▪ Multiple techniques can be employed for surgical fixation of the proximal humerus. In this chapter, we describe several current techniques. The final choice of appropriate manner of fixation should be based on the individual patient, the fracture pattern, and the surgeon's own comfort level.

Positioning

▪ The techniques discussed in this section are easiest to perform with the patient in the beach chair position. With the patient nearly seated, the hips and knees are flexed. The patient is moved as far laterally as possible on the table to allow full ROM of the shoulder. A lateral buttress is used to help keep the patient in position on the table.

▪ C-arm fluoroscopy is helpful in determining the quality of reduction. The C-arm is best positioned with the intensifier posterior to the shoulder and the arm over the patient (**FIG 2**).

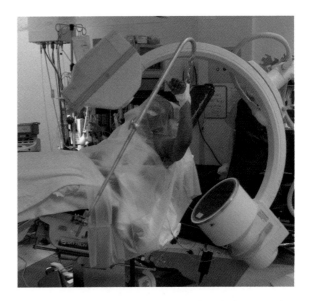

FIG 2 • Positioning of the patient in the beach chair position with fluoroscopic imaging. The C-arm intensifier should be posterior to allow for ideal visualization.

Approach

▪ The approach depends on the surgical technique to be used and is discussed further in the Techniques section.

▪ The deltopectoral approach is most commonly employed.

FIXATION OF ISOLATED TUBEROSITY FRACTURES

▪ The patient is placed in the beach chair position.

▪ An incision is made from the tip of the acromion extending laterally down the arm.

  ▪ Alternatively, an incision can be made parallel to the lateral border of the acromion, as used in open rotator cuff repair.

▪ Skin flaps are then raised.

▪ The deltoid is split in line with its fibers, and the anterior portion of the deltoid may be detached from the acromion.

  ▪ A deltopectoral approach also could be used.

  ▪ The deltoid fibers should not be split further than 5 cm below the acromion, to prevent damage to the axillary nerve. A suture at the distal aspect of the split can help prevent inadvertent extension.[10]

▪ As with all open procedures described in this chapter, the fracture should be cleaned of hematoma to facilitate reduction.

▪ The greater tuberosity usually is displaced posteriorly or superiorly. Abducting and externally rotating the shoulder will take tension off the posterosuperior rotator cuff, allowing the greater tuberosity fragment to be more easily reduced.

  ▪ Traction sutures in the rotator cuff may prove valuable in obtaining reduction.

▪ Provisional fixation can then be obtained with a K-wire (**TECH FIG 1A,B**).

▪ Cannulated screws placed over the wire may then be used for definitive fixation if placed in an acceptable location.

  ▪ Screws should be of the appropriate length to gain adequate purchase (**TECH FIG 1C,D**) but not so long that they are symptomatic.

  ▪ The use of washers may prove beneficial.

▪ Alternatively, suture fixation of the greater tuberosity back to the humerus may provide better fixation than cannulated screws in those patients with poor bone quality.

  ▪ This can be accomplished by placing two suture anchors into the fracture bed (**TECH FIG 1E**).

  ▪ Both limbs of each anchor can then be brought through drill holes in the fragment and tied over the top (**TECH FIG 1F**).

  ▪ Suture also can be placed at the bone–tendon interface of the tuberosity fragment and then through bone tunnels in the shaft, as discussed later in this section.

▪ If the anterior deltoid was detached during the approach, it must be repaired back to the acromion using nonabsorbable sutures.

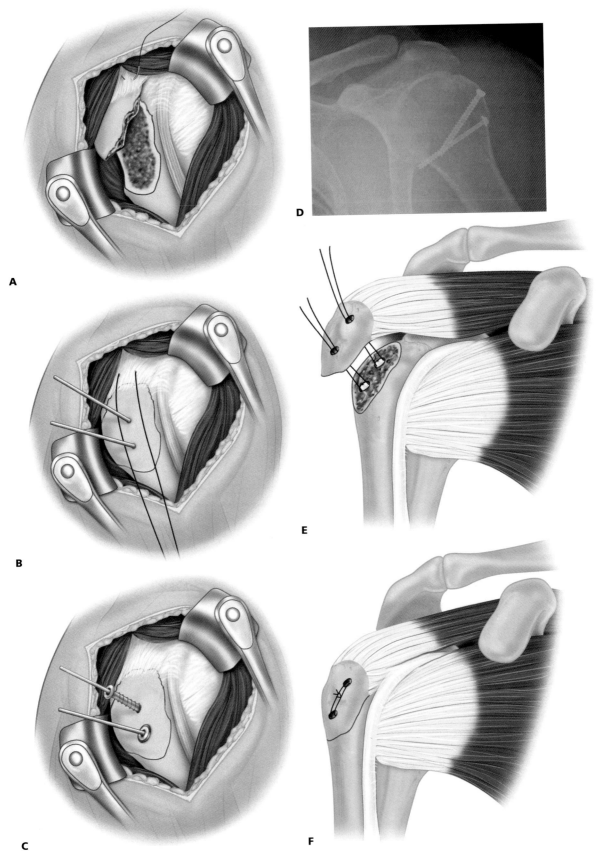

TECH FIG 1 • **A.** Traction sutures are placed through the rotator cuff tendon to aid in reduction of the displaced greater tuberosity. **B.** Wires may be used to maintain reduction of the tuberosity. **C.** Screw fixation with 4.5-mm cannulated screws. **D.** Final fixation. Screws should obtain purchase in the far cortex, but they must not be long enough to damage the axillary nerve. **E.** Placement of suture anchors into the fracture bed. **F.** Reduced fracture with sutures tied over the greater tuberosity.

OPEN REDUCTION AND SUTURE FIXATION

- The patient is placed in the beach chair position. Depending on the pattern, the fracture may be approached via the deltopectoral interval or a deltoid-splitting approach.
- The rotator interval tissue may be incised. This "interval split" allows visualization of the humeral head articular surface, if needed, in the setting of intact tuberosities and rotator cuff, as with head split patterns.
- Multiple sutures are placed through the tendons of the rotator cuff, preferably no. 5 nonabsorbable sutures or 1-mm tapes.
  - Both the subscapularis tendon and the posterosuperior cuff tendons should be incorporated[20] (**TECH FIG 2A**).

- Drill holes should be placed distal to the fracture site. The bone on either side of the bicipital groove is of excellent quality and should hold sutures well (**TECH FIG 2B,C**).
- In most cases, anatomic reduction is desired.
- With three-part fractures involving the greater tuberosity, the head fragment should first be secured to the shaft, followed by reduction of the greater tuberosity.[20]
- For high surgical neck fractures, sutures should be placed into any remaining tuberosity on the head fragment to help maintain fixation.

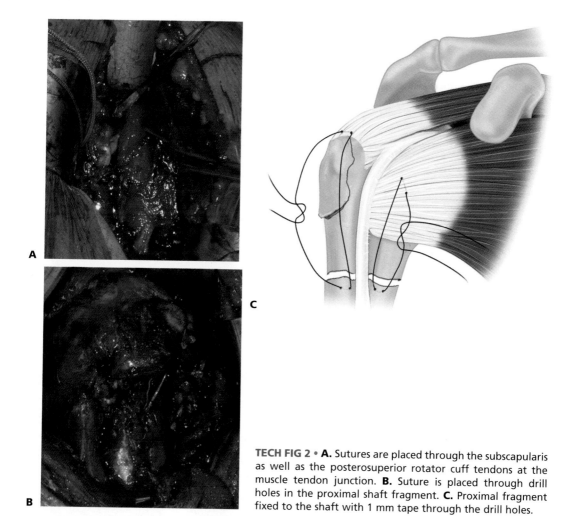

TECH FIG 2 • A. Sutures are placed through the subscapularis as well as the posterosuperior rotator cuff tendons at the muscle tendon junction. **B.** Suture is placed through drill holes in the proximal shaft fragment. **C.** Proximal fragment fixed to the shaft with 1 mm tape through the drill holes.

OPEN REDUCTION AND INTERNAL FIXATION USING ANATOMIC PLATING

Exposure

- Anatomic plating of the proximal humerus commonly is performed through the deltopectoral interval.
- With the patient in the beach chair position, an incision is made starting from above the coracoid process and extending distally as needed along the deltopectoral groove (**TECH FIG 3A**).
- The plane between the deltoid and pectoralis major is developed, mobilizing the cephalic vein.
  - Cobb elevators can be used to develop this plane, making it easier for the surgeon to identify

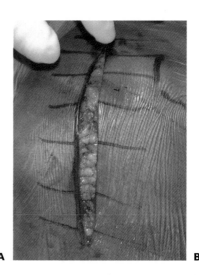
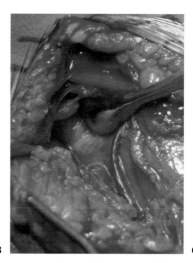
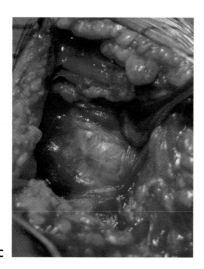

TECH FIG 3 • **A.** The incision is made extending from the coracoid process distally along the deltopectoral groove. **B.** Identifying the interval between the deltoid and pectoralis major. **C.** Using two Cobb elevators to develop the interval, bringing the cephalic vein laterally.

and ligate branches of the cephalic vein (**TECH FIG 3B,C**).

- The underlying clavipectoral fascia is identified and incised laterally to the conjoined tendon.[10]
  - The conjoined tendon is carefully retracted medially with the pectoralis major and the deltoid retracted laterally.

Reduction

- The fracture and rotator cuff are now visible. With fractures involving displaced tuberosities, we recommend obtaining control of the tuberosities with sutures placed at the bone–tendon interface (**TECH FIG 4A**).
  - Heavy sutures may be placed through the insertions of the cuff tendons and later used as supplemental fixation if necessary.
  - For fractures with minimally displaced tuberosities, sutures may not be needed before a reduction maneuver.

- A Cobb elevator placed in the fracture site will aid in reducing the fracture (**TECH FIG 4B**).
  - The pectoralis major insertion is elevated in a subperiosteal fashion if necessary. The plate should be placed lateral to the biceps tendon so as not to disrupt the blood supply to the humeral head (**TECH FIG 4C**).
  - Often, it may be necessary to release a small portion of the anterior deltoid insertion before placing the plate.

Plate Fixation

- Fluoroscopy should be used to confirm the reduction before placement of the plate, especially in regard to the superior aspect of the plate.
  - A plate positioned too high or a fracture fixed in varus may result in the plate impinging on the undersurface of the acromion. K-wires may be used to temporarily maintain fixation proximally and distally.
  - Alternatively, multiple guidewires may be placed into drill sleeves (**TECH FIG 5A**). Confirm plate location

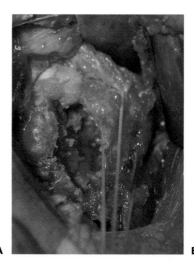
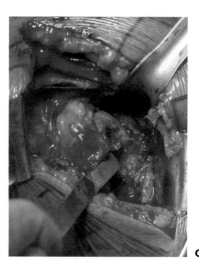
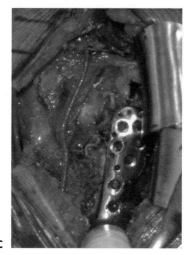

TECH FIG 4 • **A.** Traction sutures through the tendinous attachments of the rotator cuff may be helpful in correcting varus deformity. **B.** Reducing the fracture by elevating the proximal fragment. **C.** Correct placement of the plate is lateral to the biceps tendon (not seen here). Suture fixation has been used to help maintain fixation and supplement the plate.

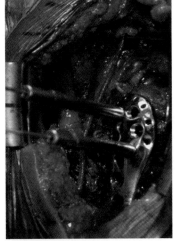
A

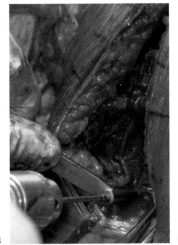
B

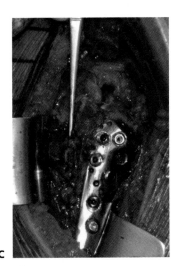
C

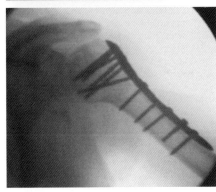
D

TECH FIG 5 • A. K-wires through drill sleeves are used to maintain plate fixation. Note the position of the superior aspect of the plate in relation to the top of the tuberosity. **B.** Once the head is secured to the plate, distal screws may be placed. **C.** Final plate fixation. **D.** Fluoroscopic image showing screw placement.

again, both proximally and distally, before placing screws.
- Locking screws usually are placed proximally into the head first, and multiple configurations of screws are possible.
  - Once the head is secured to the shaft, distal screws can be placed (**TECH FIG 5B**).
  - Final plate placement should be confirmed fluoroscopically (**TECH FIG 5C,D**).
- Sutures placed through the cuff tendons also may be secured to the plate, shaft, or other tuberosity.
  - At the completion of the procedure, the pectoralis major may be secured with sutures through holes in the plate.

- In osteoporotic bone, the tuberosities can first be attached to the shaft with sutures, following which a locking plate may be placed along the lateral aspect of the proximal humerus.
- Fixation of displaced two-part proximal humerus fractures also can be performed using a locking plate in a percutaneous fashion. With this technique, great care must be taken to prevent injury to the axillary nerve.
  - A recent cadaveric study[8] demonstrated that the axillary nerve was an average of 3 mm from the second most proximal diaphyseal screw hole, and an average of 7 mm from the third most proximal screw hole. All other screw holes were more than 1 cm from the nerve.

PEARLS AND PITFALLS

Indications	▪ An understanding of the neurovascular anatomy as well as the deforming forces present in proximal humerus fractures is vital to treating these injuries effectively.
Exposure	▪ Avoid devascularizing fracture fragments by stripping pieces minimally. ▪ Development of the "interval split" aids in fracture visualization and reduction and does not require detachment of the rotator cuff tendons. This is especially helpful when trying to fix a head-splitting fracture in a young patient.
Maintaining fixation	▪ K-wires are useful for maintaining initial fixation. ▪ With suture fixation, the strong bone along the bicipital groove of the distal fragment will hold sutures the best.
Poor bone quality	▪ With osteoporotic three-part fractures, consider suture fixation first, followed by a proximal humeral locking plate. ▪ Anatomic plating is very helpful when medial comminution is present.
Superior impingement	▪ Avoid placing the locking plate too high on greater tuberosity.

POSTOPERATIVE CARE

- Stable fixation must be obtained to allow for immediate ROM.
  - A physical therapy regimen should be established based on the stability of fixation, the fracture pattern, the quality of the bone, and individual patient factors.
  - Ideally, the fixation should allow pendulum exercises on the first postoperative day and 130 degrees of passive forward flexion and 30 degrees of passive external rotation.
  - Between 4 and 6 weeks after surgery, an overhead pulley can be added, with stretching and active motion added at 6 to 8 weeks.
  - Formal strengthening with elastic bands is not started until 10 to 12 weeks after surgery.[3]
- As with nonoperative treatment, participation in physical therapy is key to a successful outcome.
  - In a recent study looking at fixation of two- and three-part fractures, the only patients with unsatisfactory outcomes were those who were noncompliant with physical therapy.[20]

OUTCOMES

- Neer's original description called for fixation of greater tuberosity fractures when there was more than 1 cm of displacement.[17]
- One recent study had excellent or good results in 12 of 16 patients with fixation of greater tuberosity fractures displaced more than 1 cm.[7] Forward elevation averaged 170 degrees, and external rotation averaged 63 degrees.
- Some authors believe that greater tuberosity displacement of greater than 5 mm may lead to poor outcomes.
  - McLauglin[14] first suggested that patients in whom a greater tuberosity healed with residual displacement of more than 5 mm had longstanding pain with poor function. Displacement of less than 5 mm does not appear to warrant surgery.
  - Platzer et al[21] looked at minimally displaced fractures of the greater tuberosity and found no statistical significance with varying degrees of displacement less than 5 mm.
- Open reduction with suture or wire fixation can achieve acceptable fixation, especially in older patients with osteoporotic bone. The technique can be used reliably in two- and three-part fractures.
  - One study showed nearly 80% excellent results with average motion of 155 degrees of average forward flexion, 46 degrees average external rotation, and internal rotation to T11. Furthermore, there were no reported cases of osteonecrosis of the humeral head.[20]
- Early open reduction and internal fixation with a laterally placed T-plate failed to yield consistently good results, especially for four-part fractures.[12,19] Other early osteosynthesis techniques include the cloverleaf and the blade–plate, but the current trend is toward anatomic plating technology.
  - Recent studies show promise with the use of such locking plates, although this technique is not without complications.[6]

COMPLICATIONS

- Infection
- Nonunion
- Malunion
- Avascular necrosis
- Nerve injury
- Impingement secondary to fixation or residual tuberosity displacement
- Failure of fixation, including varus malposition and plate fracture with proximal humeral anatomic plating[6]

REFERENCES

1. Bernstein J, Adler LM, Blank JE, et al. Evaluation of the Neer system of classification of proximal humeral fractures with computed tomographic scans and plain radiographs. J Bone Joint Surg Am 1996; 78A:1371–1375.
2. Blom S, Dahlback LO. Nerve injuries in dislocations of the shoulder joint and fractures of the neck of the humerus. Acta Chir Scand 1970;136:461–466.
3. Cameron BD, Williams GR. Operative fixation of three-part proximal humerus fractures. Tech Shoulder Elbow Surg 2002;3:111–123.
4. Court-Brown CM, Garg A, McQueen MM. The translated two-part fracture of the proximal humerus: Epidemiology and outcome in the older patient. J Bone Joint Surg Br 2001;83B:799–804.
5. DeFranco MJ, Brems JJ, Williams GR Jr, et al. Evaluation and management of valgus impacted four-part proximal humerus fractures. Clin Orthop Relat Res 2006;442:109–114.
6. Fankhauser F, Boldin C, Schippinger G, et al. A new locking plate for unstable fractures of the proximal humerus. Clin Orthop Relat Res 2005;430:176–181.
7. Flatow EL, Cuomo F, Maday MG, et al. Open reduction and internal fixation of two-part displaced fractures of the greater tuberosity of the proximal part of the humerus. J Bone Joint Surg Am 1991;73A:1213–1218.
8. Gallo RA, Altman GT. A cadaveric study to evaluate the safety of percutaneous plating of the proximal humerus. Pennsylvania Orthopaedic Society 2006 Spring Scientific Meeting, Paradise Island, The Bahamas, May 4–6, 2006.
9. Gerber C, Schneeberger AG, Vinh T. The arterial vascularization of the humeral head. J Bone Joint Surg Am 1990;72A:1486–1494.
10. Hoppenfeld S, deBoer P. Surgical Exposures in Orthopaedics, ed 3. Philadelphia: Lippincott Williams & Wilkins, 2003.
11. Koval KJ, Gallagher MA, Marsicano JG, et al. Functional outcome after minimally displaced fractures of the proximal part of the humerus. J Bone Joint Surg Am 1997;79A:203–207.
12. Kristiansen B, Christensen SW. Plate fixation of proximal humeral fractures. Acta Orthop Scand 1986;57:320–323.
13. McKoy BE, Bensen CV, Hartsock LA. Fractures about the shoulder: Conservative management. Orthop Clin North Am 2000;31: 205–216.
14. McLauglin HL. Dislocation of the shoulder with tuberosity fractures. Surg Clin North Am 1963;43:1615–1620.
15. Moriber LA, Patterson RL Jr. Fractures of the proximal end of the humerus. J Bone Joint Surg Am 1967;49A:1018.
16. Muller ME, Nazarian S, Koch P, et al. The Comprehensive Classification of Fractures of Long Bones. Berlin: Springer-Verlag, 1990.
17. Neer CS II. Displaced proximal humeral fractures. Part I. Classification and evaluation. J Bone Joint Surg Am 1970;52A:1077–1089.
18. Neer CS II. Displaced proximal humeral fractures. Part II. Treatment of three-part and four-part displacement. J Bone and J Surg Am 1970;52A:1090–1103.
19. Paavolainen P, Bjorkenheim J, Slatis P, Paukku P. Operative treatment of severe proximal humeral fractures. Acta Orthop Scand 1983; 54:374–379.
20. Park MC, Murthi AM, Roth NS, et al. Two-part and three-part fractures of the proximal humerus treated with suture fixation. J Orthop Trauma 2003;17:319–325.
21. Platzer P, Kutscha-Lissberg F, Lehr S, et al. The influence of displacement on shoulder function in patients with minimally displaced fractures of the greater tuberosity. Injury 2005;36:1185–1189.
22. Rasmussen S, Hvass I, Dalsgaard J, et al. Displaced proximal humeral fractures: Results of conservative treatment. Injury 1992;23:41–43.

23. Sidor ML, Zuckerman JD, Lyon T, et al. The Neer Classification system for proximal humeral fractures. J Bone Joint Surg Am 1993; 75A:1745–1750.
24. Siebenrock KA, Gerber C. The reproducibility of classification of fractures of the proximal end of the humerus. J Bone Joint Surg Am 1993;75A:1751–1755.
25. Young TB, Wallace WA. Conservative treatment of fractures and fracture-dislocations of the upper end of the humerus. J Bone Joint Surg Br 1985;67B:373–377.
26. Zuckerman JD, Checroun AJ. Fractures of the proximal humerus: Diagnosis and management. In: Iannotti JP, Williams JR, eds. Disorders of the Shoulder: Diagnosis and Management. Philadelphia: Lippincott Williams & Wilkins, 1999;639–685.
27. Zyto K, Ahrengart L, Sperber A, et al. Treatment of displaced proximal humeral fractures in elderly patients. J Bone Joint Surg Br 1997;79B:412–417.
28. Zyto K. Non-operative treatment of comminuted fractures of the proximal humerus in elderly patients. Injury 1998;29:349–352.

Chapter 18

Intramedullary Fixation of Proximal Humerus Fractures

J. Dean Cole

DEFINITION

▪ From 50% to 80% of proximal humerus fractures are nondisplaced or minimally displaced and stable.[12] Early range of motion after a short period of immobilization usually is sufficient to treat these fractures and has been shown to result in satisfactory outcomes.[1] The remaining 20% to 50% of patients with proximal humerus fractures may benefit from operative management.

▪ Numerous techniques of internal fixation for proximal humerus fractures have been described and reported, including cloverleaf and blade plating,[1] Rush pinning,[15,19] spiral pinning,[18] Kirschner wire and tension band fixation,[3] suture and external fixation,[7] and intramedullary nail fixation.[8]

▪ Extensive dissection and inadequate biomechanical fixation in the context of the severe soft tissue injury and devascularization associated with these complex fracture types are the commonly cited reasons for failure of internal fixation devices.[2]

▪ Prosthetic arthroplasty traditionally has been the recommended treatment for three-part fractures with osteoporosis, four-part fractures, head-splitting fractures, and articular compression fractures that involve more than 40% of the articular surface.[1,2,11]

▪ Recently, several authors have reported satisfactory results with various types of osteosynthesis for four-part fractures, leading them to recommend an attempt at internal fixation in younger patients.[3,4,7,16] The basis of this recommendation is that subsequent published series have been unable to reproduce Neer's results with early hemiarthroplasty for four-part fractures.

▪ Various reports have been made on the use of intramedullary nails in the proximal humerus. We prefer to use an intramedullary nail that permits stable fixation of the head to the shaft of the humerus using a minimally invasive rotator cuff–splitting approach (DePuy Inc., Warsaw, IN).

  ▪ The method for treatment of proximal humeral fractures described in this chapter involves a minimally invasive anterior acromial surgical approach, an indirect method of reduction, and a unique intramedullary rod designed to permit a variety of proximal interlocking configurations.

ANATOMY

Osteology

▪ The proximal humerus includes the humeral head, the lesser tuberosity, the greater tuberosity, and the proximal humeral metaphysis.

▪ The position of the head is higher than the tuberosities, and changes in this relationship will cause impingement. The humeral head is slightly medial (3 mm) and posterior (7 mm) in relation to the humeral shaft (**FIG 1**).

▪ The humeral head is retroverted approximately 30 degrees (range 20 to 60 degrees).

▪ Minor losses in the humeral length between the head and the deltoid insertion can alter the deltoid length–tension ratio.

▪ Avulsion of the greater tuberosity indicates injury to the rotator cuff.

Vascular Supply of the Proximal Humerus

▪ The anterior and posterior humeral circumflex arteries are branches of the axillary artery.

  ▪ The arcuate artery, the terminal vessel of the ascending branch of the anterior humeral circumflex artery, supplies most of the humeral head.

    ▪ Avascularity of the humeral head can occur if this vessel is disrupted during a fracture of the anatomic neck.

  ▪ The posterior circumflex artery becomes important in patients with proximal humerus fractures.

    ▪ It may be the primary source of blood supply to the fractured head, so care should be taken to prevent additional devascularization.

▪ Traumatic and iatrogenic vascular insult may lead to devascularization of the fracture fragments, resulting in delayed union, nonunion, and avascular necrosis. Traumatic injury cannot be predicted; well-planned minimally invasive procedures should reduce the risk of further damage, however.

Innervation

▪ The brachial plexus is at risk in patients with upper extremity injury, and thorough neurologic evaluation is mandatory.

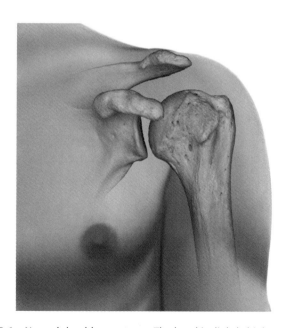

FIG 1 • Normal shoulder anatomy. The head is slightly higher than the tuberosities, slightly medial and posterior to the humeral shaft, retroverted 30 degrees. (Copyright J. Dean Cole, MD.)

- The axillary nerve courses through the quadrilateral space, where it is at risk during fracture dislocation.
- The lateral entry site for locking screw fixation (4–5 cm distal to the tip of the acromion) places the axillary nerve at risk.

PATHOGENESIS

- A blow to the anterior, lateral, or posterolateral aspect of the humerus typically is the cause.
- Axial load transmitted to the humerus may cause impacted fracture in osteoporotic bone.
- Violent muscle contractures, as in grand mal seizures and electric shock, are associated with posterior dislocation due to overpowering internal rotators and adductors.
- Pathologic causes include tumor, multiple myeloma, and metastatic or metabolic disorders.
- Osteoporosis is associated with fractures of the proximal humerus (more than any other fracture).
- In a three-part fracture with intact greater tuberosity, the humeral head is pulled by the supraspinatus and infraspinatus tendons; if the tendons are intact, the humeral head is externally rotated. The inverse is seen when the greater tuberosity is avulsed: the intact subscapularis internally rotates the humeral head (**FIG 2**).

NATURAL HISTORY

Epidemiology

- 4% to 5% of all fractures
- Increased incidence in osteoporosis, older middle-aged and elderly persons (third most common fracture in elderly)
- In persons older than 50 years of age, the female:male ratio is 4:1 (osteoporosis). Minor falls and trauma may cause comminuted fracture.
- In patients younger than 50 years of age, violent trauma, contact sports, and falls from heights are responsible for fractures.
- Surgical neck fracture is common.

Consequences of Injury

- Nondisplaced fractures may heal without major consequences.
- Acute, recurrent, or chronic dislocation

- Rotator cuff tears
- Neurovascular injury: axillary nerve, brachial plexus
- Avascular necrosis of the humeral head often results from disruption of the arcuate artery. The axillary artery also may be damaged, but less commonly, in fracture-dislocations.
- Malunion: loss of humeral length may cause deltoid weakness
- Posttraumatic arthrosis
- Adhesive capsulitis
- Chronic pain

PATIENT HISTORY AND PHYSICAL FINDINGS

- Associated injuries:
  - Rotator cuff tears
  - Dislocation
  - Forearm fractures
  - Brachial plexus, axillary, radial and ulnar nerve injuries (5%–30% of complex proximal humerus fractures)

IMAGING AND OTHER DIAGNOSTIC STUDIES

- Trauma series
  - Scapular anteroposterior (glenoid view)
  - Trans-scapular
  - Axillary
- Rotational views
- CT scan

SURGICAL MANAGEMENT

- Indications
  - Two-part proximal humerus fracture
  - Three-part proximal humerus fracture
  - Certain four-part proximal humerus fractures
- Prerequisites
  - Shoulder table, image intensification, and experienced radiology technician
  - Be aware of the learning curve (do not attempt nailing of a four-part fracture before acquiring adequate experience with two- and three-part fractures).

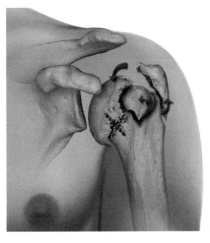
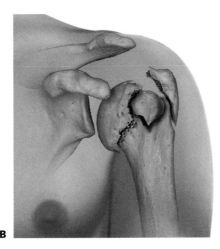
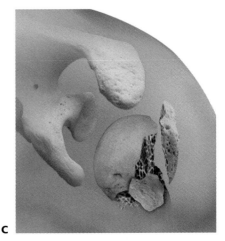

A   B   C

FIG 2 • A. Fracture pattern and deforming forces. The muscular attachments of the greater and lesser tuberosities will cause abduction, external rotation, and internal rotation, respectively. The head will follow whichever tuberosity is intact. **B,C.** In four-part fractures, the head often is in a neutrally rotated position. (Copyright J. Dean Cole, MD.)

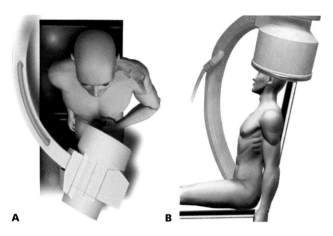

FIG 3 • Patient positioning should allow access of the C-arm to obtain orthogonal radiographs, which are critical in fracture reduction and fixation. **A.** Lateral view. **B.** Axial view. (Copyright J. Dean Cole, MD.)

■ When treating patients with complex fractures, obtain the patient's consent for a hemiarthroplasty if that is determined to be the best treatment, and have the implant available in case it is found to be necessary.

■ Contraindication: head-splitting, comminuted displaced humeral head fragment devoid of soft tissue attachment

Preoperative Planning

■ Successful intramedullary nailing of the proximal humerus fracture depends on consistent integration between image intensification and the surgical steps.

■ Patient positioning on a radiolucent table will allow the surgeon to use a minimally invasive approach.

■ Any error on the entry site will cause inevitable problems with the rest of the procedure.

■ It is crucial that the surgeon follow the surgical technique precisely.

Positioning

■ Positioning on the table must allow orthogonal and overhead axillary views.

■ The patient is placed supine in the beach chair position on a radiolucent table tilted at 60 to 70 degrees. The C-arm should be positioned on the opposite side of the table to allow the surgeon easy access to the proximal humerus (**FIG 3**).

■ A bolster is used to elevate the shoulder from the table and to allow shoulder extension. Extension of the shoulder is necessary to expose the entry site in the humeral head. Flexion of the shoulder will result in the acromion overlying the center of the humeral head in the sagittal plane, obscuring the entry site or errantly directing an entry angle. Anterior cutout of the nail in the head fragment can easily occur in an osteoporotic humeral head with an associated greater tuberosity fracture.

Approach

■ Intramedullary nailing for isolated surgical neck fractures may be performed completely percutaneously using most of the techniques described in the following paragraphs. However, when tuberosity reduction and fixation are required, a wider approach often is necessary.

■ The timing of the open approach depends on the sequencing of head, shaft, and tuberosity fixation. In the technique we describe in this chapter, head–shaft fixation is accomplished percutaneously using nailing and interlocking screws before tuberosity fixation. Alternatively, an open approach with tuberosity reduction and fixation can be performed before nail insertion.

■ The surgical approach for viewing tuberosity fractures that require fixation is a lateral deltoid-splitting approach made just below the acromion, approximately 4 cm long, that does not extend distally, to avoid injury to the axillary nerve (**FIG 4A**).

■ For a lesser tuberosity approach, a separate, small deltopectoral incision is centered just over the lesser tuberosity, and the lesser tuberosity fixation or fixation to the subscapularis tendon is performed in that plane (**FIG 4B**).

■ The rotator cuff is incised longitudinally away from the lateral watershed area of the rotator cuff and away from Sharpey's fibers and the connection of the tendon to the bone.

■ Significant rotator cuff defect is not created with this approach, as confirmed in cadaver dissection. The longitudinal incision on the rotator cuff does not weaken the cuff.

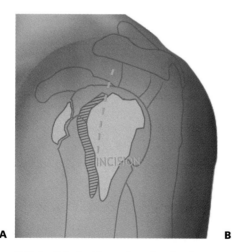
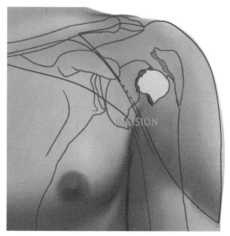

FIG 4 • Skin incisions. **A.** Deltoid-splitting incision specifically for greater tuberosity fixation. **B.** Deltopectoral incision specifically for lesser tuberosity fixation. (Copyright J. Dean Cole, MD.)

K-WIRE PLACEMENT

- Placement of K-wires allows fragment reduction and helps dictate placement of the skin incision and surgical approach. Hence, the first step involves placement of a K-wire in the subacromial space; it is inserted through the anterolateral aspect of the shoulder using the image intensifier (C-arm) and directed posteromedial toward the glenoid (**TECH FIG 1A,B**).
  - This initial pin will serve as a guide for the retroversion of the humeral head.
- Next, two K-wires are placed in the humeral head, directed lateral to medial, one anterior and one posterior to the central aspect of the head (**TECH FIG 1C,D**). The wires should be separated by enough distance to allow insertion of the nail between them (1.5 cm).

- The K-wires should be directed in the longest axis of the humeral head in the axial plane. Allowing for retroversion is important.
- Confirmation of the correct placement in the axial plane is done by the overhead axillary view. Then the C-arm is positioned to view the advancement of the pins in the coronal plane projection.
  - With longer K-wires, the surgeon's hand can be kept out of radiographs. Unfortunately, with internal rotation, extension also occurs in the humerus and the humeral head, depending on the soft tissue attachments.

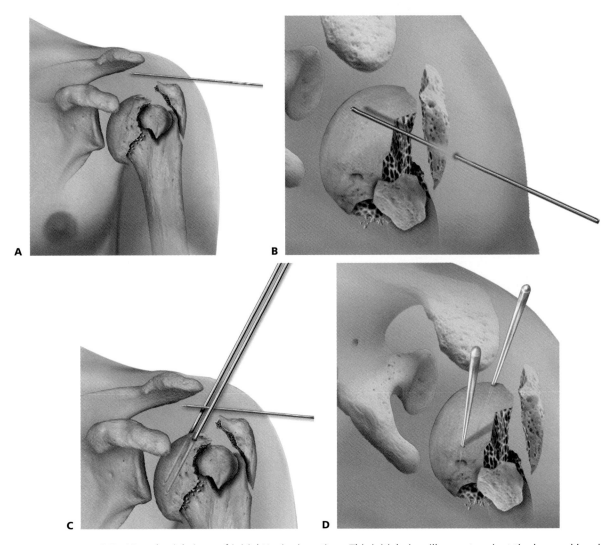

TECH FIG 1 • A,B. AP and axial views of initial K-wire insertion:. This initial pin will serve to orient the humeral head, specifically the desired degree of retroversion. **C,D.** AP and axial views of pins to control head fragment. These pins are inserted to control the head fragment in a joystick fashion. (Copyright J. Dean Cole, MD.)

FRAGMENT REDUCTION

- The K-wires can then be used in a joystick fashion to adduct and extend the head, exposing the supraspinatus tendon and optimal entry site in the head from beneath the anterior edge of the acromion (**TECH FIG 2A,B**).
- Image intensification can be used to place a K-wire through the head in line with intramedullary axis of the humerus. This maneuver includes two important aspects:
  - The first is to use the joysticks to extend and adduct the proximal humeral head, exposing the anterolateral portion of the head from under the acromion while simultaneously distracting the distal shaft, thereby aligning the longitudinal intramedullary axis of the proximal and distal fragments (**TECH FIG 2C,D**).
  - The second is to drive the K-wire into the head in a central position with reference to the medullary canal in the sagittal plane and lateral to central in reference to the canal in the frontal or coronal plane (**TECH FIG 2E**).
- To achieve fracture reduction, the joysticks in the proximal fragment must be used to rotate the head while simultaneously rotating the distal shaft manually to obtain true orthogonal views of the head in reference to the shaft.

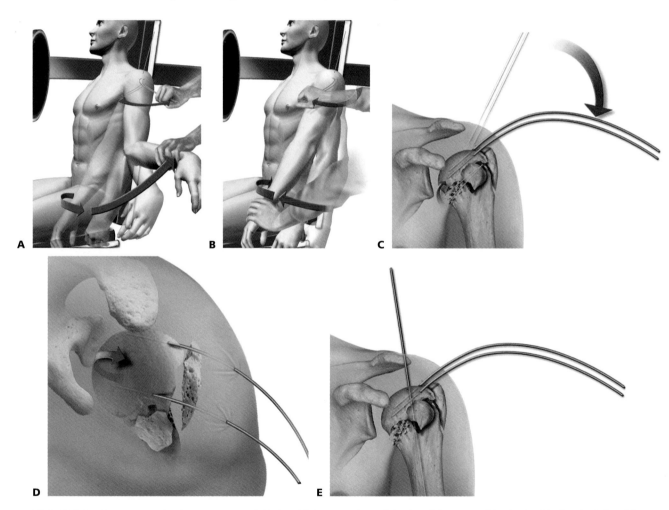

TECH FIG 2 • Fragment reduction maneuver. **A,B.** Combining rotation of the head fragment (K-wires) with the shaft (arm) is used to assist in fracture reduction. **C,D.** AP and axial views of humeral head reduction maneuver. Manipulation of the fracture fragments with the K-wires allows disimpaction of the fracture, improving the varus or valgus alignment. **E.** Pin entry site in humeral head. (Copyright J. Dean Cole, MD.)

GUIDEWIRE PLACEMENT

- The nail can be placed percutaneous just anterior to the anterior edge of the acromion.
- The anterior edge may be difficult to palpate and to differentiate from the humeral head because of edema and hematoma from the fracture. Therefore, it is helpful to locate the anterior edge of the angle of the acromion under image intensification with a K-wire where it intersects the longitudinal axis of the humerus.

- Correct placement of the guidewire is crucial; it should be centered in both frontal and sagittal planes.
- Manipulation of the proximal fragment has been the only reliable way to identify correct placement.

- This is easily accomplished in the coronal plane, but it is more difficult in the sagittal plane. Attention should be directed at the rotational alignment.

ENTRY SITE REAMING

- Reaming of the entry site should be performed carefully, as the percutaneous incision is small.
- The reamer is inserted over the guidewire, and the soft tissues are retracted and protected. The reamer is advanced through the rotator cuff in "reverse" until bone contact, then on "forward" through the humeral head. The reamer is left in place.
- The guidewire that was used to initiate the entry site is removed, and a longer guidewire is passed to the shaft

fragment. Manipulation of the shaft fragment sometimes is necessary. The reamer's sound must be used to gauge the canal diameter. It is necessary to ream 1 mm greater than the anticipated nail size.

- On some occasions, even external fixator placement from the scapular spine to the distal humerus is necessary. The external fixator is applied and distraction accomplished with manipulation of the proximal aspect of the shaft; guidewire passage usually is simple.

NAIL INSERTION

- Once the nail is inserted, confirm the rotation of the humerus in the axial plane; it is necessary to ensure proper alignment before impaction (**TECH FIG 3**).
- Usually, impaction of the distal fragment by blows against the olecranon, while supporting the proximal

humeral head indirectly through the soft tissues, is adequate.

- Large gaps are not acceptable, and it may be necessary to use filler substance.

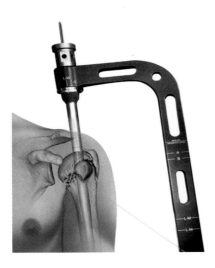

TECH FIG 3 • Nail insertion. (Copyright J. Dean Cole, MD.)

INTERLOCKING SCREW FIXATION

- We recommend that the oblique distal screw be the initial locking screw (**TECH FIG 4**). The goal of this screw is to attach the head to the shaft before fixation of the tuberosities.
- Screw placement puts the axillary nerve at risk. Careful blunt dissection to bone, drilling within the sheath, and placing the screw within the confines of the sheath are necessary. Drilling should be done very carefully, although it certainly does not completely negate the risk of drilling through the humeral head. Careful observation is important.

- It is occasionally helpful to remove the drill and then use a blunt guidewire and assure good humeral head subchondral bone contact before further drilling or screw placement.
- Central placement of the distal oblique screw in the humeral head is important. This step should flow very smoothly if the initial K-wires have been placed in the correct axial plane alignment.
  - Errant placement or acceptance of poorly positioned K-wires will result only in further deviation. If the distal oblique screw is not placed at the appropriate

- angle, the radiographs may be deceptive and may result in screw penetration.
  - Screw placement on the subchondral bone is important for fixation. However, patients with osteoporosis do have a risk of the fracture fragment settling.

- A and B screws are placed depending on goals of fixation.
  - Overdrilling to countersink the more proximal screw usually is necessary to avoid impingement.
  - These screws rarely are helpful in tuberosity fixation.

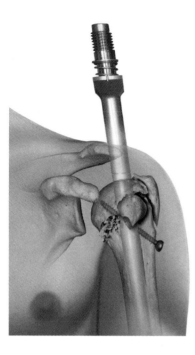
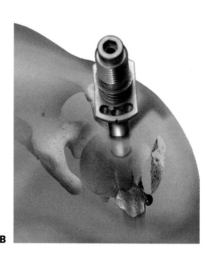

TECH FIG 4 • AP and axial views of intramedullary nail and proximal locking screw. (Copyright J. Dean Cole, MD.)

TUBEROSITY FIXATION

- The tuberosity fixation sequence is somewhat variable.
- With very displaced tuberosity fractures, if shaft-to-head fixation is performed initially with the tuberosities displaced, the guide will perforate the cuff and pin the cuff in a nonanatomic position, resulting in inability to perform reduction of the tuberosities. Therefore, if tuberosity fixation is going to be aided with the nail, the tuberosity alignment must be performed before nailing.
- Another sequence involves fixation of the head and shaft followed by later fixation of the tuberosity. Anchors can be passed through the nail with sutures used later to fix the tuberosities.

- The sequence of fixation should involve passing sutures through the musculotendinous junction of the subscapularis, infraspinatus, and supraspinatus. Sutures passed over the superior aspect of the head from the infraspinatus and subscapularis and sutures passed laterally around the head provide helpful, reliable fixation points. With practice, these maneuvers can be performed in a minimally invasive manner.
- Comminuted tuberosity fixation is challenging. It is difficult to achieve consistent fixation with screws. A headless screw has been used with some success in limited cases.

PEARLS AND PITFALLS

Indications	■ Two-part proximal humerus fracture ■ Three-part proximal humerus fracture ■ Select four-part proximal humerus fracture
Prerequisites	■ Shoulder table, image intensification, and *experienced* radiology technician ■ Be aware of the learning curve. ■ Plan B: for complex fractures, obtain consent for a hemiarthroplasty and have an implant available.
Contraindication	■ Head-splitting, comminuted displaced humeral head fragment devoid of soft tissue attachment
Positioning	■ Beach chair position to allow clear fluoroscopic images. Chair with metal extensions positioned to allow overhead axillary C-arm views.

Reduction technique	■ Humeral head is adducted; use K-wire as guide. ■ Percutaneously drill K-wires in the head fragment and use them as a "joystick" to rotate the head fragment. ■ Orthogonal views of the shoulder
Nail entry site	■ Erring at the entry site inevitably will cause problems with the rest of the procedure.
Screw placement	■ A drill guide is used to prevent injury to the axillary nerve.

POSTOPERATIVE CARE

■ The postoperative regimen depends on the stability of the fixation and the soft tissues.

■ Sling with abduction pillow that allows the proximal humerus to rest in neutral rotation and slight abduction (relax the rotator cuff and decrease tension on the greater tuberosity)

■ Gentle passive, pendulum, and active-assisted exercises of the shoulder

■ Active elbow and wrist exercises

■ Once fracture healing is detected on radiographic imaging, range of motion can be increased; weight lifting restrictions must be maintained until healing is complete.

COMPLICATIONS

■ Early
  ■ Injury to axillary nerve
  ■ Joint penetration
  ■ Loss of reduction
  ■ Infection
■ Late
  ■ Nonunion
  ■ Posttraumatic arthrosis
  ■ Avascular necrosis of humeral head
  ■ Prominent hardware

REFERENCES

1. Bigliani LU, Flatow EL, Pollock RG. Fractures of the proximal humerus: In: Rockwood CA, Green DP, Bucholz RW, et al, eds. Fractures in Adults. Philadelphia: Lippincott-Raven, 1996:1055–1107.
2. Connor PM, Flatow EL. Complications of internal fixation of proximal humeral fractures. Instr Course Lect 1997;46:25–37.
3. Darder A, Darder A Jr, Sanchis V, et al. Four-part displaced proximal humerus fractures: Operative treatment using Kirchner wires and a tension band. J Orthop Trauma 1993;7:497–505.
4. Esser RD. Open reduction and fixation of three- and four part fractures of the proximal humerus. Clin Orthop Relat Res 1994;299:244–251.
5. Goldman RT, Koval KJ, Cuomo F, et al. Functional outcome after humeral head replacement for acute three- and four-part proximal humeral fractures. J Shoulder Elbow Surg 1995;4:81–86.
6. Hawkins RJ, Switlyk P. Acute prosthetic replacement for severe fractures of the proximal humerus. Clin Orthop Relat Res 1993; 289:156–160.
7. Ko J, Yamamoto R. Surgical treatment of complex fracture of the proximal humerus. Clin Orthop Relat Res 1996;327:225–237.
8. Mouradian WI. Displaced proximal humeral fractures: seven years' experience with a modified Zickel supracondylar device. Clin Orthop Relat Res 1986;212:209–218.
9. Nayak NK, Schickendantz MS, Regan WD, et al. Operative treatment of nonunion of surgical neck fractures of the humerus. Clin Orthop Relat Res 1995;313:200–205.
10. Neer CS. Displaced proximal humeral fractures. Part I. Classification and evaluation. J Bone Joint Surg Am 1970;52A:1077–1089.
11. Neer CS. Displaced proximal humeral fractures. Part II. Treatment of three and four part displacement. J Bone Joint Surg Am 1970; 52A:1090–1103.
12. Norris TR. Fractures of the proximal humerus and dislocations of the shoulder. In: Browner BD, Jupiter JB, Levine AM, et al, eds. Skeletal Trauma: Fractures–Dislocations–Ligamentous Injuries. Philadelphia: WB Saunders, 1992:120–129.
13. Riemer BL, D'Ambrosia RD, Kellam JF, et al. The anterior acromial approach for antegrade intramedullary nailing of the humeral diaphysis. Orthopaedics 1993;16:1219–1223.
14. Robinson CM, Christie J. The two-part proximal humeral fracture: a review of operative treatment using two techniques. Injury 1993; 24:123–125.
15. Rush LV. Atlas of Rush Pin Technique: A System of Fracture Treatment. Meridian, MI: Bervion, 1955:166–167.
16. Szyszkowitz R, Seggl W, Schleifer P, et al. Proximal humeral fractures: management techniques and expected results. Clin Orthop Relat Res 1993;292:13–25.
17. Wheeler DL, Colville MR. Biomechanical comparison of intramedullary and percutaneous pin fixation for proximal humeral fracture fixation. J Orthop Trauma 1997;11:363–367.
18. Yano S, Takamura S, Kobayashi I, et al. Use of the spiral pin for fracture of the humeral neck. J Orthop Science 1981;55:1607–1619.
19. Weseley, MS, Barenfeld PA, Eisenstein AL. Rush pin intramedullary fixation for fractures of the proximal humerus. J Trauma 1977; 17:29–37.

Chapter 19

Hemiarthroplasty for Proximal Humerus Fractures

Kamal I. Bohsali, Michael A. Wirth, and Steven B. Lippitt

DEFINITION

- Proximal humerus fractures involve isolated or combined injuries to the greater tuberosity, lesser tuberosity, articular segment, and proximal humeral shaft.
- Overall, proximal humerus fractures account for 4% to 5% of all fractures.[8,13]

ANATOMY

- The proximal humerus consists of four segments: the greater tuberosity, lesser tuberosity, articular segment, and humeral shaft (**FIG 1**).
- The most cephalad surface of the articular segment is, on average, 8 mm above the greater tuberosity.[16] Humeral version averages 29.8 degrees (range 10 to 55 degrees).[23]
- The intertubercular groove lies between the tuberosities and forms the passageway for the long head of the biceps as it traverses from the intra-articular origin into the distal arm.
- The tuberosities attach to the articular segment at the anatomic neck. The greater tuberosity has three facets for the corresponding insertions of the supraspinatus, infraspinatus, and teres minor tendons; the lesser tuberosity has a single facet for the subscapularis.
- The deltoid, pectoralis major, and latissimus dorsi all insert on the humerus distal to the surgical neck. These soft tissue attachments contribute to the deforming forces sustained with proximal humerus fractures.

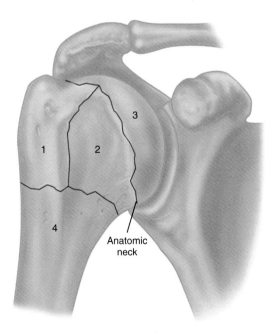

FIG 1 • Neer classification of proximal humerus fractures: *1,* greater tuberosity; *2,* lesser tuberosity; *3,* articular surface; *4,* shaft.

- The anterolateral branch of the anterior humeral circumflex artery (the arcuate artery of Laing) is the major blood supply to the humeral head. This vessel courses parallel to the lateral aspect of the long head of the biceps and enters the humeral head at the interface between the intertubercular groove and the greater tuberosity. Injury to the arcuate artery can result in osteonecrosis of the articular segment.[10,18]

PATHOGENESIS

- The incidence of proximal humerus fractures is increasing with an aging population and associated osteoporosis.
- The mechanism of injury may be indirect or direct and secondary to high-energy collisions in younger patients (eg, motor vehicle accidents, athletic injuries) or falls from standing height in elderly patients.
- Pathologic fractures from primary or metastatic disease should be included in the differential diagnosis.
- Risk factors for the development of proximal humerus fractures in the elderly patient population include low bone density, lack of hormone replacement therapy, previous fracture history, three or more chronic illnesses, and smoking.[15]

NATURAL HISTORY

- Neer's classic study in 1970 compared the results of nonoperative treatment with hemiarthroplasty for three- and four-part displaced proximal humerus fractures. No satisfactory results were found in the nonoperative group owing to inadequate reduction, nonunion, malunion, and humeral head osteonecrosis with collapse.[20]
- Stableforth[24] reaffirmed this in a study in which patients were randomized to nonoperative management or prosthetic replacement. The patients with displaced fractures treated nonoperatively had worse overall results for pain, range of motion, and activities of daily living.

PATIENT HISTORY AND PHYSICAL FINDINGS

- A thorough history and complete physical examination should be performed. History should include mechanism of injury, pre-morbid level of function, occupation, hand dominance, history of malignancy, and ability to participate in a structured rehabilitation program.[14]
- A review of systems should involve queries regarding loss of consciousness, paresthesias, and ipsilateral elbow or wrist pain.
- On physical examination, the orthopaedic surgeon should look for swelling, soft tissue injuries, ecchymosis, and deformity. Posterior fracture-dislocations will demonstrate flattening of the anterior aspect of the shoulder with an associated posterior prominence. Anterior fracture-dislocations present with opposite findings.[14]

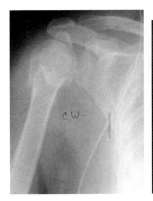
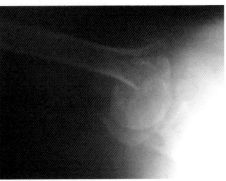

FIG 2 • AP and axillary views of a displaced three-part proximal humerus fracture without evidence of concomitant dislocation.

IMAGING AND OTHER DIAGNOSTIC STUDIES

- Appropriate radiographs include anteroposterior and axillary views of the shoulder[14] (**FIG 2**). If the axillary view cannot be obtained because of patient discomfort, alternate views such as the Velpeau trauma axillary view can be used to evaluate and classify the glenohumeral articulation.[2]
  - The Neer classification is based on the four anatomic segments of the proximal humerus: the humeral head, the greater and lesser tuberosities, and the humeral shaft (see Fig 1).[11] Number of parts is based on 45 degrees of angulation or 1 cm of displacement from neighboring segments.
  - The AO/ASIF/OTA Comprehensive Long Bone Classification system distinguishes the valgus impacted four-part proximal humerus fracture from other four-part fractures with partial preservation of the vascular inflow to the articular segment through an intact medial capsule.[17,22]
  - The current fracture classification systems have fair interobserver reliability, even with the addition of CT scans. Despite the limitations of these systems, they remain clinically useful when deciding on nonoperative versus operative treatment.[2,11]
- CT scans may be helpful in evaluating tuberosity displacement and articular surface involvement.[14]

DIFFERENTIAL DIAGNOSIS

- Acute hemorrhagic bursitis
- Traumatic rotator cuff tear
- Simple dislocation
- Acromioclavicular separation
- Calcific tendinitis [2]

NONOPERATIVE MANAGEMENT

- Nonoperative treatment usually is reserved for minimally displaced fractures of the proximal humerus, which account for nearly 80% of these injuries.
- The characteristics of the fracture (ie, bone quality, fracture orientation, concurrent soft tissue injuries), the personality of the patient (eg, compliant, realistic expectations, mental status), and surgeon experience all affect the decision to proceed with operative intervention.

- Moribund individuals and patients unable to cooperate with a postoperative rehabilitation program (eg, closed head injury) are not appropriate candidates for operative intervention.
- In general, nonoperative management of complex, displaced proximal humerus fractures has not proven as successful.
- Initial immobilization with a sling and axillary pad may be helpful. Gentle range-of-motion exercises may be started by 7 to 10 days after the fracture when pain has decreased and the patient is less apprehensive.[2]
- Intermittent biplanar radiographs are essential to determine additional displacement and the interval stage of healing.[2]
- Active and active assisted range-of-motion exercises are initiated with evidence of radiographic union. Inform the patient that he or she may never attain symmetric range of motion or strength when comparing the affected versus the uninjured side.

SURGICAL MANAGEMENT

- The goal of surgery is to anatomically reconstruct the glenohumeral joint with restoration of humeral length, placement of appropriate prosthetic retroversion, and establishment of secure tuberosity fixation.
- Prosthetic replacement is the preferred treatment of most four-part fractures, three-part fractures and dislocations in elderly patients with osteoporotic bone, head-splitting articular segment fractures, and chronic anterior or posterior humeral head dislocations with more than 40% of the articular surface involved.[25]
- Several studies have indicated that the outcome of primary hemiarthroplasty for acute proximal humerus fractures is superior to that from late reconstruction.[6,21]

Preoperative Planning

- Although some studies have suggested urgent intervention (ie, within less than 48 hours), most authors recommend preoperative planning with a careful neurovascular assessment of the injured shoulder, medical optimization of the patient, and preoperative templating with standard radiographs of the contralateral uninjured shoulder.[12]
- An interscalene block (regional anesthesia) may be used to supplement general anesthesia.
- Endotracheal intubation is recommended to allow for intraoperative muscle relaxation, but laryngeal mask intubation may be used.[12,14]

Positioning

■ The patient is placed on an operating table in the beach chair position with the arm positioned in a sterile articulating arm holder or draped free if an appropriate number of assistants are available (**FIG 3**).

Approach

■ The surgical prep site should include the entire upper extremity and shoulder region, including the scapular and pectoral regions.

■ Appropriate prophylactic intravenous antibiotics are given to the patient before skin incision.

■ A standard deltopectoral incision is used. Care is taken to minimize injury (eg, surgical detachment, contusion secondary to retractors) to the deltoid muscle. The musculocutaneous and axillary nerves are identified and protected during the procedure.

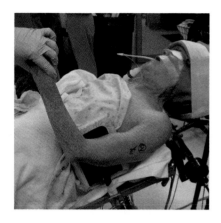

FIG 3 • Beach chair position. The patient is placed with the thorax at the end of the table. A kidney post and McConnell head holder are used to allow free and unencumbered access to the medullary canal of the humerus.

TECHNIQUES

DELTOPECTORAL APPROACH

■ The incision begins superior and medial to the coracoid process and extends toward the anterior aspect of the deltoid insertion (**TECH FIG 1A**).

■ The cephalic vein is identified, preserved, and retracted laterally with the deltoid muscle. The pectoralis major is mobilized medially. If additional exposure is necessary, the proximal 1 cm of the pectoralis major insertion is released (**TECH FIG 1B**).

■ Fracture hematoma usually is encountered once the clavipectoral fascia is incised. At this time, fracture fragments and the rotator cuff musculature become evident.

■ The axillary and musculocutaneous nerves can be identified through digital palpation of the anteroinferior aspect of the subscapularis muscle and the posterior aspect of the coracoid muscles respectively. External rotation of the humerus results in reduced tension on the axillary nerve.

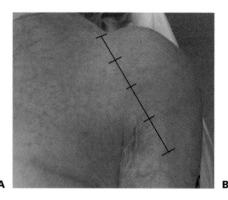

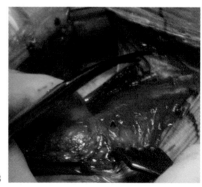

TECH FIG 1 • Skin incision and deltopectoral approach. **A.** The skin incision is centered over the anterior deltoid. The deltopectoral interval is developed with lateral retraction of the cephalic vein. **B.** For more exposure, the superior 1 cm of the pectoralis major tendon may be incised. (^, pectoralis major; #, deltoid; *, cephalic vein.)

TUBEROSITY MOBILIZATION

■ The tendon of the long head of the biceps is identified as it courses in the bicipital groove toward the rotator interval. The tendon serves as a key landmark when re-establishing the anatomic relationship between the greater and lesser tuberosities.

　■ The rotator interval and coracohumeral ligament are both released to allow for mobilization of the tuberosities (**TECH FIG 2A,B**).

■ If the fracture does not involve the bicipital groove, an osteotome or saw may be used to create a cleavage plane for tuberosity mobilization. Preservation of the coracoacromial ligament is advisable to maintain the coracoacromial arch.

■ Heavy, nonabsorbable traction sutures (eg, 1-mm cottony Dacron) are placed through the rotator cuff insertions on the tuberosities. Two or three sutures should be placed through the subscapularis tendon, and three or four sutures through the supraspinatus.

■ Tuberosity fragments vary in size and may require trimming for reduction and repair (**TECH FIG 2C,D**).

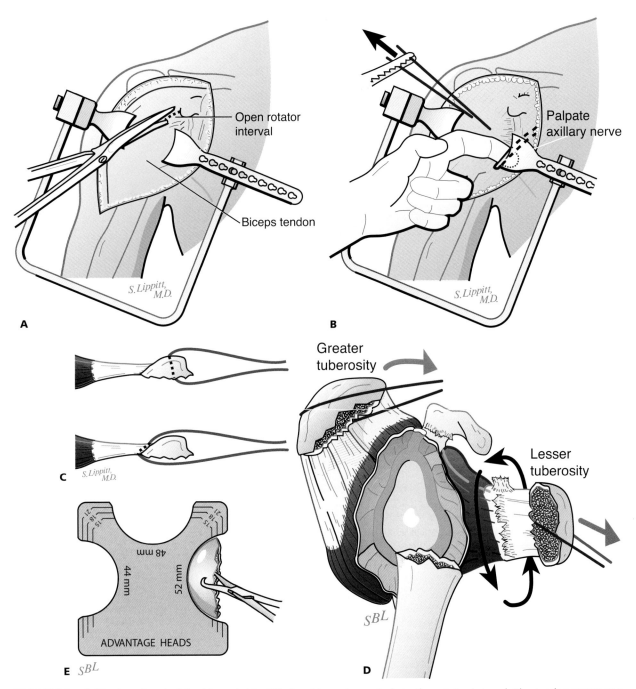

TECH FIG 2 • A. The long head of the biceps is identified and traced superiorly to the rotator interval. The tendon serves as a key landmark when re-establishing the anatomic relation between the greater and lesser tuberosities. **B.** The axillary nerve is identified at the anteroinferior border of the subscapularis. **C.** Nonabsorbable sutures are placed at the junction of the tendon–tuberosity interface and not through the tuberosities. **D.** Once the native humeral head is removed, the tuberosities with their respective rotator cuff attachments are mobilized for humeral canal preparation and later repair. **E.** Humeral head sizing. The extracted native humeral head is sized with the use of a commercially available template guide. (Copyright Steven B. Lippitt, MD.)

- With the tuberosities retracted on their muscular insertions, the humeral head and shaft fragments are removed.
- The native articular surface is removed and sized with a template for trial humeral head replacement (**TECH FIG 2E**).

- The glenoid must be examined for concomitant pathology. Hematoma and cartilaginous or bony fragments are removed with sterile saline irrigation.
- Glenoid fractures should be stabilized with internal fixation. If the glenoid exhibits significant degenerative wear or irreparable damage, a glenoid component must be used.

HUMERAL SHAFT PREPARATION

- The proximal end of the humeral shaft is delivered into the incisional wound. Loose endosteal bone fragments and hematoma are removed from the canal of the humeral shaft.
- Axial reamers, preferably without power, are used to prepare the humeral shaft for trial implantation.
- The trial humeral implant is placed with the lateral fin slightly posterior to the bicipital groove, and with the medial aspect of the trial head at least at the height of the medial calcar.
- Formerly, we used a sponge to anchor the trial stem within the intramedullary canal of the humerus. We currently use a commercially available fracture jig that can maintain the height and retroversion of the trial component through a functional range of motion (**TECH FIG 3**).[12,14]

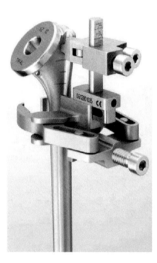
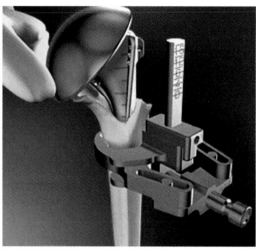

TECH FIG 3 • A commercially available fracture jig stably situates the implant at appropriate height and retroversion. (Courtesy of DePuy Orthopaedics, Warsaw, IN.)

DETERMINATION OF HUMERAL RETROVERSION

- Correct humeral retroversion is critical when recreating the glenohumeral articulation. Most techniques suggest 30 degrees as a guide during reconstruction, although native retroversion may vary from 10 to 50 degrees.
- Several methods are employed to gauge this angle:
  - External rotation of the humerus to 30 degrees from the sagittal plane of the body with the humeral head component facing straight medially
  - An imaginary line from the distal humeral epicondylar axis that bisects the axis of the prosthesis
  - Positioning of the lateral fin of the prosthesis about 8 mm posterior to the biceps groove (**TECH FIG 4**).

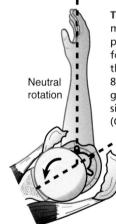

Neutral rotation

TECH FIG 4 • Retroversion assessment. The anterior fin of the prosthesis is aligned with the forearm in neutral rotation, and the lateral fin is positioned about 8 mm posterior to the biceps groove, establishing a retroversion angle of about 30 degrees. (Copyright Steven B. Lippitt, MD.)

DETERMINATION OF PROSTHETIC HEIGHT

- The prosthetic height also is critical in re-establishing appropriate muscle tension and shoulder mechanics.
- Preoperative templating may be helpful.
- Intraoperative examination of soft tissue tension, including the deltoid, rotator cuff, and the long head of the biceps, combined with fluoroscopic imaging aids in prosthetic height placement.
- Common errors involve placing the prosthesis too low, resulting in poor deltoid muscle tension and no room for the tuberosities (**TECH FIG 5**).

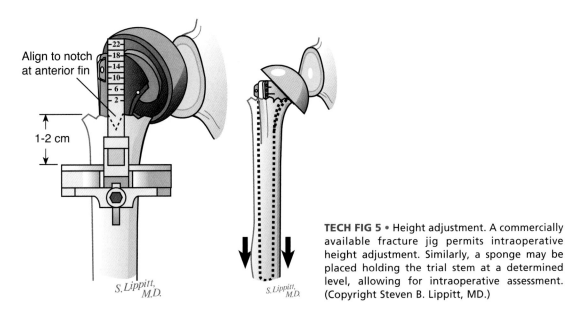

Align to notch
at anterior fin

1-2 cm

S.Lippitt,
M.D.

S.Lippitt,
M.D.

TECH FIG 5 • Height adjustment. A commercially available fracture jig permits intraoperative height adjustment. Similarly, a sponge may be placed holding the trial stem at a determined level, allowing for intraoperative assessment. (Copyright Steven B. Lippitt, MD.)

TRIAL REDUCTION

- Drill holes are placed in the proximal humerus medial and lateral to the bicipital groove, with 1-mm cottony Dacron sutures subsequently passed for fixation of the tuberosity to the shaft (**TECH FIG 6A**).
- A trial reduction is then performed with the mobilized tuberosities fitted below the head of the modular prosthesis.

- A towel clip can be used to hold the tuberosities for fluoroscopic examination and assessment of glenohumeral stability.
- Intraoperative fluoroscopy is helpful in confirming appropriate implant height and glenohumeral stability (**TECH FIG 6B**).
- The humeral head should not subluxate more than 25% to 30% of the glenoid height inferiorly.

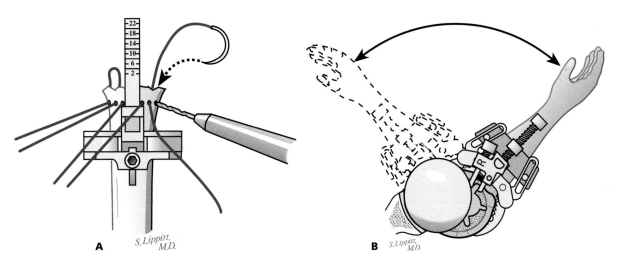

A S.Lippitt,
M.D.

B S.Lippitt,
M.D.

TECH FIG 6 • **A.** Humeral shaft preparation. Drill holes are placed in the proximal humerus medial and lateral to the bicipital groove with 1-mm cottony Dacron sutures. **B.** Trial reduction. A trial reduction may be performed with the fracture jig in place, allowing assessment of the functional range of motion. (Copyright Steven B. Lippitt, MD.)

FINAL IMPLANT PLACEMENT

- The final humeral component should be cemented in all fracture patients.
  - A cement restrictor is placed to prevent cement extravasation distally.

- Pulsatile lavage and retrograde injection of cement with suction pressurization also is used (**TECH FIG 7A**). Excess cement is removed during the curing phase.

- Spaces between the tuberosities, prosthesis, and shaft are packed with autogenous cancellous bone graft from the resected humeral head (**TECH FIG 7B**).
- A second trial reduction may be performed with a trial head after cement fixation of the humeral stem.
- The final head may be impacted before stem implantation or after the repeat trial reduction.
- A cerclage suture is placed circumferentially around the greater tuberosity and through the supraspinatus insertion, and then medial to the prosthesis and through the subscapularis insertion (lesser tuberosity). Several authors have indicated superior fixation with the cerclage

suture when compared to tuberosity-to-tuberosity and tuberosity-to-fin fixation alone.[23]
- Overreduction of the tuberosities should be avoided to prevent limitations in external (lesser tuberosity) and internal (greater tuberosity) rotation.
- Sutures are then tied, beginning with tuberosity-to-shaft reapproximation, followed by tuberosity-to-tuberosity closure using the previously placed suture limbs (**TECH FIG 7C**).
- The lateral portion of the rotator interval is closed with the arm in approximately 30 degrees of external rotation with no. 2 nonabsorbable suture (**TECH FIG 7D**).

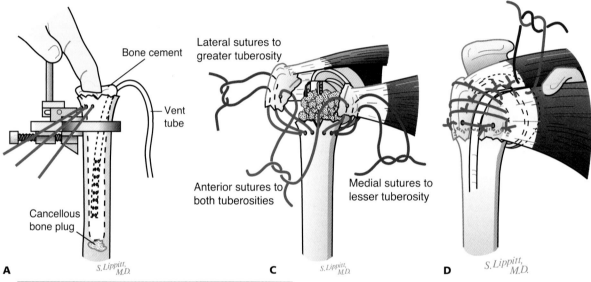

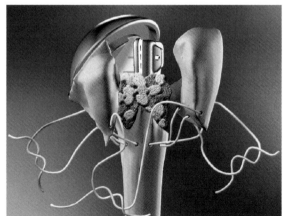

TECH FIG 7 • **A.** A cement restrictor is placed to prevent cement extravasation distally. Pulsatile lavage and retrograde injection of cement with suction pressurization is also used. **B.** Morselized cancellous bone graft is placed between the tuberosities and shaft. **C.** Tuberosity fixation. Previously placed suture limbs through the tuberosities and shaft are reapproximated. Not shown: a medial cerclage suture is placed circumferentially around the greater tuberosity and through the supraspinatus insertion, and then medial to the prosthesis and through the subscapularis insertion (lesser tuberosity) and tied. **D.** The rotator interval is closed with no. 2 nonabsorbable suture with the arm in about 30 degrees of external rotation. (**A,C,D:** Copyright Steven B. Lippitt, MD. **B:** Courtesy of DePuy Orthopaedics.)

SURGICAL WOUND CLOSURE

- The deltopectoral interval usually is not closed. Drain suction is recommended in both acute and chronic injuries to prevent hematoma formation.
- A commercially available pain pump may be used to augment postoperative analgesia and to reduce narcotic medication use.
- The subcutaneous tissues are reapproximated with 2-0 absorbable suture. Subcuticular closure is performed with 2-0 monofilament suture.
- The patient is then placed in a sling or shoulder immobilizer with 45 degrees of abduction for comfort.

PEARLS AND PITFALLS

Indications	▪ A complete history and physical examination should be performed, with particular attention paid to the neurovascular status.
Imaging studies	▪ Appropriate plain radiographs with possible CT scan supplementation aid in the surgical decision-making.
Tuberosity identification	▪ Use the long head of the biceps to define the tuberosities for mobilization. ▪ Tag this for later tenodesis before wound closure.
Implant placement	▪ Know the specifics of the implant system, including its limitations. ▪ Place the implant in appropriate retroversion (approximately 20 to 30 degrees). ▪ Check the height of the trial stem before performing cement fixation, using a fracture jig or sponge for provisional fixation. ▪ Intraoperative fluoroscopy can be used to assess appropriate implant height.
Tuberosity fixation	▪ Avoid loss of external rotation or internal rotation with overreduction of the lesser and greater tuberosities, respectively.
Postoperative rehabilitation	▪ On postoperative day 1, initiate gentle pendulum exercises, with passive forward flexion and external rotation (at 0 degrees of abduction). Always modify rehabilitation protocol based on intraoperative assessment of soft tissue compromise and patient neurologic status.

POSTOPERATIVE CARE

▪ Physician-directed therapy is initiated on postoperative day 1 with gentle, gravity-assisted pendulum exercises, as well as passive pulley-and-stick exercises to maintain forward flexion and external rotation (motion limits placed by surgeon based upon intraoperative stability).

▪ After discharge, the patient's wound is re-examined and sutures removed at 10 to 14 days. Gentle range-of-motion exercises are continued.

▪ At 6 weeks, repeat radiographs are obtained to evaluate tuberosity healing. When tuberosity healing is evident, phase 2 exercises are initiated with isometric rotator cuff exercises and active assisted elevation with the pulley.

▪ At 3 months, strength training with graduated rubber bands (phase 3) is implemented. Maximal motion and function are obtained at about 12 months from date of surgery.

OUTCOMES

▪ About 90% of patients treated with hemiarthroplasty demonstrate minimal pain, despite a wide range of function, motion, and strength.

▪ Factors that portend a poor outcome after hemiarthroplasty for fractures include tuberosity malposition, superior migration of the humeral prosthesis, stiffness, persistent pain, poor initial positioning of the implant (excessive retroversion, decreased height), and age over 75 years in women.[4]

▪ When comparing acute intervention versus late reconstruction, most authors report poorer outcomes with delayed surgical intervention (more than 2 weeks), particularly with functional results.[20,25,26]

COMPLICATIONS

▪ Complications include delays in wound healing, infection, nerve injury, humeral fracture, component malposition, instability, nonunion of the tuberosities, rotator cuff tearing, regional pain syndrome, periarticular fibrosis, heterotopic bone formation, component loosening, and glenoid arthritis.[3,7,19]

▪ The most common problems in acute fracture treatment involve stiffness, nonunion, malunion or resorption of the tuberosities.[7,19]

▪ In patients with chronic fractures treated with hemiarthroplasty, the most common problems encountered were instability, heterotopic ossification, tuberosity malunion or nonunion, and rotator cuff tears.[19]

REFERENCES

1. Beredjiklian PK, Iannotti JP, Norris TR, et al. Operative treatment of malunion of a fracture of the proximal aspect of the humerus. J Bone Joint Surg Am 1998;80:1484–1497.
2. Blaine TA, Bigliani LU, Levine WN. Fractures of the proximal humerus. In: Rockwood CA Jr, Masten FA III, Wirth MA, et al, eds. The Shoulder, ed 3. Philadelphia: Elsevier, 2004:355–412.
3. Bohsali KI, Wirth MA, Rockwood CA Jr. Current concepts review: complications of total shoulder arthroplasty. J Bone Joint Surg Am 2006;88A:2279–2292.
4. Boileau P, Krishnan SG, Tinsi L, et al. Tuberosity malposition and migration: reason for poor outcomes after hemiarthroplasty for displaced fractures of the proximal humerus. J Shoulder Elbow Surg 2002;11:401–412.
5. Boileau P, Walch G, Trojani C, et al. Surgical classification and limits of shoulder arthroplasty. In Walch G, Boileau P, eds. Shoulder Arthroplasty. Berlin: Springer-Verlag, 1999:349–358.
6. Bosch U, Skutek M, Fremery RW, et al. Outcome after primary and secondary hemiarthroplasty in elderly patients with fractures of the proximal humerus. J Shoulder Elbow Surg 1998;7:479–484.
7. Compito CA, Self EB, Bigliani LU. Arthroplasty and acute shoulder trauma. Clin. Orthop Relat Res 1994;307:27–36.
8. DeFranco MJ, Brems JJ, Williams GR Jr, et al. Evaluation and management of valgus impacted four-part proximal humerus fractures. Clin Orthop Relat Res 2006;442:109–114.
9. Frankle MA, Ondrovic LE, Markee BA, et al. Stability of tuberosity attachment in proximal humeral arthroplasty. J Shoulder Elbow Surg 2002;11:413–420.
10. Gerber C, Schneeberger A, Vinh T. The arterial vascularization of the humeral head: An anatomical study. J Bone Joint Surg Am 1990;72:1486–1494.
11. Green A. Proximal humerus fractures. In: Norris T, ed. Orthopaedic Knowledge Update: Shoulder and Elbow 2. Rosemont, IL: AAOS; 2002:209–217.
12. Green A, Lippitt SB, Wirth MA. Humeral head replacement arthroplasty. In: Wirth MA, ed. Proximal Humerus Fractures. Rosemont, IL: AAOS, 2005:39–48.
13. Green A, Norris T. Proximal humerus fractures and fracture-dislocations. In: Jupiter J, ed. Skeletal Trauma, ed 3. Philadelphia: WB Saunders; 2003:1532–1624.

14. Hartsock LA, Estes WJ, Murray CA, et al. Shoulder hemiarthroplasty for proximal humeral fractures. Orthop Clin North Am 1998; 467–475.

15. Huopio J, Kroger H, Honkanen R, et al. Risk factors for perimenopausal fractures: A prospective study. Osteoporos Int 2000; 11:219–227.

16. Iannotti JP, Gabriel JP, Schneck SL, et al. The normal glenohumeral relationships: An anatomical study of one hundred and forty shoulders. J Bone Joint Surg Am 1992;74A:491–500.

17. Jakob R, Miniaci A, Anson P, et al. Four-part valgus impacted fractures of the proximal humerus. J Bone Joint Surg Br 1991;73B: 295–298.

18. Laing P. The arterial supply of the adult humerus. J Bone Joint Surg Am 1956;38A:1105–1116.

19. Muldoon MP, Cofield RH. Complications of humeral head replacement for proximal humerus fractures. Instr Course Lect 1997: 46:15–24.

20. Neer CS. Displaced proximal humeral fractures. Part II: Treatment of 3-part and 4-part displacment. J Bone Joint Surg Am 1970;52A: 1090–1103.

21. Norris TR, Green A, McGuigan FX. Late prosthetic shoulder arthroplasty for displaced proximal humerus fractures. J Shoulder Elbow Surg 1995;4:271–280.

22. Orthopaedic Trauma Association Committee for Coding and Classification: Fracture and Dislocation Compendium. J Orthop Trauma 1996;10(suppl):1–155.

23. Pearl ML, Volk AG. Retroversion of the proximal humerus in relationship to the prosthetic replacement arthroplasty. J Shoulder Elbow Surg 1995;4:286–289.

24. Stablebforth PG. Four part fractures of the neck of the humerus. J Bone Joint Surg Br 1984;66B:104–108.

25. Zuckerman JD, Cuomo F, Koval KJ. Proximal humeral replacement for complex fractures: Indications and surgical technique. Instr Course Lect 1997;46:7–14.

Chapter 20

Plate Fixation of Humeral Shaft Fractures

Matthew J. Garberina and Charles L. Getz

DEFINITION

- Humeral shaft fractures, which account for about 3% of adult fractures, usually result from a direct blow or indirect twisting injury to the brachium.
- These injuries are most commonly treated nonoperatively with a prefabricated fracture brace. The humerus is the most freely movable long bone, and anatomic reduction is not required.
- Patients often can tolerate up to 20 degrees of anterior angulation, 30 degrees of varus angulation, and 3 cm of shortening without significant functional loss.
- There are, however, several indications for surgical treatment of humeral shaft fractures:
  - Open fracture
  - Bilateral humeral shaft fractures or polytrauma; floating elbow
  - Segmental fracture
  - Inability to maintain acceptable alignment with closed treatment (ie, angulation greater than 15 degrees)—seen more commonly with transverse fractures
  - Humeral shaft nonunion
  - Pathologic fractures
  - Arterial or brachial plexus injury
- Open reduction with internal plate fixation requires extensive dissection and operative skill. However, it offers advantages over intramedullary fixation because the rotator cuff is not violated, which leads to improved postoperative shoulder function.[3]

ANATOMY

- The humeral shaft is defined using Key's landmarks: the area between the upper margin of the pectoralis major tendon and the supracondylar ridge.[7]
- The blood supply of the humeral shaft comes from the posterior humeral circumflex vessels and branches of the brachial and profunda brachial arteries.
- The radial nerve and profunda brachial artery pass through the triangular interval (bordered superiorly by the teres major, medially by the medial head of the triceps, and laterally by the humeral shaft). The nerve then transverses from medial to lateral behind the humeral shaft and travels distally to a location between the brachialis and brachioradialis muscles.
- The musculocutaneous nerve lies on the undersurface of the biceps muscle and terminates distally as the lateral antebrachial cutaneous nerve.
- The humeral shaft has anteromedial, anterolateral, and posterior surfaces. Proximal and midshaft fractures are more amenable to plating on the anterolateral surface, whereas distal fractures often require posterior plate fixation.

PATHOGENESIS

- Humeral shaft fractures occur after both direct and indirect injuries. Direct blows to the brachium can fracture the humeral shaft in a transverse pattern, often with a butterfly fragment. Injuries with high degrees of energy often result in a greater degree of fracture comminution.
- Indirect injuries, such as those that can occur with activities such as arm wrestling, often involve a twisting mechanism and result in a spiral fracture pattern. Higher-energy injuries may result in muscle interposition between the fracture fragments, which can inhibit reduction and healing.
- A study of 240 humeral shaft fractures revealed radial nerve palsies in 42 patients, for an overall rate of 18% (17% in closed injuries). Fractures in the midshaft were more likely to have concomitant radial nerve palsy. Twenty-five of these patients had complete recovery in a range of 1 day to 10 months. Ten patients did not have radial nerve recovery. Median and ulnar nerve palsies were seen very rarely in patients with open fractures.[7]
- Concomitant vascular injuries are present in about 3% of patients with humeral shaft fractures.

NATURAL HISTORY

- Almost all humeral shaft fractures heal with nonoperative management. The most common treatment method is initial splinting from shoulder to wrist, followed by application of a prefabricated fracture brace when the patient is comfortable, usually within 2 weeks of the injury.
- Studies by Sarmiento and coauthors[10,11] have shown the effectiveness of functional bracing in the treatment of humeral shaft fractures. Nonunion rates with this method of treatment are in the 4% range, lower than seen when treating with external fixators, plates, or intramedullary nails.
- Closed fractures with initial radial nerve palsy can be observed, with expected recovery over a period of 3 to 6 months. Late-developing radial nerve palsies require surgical exploration.
- Angulation of the humeral shaft after fracture healing is expected and is well tolerated when it is less than 20 degrees. Varus deformity is most common.[10]
- Adjacent joint stiffness of the shoulder and elbow also is common. If the situation dictates treatment, physical therapy reliably restores joint motion in these patients.
- Relative contraindications to closed treatment include bilateral humeral shaft fractures or patients with polytrauma who require an intact brachium to ambulate. Transverse fractures and those with significant muscle imposition also are more amenable to operative fixation.[11]

PATIENT HISTORY AND PHYSICAL FINDINGS

- The examining physician must perform a complete examination of the affected limb to rule out concomitant injuries.
- The skin should be thoroughly evaluated for evidence of an open fracture. This includes examination of the axilla. Entry

and exit wounds are sought in gunshot victims. Swelling is common, and the patient may have an obvious deformity.

- The patient often braces the affected limb to his or her side, making evaluation of shoulder and elbow range of motion difficult. Bony prominences should be gently palpated to evaluate for other injuries, such as an olecranon fracture.
- Evaluate the appearance and skeletal stability of the forearm to rule out the presence of a co-existing both-bone forearm fracture ("floating elbow"). This finding necessitates operative fixation of humeral, radial, and ulnar fractures.
- Determine the vascular status of the upper extremity by palpating the radial and ulnar pulses at the wrist. Compare these findings with the unaffected limb. Selected cases may require Doppler arterial examination.[2]
- A complete neurologic assessment is necessary, with particular attention focused on the status of the radial nerve. This structure is at risk proximally as it passes posterior to the humeral shaft after emerging from the triangular interval, as well as distally, as it lies adjacent to the supracondylar ridge (near the location of the Holstein-Lewis distal one-third spiral humeral shaft fracture).
- Examine sensory function in the first dorsal web space, wrist extension, and thumb interphalangeal joint extension to determine the functional status of the radial nerve.

IMAGING AND OTHER DIAGNOSTIC STUDIES

- At least two plain radiographs at 90-degree angles to each other are necessary to evaluate the displacement, shortening, and comminution of the humeral shaft fracture.
- Radiographic views of the shoulder and elbow are necessary to rule out proximal extension of the shaft fracture or concomitant elbow injury (ie, olecranon fracture). This is especially important in high-energy injuries
- If swelling or evidence of skeletal instability about the forearm is present, dedicated forearm radiographs can determine the presence of a floating elbow (ie, ipsilateral humeral shaft fracture plus both-bone forearm fractures).

DIFFERENTIAL DIAGNOSIS

- Distal humerus fracture
- Proximal humerus fracture
- Elbow dislocation
- Shoulder dislocation

NONOPERATIVE MANAGEMENT

- Most isolated humeral shaft fractures can be treated nonoperatively. Initial treatment can vary with fracture location and involves splinting in either a posterior elbow or coaptation splint. The elbow is positioned in 90 degrees of flexion. An isolated humeral shaft fracture rarely necessitates an overnight hospital stay.
- In the past, definitive nonoperative treatment involved coaptation splinting or the use of hanging arm casts. Currently, functional fracture bracing provides adequate bony alignment, while local muscle compression and fracture motion promote osteogenesis. These braces provide soft tissue compression and allow functional use of the extremity.[11]
- Timing of brace application depends on the degree of swelling and patient discomfort. On average, the brace is applied about 2 weeks after the injury. A collar and cuff help

with initial patient comfort and should be worn during recumbency until the fracture heals.

- The brace often requires frequent retightening over the first 2 weeks as swelling subsides. Elbow and wrist range-of-motion exercises out of the sling are encouraged.
- Functional bracing requires that the patient be able to sit erect, and weight bearing on the humerus is not allowed. The level of humeral shaft fracture does not preclude the use of functional bracing, even if the fracture line extends above or below the brace.
- Anatomic alignment of the humerus rarely is achieved, with varus deformity most common. However, patients often are able to tolerate the bony angulation and still perform activities of daily living after injury. A cosmetic deformity rarely exists.
- Pendulum exercises are encouraged as soon as possible post-injury. Active elevation and abduction are avoided until bony healing has occurred, to prevent fracture angulation. The surgeon obtains radiographs after brace application and again 1 week later. If alignment is acceptable, repeat radiographs are obtained at 3- to 4- week intervals until fracture healing occurs.[10,11]

SURGICAL MANAGEMENT

- Certain humeral shaft fractures are not amenable to conservative treatment. Open fractures or high-energy injuries with significant axial distraction are treated with open reduction and internal fixation. Patients with polytrauma, bilateral humeral shaft fractures, vascular injury, or an inability to sit erect are best treated with operative fixation. Unacceptable fracture alignment requires abandonment of nonoperative treatment. Finally, humeral shaft nonunion is a clear indication for open reduction and internal fixation with bone grafting.[4,9]

Preoperative Planning

- The surgeon must review all radiographic images and must rule out ipsilateral elbow or shoulder injury.
- Preoperative radiographs help the surgeon estimate the required plate length. Higher-energy injuries with comminution may benefit from plating and supplemental bone grafting. The surgeon must plan for various scenarios based on these studies: moderate comminution or bone loss can be addressed with cancellous allograft or autograft bone, whereas more extensive bone defects may require strut grafting.
- Proximal and middle-third humeral shaft fractures are addressed using an anterolateral approach. Distal-third humeral shaft fractures often are treated via a posterior approach, because the distal humeral shaft is flat posteriorly, making it an ideal location for plate placement.
- Fracture patterns with extension into the proximal humerus can be exposed with a deltopectoral extension to the anterolateral humeral dissection.
- The surgeon notes any pre-existing scars that may affect the desired surgical approach, and neurovascular status is documented, with particular attention to radial nerve function.

Positioning

- Positioning depends on the intended surgical approach. For an anterolateral or medial approach, the patient is brought to the edge of the bed in the supine position. A hand table is attached to the bed and the patient's injured arm is placed on the hand table in slight abduction (**FIG 1A**).

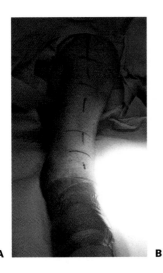

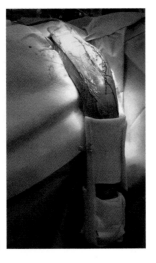

FIG 1 • **A.** Positioning for the anterolateral approach to the humeral shaft with the shoulder abducted and the arm on a hand table. **B.** Positioning for the posterior approach to the humeral shaft with the patient in the lateral decubitus position.

■ For a posterior approach, the patient can be placed prone or in the lateral decubitus position. A stack of pillows can support the brachium during the procedure (**FIG 1B**).

Approach

■ The approach depends on fracture location and the presence of any previous surgical incisions. The anterolateral and posterior approaches to the humerus are used most commonly, for proximal two-third and distal third fractures, respectively.

■ In patients who have already undergone multiple procedures to the affected extremity, Jupiter[6] recommends consideration of a medial approach to take advantage of virgin tissue planes.

ANTEROLATERAL APPROACH TO THE HUMERUS

■ The incision courses over the lateral aspect of the biceps, beginning proximally at the deltoid tubercle and terminating just proximal to the antecubital crease (**TECH FIG 1**).

■ A tourniquet rarely is used, because it often limits proximal exposure.

■ The lateral antebrachial cutaneous nerve lies in the distal aspect of the incision and must be protected during exposure.

■ Bluntly enter the interval between the biceps and brachialis by sweeping a finger from proximal to distal.

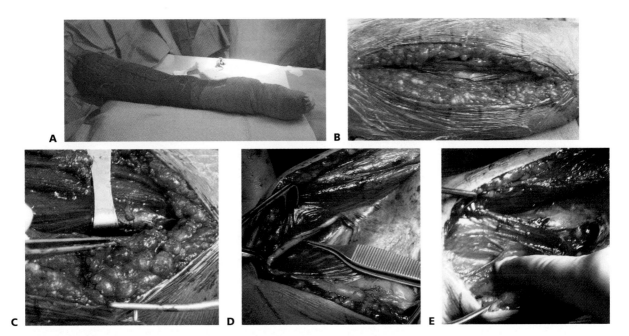

TECH FIG 1 • **A.** Anterolateral incision. **B.** Skin and subcutaneous tissue incised. **C.** Retractor on brachialis muscle, forceps on brachioradialis. **D.** Musculocutaneous nerve on undersurface of biceps muscle. **E.** Radial nerve in interval between brachialis and brachioradialis. *(continued)*

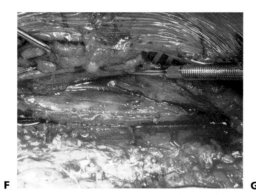
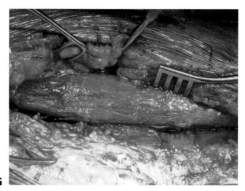

TECH FIG 1 • *(continued)* **F.** Biceps lifted to reveal brachialis muscle. **G.** Brachialis muscle split in its lateral third.

- At the level of the midhumerus, identify the musculocutaneous nerve on the undersurface of the biceps muscle. Trace this nerve out distally to protect its terminal branch, which forms the lateral antebrachial cutaneous nerve.
- Distally, the interval between the brachialis and brachioradialis is dissected to expose the radial nerve. Protect the radial nerve with a vessel loop so that it can be identified at all times.

- The brachialis is split in line with its fibers between the medial two thirds and lateral one third. This is an internervous plane between the radial nerve medially and the musculocutaneous nerve laterally.
- Identify the fracture site and proceed with reduction and fixation.

POSTERIOR APPROACH TO THE HUMERUS

- Make a generous incision over the midline of the posterior arm extending to the olecranon fossa (**TECH FIG 2**).
- Identify the interval between the long and lateral heads of the triceps proximally. Bluntly dissect this interval, taking the long head medially and the lateral head laterally.

- Distally, several blood vessels cross this plane; they require coagulation before transection.
- Identify the radial nerve proximal to the medial head of the triceps in the spiral groove. Protect the radial nerve throughout the case.
- Split the medial head of the triceps in its midline from proximal to distal to expose the fracture site.

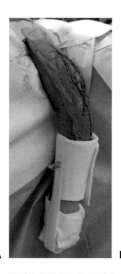
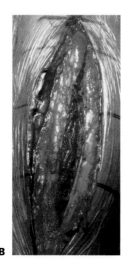
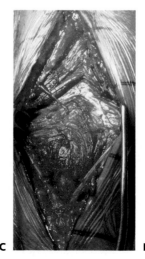
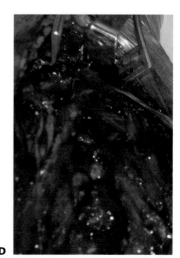

TECH FIG 2 • **A.** Incision for posterior approach. **B.** Superficial triceps split. **C.** Deep triceps split. **D.** The probe points to the radial nerve as it exits the spiral groove from medial to lateral; the fracture site is seen distally.

FRACTURE REDUCTION

- Sharp periosteal dissection exposes the fracture site. Evaluate the degree, if any, of comminution.
- Limit periosteal stripping to adequately expose the fracture. Make every attempt to leave some soft tissue attached to each fragment so as not to devascularize the fragments.
- Gentle traction and rotation often can bring the fracture fragments into better alignment.
- Anatomically reduce the fracture with one or more reduction clamps. It is advisable to reduce the fracture completely before definitive fixation, and this often requires the use of multiple reduction clamps (**TECH FIG 3**).
- After the fracture is reduced, the fragments can be provisionally fixed with Kirschner wires. Place the wires so as not to interfere with plate fixation.
- Alternatively, 3.5- or 4.5-mm interfragmentary screws can be used to hold the fracture aligned until plate fixation.
- Transverse fractures with minimal comminution often can be directly reduced with the plate and Faberge clamps.

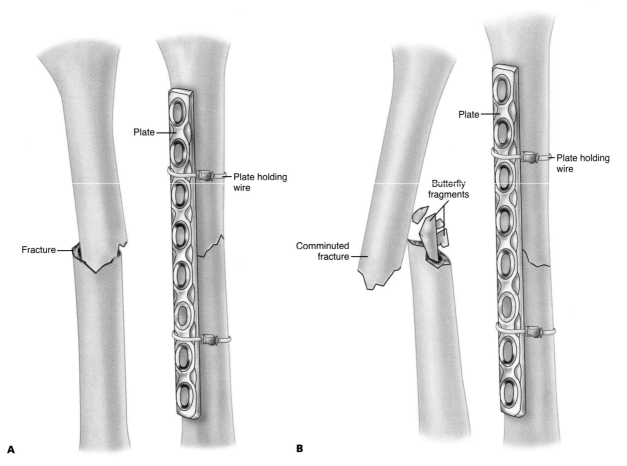

TECH FIG 3 • A. Fracture reduction maintained temporarily. **B.** Hold the plate over the reduced fracture with a plate-holding clamp.

EXPOSURE OF FRACTURE NONUNION

- Exposure of the radial nerve is more challenging, but it is very important in this situation. In many cases it is best to dissect out the nerve distally in the interval between the brachialis and brachioradialis and proximally medial to the spiral groove. The nerve is then carefully dissected free from the nonunion site.
- Pinpoint the exact location of the nonunion with a no. 15 scalpel.
- The ends of the nonunion can be brought out through the wound, and all fibrous material is extracted.
- After thorough fracture débridement, the amount of bone loss becomes clear. The surgeon can now determine whether standard cancellous bone grafting or strut grafting is necessary.

PLATE APPLICATION

- After fracture reduction, the plate length is determined.
- Humeral shaft fractures require at least six cortices of fixation above and below the fracture site.
- In larger bones, a broad 4.5-mm dynamic compression plate can provide optimal fixation. In smaller bones, a 4.5-mm limited contour dynamic compression plate often provides a better fit.
- Provisionally place the plate on a flat surface of the humerus and hold it in place with a plate-holding clamp.
- 4.5-mm cortical screws are placed through the plate holes proximal and distal to the fracture. Compression

techniques can be used, where appropriate.
- Ensure that no soft tissue, especially nerve, is trapped between the plate and the bone.
- Make sure to obtain screw purchase in at least six cortices above and below the fracture (**TECH FIG 4**).
- Cerclage wiring over the plate can add supplemental fixation, especially in weak bone.
- Rotate the arm and flex and extend the elbow to evaluate fracture stability.
- Apply cancellous bone graft into defects as needed.

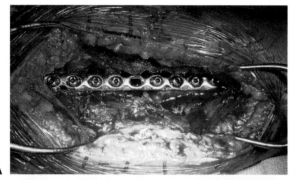

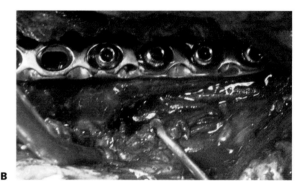

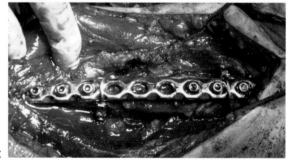

TECH FIG 4 • A. Plate spanning the fracture site with at least six cortices of fixation proximally and distally. **B.** Anterior plate with a probe pointing to the radial nerve as it exits the spiral groove posteriorly (proximal is to the right, distal to the left). **C.** Supplemental cerclage wire fixation can augment stability in weak bone.

MEDIAL APPROACH

- Positioning is similar to the anterolateral approach.
- Make an incision over the medial intermuscular septum from the axilla to 5 cm proximal to the medial epicondyle (**TECH FIG 5**).
- Mobilize the ulnar nerve.
- Resect the medial intermuscular septum; identify and coagulate the adjacent venous plexus with bipolar electrocautery.
- Mobilize the triceps posteriorly and the biceps/brachialis anteriorly.
- Expose the fracture site.
- The axillary incision raises concern for infection; there is also concern that the ulnar nerve can scar to the plate.

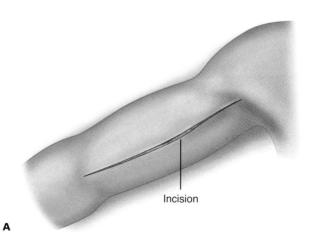

Incision

TECH FIG 5 • A. Incision for the medial approach. *(continued)*

A

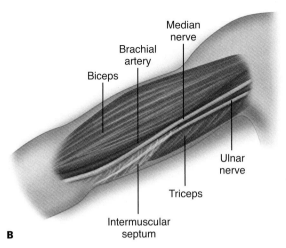

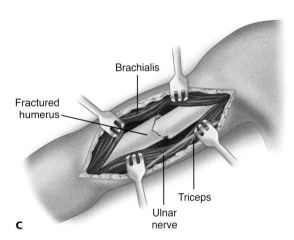

TECH FIG 5 • *(continued)* **B,C.** The brachialis and biceps are raised anteriorly, and the triceps is raised posteriorly for fracture exposure.

PEARLS AND PITFALLS

Indications	▪ Operative treatment is reserved for open fractures, patients with multiple fractures, and fractures with inadequate reduction.
Preoperative planning	▪ Review all radiographs and determine the best surgical approach. ▪ Estimate potential plate length and prepare for possible bone grafting.
Surgical exposure	▪ Locate and protect the radial nerve. ▪ Expose and reduce fracture fragments and temporarily hold them in place with pins or clamps. ▪ Alternatively, fix larger fragments with interfragmentary screws.
Plate fixation	▪ Ensure that plate length allows six cortices of fixation proximal and distal to the fracture. ▪ Use 4.5-mm dynamic compression plates or limited contact dynamic compression plates. ▪ Use compressive techniques when indicated.
Radial nerve function	▪ Preoperatively, document a detailed neurovascular examination. ▪ Ensure that the radial nerve is not trapped within the plate before closure.

POSTOPERATIVE CARE

▪ Postoperative radiographs ensure proper fracture alignment and plate placement (**FIG 2**).

▪ Initially, the patient can be placed in a sling or posterior elbow splint. This is removed and range-of-motion exercises are started when patient comfort allows (usually 1 to 2 days postoperative).

▪ Weight bearing on the affected upper extremity is allowed based on patient comfort.[12]

▪ Initial therapy consists of elbow range-of-motion and shoulder pendulum and passive self-assist exercises.

▪ The patient can come out of the sling after 2 weeks and start waist-level activities with the operative arm.

▪ At 6 weeks, elbow motion should be near normal range, and shoulder strengthening is added to the patient's physical therapy.

▪ At 3 months, radiographs should reveal some callus formation. If no callus is evident, radiographs are repeated every 6 weeks until evidence of healing appears.

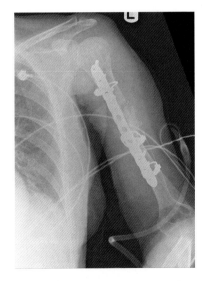

FIG 2 • Postoperative radiograph.

OUTCOMES

▪ Plate fixation leads to union in 90% to 98% of cases.

▪ Plating offers decreased complication rates compared to intramedullary nailing, especially in terms of shoulder dysfunction.[8]

▪ Iatrogenic radial nerve palsy occurs in about 2% to 5% of cases and usually resolves in 3 to 6 months. Electromyography helps monitor return of nerve function in patients with prolonged palsy. Radial nerve exploration is indicated when no nerve function returns by 6 months.

▪ Elbow and shoulder range of motion usually return to normal postoperatively.

COMPLICATIONS

▪ Infection
▪ Nonunion
▪ Malunion
▪ Hardware failure
▪ Radial nerve palsy
▪ Shoulder impingement
▪ Elbow stiffness

REFERENCES

1. Garberina MJ, Getz CL, Beredjiklian P, et al. Open reduction and internal fixation of humeral shaft nonunions. Tech Shoulder Elbow Surg 2006;7:131–138.
2. Gregory PR. Fractures of the shaft of the humerus. In Bucholz RW, Heckman JD, eds. Rockwood and Green's Fractures in Adults, ed 5, vol 1. Philadelphia: Lippincott Williams & Wilkins, 2001:973–996.
3. Gregory PR, Sanders RW. Compression plating versus intramedullary fixation of humeral shaft fractures. J Am Acad Orthop Surg 1997;5:215–223.
4. Healy WL, White GM, Mick CA, et al. Nonunion of the humeral shaft. Clin Orthop Relat Res 1987;219:206–213.
5. Hoppenfeld S, deBoer P. Surgical Exposures in Orthopaedics: The Anatomic Approach. Philadelphia: Lippincott Williams & Wilkins, 1994:51–82.
6. Jupiter JB. Complex non-union of the humeral diaphysis: Treatment with a medial approach, an anterior plate, and a vascularized fibular graft. J Bone Joint Surg Am 1990;72A:701–707.
7. Mast JW, Spiegel PG, Harvey JP Jr, et al. Fractures of the humeral shaft: A retrospective study of 240 adult fractures. Clin Orthop Relat Res 1975;112:254–262.
8. McCormack RG, Brien D, Buckley RE, et al. Fixation of fractures of the shaft of the humerus by dynamic compression plate or intramedullary nail: a prospective randomized trial. J Bone Joint Surg Br 2000;82B:336–339.
9. Ring D, Perey BH, Jupiter JB. The functional outcome of operative treatment of ununited fractures of the humeral diaphysis in older patients. J Bone Joint Surg Am 1999;81A:177–190.
10. Sarmiento A, Latta LL. Functional fracture bracing. J Am Acad Orthop Surg 1999;7:66–75.
11. Sarmiento A, Waddell JP, Latta LL. Diaphyseal humeral fractures: Treatment options. J Bone Joint Surg Am 2001;83A:1566–1579.
12. Tingstad EM, Wolinsky PR, Shyr Y, et al. Effect of immediate weightbearing on plated fractures of the humeral shaft. J Trauma 2000;49:278–280.

Chapter 21

Intramedullary Fixation of Humeral Shaft Fractures

Phillip Langer and Christopher T. Born

DEFINITION

▪ Incidence: 3% to 5% of all fractures[12]
▪ The AO/ASIF classification of humeral shaft fractures is based on increasing fracture comminution and is divided into three types according to the contact between the two main fragments:
  ▪ Type A: simple (contact > 90%)
  ▪ Type B: wedge/butterfly fragment (some contact)
  ▪ Type C: complex/comminuted (no contact)
▪ Intramedullary nailing (IMN) can be used to stabilize fractures 2 cm distal to the surgical neck to 3 cm proximal to the olecranon fossa.[12]
▪ The precise role of IMN is not defined. Proponents offer the following benefits over formal open reduction with internal fixation (ORIF): it is minimally invasive, causing limited soft tissue damage and no periosteal stripping (preservation of vascular innervation); it is biomechanically superior; it is cosmetically advantageous (smaller incision); it is capable of indirect diaphyseal fracture reduction and metaphyseal fracture approximation.
  ▪ Complications such as shoulder pain, delayed union or nonunion, fracture about the implant, iatrogenic fracture comminution, and difficulty in the reconstruction of failures, raise questions regarding the usefulness of intramedullary nailing over ORIF.
▪ Biomechanically, intramedullary nails are closer to the normal mechanical axis; consequently they act as a load-sharing device if there is cortical contact.
  ▪ Unlike plate-and-screw fixation, a load-bearing construct, intramedullary nails are subjected to lower bending forces, making fatigue failure and cortical osteopenia secondary to stress shielding less likely.

ANATOMY

▪ Comparatively, there are several anatomic differences between the long bones of the upper extremity versus the long bones of the lower extremity (femur, tibia):
  ▪ The medullary canal terminates at the metaphysis (versus diaphysis).
  ▪ Isthmus: junction is at the middle–distal third (versus proximal–middle third).
  ▪ Trumpet shape: the proximal two thirds of the humeral canal is cylindrical; distally. the medullary canal rapidly tapers to a prismatic end at the diaphysis (hard cortical bone) versus the wide flare of the metaphysis (soft cancellous bone).
▪ Because of the funnel shape of the humeral shaft, a true interference fit is difficult to obtain; therefore, proximal and distal static locking has become the standard of care for IMN of humeral fractures.
▪ Neurovascular considerations include average distances of key structures from notable bony landmarks:
  ▪ Axillary nerve to proximal humerus, 6.1 ± 0.7 cm (range 4.5 to 6.9 cm)
  ▪ Axillary nerve to surgical neck, 1.7 ± 0.8 cm (range 0.7 to 4.0 cm)
  ▪ Axillary nerve to greater tuberosity, 45.6 mm
  ▪ Axillary nerve to distal edge acromion, 5 to 6 cm
  ▪ Crossing of radial nerve at lateral intermuscular septum to proximal humerus, 17.0 ± 2.3 cm (range 13 to 22 cm)
  ▪ Crossing of radial nerve at lateral intermuscular septum to olecranon fossa, 12.0 ± 2.3 cm (range 7.4 to 16.6 cm)
  ▪ Crossing of radial nerve at lateral intermuscular septum to distal humerus, 16.0 ± 0.4 cm (range 9.0 to 20.5 cm)[1,5,9]

PATHOGENESIS

▪ Biomodal distribution[17]
  ▪ Young, male 21 to 30 years old: high-energy trauma
  ▪ Older, female 60 to 80 years old: simple fall/rotational injury
▪ 5% open[17]
▪ 63% AO/ASIF type A fracture patterns[17]
▪ Various loading modes and the characteristic fracture patterns they create
  ▪ Tension: transverse
  ▪ Compression: oblique
  ▪ Torsion: spiral
  ▪ Bending: butterfly
  ▪ High-energy: comminuted
▪ Red flags:
  ▪ Minimal trauma indicates a pathologic process
  ▪ Disconnect between history and fracture type suggests domestic abuse.

NATURAL HISTORY

▪ The humerus is well enveloped in muscle and soft tissue, hence its good prognosis for healing in most uncomplicated fractures.

PATIENT HISTORY AND PHYSICAL FINDINGS

▪ Patients with humeral shaft fractures present with arm pain, deformity, and swelling.
▪ Demographics, medical history, and information regarding the circumstance and mechanism of injury should be obtained.
▪ Particularly significant in upper extremity trauma: hand dominance, occupation, age, and pertinent comorbidities must be solicited from the patient. All of these factors play a major role in determining whether to pursue surgical versus nonsurgical treatment.
▪ On physical examination, the arm is typically shortened, angulated, or grossly deformed, with motion and crepitus on manipulation.
▪ Document the status of the skin (open versus closed fracture) and perform a careful neurovascular evaluation of the limb.

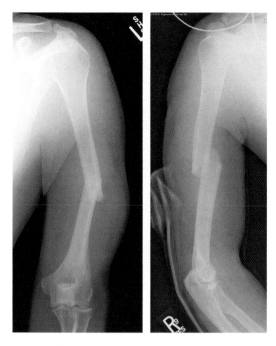

FIG 1 • AP and lateral radiographs of a displaced humeral shaft fracture, shortened and in varus angulation.

■ If indicated, Doppler pulse and compartment pressures should be checked.

■ Always examine the shoulder and elbow joint for possible associated musculoskeletal pathology.

■ Examine the radial nerve for evidence of injury by testing resistance.

IMAGING AND OTHER DIAGNOSTIC STUDIES

■ Initial studies must always include orthogonal views (anteroposterior [AP] and lateral radiographs) of the fracture site, shoulder, and elbow (**FIG 1**). To obtain these radiographs, move the patient rather than rotating the injured limb through the fracture site.

  ■ Traction radiographs may be helpful with comminuted or severely displaced fractures, and comparison radiographs of the contralateral side may be helpful for determining preoperative length.

■ CT scans rarely are indicated. Rare situations in which they should be obtained include significant rotational abnormality, precluding accurate orthogonal radiographs, and suspicion of possible intra-articular extension or an additional fracture or fractures at a different level.

■ Doppler pulse and compartment pressures should be checked if indicated following a thorough physical examination.

■ Suspicion of vascular injuries warrants an angiogram.

DIFFERENTIAL DIAGNOSIS

■ Osteoporosis
■ Pathologic fractures
■ High- or low-energy trauma
■ Open or closed fractures
■ Domestic abuse

NONOPERATIVE MANAGEMENT

■ Most non- or minimally displaced humeral shaft fractures can be successfully treated nonoperatively, with union rates of more than 90% often reported.[12]

■ Common closed techniques include hanging arm cast; coaptation splint; Velpeau dressing; abduction humeral/shoulder spica cast; functional brace; and traction.

  ■ Each of these modalities has been successfully employed, but most commonly either a hanging arm cast or coaptation splint is used for 1 to 2 weeks, followed by a functional brace, tightened as the swelling decreases.

  ■ Hanging arm casts are a very good option for displaced, midshaft humeral fractures with shortening, especially oblique or spiral fracture patterns, if the cast is able to extend 2 cm or more proximal to the fracture site.

■ For nonoperative treatment to be effective, the patient should remain upright, either standing or sitting, and avoid leaning on the elbow for support. This allows for gravitational force to assist in fracture reduction.

  ■ As soon as possible, the patient should begin range-of-motion exercises of the fingers, wrist, elbow, and shoulder to minimize dependent swelling and joint stiffness.

■ Acceptable alignment of humeral shaft fractures is considered to be 3 cm of shortening, 30 degrees of varus/valgus angulation, and 20 degrees of anterior/posterior angulation.[10]

  ■ Varus/valgus angulation is tolerated better proximally, and more angulation may be tolerated better in patients with obesity.

  ■ Patients with large pendulous breasts are at increased risk for varus angulation if treated nonsurgically.

  ■ No set values for acceptable malrotation exist, but compensatory shoulder motion allows for considerable tolerance of rotational deformity.[10]

■ Low-velocity gunshot wounds act as closed injuries after initial treatment. Following irrigation and débridement of skin at entry and exit sites, tetanus status confirmation, and prophylactic antibiotic initiation, nonoperative treatment modalities are commonly employed.[10]

SURGICAL MANAGEMENT

■ Successful nonoperative management may be impossible for various reasons:

  ■ Fracture pattern (eg, displaced, comminuted, segmental [segmental fractures are at risk of nonunion of one or both fracture sites])

  ■ Prolonged recumbency

  ■ Morbid obesity

  ■ Large, pendulous breasts (in women)

  ■ Patient's inability to maintain a semisitting or reclined position owing to polytraumatic injuries or patient noncompliance

■ Operative indications include:

  ■ Proximal humeral fractures with diaphyseal extension

  ■ Massive bone loss

  ■ Displaced transverse diaphyseal fractures

  ■ Segmental fractures

  ■ Floating elbow

  ■ Pathologic or impending pathologic fractures

  ■ Open fractures

  ■ Associated vascular injury

  ■ Intra-articular extension

- Polytrauma
- Spinal cord or brachial plexus injuries
- Poor soft tissue over the fracture site(s), such as thermal burns
- The most commonly cited overall best indication for IMN from this extensive list is a pathologic or impending pathologic fracture.
- The need for operative intervention secondary to radial nerve dysfunction after closed manipulation is controversial.
  - There are advocates for both early nerve exploration and observation.
  - This condition was once thought to be an automatic indication for surgery; however, this assumption has since been called into question.[12]
- Isolated comminution is not an indication for operative treatment.[12] However, if surgical fixation is chosen over nonoperative management, antegrade IMN currently is favored over plate fixation for comminuted fractures.[2]
- Relative contraindications include:
  - Open epiphyses
  - Narrow intramedullary canal (ie, < 9 mm)
  - Prefracture deformity of the humeral shaft
  - Open fractures with obvious radial nerve palsy and neurologic loss after penetrating stab injuries
    - The last two conditions require nerve exploration with subsequent plate-and-screw fixation.
- Chronically displaced fractures should be treated with ORIF rather than IMN to prevent traction-induced brachial plexus palsy and radial nerve injury.

Preoperative Planning

- When selecting implant size, consider canal diameter, fracture pattern, patient anatomy, and postoperative protocol.
  - Nail length and diameter should take into account the distal narrowing of the humerus.
- Estimations of the nail diameter, length, and necessity of reaming can be made using preoperative roentgenograms of the uninjured humerus.
- Alternatively, the length and diameter of the medullary canal can be ascertained intraoperatively using a radiopaque gauge and C-arm imaging of the intact humerus. Use of a radiolucent table top will substantially improve the quality of the image as well as the ability to obtain accurate C-arm images.
  - Position the gauge anterior to the unaffected humerus with its distal end 2.5 cm or more proximal to the superior edge of the olecranon fossa and 1 cm distal to the superior edge of the articular surface.
  - Move the C-arm to the proximal end of the humerus and read the correct length directly from the stamped measurements on the nail length gauge. The IMN should end approximately 1 to 2 cm proximal to the olecranon fossa.
- Measure the length of the IMN to allow the proximal end to be buried. This will reduce the incidence of subacromial impingement if an antegrade technique is used, or encroachment on the olecranon fossa and blocked elbow extension if a retrograde approach is chosen.
  - In comminuted fractures, carefully chose the length to avoid distracting the humerus, which predisposes the patient to delayed union or nonunion.
- Measure the diameter of the medullary canal at the narrowest part that will contain the nail.

- In retrograde nailing, it is important to determine the relation between alignment of the humeral canal and the entry point of the nail by measuring the anterior deviation/distal humeral offset of the distal canal on the preoperative lateral radiograph.
  - Based on these calculations, if the deviation is small, make a distal, long entry portal that includes the superior border of the olecranon fossa.
  - If the anterior deviation is large, however, make the entry portal more proximal and shorter in length.

Positioning

- The patient's position for surgery is determined based on the method chosen for fixation.

Antegrade Intramedullary Nailing

- Place the patient in either a beach chair or supine position on a radiolucent table with the head of the bed elevated 30 to 40 degrees (**FIG 2**).
- Put a small roll between the medial borders of the scapula and rotate the head to the contralateral side to increase exposure of the shoulder.
- Certain fracture patterns may call for skeletal traction.
  - If it is used, place an olecranon pin and apply intermittent traction to avoid brachial plexus palsy.
- Clinically assess the rotational alignment by placing the shoulder in an anatomic position and rotating the distal fragment of the fracture humerus so that the arm and hand point toward the ceiling and the elbow is flexed 90 degrees.
- Prepare the affected extremity and drape the arm free in the typical manner. The operative area should encompass the shoulder proximal to the nipple line, the midline of the chest to the nape of the neck, and the entire affected extremity to the fingertips.
- Bring the patient to the edge of the radiolucent table to improve the ability to obtain orthogonal C-arm images of the affected extremity.
  - It may be necessary to have the patient lying partially off the table on a radiolucent support.
- Cover the C-arm imager with a sterile isolation drape. Most commonly, the C-arm is brought in directly lateral on the injured side, although some surgeons favor coming in from the contralateral side.
  - Regardless of which direction the C-arm is brought into the field, it is imperative to obtain orthogonal views of the entire humerus before the first incision is made.

Retrograde Intramedullary Nailing

- Put the patient in the lateral decubitus or prone position with dorsum placed near the edge of the operating table.
  - If the patient is in the prone position, the affected arm may be supported on a radiolucent arm board, or placed over a bolster or paint roller upper extremity support. The latter two options facilitate access to the olecranon fossa and prevent a traction injury to the brachial plexus. The arm should be positioned in 80 degrees of abduction with the elbow flexed at least 90 degrees.
  - If the lateral decubitus position is used, suspend the fractured extremity, taking care not to distract the fracture site or cause neurovascular compromise. Suspension can be aided by an olecranon pin.

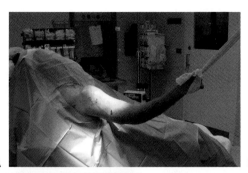
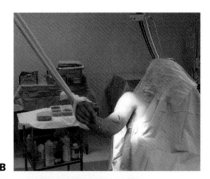
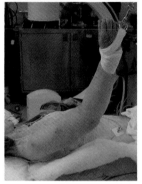
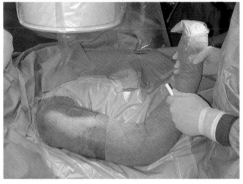

FIG 2 • **A.** Beach chair position for antegrade intramedullary nailing. **B.** Beach chair position for antegrade intramedullary nailing using a McConnell positioner (McConnell Orthopedic Mfg. Co, Greenville, TX). **C.** Supine position. Note the bump under the scapula and the C-arm image intensifier ready to come in from the contralateral side. **D.** C-arm imaging from the contralateral side. The patient is in the supine position.

■ Prepare the affected extremity and drape the arm free in the typical manner. Include the distal clavicle, the acromion, the medial scapula, and the entire arm and hand in the operative field.

■ Cover the C-arm imager with a sterile isolation drape. Bring the C-arm from the ipsilateral side and make sure that adequate orthogonal C-arm images are possible before making the surgical approach.

Approach

■ Standard locked intramedullary humeral nails can be inserted either antegrade or retrograde.

ANTEGRADE INTRAMEDULLARY NAILING

Approach

■ The antegrade approach, which has been the traditional method of IMN, typically involves a starting point at the proximal humerus—either through the rotator cuff, where the tissue is less vascular, or just lateral to the articular surface, where the blood supply is higher (**TECH FIG 1**).

■ Palpate and outline the surface anatomy of the acromion, clavicle, and humeral head.
  ■ Feel the anterior and posterior borders of the humeral head to locate and mark the midline.
  ■ Make a small longitudinal incision at the anterolateral corner of the acromion centered over the top of the greater tuberosity. Extend it distally 3 cm.

■ The C-arm can be used to locate the exact entry point before performing the anterior acromial approach.
  ■ Place a K-wire into the ideal entry point under C-arm imaging guidance. Confirm the location on orthogonal images.
  ■ Leave the K-wire intact while making an anterior acromial approach.

■ Split the deltoid fibers in line with the longitudinal cutaneous incision.
  ■ Do not extend the incision distally more than 4 or 5 cm in the deltoid muscle, to avoid damage to the axillary nerve.

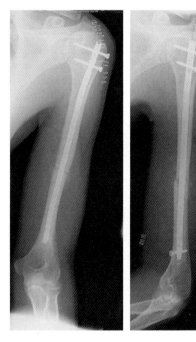

TECH FIG 1 • Postoperative AP and lateral radiographs of antegrade intramedullary nailing for a midshaft humerus fracture.

- Excise any visible subdeltoid bursae to improve your visualization of the rotator cuff.
- Longitudinally incise the supraspinatus in line with the deltoid/cutaneous incision for 1 to 2 cm, just posterior to the bicipital tuberosity.
  - Placing suture tags at the margins of the supraspinatus will help retract its edges during the remainder of the procedure and assist in achieving an optimal rotator cuff repair during wound closure.
- There is insufficient evidence to indicate that a larger incision, in cases in which the rotator cuff is identified and purposely incised, is superior to a smaller incision made with the aid of C-arm imaging.[13]

Entry Hole

- Make the entry hole medial to the tip of the greater tuberosity, just lateral to the articular margin and approximately 0.5 cm posterior to the bicipital groove to minimize damage to the supraspinatus.
  - Linear access to the humeral medullary canal is possible only though an entry portal made in this sulcus between the greater tuberosity and the articular surface.
  - Make sure the entry portal is centered on AP and lateral C-arm images to ensure the nail will be in the midplane of the humerus.
  - If the entry hole is too medial, it will violate the supraspinatus; if the entry portal is too lateral, it will cause some degree of varus angulation (in proximal fractures) or substantially increase the risk of an iatrogenic fracture during nail insertion.
  - Proximal third fractures may require a more medially located entry hole to avoid varus angulation at the fracture site.

Entrance into Medullary Canal

- After establishing the entry hole, insert a K-wire through the portal into the medullary canal to the level of the lesser tuberosity.
- Next, to open the medullary canal, either use a cannulated awl or pass a cannulated drill bit over the K-wire, through a protection sleeve, and drill to the depth of the lesser tuberosity.
  - Adduct the proximal component of the fractured humerus and extend the shoulder to improve clearance of the acromion and facilitate awl or starter reamer access to the correct portal location.
- Once the medullary canal has been opened, remove the guidewire and insert a long, ball-tipped guidewire. Bending the tip of the guidewire may aid in its passage across the fracture site.

Provisional Reduction/Guidewire Passage

- Manipulate the extremity to reduce the fracture. In many cases, reduction is obtained through a combination of adduction, neutral forearm rotation, and longitudinal traction.
- While advancing the guidewire down the canal, rotate the arm about its longitudinal axis and take several C-arm images to confirm that the guidewire remains contained in the canal.

- This is especially important if the humerus is substantially comminuted.
- Slowly and deliberately pass the guidewire across the fracture site.
  - Difficult passage may be a tip-off that soft tissue may be interposed (possibly the radial nerve).
  - An open fracture is advantageous in this situation because it provides the opportunity to directly visualize and clear the fracture site of any problematic soft tissue.
- After crossing the fracture site, advance the ball-tipped guidewire into the center of the distal fragment until the tip is 1 to 2 cm proximal to the olecranon fossa.
- Avoid shortening or distracting the fracture site while firmly securing the guidewire into the distal fragment.

Determining Nail Length

- Determine the correct nail length by one of two methods:
  - Guide rod method: with the distal end of the rod 1 to 2 cm proximal to the olecranon fossa, overlap a second guide rod extending proximally from the humeral entry portal. Subtract the length in mm of the overlapped guide rod from the total length of an identical guidewire to determine the correct nail length.
  - Nail length gauge: position the radiopaque gauge anterior to the fractured humerus. Move the C-arm to the proximal end of the humerus and read the length from the stamped measurements on the gauge.
- The ideal length of an IMN should be measured 1 cm distal to the articular surface of the humeral head to a point 1 to 2 cm proximal to the olecranon fossa.
  - If the calculated length falls between two standardized nail lengths of the chosen implant, always choose the smaller size.
  - Long nails are a risk factor for subacromial impingement and fracture site distraction.
    - Burying a long nail proximally below the subchondral surface has the potential to iatrogenically split the distal humerus or create a supracondylar fracture when the tip of the nail is wedged too close to the olecranon fossa.

Reaming the Humeral Shaft

- Reaming the humeral shaft usually is avoided, especially in comminuted fractures, to avoid reaming injury to the radial nerve or the rotator cuff.
- If it is warranted, slowly ream the entire humerus over the ball-tipped reamer guidewire in 0.5-mm increments.
  - Exercise greater caution when reaming the humerus than when reaming the long bones of the lower extremity, because the cortical thickness of the humerus is substantially less than that of the tibia or femur.
- Ream 0.5 mm to 1 mm larger than the selected nail diameter. Ream minimally until the sound of cortical chatter becomes audible.
- Choose a nail 1 mm smaller in diameter than the last reamer used.
- Some implant systems require that the ball-tipped guidewire be replaced with a rod that does not have a tip.
  - Use the medullary exchange tube when replacing the guidewire to maintain fracture reduction.

Inserting the Nail

- Once the correct nail length and the diameter of the selected implant have been verified, attach the nail adapter, place the nail-holding screw through the nail adapter, and then attach the radiolucent targeting device onto the nail adapter.
- Verify that this assembly is locked in the appropriate position and that its alignment is correct by inserting a drill bit through the assembled tissue protection/drill sleeve placed in the required holes of the targeting device.
- Insert the nail with sustained manual pressure.
  - Aggressive placement can result in iatrogenic fractures or displacement of the fracture fragments.
  - Use the C-arm image intensifier to identify the source of the problem if the IMN does not easily advance.
- Insert the nail at least to the first circumferential groove on the nail adapter but no deeper than the second groove.
  - Ideally, the IMN should be countersunk about 5 mm below the articular surface to avoid subacromial impingement.
  - Sinking the nail more than 1 cm below the articular surface may place the proximal interlocking screws at the level of the axillary nerve.
  - If the proximal end of the nail is properly countersunk, the incidence of shoulder pain is reportedly less than 2%.[4]
- Attach a strike plate to the targeting device and use a mallet to impact the proximal jig assembly to eliminate any fracture gap or advance the IMN.
  - Do not hit the targeting device or the nail-holding screw directly.
- The distal end of the IMN should come to lie about 2 cm proximal to the olecranon fossa.
- Remove the guidewire.

Compression

- Before proximal interlock insertion, make sure that optimal fracture site compression is present.
- Proximal compression locking can be used for transverse or short oblique fracture patterns. Severe osteopenia is a contraindication to its use.
  - Explore the radial nerve before compression locking if any possibility of radial nerve entrapment exists.
  - The nail must be overinserted by the same distance of anticipated interfragmentary travel because otherwise, during compression, the nail will back out and cause subacromial impingement.
  - Additionally, if the fracture is suitable for compression, the chosen implant should be 6 to 10 mm shorter than the calculated measurement to avoid proximal migration of the nail beyond the insertion site.
- Proximal locking screw placement
  - Oblique proximal locking screws are preferred because their insertion point is cephalad to axillary nerve.
  - Only lateral-to-medial placement is recommended for proximal interlocking screws.
  - It is important to make sure that these screws are inserted above the level of the humeral neck to avoid axillary nerve injury.

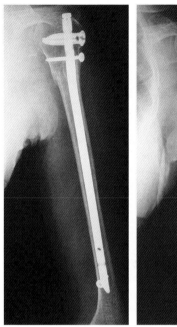
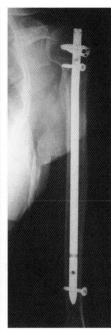

TECH FIG 2 • Postoperative AP and lateral radiographs of antegrade intramedullary nailing for a midshaft humerus fracture. A spiral blade has been used for proximal interlock fixation.

- Lateral screws placed too proximal can produce subacromial impingement with terminal arm elevation.
- Some implant systems may offer a spiral blade fixation as an option for proximal interlocking. In theory, it creates a fixed angle construct and has a higher resistance (versus screws) against loosening (ie, "windshield wiper" effect; **TECH FIG 2**).

Determining Rotation

- Confirm rotational alignment before placing distal interlock screws. Rotational alignment can be ascertained clinically and radiographically.
  - Magnified C-arm AP images of the fracture site can be used to judge the medial and lateral cortical width of the most proximal and most distal aspects of the fracture site.
  - Proper rotation is achieved when these widths are identical.

Distal Locking Screws

- Place anterior, then posterior and/or lateral, then medial directed distal interlocking screws.
- Insert distal interlocking screws using a freehand technique.
  - To place AP-directed screws, advance the C-arm over the distal humerus until the oval slot is seen to be in maximal relief—that is, "perfect circle."
  - Under C-arm imaging, place a scalpel over the skin to precisely determine the location of the incision. Make every attempt to keep this incision just lateral to the biceps tendon. This will decrease the risk to brachial artery, median nerve, and musculocutaneous nerve.

- Carefully make the incision though the skin and use a blunt hemostat to spread under the brachialis muscle down to the bone.
- Insert a short drill bit through a soft tissue protector.
  - Center the drill bit in the locking hole and then position it perpendicular to the nail.
  - Ideally, place the drill bit distally in the oval hole to allow axial compression to occur postoperatively.
- Attach the drill and penetrate the near cortex. Then detach the drill bit from the drill and use a mallet to gently advance the drill bit through the nail up to the far cortex.
  - An orthogonal C-arm image may be used to verify that the position of the drill bit is satisfactory.
- Reattach the drill and penetrate the far cortex.
- A depth gauge can now be inserted to ascertain the length of the interlock screw.
  - The distal screws usually are 24 mm in length.
- Use C-arm image intensification to confirm screw position through the nail as well as screw length.
  - Avoid articular penetration into the glenohumeral joint.
- Lateral-to-medial directed distal locking screws
  - Either in combination with or as an alternative to anterior-to-posterior screws, insert lateral-to-medial screws.

- Make a generous 5 cm incision to decrease the risk to the radial nerve.
- Use the same technique employed when placing AP-directed screws: blunt dissection, a protecting drill/screw insertion sleeve, and perfect circle freehand technique.
- Finally, confirm the IMN position, fracture reduction, and interlocking screw(s) placement with multiple orthogonal C-arm images.
- After orthogonal C-arm images demonstrate satisfactory reduction and hardware implantation, remove the proximal targeting device and place an end cap (this last step is optional, depending on surgeon preference).
  - Carefully select the length of the end cap to avoid impingement.

Wound Closure

- Copiously irrigate all wounds before they are closed.
- During closure of the proximal insertion site, formally repair the surgically incised rotator cuff and deltoid raphe; side-to-side nonabsorbable sutures commonly are recommended.

RETROGRADE INTRAMEDULLARY NAILING

Approach

- Make a limited posterior approach centered over the distal humerus, starting at the olecranon tip to a point 6 cm proximal.
- Longitudinally split the triceps in line with its fibers to the cortical surface of the humerus and identify the olecranon fossa.
- Make every attempt to avoid entering the elbow joint, to decrease the possibility of periarticular scarring.

Starting or Entry Portals

- As previously discussed in the Approach section, the coronal deviation of the distal humerus is variable, and, therefore, two potential starting portals exist:
  - Traditional metaphyseal entry portal: created by reaming in the midline of the distal metaphyseal triangle 2.5 cm proximal to the olecranon fossa.
  - Olecranon fossa entry portal: established by reaming the proximal slope of the olecranon at the superior border of the olecranon fossa.
- The more distal location of the nontraditional olecranon fossa entry portal increases the effective working length of the distal segment and provides a straighter alignment with the medullary canal.
  - However, biomechanical investigation has found that the olecranon fossa entry portal provides greater reduction in torque resistance and load to failure, which may increase the probability of an iatrogenic or postoperative fracture.[16]
- When making either entry portal, pay careful attention to the relation between the olecranon fossa and the

longitudinal axis of the humerus in order to place the entry portal in line with the humeral shaft. The axis of the humerus usually is colinear with the lateral aspect of the olecranon fossa.
- Make the initial entry portal in one of two ways:
  - Open the near cortex with a 4.5-mm drill bit. Continue drilling while progressively lowering the drill toward the arm until the drill bit is in line with the medullary canal on the lateral C-arm images.
  - Drill three small pilot holes in a triangular configuration perpendicular to the cortical surface. Connect these holes with a large drill bit and small rongeur or enlarge the triangular site with a small curved awl to create a long, oval hole 1 cm wide × 2 cm long that leads directly into the medullary canal.
- Undercut the internal aspect of the posterior cortex in addition to the medial and lateral walls of the entry portal to create a distal bevel along the path of nail insertion.
  - This will facilitate easy passage of the guidewire, optional reamer, and final implant.

Provisional Reduction and Guidewire Passage

- Now follow the same steps outlined in the antegrade IMN technique section to pass the guidewire, reduce the fracture, ream (optional), measure the desired nail length and diameter, and insert the chosen implant.
  - Reduction of the fracture usually involves gentle longitudinal traction on the distal humerus and correction of the varus–valgus displacement.

Reaming (Optional)

- If it is necessary to ream, carefully select the reamer size to avoid damage to the posterior cortex. In addition, slowly advance the reamer under C-arm image guidance to avoid excessive reaming of the anterior humeral cortex.
  - Both of these steps decrease the risk of possible iatrogenically induced fractures.

Distal Locking Screws

- Next, distally lock the nail to prevent backing out, that is, blocked elbow extension.
  - Place the distal locking screws from posterior to anterior using a guide.
  - Make an indentation with the guide, incise the cutaneous layer, and then use a blunt hemostat to spread down to the bone.
  - Follow the remaining steps unique to the chosen implant.

- After distal interlocking, gently tap the insertion bolt with a mallet to compress the fracture site. Assess the reduction with C-arm images.

Proximal Locking Screws

- Next, place a proximal interlocking screw, either anterior to posterior, posterior to anterior, or lateral to medial.
- Incise the skin and use a blunt hemostat to spread down to bone to protect the biceps tendon (anterior-to-posterior directed screws) or axillary nerve (posterior-to-anterior and lateral-to-medial directed screws).
- Use C-arm image intensification to confirm screw position through the nail as well as screw length.

Wound Closure

- Copiously irrigate each wound before closing it. Close triceps split with interrupted nonabsorable sutures.

PEARLS AND PITFALLS

IMN contraindications	■ Pre-existing shoulder pathology (eg, impingement, rotator cuff) ■ Permanent upper extremity weight bearers (eg, para- or tetraplegics) ■ Narrow-diameter (<9 mm) canals: excessive reaming is not desirable in the humerus because of the risk of thermal necrosis or radial nerve injury.
Antegrade IMN entry site	■ If the entry portal is too far lateral, the lateral wall of the proximal humerus can be reamed out or fractured during nail insertion. ■ Pushing the reamer shaft medially may prevent this complication.
Nail insertion	■ If any resistance is met while attempting to pass the nail, either antegrade or retrograde, make a small incision to ensure that the radial nerve is not entrapped in the fracture site.
Interlock screws	■ In most cases, soft tissues should be bluntly spread down to the bone with a hemostat before holes are drilled for any interlocking screw, to minimize neurovascular injury. ■ Antegrade IMN distal interlock screws: An alternate and possibly safer method involves placing the screw posteroanteriorly to avoid neurovascular risk when AP (musculocutaneous nerve, brachial artery) or LM (radial nerve) direction is used. When placing interlock screws using the freehand technique, tie an absorbable suture to the screw so that if the screw becomes dislodged from the screwdriver, it will not be displaced in the soft tissues. ■ Antegrade IMN: rotate the C-arm 180 degrees, so the top can be used as a table to support the arm for placing the distal locking screws.
Nail length	■ Always err on the side of a shorter nail: do not distract the fracture site or cause iatrogenic fractures by trying to impact a nail that is excessively long. ■ The retrograde IMN must be long enough to engage the cancellous part of the humeral head; the wide medullary flare of the proximal one third of the shaft does not provide sufficient stability to the inserted nail.
Open fractures: reaming	■ After a thorough irrigation and débridement is performed and the guidewire is successfully passed across the fracture site, close the deep muscle layer around the fracture site to keep the osteogenic reaming debris from washing away.

POSTOPERATIVE CARE

- Tailor the postoperative rehabilitation regimen to the method of nailing (antegrade versus retrograde), stability of the fracture, overall patient health, and preinjury level of activity/workplace demands.
- Antegrade IMN
  - Place the affected arm in a sling or shoulder immobilizer at the end of surgery.

- Postoperative day 2: remove the dressing and begin gentle shoulder pendulum and elbow ROM exercises.
- Postoperative days 10 to 14: remove the sutures. Institute a structured, supervised physical therapy program. Close patient monitoring and formal therapy are key components to achieving maximum postoperative function.
- Subsequently, schedule follow-up visits at 4- to 6-week intervals, depending on the patient's clinical and radiographic progression. Healing often takes 12 weeks or longer.

▪ As union progresses, the therapist may begin supervised exercises to recover upper extremity strength. Caution the therapist against instituting programs or exercises that create large rotational stresses to the arm until radiographic healing becomes evident.

▪ Retrograde IMN

  ▪ Initial postoperative management is identical to treatment following antegrade nailing, unless weight bearing is necessary for wheelchair transfers, walkers, or crutch ambulation. Use a posterior splint and platform attachment if crutches are necessary.

  ▪ It is important to institute early elbow active ROM or gentle passive ROM by the patient to prevent elbow stiffness.

▪ Avoid

  ▪ Aggressive PROM or stretching to decrease the risk of myositis ossificans formation

  ▪ Resisted elbow extension for the first 6 weeks after surgery to protect the repair of the triceps split.

OUTCOMES

▪ Randomized clinical trials comparing IMN to compression plating show a higher reoperation rate and greater shoulder morbidity with the use of nails.[11]

▪ Locked antegrade IMN has resulted in loss of shoulder motion in 6% to 37% of cases.[13]

▪ Recent antegrade nails designed to eliminate insertion site shoulder morbidity though an extra-articular start point have been introduced, and prospective randomized trials are pending.

▪ Retrograde IMN union rates range from 91% to 98%, and the mean healing time is 13.7 weeks.[15]

▪ Retrospective reviews of retrograde IMN have found shoulder function to be excellent in 92.3% of patients and elbow function excellent in 87.2% of patients after fracture consolidation.[15]

  ▪ Functional end results were excellent in 84.6% of patients, moderate in 10.3% of patients, and bad in 5.1% of patients.

▪ Biomechanical studies have shown that, for midshaft fractures, both antegrade and retrograde nailing showed similar initial stability and bending and torsional stiffness—20% to 30% of normal humeral shafts.[8]

  ▪ In proximal fractures (ie, 10 cm distal to the greater tuberosity tip), antegrade nails demonstrated significantly more initial stability and higher bending and torsional stiffness, as was true for distal fractures with retrograde nailing.

COMPLICATIONS

▪ Nonunion[3]

  ▪ Antegrade IMN: 11.6%

  ▪ Retrograde IMN: 4.5%

▪ Infection: 1% to 2%

▪ Insertion site morbidity

  ▪ Antegrade IMN: shoulder pain, impingement, stiffness, and weakness

  ▪ Retrograde IMN: elbow pain, stiffness, and triceps weakness

▪ Iatrogenic fractures[3]

  ▪ Antegrade IMN: 5.1%

  ▪ Retrograde IMN: 7.1%

▪ Iatrogenic comminution and distraction at the fracture site

▪ Neurovascular risk

  ▪ Risk to the radial nerve in the spiral groove from canal preparation and nail insertion

  ▪ Risk to the axillary nerve from proximal interlocking

  ▪ Risk to the radial, musculocutaneous, and median nerves or brachial artery from distal interlocking

▪ Heat-induced segmental avascularity after reaming

REFERENCES

1. Bono CM, Grossman MG, Hochwald N, et al. Radial and axillary nerves. Anatomic considerations for humeral fixation. Clin Orthop Relat Res 2000;373:259–264.
2. Chen AL, Joseph TN, Wolinsky PR, et al. Fixation stability of comminuted humeral shaft fractures: locked intramedullary nailing versus plate fixation. J Trauma 2002;53:733–737.
3. Court-Brown C. Paper presented at the Orthopaedic Trauma Association Specialty Day Meeting; February 26, 2005; Washington, DC.
4. Crates J, Whittle AP. Antegrade interlocking nailing of acute humeral shaft fractures. Clin Orthop Relat Res 1998;350:40–50.
5. Farragos AF, Schemitsch EH, McKee MD. Complications of intramedullary nailing for fractures of the humeral shaft: a review. J Orthop Trauma 1999;13:258–267.
6. Foster RJ, Swiontkowski MF, Back AW, et al. Radial nerve palsy caused by open humeral shaft fractures. J Hand Surg Am 1993;18:121–124.
7. Green AG, Reid JS, Carlson DA. Fractures of the humerus. In: Baumgaertner MR, Tornetta P, eds. Orthopaedic Knowledge Update: Trauma. Rosemont, IL: American Academy of Orthopaedic Surgeons, 2005:163–180.
8. Lin J, Inoue N, Valdevit A, et al. Biomechanical comparison of antegrade and retrograde nailing of humeral shaft fracture. Clin Orthop Relat Res 1998;351:203–213.
9. Lin J, Hou SM, Inoue N, et al. Anatomic considerations of locked humeral nailing. Clin Orthop Relat Res 1999;368:247–254.
10. Lyons RP, Lazarus MD. Shoulder and arm trauma: bone. In: Orthopaedic Knowledge Update 8. Rosemont, IL: American Academy of Orthopaedic Surgeons, 2005:275–277.
11. McCormack RG, Brien D, Buckley RE, et al. Fixation of fractures of the shaft of the humerus by dynamic compression plate or intramedullary nail: A prospective randomized trial. J Bone Joint Surg Br 2000;82B:336–339.
12. McKee MD. Fractures of the shaft of the humerus. In: Bucholz RW, Heckman JD, Court-Brown C, eds. Rockwood and Green's Fractures in Adults, ed 6. Philadelphia: Lippincott Williams & Wilkins, 2006:1117–1157.
13. Riemer BL, Foglesong ME, Burke CJ. Complications of Seidel intramedullary nailing of narrow diameter humeral diaphyseal fractures. Orthopedics 1994;17:19–29.
14. Roberts CS, Walz BM, Yerasimides JG. Humeral shaft fractures: Intramedullary nailing. In: Wiss D, ed. Master Techniques in Orthopaedic Surgery: Fractures, ed 2. Philadelphia: Lippincott Williams & Wilkins, 2006:81–95.
15. Rommens PM, Verbruggen J, Broos PL. Retrograde locked nailing of humeral shaft fractures. A review of 39 patients. J Bone Joint Surg Br 1995;77B: 84–89.
16. Strothman D, Templeman DC, Varecka T, et al. Retrograde nailing of humeral shaft fractures: a biomechanical study of its effects on strength of the distal humerus. J Orthop Trauma 2000;14:101.
17. Tytherleigh-Strong G, Walls N, McQueen MM. The epidemiology of humeral shaft fractures. J Bone Joint Surg Br 1998;80B:249–253.

Chapter 22

Open Reduction and Internal Fixation of Nonarticular Scapular Fractures

Brett D. Owens and Thomas P. Goss

DEFINITION

■ Nonarticular scapular fractures include fractures of the glenoid neck, scapular spine and body, acromial process, and coracoid process. They account for 90% of scapular fractures.[6]

■ Most nonarticular scapular fractures can be treated nonoperatively, including all isloated scapular body–spine fractures.

■ Significant displacement at one or more of these sites, alone or in conjunction with ligamentous disruptions of the superior shoulder suspensory complex, require evaluation for surgical intervention.[1,10]

ANATOMY

■ The scapula is a flat triangular bone with three processes laterally: the glenoid process, the acromial process, and the coracoid process.

■ The glenoid proocess consists of the glenoid fossa, the glenoid rim, and the glenoid neck.

■ The superior shoulder suspensory complex is a bone and soft tissue ring at the end of a superior and an inferior bony strut (**FIG 1**). This ring is composed of the glenoid process, the coracoid process, the coracoclavicular ligament, the distal clavicle, the acromioclavicular joint, and the acromial process. The superior strut is the middle third of the clavicle, whereas the inferior strut is the junction of the most lateral portion of the scapular body and the most medial portion of the glenoid neck.[1]

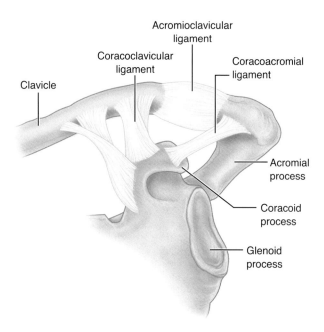

Acromioclavicular ligament

Coracoclavicular ligament

Coracoacromial ligament

Clavicle

Acromial process

Coracoid process

Glenoid process

FIG 1 • Superior shoulder suspensory complex.

PATHOGENESIS

■ Scapular fractures usually are the result of high-energy trauma and have a high rate of associated musculoskeletal and underlying thoracic injuries.[3]

■ Fractures of the acromion process may be the result of direct trauma due to its subdermal location, whereas coracoid process fractures may be due to a sudden muscular contraction.[4]

NATURAL HISTORY

■ The results of nonoperative treatment of nonarticular scapular fractures generally are good. Nonunion is rare because the area has a rich blood supply. Angular deformities often are well compensated for by the wide range of motion of the glenohumeral joint and scapulothoracic articulation.

PATIENT HISTORY AND PHYSICAL FINDINGS

■ In addition to the specifics of the injury, it is helpful to obtain an understanding of the functional demands on the extremity. Hand dominance, occupation, and sports participation are all relevant.

■ A thorough neurovascular examination must be performed and deficits evaluated with angiography and electromyography, as necessary.

■ A thorough soft tissue examination also is warranted, as wounds may represent an open fracture and warrant exploration. Blisters or swelling may delay surgery.

IMAGING AND OTHER DIAGNOSTIC STUDIES

■ Nonarticular scapular fractures usually are identified on routine shoulder trauma series radiographs: a true anteroposterior (AP) view of the shoulder with the arm in neutral rotation, a true axillary view of the glenohumeral joint, and a true lateral scapular view. An AP weight-bearing view may be indicated.

■ CT scans and three-dimensional reconstructions can be helpful for identification and classification of fractures owing to the complex bony anatomy in this region. In addition, the bony relationships should be evaluated for evidence of any ligamentous disruption.

DIFFERENTIAL DIAGNOSIS

■ Nonarticular scapular fractures
■ Intra-articular scapular fractures
■ Double disruptions of the superior shoulder suspensory complex including a floating shoulder (ie, glenoid neck fracture with ipsilateral middle third clavicle fracture)
■ Scapulothoracic dissociation

NONOPERATIVE MANAGEMENT

▪ Most (over 90%) scapular fractures can be treated nonoperatively.

▪ Glenoid fossa and rim fractures may require operative management and are discussed in Chapter SE-23.

▪ Glenoid neck fractures with more than 40 degrees of angulation in the coronal or sagittal plane or translational displacement of 1 cm or more require surgical management. Anatomic neck fractures (lateral to the coracoid process) are inherently unstable and should also be considered for operative intervention.[2]

▪ Isolated acromial and coracoid process fractures usually are minimally displaced and can be managed nonoperatively. Significant displacement or fractures in conjunction with other bony and soft tissue injuries to the shoulder girdle may require surgical stabilization.[4]

SURGICAL MANAGEMENT

Preoperative Planning

▪ Imaging studies should be reviewed and available for reference in the operating room. A draped fluoroscopy unit

and competent technician should be available during the surgery.

Positioning

▪ Open reduction with internal fixation (ORIF) of scapular fractures requires wide access to the entire shoulder girdle. The patient may be placed in either the lateral decubitus position (**FIG 2A**) or in the beach chair position (**FIG 2B**), but care must be taken to allow adequate exposure of the entire scapula and clavicle.

▪ The shoulder girdle is prepped and draped widely, and the entire upper extremity is prepped and draped "free."

▪ Alternatively, a staged procedure can be performed using separate positions, sterile preparations, and separate exposures.[9]

Approach

▪ Glenoid neck fractures are approached posteriorly.

▪ A superior approach can added for control and positioning of a difficult-to-control glenoid fragment.

▪ An anterior approach is used for coracoid process fractures.

▪ A superior approach is used for access to acromial process fractures.

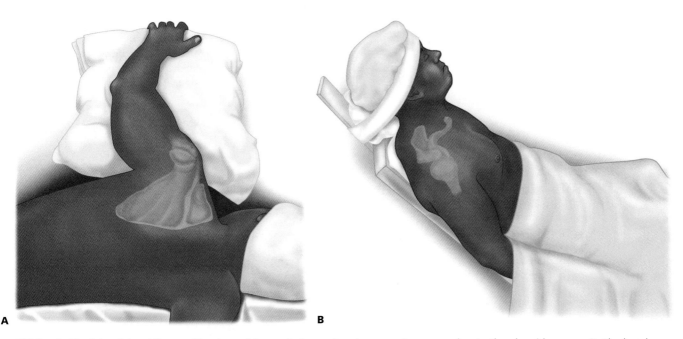

FIG 2 • **A.** The lateral decubitus position is used for posterior and posterosuperior approaches to the glenoid process. **B.** The beach chair position.

POSTERIOR APPROACH TO GLENOID NECK

▪ Bony landmarks are outlined with marking pen (**TECH FIG 1A**).

▪ An incision is made along the scapular spine and acromion and down the lateral aspect of the shoulder, as needed.

▪ The origins of the posterior and middle heads of the deltoid muscle are sharply detached from the scapular spine–acromial process and retracted distally (**TECH FIG 1B**).

▪ The interval between infraspinatus and teres minor is developed.

▪ If access to the glenoid fossa is necessary, the infraspinatus tendon and underlying posterior glenohumeral joint capsule are incised 2 cm lateral to their insertion on the greater tuberosity and reflected laterally (**TECH FIG 1C,D**).

▪ Mobilization of the teres minor muscle allows access to the lateral scapular border.

TECHNIQUES

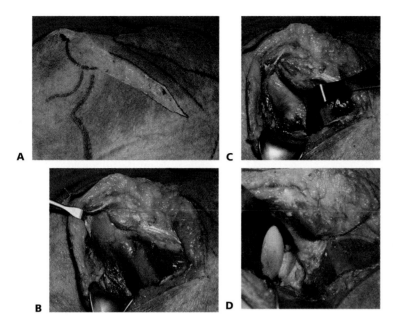

TECH FIG 1 • A. The standard posterior incision extends along the inferior margin of the scapular spine and the acromion. At the lateral tip of the acromion, the incision continues in the midlateral line for 2.5 cm. **B.** The posterior and middle heads of the deltoid muscle have been detached from the scapular spine–posterior acromial process and retracted distally to expose the infraspinatus musculotendinous unit. **C.** The infraspinatus–teres minor interval has been developed, with the infraspinatus retracted superiorly and the teres minor retracted inferiorly to expose the posterior glenohumeral joint capsule (the inferior portion of the infraspinatus insertion has been released). **D.** The infraspinatus tendon and underlying posterior glenohumeral joint capsule are incised 2 cm from insertion on the greater tuberosity to allow access to the glenohumeral joint. (From Goss TP. Glenoid fractures: Open reduction and internal fixation. In Wiss DA, ed. Master Techniques in Orthopaedic Surgery: Fractures. Philadelphia: Lippincott–Raven, 1998.)

- Reduction of the fracture is performed with lateral traction on the draped arm and manipulation of the fracture site.
- Temporary fixation may be obtained with K-wires.
- Rigid fixation may be obtained with a contoured reconstruction plate and 3.5-mm cortical screws (**TECH FIG 1D**).

- Care must be taken to avoid violating the glenoid fossa with the screws in the glenoid fragment.
- Meticulous repair of the deltoid origin to the scapular spine–acromion should be performed with permanent sutures through drill holes.

SUPERIOR APPROACH TO GLENOID NECK

- The superior approach to the glenoid neck is made in an extensile fashion by extending the posterior incision superiorly.
- The trapezius and underlying supraspinatus muscles are split in the line of their fibers (**TECH FIG 2**).

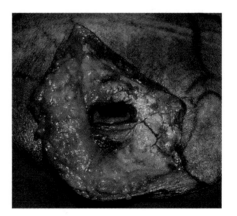

TECH FIG 2 • In the interval between the clavicle and the scapular spine–acromial process, the trapezius and supraspinatus tendon have been split in line of their fibers for exposure. (From Goss TP. Glenoid fractures: Open reduction and internal fixation. In Wiss DA, ed. Master Techniques in Orthopaedic Surgery: Fractures. Philadelphia: Lippincott–Raven, 1998.)

ORIF OF ACROMIAL PROCESS FRACTURE

- Incision directly over the acromial process
- Subperiosteal dissection to expose the superior surface of the acromion
- Anatomic fracture reduction under direct visualization

- Proximal fractures: fixation with a contoured 3.5-mm reconstruction plate (**TECH FIG 3A**)
- Distal fractures: fixation with a tension band construct (**TECH FIG 3B**)

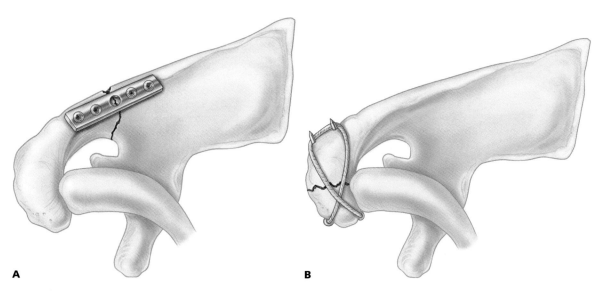

A   **B**

TECH FIG 3 • Fixation techniques for acromion process fractures. **A.** Plate-and-screw construct for a fracture of the base of the acromion. **B.** Tension band wire construct.

ORIF OF CORACOID PROCESS FRACTURE

- Vertical incision 1 cm lateral to coracoid process (**TECH FIG 4A**)
- Development of deltopectoral interval or split of the deltoid muscle in line with its fibers directly over the coracoid process
- Exposure of the fracture site (may need to open the rotator interval)

- If coracoid tip has sufficient stock, cannulated screw fixation can be performed (**TECH FIG 4B**).
- If not, fragment excision and suture fixation of conjoint tendon to remaining coracoid is performed (**TECH FIG 4C**).
- Coracoid base fractures are fixed with a single cannulated cortical screw (**TECH FIG 4D**).

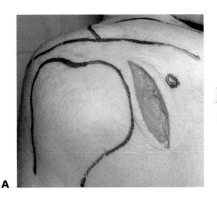

A

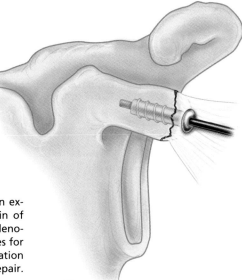

TECH FIG 4 • **A.** Standard anterior incision extends from the superior to inferior margin of the humeral head, centered over the glenohumeral joint. **B–D.** Three repair techniques for coracoid fractures. **B.** Cannulated screw fixation of tip avulsion with sufficient bone to repair. *(continued)*

B

TECHNIQUES

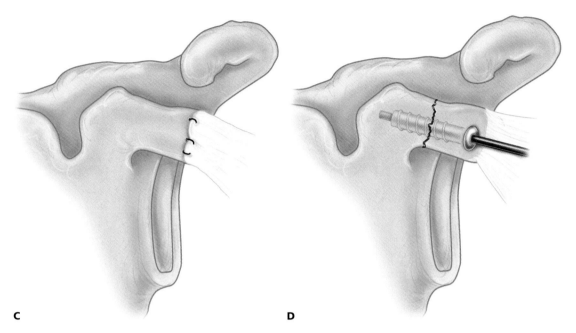

C

D

TECH FIG 4 • *(continued)* **C.** Suture fixation of conjoint tendon when insufficient bone is available to repair. **D.** Cannulated screw fixation for proximal fracture. (**A:** From Goss TP. Open reduction and internal fixation of glenoid fractures. In: Craig EV, ed. Master Techniques in Orthopaedic Surgery: The Shoulder, 2nd ed. Philadelphia: Lippincott Williams & Wilkins, 2004.)

PEARLS AND PITFALLS

Indications	■ CT can help define the fracture, assess possible intra-articular involvement, and identify concomitant injuries. ■ Most nonarticular injuries and all scapular body–spine fractures are treated nonoperatively.
Approach	■ Deltoid detachment and reflection provides maximal visualization and is recommended for surgeons unfamiliar with the posterior approach. ■ During the posterior approach, the internervous plane is between the infraspinatus (a bipennate muscle) superiorly and the teres minor inferiorly.
Reduction	■ K-wires can be placed to serve as "joysticks" to assist with fracture reduction.
Fixation	■ K-wires should be avoided for permanent fixation. However, they can be placed percutaneously and used for temporary or supplemental fixation, being removed at 4 to 6 weeks. ■ Reconstruction plates may be pre-contoured using a scapula model.
Closure	■ Meticulous repair of the deltoid to the scapular spine–acromial process is necessary, using nonabsorbable sutures placed through drill holes.

POSTOPERATIVE CARE

■ How aggressive the rehabilitation program following ORIF of nonarticular scapular fractures must be is determined by the rigidity of the fixation construct and the adequacy of the soft tissue repair.[5]

■ Patients are immobilized in a sling and swathe binder and started on gentle pendulum exercises during the first 2 weeks.

■ Progressive passive and active-assisted range of motion exercises are emphasized during weeks 2 through 6 postoperatively.

■ All protection is discontinued by 6 weeks postoperatively.

■ Strengthening is begun after 6 weeks postoperatively and after range of motion is satisfactory.

■ Return to sports or labor is restricted until 4 to 6 months postoperatively.

OUTCOMES

■ Relatively few outcome studies detailing the results of scapular fractures treated operatively are available.

■ While most nonarticular scapular fractures are treated non-operatively, those that warrant surgical intervention appear to benefit from this treatment.[7,8]

COMPLICATIONS

■ When neurologic complications occur, they most commonly are caused by overly aggressive retraction or misdirected dissection.

■ The musculocutaneous and axillary nerves are vulnerable in the anterior approach, the suprascapular nerve in the superior approach, and the axillary and suprascapular nerves in the posterior approach.[9]

REFERENCES

1. Goss TP. Double disruptions of the superior shoulder complex. J Orthop Trauma 1993;7:99.
2. Goss TP. Fractures of the glenoid neck. J Shoulder Elbow Surg 1994;3:42–61.
3. Goss TP. Scapular fractures and dislocation: diagnosis and treatment. J Am Acad Orthop Surg 1995;3:22.
4. Goss TP. The scapula: Coracoid, acromial and avulsion fractures. Am J Orthop 1996;25:106.
5. Goss TP. Glenoid fractures: Open reduction and internal fixation. In: Wiss DA, ed. Master Techniques in Orthopaedic Surgery: Fractures, 2nd ed. Philadelphia: Lippincott Williams & Wilkins, 2006.
6. Goss TP, Owens BD. Fractures of the scapula: Diagnosis and treatment. In: Iannotti JP, Williams GR, eds. Disorders of the Shoulder: Diagnosis and Management, 2nd ed. Philadelphia: Lippincott Williams & Wilkins, 2007.
7. Hardegger FH, Simpson LA, Weber BG. The operative treatment of scapular fractures. J Bone Joint Surg Br 1984;66B:725.
8. Kavanagh BF, Bradway JK, Cofield RH. Open reduction of displaced intra-articular fractures of the glenoid fossa. J Bone Joint Surg Am 1993;75A:479.
9. Owens BD, Goss TP. Surgical approaches for glenoid fractures. Tech Shoulder Elbow Surg 2004;5:103–115.
10. Owens BD, Goss TP. The floating shoulder. J Bone Joint Surg Br 2006;88(11):1419–1424.

Chapter 23

Open Reduction and Internal Fixation of Intra-articular Scapular Fractures

Brett D. Owens, Joanna G. Branstetter, and Thomas P. Goss

DEFINITION

▪ Intra-articular scapular fractures include fractures of the glenoid cavity, which includes the glenoid rim and the glenoid fossa. They account for 10% of scapular fractures.[6] Most scapular fractures are extra-articular, and 50% involve the body and spine.

▪ Over 90% of fractures of the glenoid cavity are insignificantly displaced and are managed nonoperatively.[3]

▪ Significant displacement requires evaluation for surgical intervention to achieve the best possible outcome.

ANATOMY

▪ The scapula is a flat triangular bone with three processes: the glenoid process, the acromial process, and the coracoid process.

▪ The glenoid process consists of the glenoid cavity (the glenoid rim and glenoid fossa) and the glenoid neck.

▪ The glenoid cavity provides a firm concave surface with which the convex humeral head articulates. The average depth of the articular cartilage is 5 mm.

▪ Glenoid cavity fractures are classified according to whether they involve the glenoid rim or the glenoid fossa and the direction of the fracture line (**FIG 1**).

PATHOGENESIS

▪ Scapular fractures usually are the result of high-energy trauma and have a high rate (90%) of associated bony and soft tissue injuries, both local and distant.[5]

▪ Fractures of the glenoid rim occur when the humeral head strikes the periphery of the glenoid cavity. They are true fractures, not avulsion injuries caused by indirect forces applied to the periarticular soft tissues by the humeral head.

▪ Fractures of the glenoid fossa occur when the humeral head is driven into the center of the concavity. The fracture then promulgates in a number of different directions, depending on the characteristics of the humeral head force.

NATURAL HISTORY

▪ The results of nonoperative treatment of intra-articular scapular fractures usually are good if the fracture displacement is minimal and the humeral head lies concentrically within the glenoid cavity.

▪ Significant displacement can result in posttraumatic degenerative joint disease, glenohumeral instability, and even nonunion.[2]

PATIENT HISTORY AND PHYSICAL FINDINGS

▪ In addition to the specifics of the injury, it is helpful to obtain an understanding of the functional demands on the extremity. Hand dominance, occupation, and sports participation are all relevant.

▪ A thorough neurovascular examination must be performed. Deficits are evaluated with angiography and electromyography, as necessary.

▪ A thorough soft tissue examination also is warranted. Wounds may represent an open fracture and warrant exploration. Blisters or swelling may delay surgery.

IMAGING AND OTHER DIAGNOSTIC STUDIES

▪ Intra-articular scapular fractures initially are evaluated with a routine scapula trauma radiographic series (a true anteroposterior view of the shoulder with the arm in neutral rotation, a true axillary view of the glenohumeral joint, and a true lateral scapular view; **FIG 2A**).

▪ CT scans and three-dimensional studies with reconstructions can be helpful in evaluating articular congruity and fracture displacement (**FIG 2B–D**). In addition, the bony relationships should be evaluated for evidence of ligamentous disruption(s) or instability.

DIFFERENTIAL DIAGNOSIS

▪ Intra-articular scapular fractures
▪ Nonarticular scapular fractures
▪ Scapulothoracic dissociation
▪ Double disruptions of the superior shoulder suspensory complex, including a floating shoulder (a glenoid neck fracture with an ipsilateral middle third clavicle fracture)

NONOPERATIVE MANAGEMENT

▪ Most (over 90%) intra-articular scapular fractures are insignificantly displaced and are managed nonoperatively.

▪ Significantly displaced glenoid fossa and glenoid rim fractures require operative management.

SURGICAL MANAGEMENT

▪ Surgical indications are as follows:
  ▪ Rim fractures: 25% or more of the glenoid cavity anteriorly or 33% or more of the glenoid cavity posteriorly and displacement of the fragment 10 mm or more
  ▪ Fossa fractures: an articular step-off of 5 mm or more, significant separation of the fracture fragments, or failure of the humeral head to lie in the center of the glenoid cavity

Preoperative Planning

▪ Imaging studies should be reviewed before the surgery and should be available for reference in the operating room. A draped fluoroscopy unit and a competent technician should be available. An examination for instability can be performed while under anesthesia.

Positioning

▪ Open reduction with internal fixation (ORIF) of intra-articular scapular fractures requires wide access to the entire

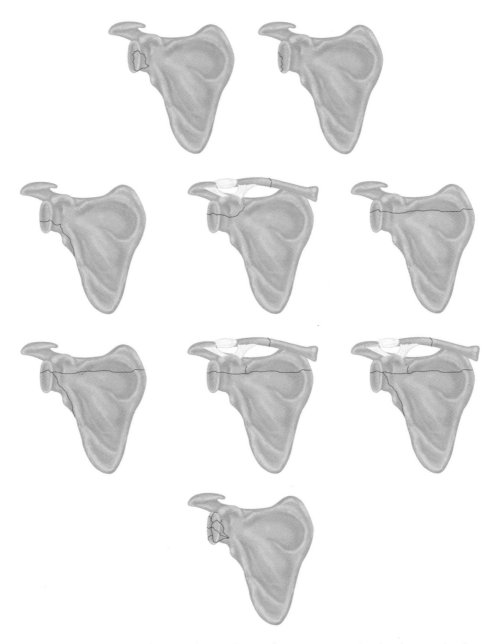

FIG 1 • Goss-Ideberg classification of glenoid cavity fractures. Ia, anterior rim; Ib, posterior rim; II, inferior glenoid; III, superior glenoid; IV, transverse through the body; V; combination II-IV; VI, comminuted.

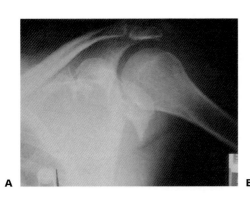

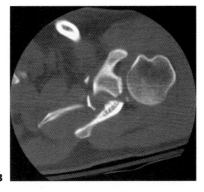

FIG 2 • **A.** The AP radiograph shows a type Vc glenoid cavity fracture. **B.** Axillary CT image shows a large anterosuperior glenoid cavity fragment including the coracoid process. *(continued)*

A

B

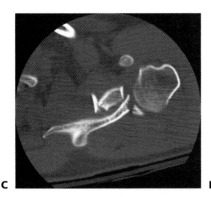
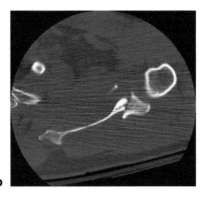

FIG 2 • *(continued)* **C.** Axillary CT image shows the lateral aspect of the scapular body lying between the two glenoid cavity fragments and abutting the humeral head. **D.** Axillary CT image shows a large posteroinferior cavity fragment. (From Goss TP, Owens BD. Fractures of the scapula: Diagnosis and treatment. In: Iannotti JP, Williams GR, eds. Disorders of the Shoulder: Diagnosis and Management, 2nd ed. Philadelphia: Lippincott Williams & Wilkins, 2007:793–840.)

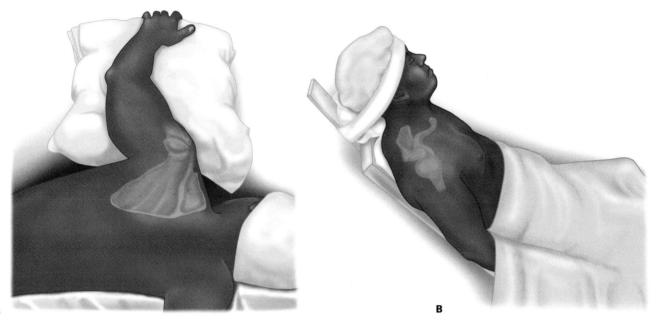

FIG 3 • Patient position: lateral decubitus (**A**) and beach chair (**B**).

shoulder girdle. Depending on the particular fracture, the patient is placed in either the lateral decubitus position (**FIG 3A**) or the beach chair position (**FIG 3B**).

▪ Care must be taken to allow adequate exposure of the entire scapula and clavicle. The shoulder girdle is prepped and draped widely, and the entire upper extremity is prepped and draped "free."

▪ In some cases, a staged procedure may be necessary using separate positions, sterile preparations, and exposures.[10]

Approach

▪ The posterior approach is used for fractures of the posterior glenoid rim and most fractures of the glenoid fossa.

▪ The superior approach is used, in conjunction with a posterior approach, for fractures of the glenoid fossa with a difficult-to-control superior fragment.

▪ The anterior approach is used for fractures of the anterior glenoid rim and some fractures involving the superior aspect of the glenoid fossa.

POSTERIOR APPROACH TO THE GLENOID CAVITY

▪ Bony landmarks are outlined with a marking pen.

▪ An incision is made along the scapular spine and acromion and down the midlateral aspect of the shoulder, as needed (**TECH FIG 1A**).

▪ Origins of the posterior and middle heads of the deltoid muscle are sharply detached from the scapular spine–acromial process, and the deltoid muscle is split in the line of its fibers for 2.5 cm in the midlateral line. It is then retracted distally (**TECH FIG 1B**).

▪ The interval between infraspinatus and teres minor is developed (**TECH FIG 1C**). To gain access to the glenoid fossa, the infraspinatus tendon and underlying posterior glenohumeral joint capsule are incised 2 cm lateral to their insertion on the greater tuberosity and reflected posteriorly (**TECH FIG 1D**).

▪ Subperiosteal mobilization of the teres minor muscle allows access to the lateral scapular border.

TECHNIQUES

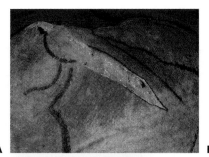 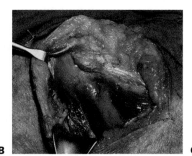 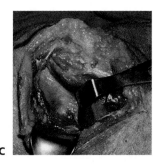

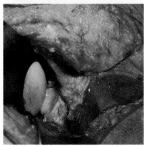

TECH FIG 1 • A. Posterior approach using a skin incision along the scapular spine and acromion. **B.** The posterior and posteromedial heads of the deltoid are detached from the scapular spine and acromial process. **C.** Interval developed between the infraspinatus and teres minor. **D.** The infraspinatus tendon and underlying posterior glenohumeral capsule are incised 2 cm from insertion on the greater tuberosity to allow access to the glenohumeral joint. (From Goss TP. Glenoid fractures: open reduction and internal fixation. In Wiss DA, ed. Master Techniques in Orthopaedic Surgery: Fractures. Philadelphia: Lippincott–Raven, 1998.)

SUPERIOR APPROACH TO THE GLENOID CAVITY

- The superior approach to the glenoid cavity is made by extending the posterior incision superiorly.
- The trapezius and underlying supraspinatus muscles are split in the line of their fibers (**TECH FIG 2**).

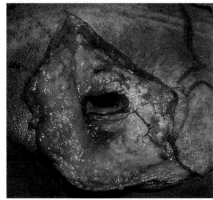

TECH FIG 2 • Superior approach. The trapezius and underlying supraspinatus muscles are split in line with their fibers. (From Goss TP. Glenoid fractures: open reduction and internal fixation. In Wiss DA, ed. Master Techniques in Orthopaedic Surgery: Fractures. Philadelphia: Lippincott–Raven, 1998.)

ANTERIOR APPROACH TO THE GLENOID CAVITY

- The incision is made in Langer's lines and centered over the glenohumeral joint from the superior to inferior level of the humeral head (**TECH FIG 3A**).
- The deltoid muscle is split in the line of its fibers over the palpable coracoid process and retracted medially and laterally.
- The conjoined tendon is retracted medially after division of the overlying fascia along its medial border (**TECH FIG 3B**).
- Care must be taken to protect all neurovascular structures from injury.

- Incise the subscapularis tendon vertically 2.5 cm medial to its insertion on the lesser tuberosity and along its superior and inferior borders.
  - Dissect it off the underlying anterior glenohumeral capsule.
- Tag the corners of the subscapularis unit and turn it back medially (**TECH FIG 3C**).
- Incise the anterior glenohumeral capsule in the same fashion, tag its corners, and turn it back medially to gain access to the glenohumeral joint.

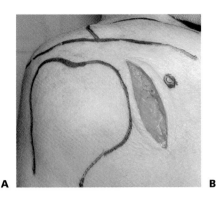
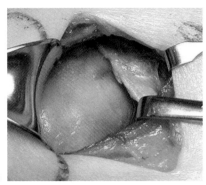
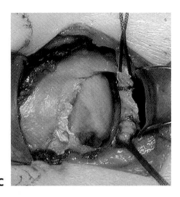

TECH FIG 3 • A. Anterior approach using a skin incision made in Langer's lines and centered over the glenohumeral joint. **B.** The conjoined tendon is retracted medially. **C.** Incise the subscapularis tendon 2 cm from its insertion on the lesser tuberosity, dissect it off the glenohumeral capsule, incise the capsule similarly, and turn both of them back medially to gain access to the glenohumeral joint. (From Goss TP. Open reduction and internal fixation of glenoid fractures. In: Craig EV, ed. Master Techniques in Orthopaedic Surgery: The Shoulder, 2nd ed. Philadelphia: Lippincott Williams & Wilkins, 2004.)

FIXATION TECHNIQUES

- The fracture is reduced as anatomically as possible.
- Temporary fixation may be obtained with K-wires.
- Rigid fixation may be obtained with a contoured reconstruction plate and 3.5-mm cortical screws or with cannulated interfragmentary compression screws, depending on the characteristics of the fracture.
- Care must be taken to avoid violating the glenoid fossa with any screws placed in the glenoid fragment (**TECH FIG 4A,B**).

- If severe comminution is present, an iliac crest tricortical bone graft is an option (**TECH FIG 4C**).
- All soft tissues divided to gain access to the fracture site must be meticulously repaired. With posterior approaches, the deltoid must be securely reattached to the acromion and scapular spine with permanent sutures through drill holes.

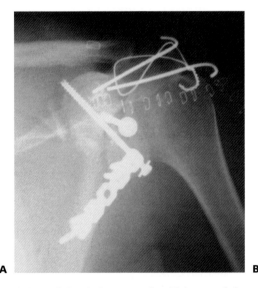
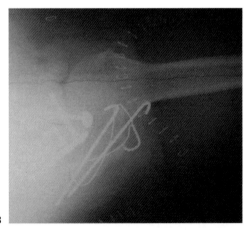

TECH FIG 4 • A. Postoperative AP image of the patient shown in Tech Fig 1. **B.** Axillary radiograph showing the glenoid cavity fragments secured together with cannulated screws and the glenoid unit secured to the scapular body with a malleable reconstruction plate (the acromial fracture was reduced and stabilized with a tension band construct). *(continued)*

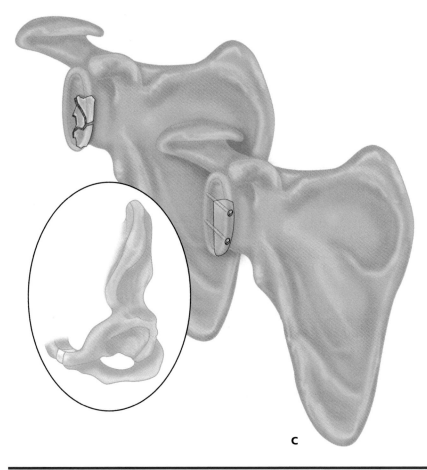

C

TECH FIG 4 • *(continued)* **C.** If severe comminution is present, an iliac crest tricortical bone graft is an option. (**A,B:** From Goss TP, Owens BD. Fractures of the scapula: diagnosis and treatment. In: Iannotti JP, Williams GR, eds. Disorders of the Shoulder: Diagnosis and Management, 2nd ed. Philadelphia: Lippincott Williams & Wilkins, 2007:793–840.)

PEARLS AND PITFALLS

Indications	▪ Rim fractures: 25% or more of the glenoid cavity anteriorly or 33% or more of the glenoid cavity posteriorly and displacement of the fragment 10 mm or more ▪ Fossa fractures: an articular step-off of 5 mm or more, significant separation of the fracture fragments, or failure of the humeral head to lie in the center of the glenoid cavity
Approach	▪ Incising the rotator interval and leaving the subscapularis unit intact may allow adequate exposure for injuries involving a displaced superior glenoid fragment. ▪ Some injuries require combined anteroposterior or posterosuperior approaches. ▪ Deltoid detachment and retraction provide maximal posterior exposure and access. ▪ During the posterior approach, develop the internervous plane in between the infraspinatus (a bipennate muscle) superiorly and the teres minor inferiorly.
Reduction	▪ K-wires can be placed to serve as "joysticks" to assist with fracture reduction. They also can be driven across the fracture site to provide temporary or permanent fixation.
Fixation	▪ Bone stock capable of allowing internal fixation is at a premium in the scapula. The four satisfactory areas include the glenoid neck, the acromion–scapular spine, the lateral scapular border, and the coracoid process. Reconstruction plates may be pre-contoured using a scapula model and flash-sterilized. If severe comminution is present, an iliac crest tricortical bone graft is an option. Cannulated interfragmentary screws can be inserted using previously placed K-wires as guidewires.
Closure	▪ If the deltoid muscle is detached, meticulous repair to the scapular spine–acromial process is necessary using nonabsorbable sutures placed through drill holes.

POSTOPERATIVE CARE

▪ The aggressiveness of the rehabilitation program following ORIF of intra-articular scapular fractures is determined by the rigidity of the fixation construct and the adequacy of the soft tissue repair.[4]

▪ Patients are immobilized in a sling and swathe binder and started on gentle pendulum exercises during the first 2 weeks.
▪ Progressive passive and active-assisted range-of-motion exercises emphasizing forward flexion and internal–external rotation are prescribed during weeks 2 through 6 postoperatively.

- All protection is discontinued at 6 weeks postoperatively.
- Strengthening is begun after 6 weeks postoperatively and when range of motion is satisfactory.
- Return to sports or physical labor is restricted until 3 to 6 months postoperatively.
- Close outpatient follow-up with radiographs, especially early in recovery, and a well-defined, closely monitored physical therapy program are extremely important.

OUTCOMES

- Good results have been reported for the operative management of glenoid rim fractures.[9,12]
- Bauer et al[1] reviewed six patients treated surgically for glenoid cavity fractures. Four patients with an anatomic reduction had good results; two patients with nonanatomic reductions developed arthritic changes.
- Kavanaugh and colleagues[7] presented their experience at the Mayo Clinic in which 10 displaced intra-articular fractures of the glenoid cavity were treated with ORIF. They found ORIF to be "a useful and safe technique" that "can restore excellent function of the shoulder." In their series, the major articular fragments were displaced 4 to 8 mm.
- Schandelmaier and coauthors[11] reported a series of 22 fractures of the glenoid fossa treated with ORIF with good results.
- Leung and colleagues[8] reviewed 14 displaced intra-articular fractures of the glenoid treated with ORIF (30.5-year average follow-up) and reported 9 excellent and 5 good results.
- On the basis of these reports, it seems reasonable to conclude that there is a definite role for surgical management in the treatment of glenoid cavity fractures.

COMPLICATIONS

- Neurologic complications most commonly are caused by overly aggressive retraction or misdirected dissection.
  - The musculocutaneous and axillary nerves are vulnerable in the anterior approach.

- The suprascapular nerve is at risk in the superior approach, and the axillary and suprascapular nerves are vulnerable in the posterior approach.[10]
- A variety of other complications can occur as a result of poor surgical technique, inadequately directed or managed rehabilitation, and poor patient compliance.

REFERENCES

1. Bauer G, Fleischmann W, DuBler E. Displaced scapular fractures: Indication and long term results of open reduction and internal fixation. Arch Orthop Trauma Surg 1995;14:215.
2. DePalma AF. Surgery of the Shoulder, 3rd ed. Philadelphia: JB Lippincott, 1983.
3. Goss TP. Fractures of the glenoid cavity. J Bone Joint Surg Am 1992;74:299–305.
4. Goss TP. Glenoid fractures—open reduction and internal fixation. In Wiss DA, ed: Master Techniques in Orthopaedic Surgery: Fractures. Philadelphia: Lippincott-Raven, 1998.
5. Goss TP. Scapular fractures and dislocation: diagnosis and treatment. J Am Acad Orthop Surg 1995;25:106.
6. Goss TP, Owens BD. Fractures of the scapula: Diagnosis and treatment. In: Iannotti JP, Williams GR, eds. Disorders of the Shoulder: Diagnosis and Management, 2nd ed. Philadelphia: Lippincott Williams & Wilkins, 2007:793–840.
7. Kavanagh BF, Bradway JK, Cofield RH. Open reduction of displaced intra-articular fractures of the glenoid fossa. J Bone Joint Surg Am 1993;75A:479.
8. Leung KS, Lam TB, Poon KM. Operative treatment of displaced intra-articular glenoid fractures. Injury 1993;24:324.
9. Niggebrugge AHP, van Heusden HA, Bode PJ, van Vugt AB. Dislocated intra-articular fracture of the anterior rim of glenoid treated by open reduction and internal fixation. Injury 1993;24:130.
10. Owens BD, Goss TP. Surgical approaches for glenoid fractures. Tech Shoulder Elbow Surg 2004;5:103–115.
11. Schandelmaier P, Blauth M, Schneider C, Krethek C. Fractures of the glenoid treated by operation. A 5- to 23-year follow-up of 22 cases. J Bone Joint Surg Br 2002;84B:173–177.
12. Sinha J, Miller AJ. Fixation of fractures of the glenoid rim. Injury 1992;23:418.

Chapter 24

Glenohumeral Arthrodesis

Brent B. Wiesel and Robin R. Richards

DEFINITION

▪ Despite significant advances in shoulder arthroplasty and other reconstructive procedures, glenohumeral arthrodesis remains an important treatment option in appropriately selected patients.

▪ The goal of glenohumeral arthrodesis is to provide a stable base for the upper extremity to optimize elbow and hand function.

▪ Given the tremendous normal range of motion of the glenohumeral joint and the relatively small amount of surface area available for fusion, particularly on the scapular side, successful arthrodesis is technically demanding and requires meticulous surgical technique.

ANATOMY

▪ The surface area of the glenoid is too small to allow for predictable fusion. Therefore, to increase the area available for fusion, the glenohumeral articular surface and the articulation between the humeral head and undersurface of the acromion are decorticated (**FIG 1**).

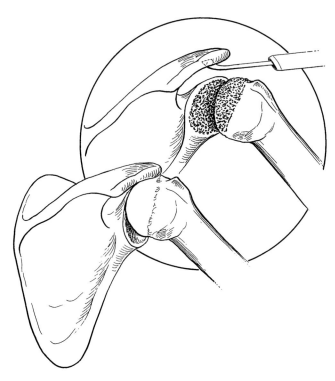

FIG 1 • The glenohumeral joint and the articulation between the humeral head and acromion are decorticated to increase the area available for fusion. (From Iannotti JP, Williams GR, eds. Disorders of the Shoulder: Diagnosis and Management, ed 2. Philadelphia: Lippincott Williams & Wilkins, 2007:684.)

▪ The bone of the scapula is extremely thin, with only the glenoid fossa and base of the coracoid providing sufficient strength for fixation.

▪ The optimal position for glenohumeral arthrodesis has been controversial.[1,4]

▪ We use a position of 30 degrees of abduction, 30 degrees of forward flexion, and 30 degrees of internal rotation.

▪ This position brings the hand to the midline anteriorly, allowing the patient to reach his or her mouth with elbow flexion.

PATIENT HISTORY AND PHYSICAL FINDINGS

▪ The history and physical findings are specific to the underlying condition requiring arthrodesis.

▪ All patients will exhibit symptomatic dysfunction at the glenohumeral joint that prevents them from effectively using the involved extremity.

IMAGING AND OTHER DIAGNOSTIC STUDIES

▪ Standard radiographs, including an anteroposterior, lateral, and axillary view, are used to assess any deformities as well as the bone stock available for fusion.

▪ If there is concern regarding bone loss on the glenoid side, especially in the setting of failed arthroplasty, this is better evaluated with a CT scan.

▪ When the neurologic condition of the shoulder girdle muscles is unclear, an electromyelogram of the scapular muscles is indicated.

SURGICAL MANAGEMENT

Indications

▪ The presence of a flail shoulder is an indication for glenohumeral arthrodesis.

▪ Paralysis in patients with a flail shoulder can be the result of anterior poliomyelitis, severe proximal root or irreparable upper trunk brachial plexus lesions, or isolated axillary nerve paralysis.

▪ Many patients with flail shoulders develop a painful inferior subluxation that responds well to arthrodesis.

▪ The need for fusion following isolated axillary nerve injury depends on the level of impairment. Many patients, especially those with partial paralysis, have reasonable function; however, complete injury often leads to significant limitation of shoulder function.

▪ Glenohumeral arthrodesis is useful following en bloc resection of periarticular malignant tumors requiring resection of the deltoid, rotator cuff, or both.

▪ Fusion is useful for the treatment of joint destruction following septic arthritis of the shoulder, particularly in young patients.

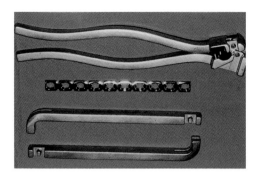

FIG 2 • Handheld bending irons and a plate press are needed to contour the 4.5-mm pelvic reconstruction plate. (From Iannotti JP, Williams GR, eds. Disorders of the Shoulder: Diagnosis and Management, ed 2. Philadelphia: Lippincott Williams & Wilkins, 2007:684.)

▪ Arthrodesis is a salvage option for patients with multiple failed total shoulder arthroplasties who have insufficient bone stock or soft tissue for revision arthroplasty.
▪ Symptomatic, uncontrolled shoulder instability that is recalcitrant to soft tissue or bony reconstructive procedures can be managed with fusion.
▪ Rarely, arthrodesis is indicated in young laborers with severe osteoarthritis who are poor candidates for arthroplasty because of their young age and high activity levels.

Contraindications

▪ The primary contraindication to glenohumeral arthrodesis is weakness or paralysis of the periscapular muscles, especially the trapezius, levator scapula, and serratus anterior.
  ▪ Progressive neurologic disorders that are likely to lead to paralysis of these muscles also are a contraindication.
▪ Arthrodesis of the opposite shoulder is a contraindication to fusion.
▪ Shoulder fusion requires a significant effort by the patient to rehabilitate the shoulder and is contraindicated in patients unwilling or unable to participate in such a program.

Preoperative Planning

▪ Preoperative radiographs should be evaluated for any bone defects that may require bone grafting.

▪ The surgeon should make sure that the pelvic reconstruction plate and a set of handheld bending irons are available (**FIG 2**).

Positioning

▪ The patient is placed in the beach chair position with the back of the table elevated 30 to 45 degrees.
▪ A folded sheet is placed medial to the scapula to elevate it from the table.
▪ The drapes are applied as medial as possible, allowing access to the scapula and the anterior chest wall. The arm is draped free (**FIG 3**).
▪ We do not routinely use intraoperative fluoroscopy; however, early in their experience with this procedure, surgeons may find fluoroscopy useful to confirm the position of the hardware.

Approach

▪ We perform glenohumeral arthrodesis using a 10-hole, 4.5-mm pelvic reconstruction plate.
▪ Compression across the glenohumeral articular surface is achieved by placing the initial screws from the plate through the proximal humerus and into the glenoid fossa.
▪ The plate is then anchored to the spine of the scapula by a screw directed into the base of the coracoid.

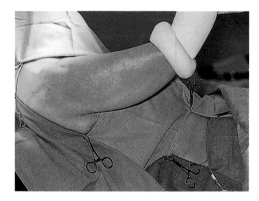

FIG 3 • The drapes are applied, taking care to allow sufficient access to the scapula spine. (From Craig EV, ed. Master Techniques in Orthopaedic Surgery: The Shoulder, ed 2. Philadelphia: Lippincott Williams & Wilkins, 2007:647.)

EXPOSURE

- An S-shaped skin incision begins over the scapular spine, transverses anteriorly over the acromion, and extends down the anterolateral aspect of the arm (**TECH FIG 1A**).
- The skin and subcutaneous tissue are incised down to the fascia along the entire length of the incision.
- The spine of the scapula and acromion are exposed first by electrocautery, and then by subperiosteal dissection (**TECH FIG 1B**).
- Anteriorly, the deltopectoral arterval is developed, and the deltoid is subperiosteally elevated off the acromion,

beginning at the medial aspect of the anterior head and progressing laterally and posteriorly to the posterolateral corner of the acromion.
  - Alternatively, if the deltoid is de-innervated, as may occur following brachial plexus injury, it can be split between the anterior and lateral heads. The anterior head is then elevated medially and the lateral head laterally to provide wide exposure of the proximal humerus.
- Distally, the biceps tendon is identified and tenodesed to the upper border of the pectoralis major tendon.

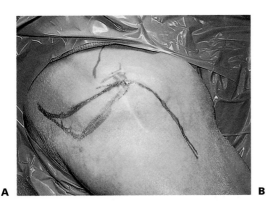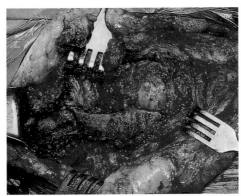

TECH FIG 1 • **A.** An S-shaped skin incision begins over the spine of the scapula. **B.** The spine of the scapula and acromion are exposed by subperiosteal dissection. (From Craig EV, ed. Master Techniques in Orthopaedic Surgery: The Shoulder, ed 2. Philadelphia: Lippincott Williams & Wilkins, 2007:647, 648.)

PERFORMING THE GLENOHUMERAL ARTHRODESIS

- The rotator cuff is resected from the proximal humerus, beginning at the inferior border of the subscapularis and proceeding superiorly and then posteriorly and inferiorly to the level of the teres minor.
- A ring or Hohmann retractor is placed on the posterior lip of the glenoid, and the humeral head is retracted posteriorly to expose the glenoid.
- The glenoid cartilage is removed using a ⅜-inch curved osteotome or burr (**TECH FIG 2A**). The glenoid labrum also is removed.
- The retractors are then removed, and the arm is extended, adducted, and externally rotated to expose the humeral head.
- A ½-inch curved osteotome or burr is used to remove the articular surface of the humerus in its entirety.
- The undersurface of the acromion is decorticated with a ¾-inch curved osteotome or burr.
- The arm is placed in 30 degrees of flexion, 30 degrees of abduction, and 30 degrees of internal rotation, and the humerus is brought proximally to appose the decorticated surface of the acromion (**TECH FIG 2B**).
  - The arm is maintained in this position by placing folded sheets between the thorax and the extremity and having an assistant stand on the opposite side of the table to support the forearm and hand.
- The 4.5-mm, 10-hole pelvic reconstruction plate is contoured to run along the spine of the scapula,

over the acromion and down the shaft of the humerus (**TECH FIG 2C**).
- The plate is bent 60 degrees between the third and fourth holes and then twisted 20 to 25 degrees just distal to the bend so it apposes the shaft of the humerus.
- With the arm supported in the appropriate position and the plate held against the scapula and humerus, a hole is drilled through the plate, through the humerus, and into the glenoid using a 3.2-mm drill bit.
- The screw length is measured; usually it is between 65 and 75 mm.
- The humeral cortex is tapped with a 6.5-mm tap.
- A short-thread 6.5-mm cancellous screw is inserted as a lag screw into the glenoid.
- Depending on glenoid bone stock, one or two more screws are placed in a similar manner.
- The plate is then anchored to the scapula by placing one or two fully threaded cancellous screws from the plate through the spine of the scapula and into the base of the coracoid.
- Another cancellous screw is placed across the acromiohumeral fusion site.
- Distally, the remaining holes are filled with cortical screws (**TECH FIG 2D**).
- The wound is closed in standard fashion over two ⅛-inch suction drains. Care is taken to reattach the deltoid to the acromion in an effort to cover as much of the plate as possible.

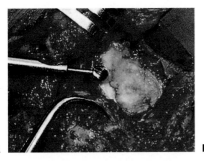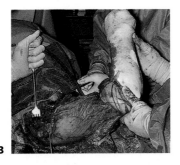

TECH FIG 2 • **A.** The glenoid articular surface is removed using a burr or 3/8-inch curved osteotome. **B.** The arm is placed in the arthrodesis position: 30 degrees of flexion, 30 degrees of abduction, and 30 degrees of internal rotation. This position allows the patient to reach his or her mouth with elbow flexion. *(continued)*

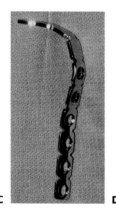
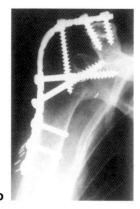

C **D**

TECH FIG 2 • *(continued)* **C.** The 10-hole, 4.5-mm pelvic reconstruction plate is bent 60 degrees between the third and fourth holes and then twisted 20 to 25 degrees in the sagittal plane. **D.** AP radiograph following glenohumeral arthrodesis with a 10-hole, 4.5-mm pelvic reconstruction plate. The two 6.5-mm partially threaded screws are placed first to achieve compression at the glenohumeral joint. (**A,B:** From Craig EV, ed. Master Techniques in Orthopaedic Surgery: The Shoulder, ed 2. Philadelphia: Lippincott Williams & Wilkins, 2007:648, 649. **C,D:** From Iannotti JP, Williams GR, eds. Disorders of the Shoulder: Diagnosis and Management, ed 2. Philadelphia: Lippincott Williams & Wilkins, 2007:683, 685.)

BONE GRAFTING

- We do not routinely use bone graft when performing glenohumeral arthrodesis.
- Bone grafting is indicated to fill large defects in patients who are undergoing arthrodesis for complex and revision problems as well as following tumor resection.
- Nonstructural autogenous bone graft can be obtained from the ipsilateral iliac crest and is combined with revision of the internal fixation for the treatment of nonunited fusions.
- Tricortical iliac crest graft can be placed between the humerus and glenoid when structural bone graft is needed (**TECH FIG 3A**).
  - This type of graft commonly is needed to treat bone deficiency following failed shoulder arthroplasty.
  - The graft is placed underneath the plate so that the compression screws pass first through the plate and any remaining proximal humerus and then through the graft and into the glenoid.
- When an intercalary defect larger than 6 cm is present, the surgeon should consider a vascularized fibular bone graft (**TECH FIG 3B**).
  - The vascularized graft should be fixed at each end with minimal internal fixation.
  - The entire defect is then spanned with a very long plate.
  - The vascular anastomosis is performed between the peroneal artery and its vena comitantes and a branch of either the axillary or brachial artery.
  - Nonstructural autogenous graft is placed at each end of the vascularized graft to maximize the likelihood of fusion occurring.

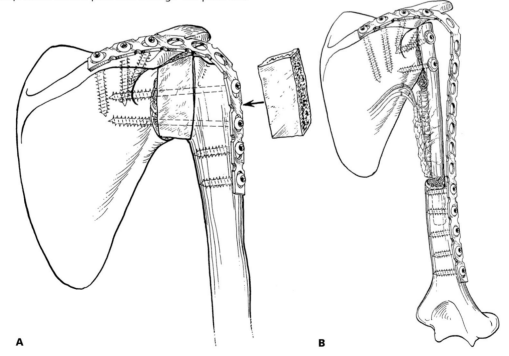

A **B**

TECH FIG 3 • **A.** Tricortical bone graft can be placed between the humerus and glenoid when there is proximal humeral deficiency. **B.** Vascularized graft is used for defects greater than 6 cm. (From Iannotti JP, Williams GR, eds. Disorders of the Shoulder: Diagnosis and Management, ed 2. Philadelphia: Lippincott Williams & Wilkins, 2007:689.)

PEARLS AND PITFALLS

Preoperative counseling	■ The concept of shoulder arthrodesis is difficult for most patients to understand. The most practical way to help them understand is to have them speak with a patient who has undergone the procedure.
Position of fusion	■ It is important not to place the arm in excessive abduction, because this can lead to increased periscapular pain when the patient rests the arm at the side. ■ Excessive internal rotation can prevent the patient from reaching his or her mouth or pocket.
Increasing fusion rates	■ When positioning the arm for arthrodesis, it is important to move the humerus proximal to maximize contact between the undersurface of the acromion and proximal humerus, thereby increasing the surface area available for fusion. ■ Partially-threaded screws are placed from the plate, through the humerus, and into the glenoid using lag screw technique to increase compression at the glenohumeral joint.
Prominent hardware	■ The acromion can be notched laterally to decrease any prominence of the hardware in this area. ■ Even in the presence of extensive deltoid atrophy, the muscle fibers help to protect the hardware, so it is important to reattach the deltoid to the acromion and cover as much of the plate as possible. ■ If the hardware is removed, the patient should be informed that there is an initial risk of humeral fracture because of the increase in stress on the screw holes.

POSTOPERATIVE CARE

■ In the operating room, after the procedure, a pillow is placed between the patient's arm and chest, and the arm is then wrapped to the chest with a swathe.

■ A radiograph is obtained in the recovery room to verify position of the internal fixation.

■ A thermoplastic orthosis is applied on the day after surgery and adjusted as needed.

■ Patients usually are discharged from the hospital on the second postoperative day and maintained in the orthosis for 6 weeks.

■ If, at 6 weeks, there are no radiographic signs of loosening of the hardware, the patient may progress to a sling.

■ Another radiograph is obtained at 3 months. If there are no signs of loosening, thoracoscapular strengthening and mobilization exercises are initiated.

■ Glenohumeral arthrodesis places significant stress on the periscapular musculature. The rehabilitation process is slow, and a recovery period of 6 to 12 months should be expected.

OUTCOMES

■ After successful arthrodesis, the patient usually can reach the mouth, opposite axilla, belt buckle, and side pocket. The patient cannot work or reach overhead, and cannot reach the back pocket or a bra strap, and perineal care often is very difficult using the fused shoulder.

■ Richards et al.[3] assessed the ability to perform specific activities of daily living in 33 patients following glenohumeral arthrodesis.

■ Patient satisfaction was highest in those patients undergoing the procedure for a brachial plexus injury, osteoarthritis, and failed total shoulder arthroplasty.

■ Cofield and Briggs[4] reported their results for glenohumeral fusion with internal fixation in 71 patients. Eighty-two percent of the patients felt that they benefited from the procedure, and 75% were able to perform activities that involved reaching their trunk.

■ Scalise and Iannotti[5] analyzed the results of arthrodesis in seven patients following failed prosthetic arthroplasty. Five of the seven patients eventually achieved fusion. Four patients required additional bone-grafting procedures in an attempt to achieve union, and two of these patients ultimately had a persistent nonunion despite the additional procedures.

COMPLICATIONS

■ Nonunion
■ Prominent hardware
■ Malposition
■ Infection
■ Humeral shaft fracture

REFERENCES

1. Barr J, Freiberg JA, Colonna PC, et al. A survey of end results on stabilization of the paralysed shoulder. Report of the Research Committee of the American Orthopaedic Association. J Bone Joint Surg 1942;24:699–707.
2. Cofield RH, Briggs BT. Glenohumeral arthrodesis. J Bone Joint Surg Am 1979;61A:668–677.
3. Richards RR, Beaton DE, Hudson AR. Shoulder arthrodesis with plate fixation: A functional outcome analysis. J Shoulder Elbow Surg 1993;2:225–239.
4. Rowe CR. Re-evaluation of the position of the arm in arthrodesis of the shoulder in the adult. J Bone Joint Surg Am 1974;56A:913–922.
5. Scalise JJ, Iannotti JP. Glenohumeral arthrodesis after failed prosthetic shoulder arthroplasty. J Bone Joint Surg Am 2008;90A:70–77.

Chapter 25

Hemiarthroplasty, Total Shoulder Arthroplasty, and Biologic Glenoid Resurfacing for Glenohumeral Arthritis With an Intact Rotator Cuff

Gerald R. Williams

DEFINITION

▪ Glenohumeral arthritis is characterized by loss of articular cartilage and varying degrees of soft tissue contracture, rotator cuff dysfunction, and bone erosion, depending on the underlying arthritic condition.

▪ The results of surgical treatment are largely dependent on the integrity of the rotator cuff; therefore, glenohumeral arthritides are often subdivided on this basis.

▪ Common arthritic and related conditions that generally involve an intact or reparable rotator cuff include osteoarthritis, posttraumatic arthritis, and avascular necrosis.

▪ Although some patients with inflammatory arthritides such as rheumatoid arthritis have intact or reparable rotator cuffs, the rotator cuff is torn or dysfunctional in many patients. When reference is made to patients with inflammatory arthritis in this section, it pertains to the subset of patients in whom the cuff is intact or reparable.

ANATOMY

▪ The pertinent surgical anatomy can be divided into bone, ligaments, muscles, and neurovascular structures.

▪ Normal osseous relationships include humeral head center, thickness, and radius of curvature, humeral neck–shaft angle, humeral head offset, glenohumeral offset, greater tuberosity-to-acromion distance, greater tuberosity-to-humeral-head distance, glenoid radius of curvature, glenoid size, glenoid version, and glenoid offset (**FIG 1**).[14,22]

▪ Humeral head radius and thickness are variable and correlate with patient size. Mean humeral head radius is about 24 mm, with a range of 19 to 28 mm. Mean humeral head thickness is about 19 mm, with a range of 15 to 24 mm.[14,22]

▪ The ratio of humeral head thickness to humeral head radius of curvature is remarkably constant at about 0.7 to 0.9, regardless of patient height or humeral shaft size.[14,22]

▪ The center of the humeral head does not coincide with the projected center of the humeral shaft. The distance between the center of the humeral head and the central axis of the intramedullary canal is defined as the humeral head offset and is about 7 to 9 mm medial and 2 to 4 mm posterior (**FIG 2**).[2,22]

▪ Humeral retroversion averages 20 to 30 degrees, with a wide range of about 20 to 55 degrees.[2,14,22] The vertical distance between the highest point of the humeral articular surface and the highest point of the greater tuberosity (ie, head to greater tuberosity height) is about 8 mm and shows a relatively small range of interspecimen variability.[14]

▪ Humeral neck–shaft angle is defined as the angle subtended by the central intramedullary axis of the humeral shaft and the base of the articular segment and shows substantial individual variation. The average neck–shaft angle is 40 to 45 degrees (130–135) degrees, with a range of 30 to 55 (120–145) degrees.[2,14,22]

▪ Pertinent musculotendinous anatomy includes the deltoid, pectoralis major, conjoined tendon of the coracobrachialis and short head of the biceps, rotator cuff, and long head of the biceps.

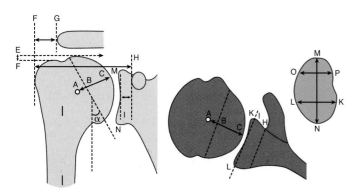

FIG 1 • The normal glenohumeral anatomical relationships. (Adapted from Iannotti JP, Gabriel JP, Schneck SL, et al. The normal glenohumeral relationships: an anatomical study of one hundred and forty shoulders. J Bone Joint Surg Am 1992;74A:491–500.)

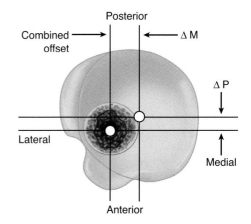

FIG 2 • The humeral head center, on average, lies 2 to 4 mm posterior and 7 to 9 mm medial to the projected center of the intramedullary canal. (Adapted from Boileau P, Walch G. The three-dimensional geometry of the proximal humerus: implications for surgical technique and prosthetic design. J Bone Joint Surg Br 1997;79B:857–865.)

■ Ligamentous structures that are potentially important in the surgical management of glenohumeral arthritis include the coracoacromial ligament and the glenohumeral capsular ligaments. In many cases of glenohumeral arthritis with an intact cuff, the anterior and inferior capsular ligaments are contracted, resulting in restriction of external rotation and posterior humeral head subluxation.

■ Neurovascular structures are abundant and subject to potential injury during shoulder arthroplasty. The axillary artery and all of its branches, especially the anterior humeral circumflex, posterior humeral circumflex, and the subscapular arteries, are particularly vulnerable.

■ The entire brachial plexus traverses the anterior aspect of the shoulder and is subject to traction and other injuries. The two most pertinent nerves are the axillary nerve and the musculocutaneous nerve.

■ The axillary nerve is a terminal branch of the posterior cord of the brachial plexus and is composed primarily of motor fibers from the fifth and sixth cervical roots. It descends the anterior surface of the subscapularis to the inferior aspect of the joint capsule, where it courses through the quadrilateral space to enter the posterior aspect of the shoulder.

■ The musculocutaneous nerve is one of the terminal branches of the lateral cord of the brachial plexus that is anterior and lateral to the axillary nerve. It typically pierces the conjoined tendon of the coracobrachialis and short head of the biceps about 5 cm distal to the tip of the coracoid. However, this course is variable and the entry point into the conjoined tendon can be as proximal as 2 cm.

PATHOGENESIS

■ The biologic basis for glenohumeral arthritis is not known. However, the loss of articular cartilage associated with primary osteoarthritis, posttraumatic arthritis, avascular necrosis, and other arthritides is, in some way, the result of imbalance in the normal cycle of cartilage damage and repair.

■ In some cases of posttraumatic arthritis, catastrophic cartilage damage associated with single-event or repetitive trauma overwhelms the shoulder's cartilage repair mechanisms and arthritis ensues.

■ Primary osteoarthritis may be associated with mechanical factors such as glenoid hypoplasia and increased retroversion. However, in many cases, no cause is evident. The final common pathway involves a release of degradative enzymes such as collagenase, gelatinase, and stromelysin, and a variety of inflammatory mediators, which further damage the cartilage and eventually the underlying bone.

■ A detailed discussion of the pathogenesis of avascular necrosis is beyond the scope of this chapter. However, the development of glenohumeral arthritis in this condition is likely the result of advanced cartilage damage following collapse of the humeral head. Involvement of glenoid articular cartilage does not occur until the later stages of the disease, when the irregular humeral head has been articulating with the previously normal glenoid surface.

■ Rheumatoid arthritis is characterized by activation of the immune system that leads to an influx of lymphocytes into the joint and synovial tissue, with subsequent release of a variety of cytokines, destructive enzymes, and mediators of inflammation such as interleukins and tumor necrosis factor. This autoimmune response is thought to be important in perpetuating joint destruction.[25]

NATURAL HISTORY

■ Glenohumeral arthritis of any type is characterized by progressive stiffness, pain, and loss of function.

■ Patients with primary osteoarthritis and many types of posttraumatic arthritis develop progressive loss of external rotation, posterior subluxation, and posterior glenoid bone loss. Large osteophyte formation, especially on the inferior humeral neck, is common. Full-thickness rotator cuff tears are distinctly uncommon and occur in 5% to 10% of patients.

■ Rheumatoid arthritis results in progressive regional osteopenia, central glenoid bone erosion, and rotator cuff tears. The prevalence of full-thickness rotator cuff tears in patients with rheumatoid arthritis of the shoulder is 25% to 40%.[27] However, rotator cuff dysfunction and substantial partial tearing are extremely common.

PATIENT HISTORY AND PHYSICAL FINDINGS

■ Patients with glenohumeral arthritis will give a history of chronic (years) shoulder pain and restricted motion, often with a recent (months) exacerbation. Posttraumatic arthritis is typically associated with a history of prior injury, such as fracture or dislocation, or surgery.

■ Pain is often worse with activity and usually interferes with sleep. Neck pain, distal radiation below the elbow, and numbness and paresthesias in the fingers and hand are uncommon and should suggest other potential causes of shoulder pain, such as cervical stenosis or cervical radiculopathy.

■ Bilateral involvement is common in primary osteoarthritis. Contralateral symptoms are often present, but to a lesser extent.

■ Physical findings in patients with glenohumeral arthritis and an intact rotator cuff include:
  ■ Posterior joint line tenderness, especially in osteoarthritis associated with posterior subluxation[20]
  ■ Generalized atrophy or flattening of the shoulder from long-term lack of function
  ■ Posterior prominence of the humeral head in cases of posterior subluxation
  ■ Symmetrical loss of active and passive range of motion (**FIG 3**)
  ■ Disproportionate loss of external rotation in comparison to other motions, especially in osteoarthritis or after capsulorrhaphy arthropathy[20]
  ■ Increased pain with passive stretch of the capsule at the end range of motion, especially external rotation
  ■ Intact neurologic function, except in rare patients with prior neurologic injury from trauma or surgery

IMAGING AND OTHER DIAGNOSTIC STUDIES

■ Glenohumeral arthritis is a radiographic diagnosis. Routine radiographs should include anteroposterior (AP) views in internal and external rotation and an axillary view.

■ Radiographic findings in primary osteoarthritis include subchondral sclerosis and cyst formation, osteophyte formation, and asymmetrical posterior joint space narrowing (**FIG 4A,B**).[20]

■ In cases of posttraumatic arthritis, radiographs may reveal retained hardware.

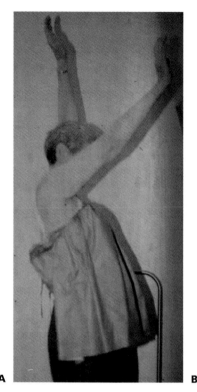

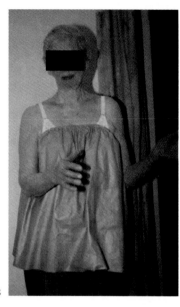

A   **B**

FIG 3 • The hallmark of glenohumeral osteoarthritis is symmetrical loss of both active and passive range of motion (**A**), especially external rotation (**B**).

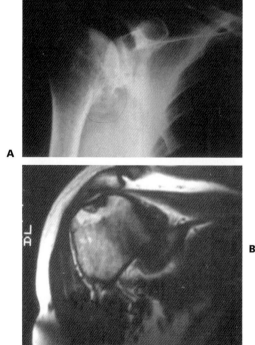

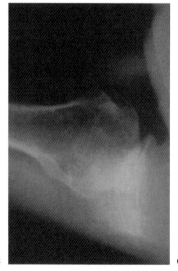

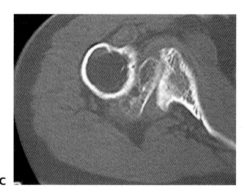

A

D

B   **C**

FIG 4 • Radiographic findings in osteoarthritis include osteophyte formation, especially on the inferior humerus as seen on the AP view (**A**), and asymmetrical posterior glenoid wear with posterior subluxation, as seen on the axillary view (**B**). **C.** CT scan reveals a large inferior humeral osteophyte and a type C glenoid, with increased glenoid retroversion. **D.** Coronal MR image in a patient with rheumatoid arthritis reveals an intact but very thin rotator cuff with erosion of the humeral attachment site, and evidence of rotator cuff dysfunction (ie, proximal humeral migration).

- Glenoid deformity in osteoarthritis has been classified by Walch[29] according to the presence of posterior subluxation and posterior bone deformity:
  - Type A: centered
  - Type B: posteriorly subluxated (B1) and posteriorly subluxated with posterior erosion (B2)
  - Type C: posteriorly subluxated with increased retroversion (hypoplasia)
- Computed tomographic (CT) scans are helpful in quantifying bone loss in patients with posterior subluxation (**FIG 4C**).
- MRI is useful in patients with rheumatoid arthritis to determine rotator cuff integrity (**FIG 4D**).
- Electromyography may be used in patients suspected of having posttraumatic or postsurgical nerve injuries.
- Medical consultation is warranted in patients with substantial comorbidities.

DIFFERENTIAL DIAGNOSIS

- Frozen shoulder
- Posttraumatic or postsurgical infection
- Cervical stenosis
- Cervical radiculopathy
- Neoplasm

NONOPERATIVE MANAGEMENT

- Avoiding activities that are painful or place an undue strain on the shoulder, such as weight lifting, is important.
- Nonsteroidal anti-inflammatory medications may be helpful in reducing pain and inflammation.
- In patients with rheumatoid arthritis, rheumatologic consultation for maximizing medical treatment is helpful.
- Glucosamine chondroitin and other nutritional supplements may reduce the pain associated with arthritis, despite the relative lack of standardized data.
- Intra-articular corticosteroid injections are almost always helpful, but the relief is often only temporary.
- Hyaluronic acid derivatives are not yet approved by the U.S. Food and Drug Administration for use in the shoulder but may be of benefit in the future.
- Therapeutic exercises should be used judiciously. Stretching to maintain flexibility may be helpful, but vigorous exercises may increase pain.

SURGICAL MANAGEMENT

- Surgical options are considered when pain and dysfunction justify surgical intervention, nonoperative management has failed, medical comorbidities do not preclude surgery, and the patient is willing to accept the risks of surgery and the responsibility of postoperative rehabilitation and activity limitations.
- Nonprosthetic options such as arthroscopic or open débridement are indicated in patients who are too young and active for any type of prosthetic replacement.
- Prosthetic options include hemiarthroplasty, hemiarthroplasty plus biologic resurfacing, and total shoulder replacement.
- Total shoulder replacement with a polyethylene glenoid component provides the most predictable pain relief but has the disadvantage of progressive polyethylene wear and eventual component loosening.[26]
- Hemiarthroplasty can be successful in providing pain relief, especially with minimal glenoid involvement or concentric

glenoid wear. However, progressive glenoid erosion is likely and may require revision to total shoulder replacement.
- Hemiarthroplasty with resurfacing of the glenoid with biologic materials such as meniscal allograft, capsular or fascia lata autograft, fascia lata allograft, dermal allograft, Achilles tendon allograft, or xenograft materials has been performed, particularly in patients too young or active for a polyethylene glenoid component.[3,21,30]
- The additional benefit of biologic resurfacing of the glenoid over hemiarthroplasty alone has not been clearly demonstrated, nor has its durability been confirmed.[10]
- Hemiarthroplasty may be accomplished by replacement or resurfacing of the humeral head.
- Replacement of the humeral head is most commonly accomplished with a prosthetic head that is anchored to the shaft with a stem. However, more recently, humeral head replacements have been developed that are fixed to the metaphysis without violation of the diaphyseal canal.
- The relative indications for hemiarthroplasty, hemiarthroplasty with biologic resurfacing, and total shoulder arthroplasty are controversial, vary among surgeons, and must be individualized according to patient age, activity level, and bone deformity, among other factors.
- Similarly, the type of implant can be individualized according to patient factors and surgeon preference.
- Concentricity of the joint, without subluxation, likely improves prosthetic performance in all circumstances. Therefore, fixed subluxation should be corrected when possible. Options include contracture release and correction of bone deformity with some combination of asymmetric reaming, bone grafting, and specialized components.
- General principles that summarize procedural and implant indications in patients with glenohumeral arthritis and an intact or reparable cuff include the following:
  - Total shoulder arthroplasty is preferred with adequate glenoid bone, age greater than 50, and sedentary or moderate activity levels.
  - Hemiarthroplasty is favored in patients with normal or minimally involved glenoids, inadequate glenoid bone, age of 50 or under, and activity levels that include weight lifting or other strenuous activity.
  - Biologic resurfacing of the glenoid may be added to hemiarthroplasty but may also fail in patients who participate in heavy weight lifting or other strenuous activity.
  - When substantial reaming or resurfacing of the glenoid is planned, the procedure is facilitated by removing the humeral head rather than resurfacing it. Currently stemmed implants are most popular, but implants with metaphyseal fixation may be useful in patients with adequate bone quality.
  - Humeral resurfacing is useful when hemiarthroplasty is indicated in the absence of substantial glenoid deformity. Resurfacing preserves humeral bone and obviates the need to address humeral head–humeral canal offset.
  - These principles are merely guidelines and should be individualized.
- The following sections will cover the technical aspects of humeral resurfacing, humeral replacement, humeral replacement combined with biologic glenoid resurfacing with allograft lateral meniscus, and total shoulder arthroplasty. Glenoid bone grafting is beyond the scope of this chapter and will not be covered.

Preoperative Planning

■ Preoperative radiographs and CT scans should be reviewed to quantify humeral subluxation (especially posterior in osteoarthritis) and glenoid bone loss. This will identify the need for asymmetric glenoid reaming.

■ If the goals of asymmetric reaming are to correct glenoid deformity and to contain all fixation appendages of the glenoid component within the glenoid vault, the extent of reaming should be limited to about 5 mm or 15 degrees. If greater correction is desired, arrangements for glenoid bone grafting should be made.

■ Preoperative radiographs should be templated to gain an appreciation of the humeral head size, canal diameter, and neck–shaft angle. In patients with highly varus (115–120 degrees) or valgus (145–150 degrees) neck–shaft angles in whom cementless fixation of a stemmed implant is planned, alterations in the level of the humeral cut or the use of a prosthesis with neck–shaft angle variability will be required.

■ MRI scans should be read for substantial rotator cuff abnormalities in rheumatoid patients and others suspected of having rotator cuff tears.

■ All other relevant preoperative data should be reviewed, including consultations from medical colleagues. The presence of all surgical implants and instruments should be verified.

■ Passive range of motion should be measured intraoperatively, before positioning, to determine the need for contracture release. In particular, the degree of passive external rotation loss may dictate the method of subscapularis reflection and repair.

■ Subscapularis shortening is typically not a substantial factor in passive external rotation loss, unless the patient has had a prior subscapularis shortening or tightening procedure (eg, Putti-Platt or Magnuson-Stack) or the contracture is particularly severe (eg, external rotation of –30 degrees or more) and longstanding.

■ Methods of managing the subscapularis include intratendinous incision and anatomic repair, lesser tuberosity osteotomy and anatomic repair, lateral tendinous release with medial advancement, and Z-lengthening.

■ Recent evidence suggests that lesser tuberosity osteotomy is associated with better subscapularis function than soft tissue reflection and repair.[12,23] However, randomized comparison data are not currently available. In addition, a recent study documents good postoperative subscapularis function with tenotomy and soft tissue repair.[4]

■ My current preference for subscapularis management in primary shoulder arthroplasty is lesser tuberosity osteotomy and anatomic repair, with the following exceptions:

■ Rheumatoid arthritis with substantial erosion of the subscapularis attachment site on MRI

■ History of a subscapularis shortening or tightening procedure (eg, Putti-Platt or Magnuson-Stack procedure)

■ Passive external rotation of less than –30 degrees

■ If lesser tuberosity osteotomy is not performed, lateral detachment with medial reattachment is most often adequate. Subscapularis Z-lengthening is rarely required.

Positioning

■ Shoulder arthroplasty is performed with the patient in the semirecumbent position (**FIG 5A**). The hips should be flexed about 30 degrees to prevent the patient from sliding down the table; the knees should be flexed about 30 degrees to relax tension on the sciatic nerves; the back should be elevated 35 to 40 degrees.

■ The entire shoulder should be lateral to the edge of the table to allow adduction and extension of the arm (**FIG 5B**). This is

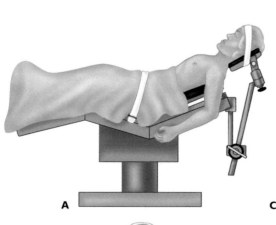
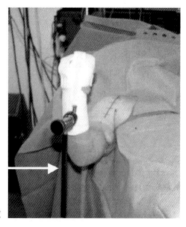
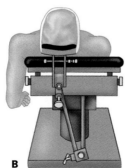

FIG 5 • **A.** Shoulder arthroplasty is carried out with the patient in the semirecumbent position; a special horseshoe-shaped headrest may improve access to the superior aspect of the shoulder. **B.** Positioning should allow unrestricted adduction and extension to allow access to the humeral shaft. **C.** A mechanical arm-holding device may be used to help position the arm throughout the procedure.

required for safe access to the humeral canal and can be accomplished by positioning the patient as far toward the operative side of the table as possible or by using a specialized table with removable cutouts behind the shoulders.

■ A specialized padded, horseshoe-shaped headrest may be helpful in facilitating access to the superior aspect of the shoulder.

■ An adjustable mechanical arm holder (McConnell Orthopedic Mfg. Co., Greenville, TX, or Tenet Medical Engineering, Inc., Calgary, Alberta, CA) is helpful for positioning the arm. Alternatively, a padded Mayo stand can also be used (**FIG 5C**).

Approach

■ The most common approach for shoulder arthroplasty is the deltopectoral approach popularized by Neer.[20] The advantages are preservation of the deltoid origin and insertion, extensibility, and excellent humeral exposure. The need for posterior deltoid retraction, especially in muscular men, can make posterior glenoid exposure difficult and can lead to injury of the cephalic vein, the deltoid itself, or the brachial plexus.

■ The superior or anterosuperior approach was popularized by MacKenzie[19] and involves access to the shoulder by reflecting the anterior deltoid from the acromion. Advantages include excellent anterior and posterior glenoid exposure and a lower incidence of axillary nerve traction injuries than the traditional deltopectoral approach. Disadvantages include nonextensibility, difficult medial and inferior humeral exposure, and potential deltoid dehiscence.

■ Modifications of these exposures include the addition of a clavicular osteotomy and extensive takedown of the deltoid origin to aid in exposure for difficult cases.[13,24]

■ The deltopectoral approach is the most commonly used approach for primary arthroplasty with an intact or reparable cuff and will be used in all subsequent sections of this chapter.

HUMERAL RESURFACING

Superficial Dissection

■ A deltopectoral incision is made from the tip of the coracoid toward the deltoid insertion.

■ The cephalic vein is taken laterally with the deltoid and the pectoralis major is taken medially.

■ The upper 1 cm of the pectoralis major may be released to improve visualization of the inferior aspect of the joint, but this is not always needed.

Deep Dissection

■ The clavipectoral fascia is incised lateral to the conjoined tendon of the short head of the biceps and coracobrachialis and is carried superiorly to the coracoacromial ligament, which does not require excision or release to attain adequate exposure.

■ Digital palpation is used to verify the position of the axillary nerve, which is protected throughout the procedure. The musculocutaneous nerve is usually not easily palpable within the surgical field but can be palpated when its entrance is close to the tip of the coracoid. This should be noted so that excessive retraction of the conjoined tendon can be avoided.

■ With the conjoined tendon retracted medially and the deltoid laterally, the arm is placed in slight external rotation to expose the anterior humeral circumflex artery and veins. These are clamped and coagulated or ligated to avoid inadvertent injury and bleeding during the case.

■ The arm is placed in slight internal rotation and the long head of the biceps is exposed from the superior border of the pectoralis major to the supraglenoid tubercle by incising its investing soft tissue envelope and the rotator interval capsule. The long head of the biceps is tenodesed to the upper border of the pectoralis major using two nonabsorbable sutures and is then released proximal to this tenodesis site and excised from the supraglenoid tubercle.

Lesser Tuberosity Osteotomy

■ A large (2 inch) curved osteotome is used to perform a lesser tuberosity osteotomy (**TECH FIG 1A**). The goal is to obtain a 0.5- to 1-cm-thick, noncomminuted fragment with which to reflect the subscapularis.

■ This is most easily accomplished by placing the blade of the osteotome at the base of the bicipital groove with one hand, palpating the most anterior extent of the tuberosity with the index finger of the other hand, and allowing an assistant to strike the osteotome while the surgeon directs it.

■ Once the osteotomy is completed, a large straight osteotome is placed in the osteotomy and is rotated about its long axis to free the osteotomy fragment from any adjacent soft tissue attachments.

■ A large Cobb elevator is then placed in the osteotomy to lever the fragment anteriorly. This further frees the fragment from the underlying capsule and allows sectioning of the superior glenohumeral ligament attachment.

■ The fragment should now be freely mobile. Three 1-mm nonabsorbable sutures are passed around the lesser tuberosity fragment through the bone–subscapularis tendon junction for traction and later reattachment (**TECH FIG 1B,C**).

■ The arm is externally rotated to expose the most inferior portion of the subscapularis muscle. This may require a right-angle retractor for the pectoralis major. The muscle belly is incised superficially, in line with its fibers, about 1 cm superior to its most inferior border.

■ A blunt elevator is used to dissect the interval between the subscapularis and the underlying capsule. Once this interval is adequately developed, a scalpel is placed between the subscapularis and capsule. With the lesser tuberosity pulled anteriorly, the scalpel is passed laterally so that is exits inferior to the fragment. This is continued from inferior to superior to release the subscapularis and

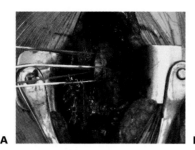

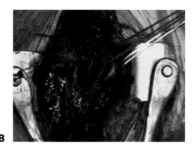

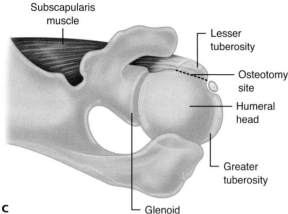

TECH FIG 1 • A. A lesser tuberosity osteotomy is performed using a large curved osteotome placed in the base of the bicipital groove and driven medially to produce a lesser tuberosity fragment about 0.5 to 1.0 cm thick. **B,C.** A lesser tuberosity osteotomy has been performed in this right shoulder. **B.** After the fragment has been mobilized from the surrounding soft tissues, three heavy nonabsorbable sutures are placed around the fragment at the bone–tendon junction. **C.** The fragment is then reflected medially and the subscapularis and the accompanying lesser tuberosity are separated from the underlying capsule and retracted medially. (**A**: Adapted from Gerber C, Pennington SD, Yian EH, et al. Lesser tuberosity osteotomy for total shoulder arthroplasty: surgical technique. J Bone Joint Surg Am 2006; 88A[Suppl 1]:170–177.)

lesser tuberosity from the underlying anterior and inferior capsule.

Capsular Release and Osteophyte Excision

- Once released, the subscapularis and attached lesser tuberosity are retracted medially to expose the anterior capsule. A blunt elevator is passed between the remaining inferior 1 cm of subscapularis and the inferior capsule to create a space for a blunt Hohmann retractor. This is used to retract and protect the axillary nerve during inferior capsular release and excision.
- The anterior capsule is released from the anatomic neck of the humerus, starting superiorly and extending inferiorly, well past the 6 o'clock position. This is facilitated by gradually flexing and externally rotating the adducted humerus.
- The humerus is then delivered into the wound with simultaneous adduction, extension, and external rotation (**TECH FIG 2A**). All humeral osteophytes are removed using a combination of rongeurs and osteotomes (**TECH FIG 2B**). This allows identification of the anatomic neck and the peripheral extent of the native articular surface.

Humeral Preparation

- Accurate placement of the central guide pin is the most important portion of the resurfacing procedure. This guide pin fixes the center and inclination of the articular surface in all planes. Once the guide pin is anatomically positioned, the remainder of the procedure is only a matter of choosing the appropriately sized head and placing it at the appropriate depth.

- The pin should penetrate the head at its geometric center and should be advanced slightly through the lateral cortex at an angle that is perpendicular to the plane defined by the periphery of the native articular margin (ie, the anatomic neck).

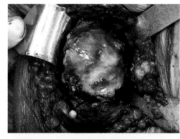

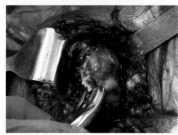

TECH FIG 2 • A. The humerus is delivered into the wound with simultaneous adduction, extension, and external rotation in this right shoulder. Retractors include a Brown deltoid retractor superiorly, a large Darrach retractor medially, and a blunt Hohmann retractor anteroinferiorly on the calcar. **B.** All humeral osteophytes are removed at this stage to identify the anatomic neck.

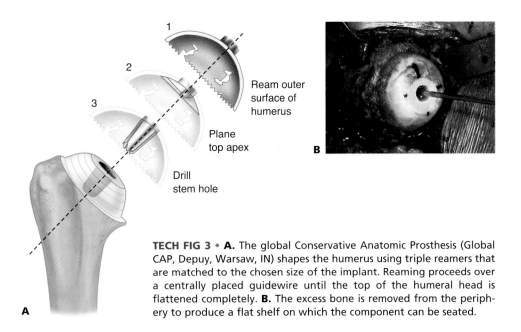

TECH FIG 3 • A. The global Conservative Anatomic Prosthesis (Global CAP, Depuy, Warsaw, IN) shapes the humerus using triple reamers that are matched to the chosen size of the implant. Reaming proceeds over a centrally placed guidewire until the top of the humeral head is flattened completely. **B.** The excess bone is removed from the periphery to produce a flat shelf on which the component can be seated.

- In some systems, there are guides that can assist in accurate pin placement. The guides usually are hemispherical and cannulated centrally so that the edge of the guide is positioned parallel to the articular margin in the visual center of the head.
- Once the surgeon is satisfied with pin placement, shaping of the humeral head to fit the deep surface of the resurfacing implant can commence.
- Reamers are selected based on the anticipated size of the prosthetic humeral head, which is, in turn, decided through a combination of preoperative templating and intraoperative measurements.
- Proper selection of humeral head radius and thickness (ie, neck length) is critical and there is a tendency to choose a head that is too large.
- The appropriate reamer is selected and the humerus is reamed until the reamer bottoms out on the humerus (**TECH FIG 3**). There is a tendency to underream. Reaming can continue to within 2 to 3 mm of the rotator cuff reflection superiorly.
- Trial implants are placed over the guide pin onto the reamed humeral surface. Circumferential contact is verified.
- The central punch is placed over the guide pin and driven into the humeral metaphysis to prepare it for the central peg of the prosthetic head.

Glenoid Inspection, Capsular Excision, and Release

- The guide pin is removed and the glenoid is exposed by placing a humeral head retractor within the joint and retracting the humeral head posteriorly. Care should be taken not to damage the reamed surface of the humerus.
- The axillary nerve is protected and the anteroinferior capsule is excised. If the labrum is present, it is left in place. The posterior capsule is released.

- Substantial glenoid reaming should not be required, as these patients are treated with humeral head resection and a stemmed implant in my practice.

Humeral Component Placement and Lesser Tuberosity Repair

- The humerus is redelivered into the wound and the appropriate humeral resurfacing implant is placed and impacted into position (**TECH FIG 4**). Care should be taken to ensure that the implant is completely seated. This requires removal of excess bone from around the periphery of the projected seating point of the implant.
- Two small bone anchors are placed in the humerus medial to the osteotomy but lateral to the humeral prosthetic edge. The sutures on the anchors are passed in a mattress configuration through the subscapularis tendon from deep to superficial at the bone–tendon junction. The sutures are clamped but not tied yet.
- With the humerus reduced and the arm in neutral rotation, the deep limbs of the three sutures previously passed around the lesser tuberosity are passed through the cancellous bone of the osteotomy bed as far laterally

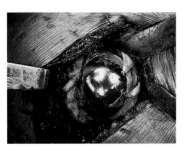

TECH FIG 4 • The final implant is impacted onto the prepared humeral surface and complete seating is verified by visualizing the periphery of the implant sitting flush against the peripheral shelf created on the humerus by the reaming process.

as possible, deep to the bicipital groove and out the lateral cortex of the humerus using a large, cutting free needle. A new needle is used for each pass and the sutures are clamped but not tied.

- The clamps on these three sutures are pulled laterally to hold the lesser tuberosity in a reduced position. The rotator interval is then closed laterally with a 1-mm nonabsorbable suture.
- After the rotator interval suture is tied, the three interfragmentary sutures are tied, followed by the sutures from the anchors. This provides a secure lesser tuberosity and subscapularis repair.

- Passive motion achievable without undue tension on the subscapularis repair is noted for guidance of postoperative rehabilitation.

Wound Closure

- A drain is placed deep to the deltoid and is brought out through a separate stab wound, distal to the axillary nerve.
- The wound is closed in layers with interrupted absorbable sutures in the subcutaneous tissues and a running subcuticular monofilament suture.

HEMIARTHROPLASTY

- Hemiarthroplasty with head resection is performed when concentric glenoid reaming is required.
- The techniques of superficial and deep dissection, lesser tuberosity osteotomy, capsular release, and osteophyte excision are the same as described previously.

Humeral Head Resection

- The humeral head is removed with a saw at or near the anatomic neck (**TECH FIG 5A**). This can be accomplished freehand or with intramedullary or extramedullary guides.
- Retroversion of the cut in my practice is prescribed by the plane of the periphery of the native articular surface (ie, native retroversion). A small amount of bone (2 to 3 mm) can be left medial to the supraspinatus insertion (**TECH FIG 5B**).

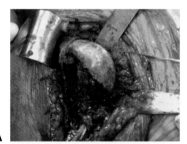
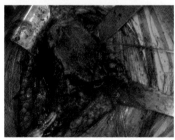

TECH FIG 5 • A. After removal of all osteophytes, the location of the anatomic neck is marked with an electrocautery. This can be done freehand or using an external guide. **B.** The humerus is cut in native retroversion, leaving 2 to 3 mm of bone medial to the supraspinatus insertion.

- The neck–shaft angle of the humeral cut is determined by the type of implant used.
- With fixed neck–shaft angle devices, the cut should precisely fit the neck–shaft angle of the selected device.
- With variable neck–shaft angle implants there is more flexibility in osteotomy angle, especially if the variability of the implant neck–shaft angle is infinite within a range.
- Preoperative templating should identify the patient with an extreme varus (less than 125) or valgus (greater than 145 degrees) neck–shaft angle.
- In cases of extreme varus, use of a fixed-angle cementless stem will require a humeral cut that is more valgus than the native neck–shaft angle.
  - The cut exits superiorly 2 to 3 mm medial to the cuff reflection and inferiorly through the native head. This will leave a small portion of the native head in place, even after the inferior osteophyte is removed.
- In cases of extreme valgus, use of a fixed-angle cementless stem will require a humeral cut that is more varus than the native neck–shaft angle.
  - The cut exits inferiorly at the native articular margin and superiorly through the native head. This will leave a small portion of the native head medial to the cuff reflection.
- Alternatively, the cut can be made along the native neck–shaft angle and a variable neck–shaft angle device can be used to fit the native neck–shaft angle.
- The size of the humeral head is estimated by placing trial humeral heads on the cut surface of the osteotomy.

Glenoid Exposure, Capsular Excision, and Surface Preparation

- With the humeral head resected, a Fukuda ring retractor is placed within the joint and the humerus is retracted posteriorly.
- A reverse, double-pronged Bankart retractor is placed on the scapular neck anteriorly, between the anterior capsule and the subscapularis.
- A blunt Hohmann retractor is placed along the anteroinferior portion of the scapular neck to retract and protect the axillary nerve, and the anterior and inferior capsule is excised.

- The posterior capsule is released unless preoperative posterior humeral subluxation of greater than 25% was present, in which case the posterior capsule is preserved.
- The labrum is excised circumferentially to expose the entire periphery of the glenoid. If greater than 25% posterior humeral subluxation was present preoperatively, care is taken to preserve the posterior capsular attachment to the glenoid.
- The glenoid is sized with a sizing disk. The previously estimated humeral head size may give some idea of the glenoid size.
- The center of the glenoid is marked and a centering drill hole for the glenoid reamer is drilled.
- The orientation of this drill hole should be perpendicular to the estimated reamed surface. This can be estimated using preoperative CT measurements of the amount of posterior glenoid bone loss.
- The glenoid is reamed until a concentric surface is obtained.

Humeral Preparation and Component Placement

- The humerus is redelivered into the wound and the humeral canal is reamed with sequentially larger reamers until light purchase is obtained within the intramedullary canal.
- A box osteotome that corresponds to the final reamer size is passed into the humerus to cut the footprint of the humeral implant.
- A broach that corresponds to the size of the box osteotome and final canal reamer is placed to the appropriate depth.
- The system I use allows either a fixed 135-degree neck–shaft angle or an infinitely variable neck–shaft angle within 120 to 150 degrees (Global AP, Depuy, Warsaw, IN).
- Therefore, a collar is screwed into the broach that creates a 135-degree neck–shaft angle. A calcar reamer is placed over the collar and, if the reamer is nearly parallel to the osteotomy surface, it is used to plane the surface to 135 degrees so that an implant with a fixed neck–shaft angle of 135 degrees can be used.
- A trial humeral head is placed over the collar, it is rotated into the offset position that provides the most symmetrical coverage of the humeral metaphysis, and the collar is locked to the broach.
- If the planes of the calcar reamer and the osteotomy surface are not nearly parallel, a variable neck–shaft angle implant will be used. The 135-degree collar is removed and a trial ball taper fitted with a humeral head trial is inserted into the broach. The trial head and ball taper are placed into the position that provides symmetrical coverage of the humeral metaphysis, and the taper is locked to the broach.
- With the trial humeral head locked into position, the remaining humeral osteophytes are removed so that the humeral bone is flush with the humerus around the entire periphery.
- Assuming the humerus has been reduced and adequate soft tissue tension and stability have been verified, the

trial broach is removed and the real implant is assembled with either a fixed 135-degree taper or a variable ball taper in the same position as the trial.
- A nonabsorbable suture is passed around the neck of the prosthesis and the prosthesis is impacted into the humerus with the two ends of the suture protruding anteriorly.
- The humerus is then reduced.

Lesser Tuberosity Repair

- The technique for lesser tuberosity repair is the same as described for humeral resurfacing, except that the suture that was placed around the prosthetic neck before impaction into the humerus takes the place of the suture anchors that were placed in the anterior humerus between the osteotomy bed and the lateral extent of the resurfacing prosthesis (**TECH FIG 6A**).
- Therefore, the osteotomy is stabilized with three suture groups:
    - The three interfragmentary sutures from the lesser tuberosity to the osteotomy bed
    - The rotator interval closure suture at the superior aspect of the osteotomy
    - The suture from the prosthetic through the bone–tendon junction (**TECH FIG 6B**)
- The technique for wound closure is identical to that described for humeral resurfacing.

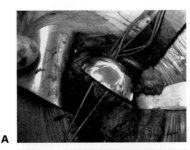
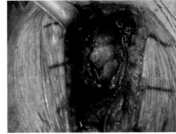

TECH FIG 6 • A. The final implant is seated and any remaining bone prominences are removed. The three interfragmentary sutures around the lesser tuberosity are visible posterior to the prosthesis. The strands from the suture that was placed around the neck of the prosthesis can be seen exiting the space between the prosthetic humeral head and the anterior humeral metaphysis. **B.** The lesser tuberosity has been repaired with a superior side-to-side suture in the lateral rotator interval, the three interfragmentary sutures tied over the bicipital groove, and the medial suture passed from the prosthetic neck through the bone–tendon junction.

HEMIARTHROPLASTY WITH BIOLOGIC RESURFACING (LATERAL MENISCAL ALLOGRAFT)

- All techniques are the same as described earlier for humeral resurfacing and hemiarthroplasty, except that placement of the allograft requires maximum glenoid exposure.
- The allograft can be grossly sized using glenoid sizing disks. It is prepared by suturing the anterior and posterior horns together.
- The glenoid surface should be concentric in order for biologic resurfacing with meniscal allograft to be successful. Therefore, reaming to correct glenoid bone deficiency (eg, posterior wear) should be performed before placing the allograft.
- If the labrum can be preserved, it can be used to anchor the allograft to the glenoid.
- Often, the labrum is absent or too degenerative to dependably hold sutures. Under these circumstances,

absorbable suture anchors are used to attach the allograft around the periphery of the glenoid. Four to six anchoring points should be used, depending on the size of the glenoid (**TECH FIG 7A**).
- The sutures are passed into the periphery of the ring-shaped allograft above the wound at appropriate positions (**TECH FIG 7B**). The allograft is then shuttled down the sutures onto the glenoid surface and the sutures are tied (**TECH FIG 7C**).[30]
- If there is no bleeding bone exposed from reaming, drilling a few holes through the subchondral surface into the glenoid cavity may assist in decompressing the glenoid vault and providing progenitor cells that can assist in healing.

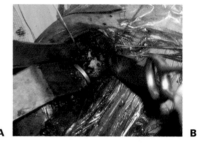
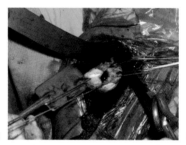
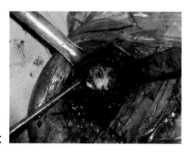

A   B   C

TECH FIG 7 • A. The glenoid in this right shoulder is exposed with a Fukuda retractor posteriorly, a large Darrach retractor anteriorly on the neck of the scapula, and a single-prong Bankart retractor posterosuperiorly. Anchors have been placed in the four quadrants of this small glenoid. **B.** The meniscal allograft has been sutured into a ring and sutures from the previously placed anchors are passed through the meniscal allograft above the joint. **C.** The allograft is then transported down the sutures onto the glenoid surface and the sutures are tied. (From Williams G. Hemiarthroplasty and biological resurfacing of the glenoid. In: Zuckerman JD, ed. Advanced Reconstruction: Shoulder. Rosemont, IL: AAOS, 2007:545–556.)

TOTAL SHOULDER ARTHROPLASTY

- All techniques are the same as described earlier for humeral resurfacing and hemiarthroplasty except for placement of the glenoid component.
- Concentric glenoid reaming is an important step in glenoid resurfacing that improves initial seating and stability. This is accomplished by drilling a pilot hole in the center of the glenoid (**TECH FIG 8A**). Special glenoid reamers are used to ream concentrically around the center pilot hole (**TECH FIG 8B**).
- After the surface of the glenoid has been reamed concentrically, the anchoring holes for the glenoid component are created. Both pegged and keeled components are available. The technique described is for an off-axis pegged system (anchor peg glenoid, Depuy, Warsaw, IN).
- The center hole for the larger fluted central peg is drilled, followed by the holes for the three peripheral

pegs (**TECH FIG 8C**). Penetration of any of the peripheral holes is uncommon but should be noted so that a bone plug from the humeral head can be placed before filling the hole with cement.
- A trial glenoid component is placed and complete seating and stability are verified.
- The holes are irrigated and dried.
- Bone cement is placed into the three peripheral holes using a syringe to pressurize the cement column. Any holes that required bone grafting from drill perforation should not receive pressurized cement.
- The glenoid component is impacted into position and can be held with digital pressure until the cement hardens (**TECH FIG 8D**).

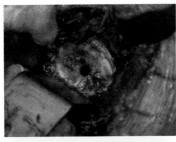
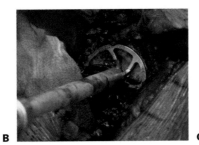
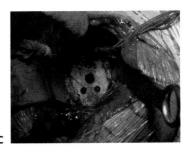
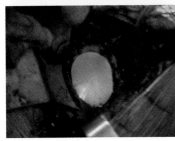

TECH FIG 8 • A center pilot hole is drilled in the glenoid surface (**A**) and a spherical reamer is used to create a concentric surface (**B**). **C.** The centering hole is enlarged and the three peripheral anchoring holes are drilled in the glenoid surface. **D.** A polyethylene glenoid component is then cemented into place.

PEARLS AND PITFALLS

Imaging	▪ Radiographic evaluation must include a quantification of glenoid version, asymmetrical wear, and available bone stock. This requires either a perfect axillary lateral or cross-sectional study, preferably a CT scan.
Patient selection	▪ Glenoid components should be used cautiously if at all in young (ie, under 50) or active patients. The use of biologic resurfacing is controversial and may not offer any advantage over hemiarthroplasty alone.
Patient positioning	▪ Safe access to the humerus during humeral preparation and component placement requires maximum humeral adduction. Therefore, patient positioning must prevent interference from the edge of the operating table.
Glenoid exposure	▪ Adequate glenoid exposure requires accurate humeral resection, humeral osteophyte excision, and adequate capsular excision and releases.
Humeral preparation	▪ Do not over-externally rotate or overream. This may lead to periprosthetic fracture.
Nerve management	▪ Know the position of the axillary nerve and protect it throughout the procedure. Avoid excessive traction on the conjoined tendon, especially if the musculocutaneous nerve is close to the tip of the coracoid. Take the arm out of extreme positions whenever possible.

POSTOPERATIVE CARE

- Early rehabilitation (6 weeks)
  - The goals of rehabilitation during the first 6 weeks after surgery are to maximize passive range of motion and to allow healing of the subscapularis or lesser tuberosity.
  - The safe range of glenohumeral motion that prevents excessive tension on the subscapularis is identified intraoperatively.
  - This range of passive motion is performed starting the first postoperative day.
  - In general, uncomplicated shoulder arthroplasty will allow passive elevation to 140 degrees and passive external rotation to 40 degrees. If there is concern for the subscapularis repair, elevation and external rotation can be dropped to 130 and 30 degrees, respectively. If the tissue is poor quality, one may even drop the limits to 90 degrees of elevation and 0 degrees of external rotation.
  - These exercises are performed for 6 weeks postoperatively, in combination with pendulum exercises.
  - The sling may be discontinued at home after the first week or 10 days, when the hand can be used as a helping hand for daily activities.
  - Active elevation above 90 degrees is delayed until 6 weeks postoperatively.
- Midterm rehabilitation (6 to 12 weeks)
  - During midterm rehabilitation, active range of motion is encouraged, passive stretching is instituted, and strengthening exercises for the rotator cuff, deltoid, and scapular stabilizers are pursued.
  - Active assisted range of motion within the limits of pain is accomplished with an overhead pulley and 3-foot stick.
  - This is progressed to active range of motion as tolerated.
  - End-range stretching in all planes is begun and progressed.
  - Strengthening exercises with the Theraband commence when active range of motion is maximized.
- Late rehabilitation (12 to 24 weeks)
  - Strengthening exercises for the rotator cuff, deltoid, and scapular stabilizers continue throughout the late stage of rehabilitation.
  - Patients will be functional with most daily activities, except at the extremes of motion.
  - Total arm strengthening and gradual return to activities are encouraged.

▪ Although improvement in function will continue for about 1 year, the vast majority of improvement from formal rehabilitation will be seen in the first 24 weeks (6 months).

OUTCOMES

▪ Resurfacing

▪ Reports of resurfacing arthroplasty are relatively sparse. Most data come out of a single institution.

▪ In general, the results parallel the results of hemiarthroplasty. In one series of 103 patients with 5 to 10 years of follow-up, constant scores for patients with osteoarthritis undergoing total shoulder arthroplasty and hemiarthroplasty were 93.7% and 73.5% respectively. Lucency around the humeral component was 30.7%, and 1.9% required revision.[17]

▪ In another series of patients with osteoarthritis undergoing resurfacing, hemiarthroplasty was found to be similar to total shoulder replacement.[16]

▪ Hemiarthroplasty

▪ Neer's original article on replacement for osteoarthritis in 1974 included primarily hemiarthroplasties. Over 90% of patients had good or excellent results.[20]

▪ The addition of concentric glenoid reaming to encourage the formation of a biologic membrane to resurface the glenoid has been reported by Matsen et al.[8,18] The authors note that similar pain relief and function are possible with this procedure but that patients may take longer than total shoulder replacement patients to reach maximum improvement. In addition, in one of their series, 3 of 37 patients were no better or worse after the surgery.[18]

▪ Additional studies have stressed the importance of concentricity of the glenoid in attaining a successful result as well as the relative difficulty in converting a painful hemiarthroplasty to total shoulder replacement.[5]

▪ In addition, progressive, painful glenoid erosion can be associated with hemiarthroplasty.

▪ Survivorship of hemiarthroplasty in one series decreased substantially with increasing follow-up, with 92%, 83%, and 73% survival at 5, 10, and 15 years, respectively.[26]

▪ Hemiarthroplasty with biologic resurfacing

▪ Although descriptions of this procedure exist before 1993, Burkhead popularized the concept of combining hemiarthroplasty with biologic glenoid resurfacing.[3]

▪ A more recent report from Krishnan et al[15] with long-term follow-up revealed only 5 of 39 patients with unsatisfactory results. Moreover, the patient population was relatively young and active.

▪ Elhassan et al[10] reported poor results in 13 patients undergoing hemiarthroplasty with biologic glenoid resurfacing. Ten of 13 patients required revision to total shoulder arthroplasty at a mean of 14 months after hemiarthroplasty.

▪ Two additional studies,[21,30] one with a minimum 2-year follow-up,[30] confirm good early pain relief and return of function in young active patients undergoing hemiarthroplasty and glenoid resurfacing with lateral meniscal allograft. Both emphasize the importance of articular concentricity and offer data that may be interpreted to question the durability of the allograft.

▪ Total shoulder arthroplasty

▪ Many studies document consistent improvement in pain and function with total shoulder arthroplasty.

▪ Several studies document better pain relief and, in some cases, better function with total shoulder arthroplasty in comparison to hemiarthroplasty. Survivorship of total shoulder arthroplasty in patients with an intact or reparable cuff is 84% to 88% at 15 years.[9,26]

COMPLICATIONS

▪ The reported complication rate after shoulder arthroplasty is 12% to 14.7%.[1,6,31] One series reports a decrease in the complication rate with time, which may be explained by glenoid and humeral component loosening in only one shoulder.[6]

▪ Complications include:

▪ Instability
▪ Rotator cuff tear
▪ Ectopic ossification
▪ Glenoid component loosening
▪ Intraoperative fracture
▪ Nerve injury
▪ Infection
▪ Humeral component loosening

REFERENCES

1. Bohsali KI, Wirth MA, Rockwood CA Jr. Complications of total shoulder arthroplasty. J Bone Joint Surg Am 2006;88A:2279–2292.
2. Boileau P, Walch G. The three-dimensional geometry of the proximal humerus: implications for surgical technique and prosthetic design. J Bone Joint Surg Br 1997;79:857–865.
3. Burkhead WZ Jr. Hemiarthroplasty with biologic resurfacing of the glenoid for glenohumeral arthritis. J Shoulder Elbow Surg 1993;2:29.
4. Caplan JL, Whitfield B, Neviaser RJ. Subscapularis function after primary tendon to tendon repair in patients after replacement arthroplasty of the shoulder. J Shoulder Elbow Surg 2009;18:193–198.
5. Carroll RM, Izquierdo R, Vazquez M, Blaine TA, et al. Conversion of painful hemiarthroplasty to total shoulder arthroplasty: long-term results. J Shoulder Elbow Surg 2004;13:599–603.
6. Chin PY, Sperling JW, Cofield RH, et al. Complications of total shoulder arthroplasty: are they fewer or different? J Shoulder Elbow Surg 2006;15:19–22.
7. Clavert P, Millett PJ, Warner JJ. Glenoid resurfacing: what are the limits to asymmetric reaming for posterior erosion? J Shoulder Elbow Surg 2007;16:843–848.
8. Clinton J, Franta AK, Lenters TR, et al. Nonprosthetic glenoid arthroplasty with humeral hemiarthroplasty and total shoulder arthroplasty yield similar self-assessed outcomes in the management of comparable patients with glenohumeral arthritis. J Shoulder Elbow Surg 2007;16:534–538.
9. Deshmukh AV, Koris M, Zurakowski D, et al. Total shoulder arthroplasty: long-term survivorship, functional outcome, and quality of life. J Shoulder Elbow Surg 2005;14:471–479.
10. Elhassan B, Ozbaydar M, Diller D, et al. Soft-tissue resurfacing of the glenoid in the treatment of glenohumeral arthritis in active patients less than fifty years old. J Bone Joint Surg Am 2009;91A:419–424.
11. Gerber C, Pennington SD, Yian EH, et al. Lesser tuberosity osteotomy for total shoulder arthroplasty: surgical technique. J Bone Joint Surg Am 2006;88A(Suppl 1 Pt 2):170–177.
12. Gerber C, Yian EH, Pfirrmann CA, et al. Subscapularis muscle function and structure after total shoulder replacement with lesser tuberosity osteotomy and repair. J Bone Joint Surg Am 2005;87A:1739–1745.
13. Gill DR, Cofield RH, Rowland C. The anteromedial approach for shoulder arthroplasty: the importance of the anterior deltoid. J Shoulder Elbow Surg 2004;13:532–537.
14. Iannotti JP, Gabriel JP, Schneck SL, et al. The normal glenohumeral relationships: an anatomical study of one hundred and forty shoulders. J Bone Joint Surg Am 1992;74A:491–500.
15. Krishnan SG, Nowinski RJ, Harrison D, et al. Humeral hemiarthroplasty with biologic resurfacing of the glenoid for glenohumeral arthritis: two to fifteen-year outcomes. J Bone Joint Surg Am 2007; 89A:727–734.

16. Levy O, Copeland SA. Cementless surface replacement arthroplasty (Copeland CSRA) for osteoarthritis of the shoulder. J Shoulder Elbow Surg 2004;13:266–271.

17. Levy O, Copeland SA. Cementless surface replacement arthroplasty of the shoulder: 5- to 10-year results with the Copeland mark-2 prosthesis. J Bone Joint Surg Br 2001;83B:213–221.

18. Lynch JR, Franta AK, Montgomery WH Jr, et al. Self-assessed outcome at two to four years after shoulder hemiarthroplasty with concentric glenoid reaming. J Bone Joint Surg Am 2007;89A: 1284–1292.

19. MacKenzie D. The antero-superior exposure for total shoulder replacement. Orthop Traumatol 1993;2:71–77.

20. Neer CS. Replacement arthroplasty for glenohumeral osteoarthritis. J Bone Joint Surg Am 1974;56A:1–13.

21. Nicholson GP, Goldstein JL, Romeo AA, et al. Lateral meniscus allograft biologic glenoid arthroplasty in total shoulder arthroplasty for young shoulders with degenerative joint disease. J Shoulder Elbow Surg 2007;16(5 Suppl):S261–S266.

22. Pearl ML, Volk AG. Coronal plane geometry of the proximal humerus relevant to prosthetic arthroplasty. J Shoulder Elbow Surg 1996;5:320–326.

23. Qureshi S, Hsiao A, Klug RA, et al. Subscapularis function after total shoulder replacement: results with lesser tuberosity osteotomy. J Shoulder Elbow Surg 2008;17:68–72.

24. Redfern TR, Wallace WA, Beddow FH. Clavicular osteotomy in shoulder arthroplasty. Int Orthop 1989;13:61–63.

25. Rodnan G, Schumacher H, Zvaifler N. Rheumatoid arthritis. In Rodnan GP, Schumacher H, Zvaifler N, eds. Primer on the Rheumatic Diseases. Atlanta: Arthritis Foundation, 1983: 38–48.

26. Sperling JW, Cofield RH, Rowland CM. Neer hemiarthroplasty and Neer total shoulder arthroplasty in patients fifty years old or less: long-term results. J Bone Joint Surg Am 1998;80: 464–473.

27. Thomas BJ, Amstutz HC, Cracchiolo A. Shoulder arthroplasty for rheumatoid arthritis. Clin Orthop Relat Res 1991;265: 125–128.

28. Torchia ME, Cofield RH, Settergren CR. Total shoulder arthroplasty with the Neer prosthesis: long-term results. J Shoulder Elbow Surg 1997;6:495–505.

29. Walch G, Badet R, Boulahia A, et al. Morphologic study of the glenoid in primary glenohumeral osteoarthritis. J Arthroplasty 1999;14(6):756–760.

30. Wirth MA. Humeral head arthroplasty and meniscal allograft resurfacing of the glenoid. J Bone Joint Surg Am 2009;91A: 1109–1119.

31. Wirth MA, Rockwood CA Jr. Complications of shoulder arthroplasty. Clin Orthop Relat Res 1994;307:47–69.

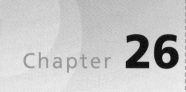

Chapter 26

Hemiarthroplasty and Total Shoulder Arthroplasty for Glenohumeral Arthritis With an Irreparable Rotator Cuff

Frederick A. Matsen III, Steven B. Lippitt, and Ryan T. Bicknell

DEFINITION

▪ *Glenohumeral arthritis* is defined as loss of the normal articular cartilage covering of the humeral head and glenoid fossa.

▪ An irreparable rotator cuff defect is one in which a durable attachment of detached cuff tendons to the tuberosity cannot be re-established.

▪ The association of glenohumeral arthritis and irreparable rotator cuff defects occurs in several distinct clinical situations, each of which has unique features and specific treatment options.

▪ The key points in managing these conditions are to define the following:
  ▪ The pathology
  ▪ The deficits in comfort and function experienced by the patient
  ▪ The options for reconstruction
  ▪ The benefits and risks of each of the treatment options

ANATOMY

▪ The glenohumeral articulation normally is covered with hyaline articular cartilage. The glenoid fossa is a spherical concavity that is deepened because the cartilage is thicker at the periphery and the glenoid rim is surrounded by a fibrocartilaginous labrum. The humeral head is a convexity that fits into this concavity.

▪ The rotator cuff is a synthesis of the tendons of the subscapularis, supraspinatus, infraspinatus, and teres minor with the subjacent glenohumeral capsule.

▪ The rotator cuff tendons insert into the humerus just lateral to the articular cartilage and at the base of the tuberosities.
  ▪ The spherical proximal humeral convexity is formed by the smooth blending of the cuff tendons with the tuberosities.
  ▪ The radius of the proximal humeral convexity is the radius of the humeral head plus the thickness of the rotator cuff tendons.

▪ The coracoacromial arch is a spherical concavity consisting of the undersurface of the acromion and the coracoacromial ligament. The proximal humeral convexity fits into this concavity.

▪ The glenohumeral joint is normally stabilized by the concavity compression mechanism:
  ▪ The rotator cuff muscles compress the humeral head into the glenoid fossa.
  ▪ The deltoid compresses the proximal humeral convexity into the coracoacromial arch.

PATHOGENESIS

▪ Loss of glenohumeral articular cartilage can be caused by osteoarthritis, rheumatoid arthritis, neurotrophic arthritis, septic arthritis, traumatic arthritis, avascular necrosis, and iatrogenic arthritis.

▪ It also can arise from abrasion of the unprotected humeral head on the undersurface of the coracoacromial arch in chronic rotator cuff deficiency, a situation that often is referred to as *rotator cuff tear arthropathy*.

▪ Defects in the rotator cuff tendons arise when loads are applied to the tendon insertion that are greater than the strength of the tendon attachment to the tuberosity.
  ▪ These defects typically begin at the anterior undersurface of the supraspinatus tendon.
  ▪ Age, systemic disease, corticosteroid injections, and smoking are among the factors that weaken the insertional strength of the rotator cuff tendons, making them more susceptible to tearing and wear.

▪ When the superior rotator cuff is deficient, the radius of the proximal humeral convexity is decreased by the thickness of the cuff tendon.

▪ The loss of the spacer effect of the cuff tendon allows the humeral head to translate superiorly under the active pull of the deltoid until the uncovered head contacts the coracoacromial arch.

▪ The intact coracoacromial arch can provide secondary superior stability to the uncovered humeral head.
  ▪ The upward translation of the humeral head necessary to contact the arch slackens the deltoid, however, reducing its effectiveness in elevation of the arm.

▪ The coracoacromial arch can be compromised by progressive abrasion with the uncovered humeral head. It also can be compromised by acromioplasty and section of the coracoacromial ligament.

▪ Compromise of the coracoacromial arch coupled with a substantial rotator cuff defect permits anterosuperior escape of the humeral head on deltoid contraction.
  ▪ This anterosuperior escape eliminates the fulcrum needed for the deltoid to elevate the arm.

▪ The inability of a functioning deltoid to elevate the arm because of slackening and lack of a fulcrum is known as *pseudoparalysis*.

NATURAL HISTORY

▪ Rotator cuff deficiency and arthritis can occur individually or together.
  ▪ In most cases of osteoarthritis, the rotator cuff is functionally intact.
  ▪ In most cases of rheumatoid arthritis, the rotator cuff may be thinned but usually is functionally intact.

▪ In rotator cuff tear arthropathy, the integrity of the cuff, the articular cartilage, and the coracoacromial arch all characteristically degenerate in a progressive manner.

- Some surgeons attempt to improve the comfort and functions of individuals with rotator cuff problems by performing an acromioplasty and coracoacromial ligament section.
  - Unless cuff function is durably restored, this sacrifice of the coracoacromial arch predisposes the shoulder to anterosuperior escape.
- The rotator cuff mechanism can be damaged in the process of humeral head resection during shoulder arthroplasty.
- Individuals who have had a shoulder arthroplasty may tear their rotator cuff in a fall or while lifting.
- When a prosthesis is used to reconstruct a complex proximal humeral fracture, the tuberosities may fail to unite, resulting in the functional equivalent of rotator cuff deficiency.

PATIENT HISTORY AND PHYSICAL FINDINGS

- Rotator cuff tendons fail by some combination of applied load and degeneration ("tear" and "wear").
  - There need be no history of a traumatic episode, especially in older individuals who give a history of progressive loss of comfort, strength, and ability to perform functions of their daily living. These are the persons whose condition may progress to cuff tear arthropathy.
  - By contrast, individuals with acute traumatic rotator cuff tears from the application of substantial load do not typically progress to cuff tear arthropathy.
- In patients with massive atraumatic cuff deficiency, it is important to seek historical evidence of factors that may weaken the cuff, such as systemic disease, cortisone injections, antimetabolic medications, and smoking.
  - Osteoarthritis often presents without a history of injury. Instead, it presents as progressive stiffness, pain, and loss of function.

- Rheumatoid arthritis of the shoulder presents in the context of this systemic condition.
- Important elements of the history are the patient's self-assessment of shoulder comfort and function (such as the simple shoulder test) and an assessment of the patient's goals for treatment.
- The integrity of the principal rotator cuff tendons is determined by the isometric strength of each of the three primary muscles in defined positions.
  - Supraspinatus integrity: weakness (ie, strength grade 3 or less) indicates a full-thickness supraspinatus tear.
  - Infraspinatus integrity: weakness (ie, strength grade 3 or less) indicates a large, full-thickness rotator cuff tear, extending into the infraspinatus.
  - Subscapularis integrity: weakness (ie, strength grade 3 or less) indicates a full-thickness subscapularis tear.
- Defects in the rotator cuff often can be palpated just anterior to the acromion while the shoulder is passively rotated.
- Chronic cuff defects usually are accompanied by atrophy of the muscles attached to the deficient tendons.
- Cuff degeneration often is associated with subacromial crepitus on passive rotation of the humerus beneath the coracoacromial arch.
- Cuff tear arthropathy often is associated with a substantial subacromial effusion.
- Superior instability is demonstrated by having the patient relax the shoulder, hanging it at the side, and then actively contracting the deltoid while the examiner notes superior translation of the humeral head until it contacts the coracoacromial arch (**FIG 1A,B**).
- Anterosuperior escape is the exaggerated form of superior instability that results when the coracoacromial arch is compromised (**FIG 1C,D**).

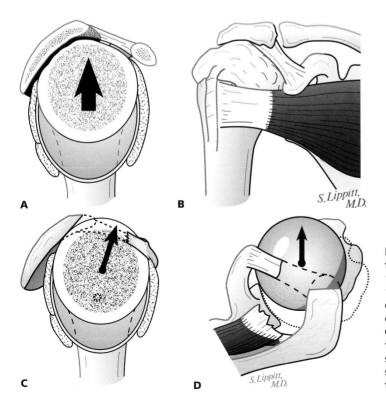

FIG 1 • **A,B.** Characteristic findings of cuff tear arthropathy, including superior displacement of the humeral head, "femoralization" of the proximal humerus, and "acetabularization" of the coracoacromial arch. In such a case, a conventional hemiarthroplasty, possibly using a special cuff tear arthropathy (CTA) head, may be considered. **C,D.** Anterosuperior escape of the humeral head resulting from surgical compromise of the coracoacromial arch. In such a case, a conventional arthroplasty will not provide stability, and a Delta (DePuy, Warsaw, IN) or reverse prosthesis may be considered. (Copyright Steven B. Lippitt, MD.)

IMAGING AND OTHER DIAGNOSTIC STUDIES

- An anteroposterior plain radiograph in the plane of the scapula may reveal:
  - Decreased acromio–humeral distance, signaling the absence of the normally interposed supraspinatus tendon
  - "Femoralization" of the proximal humerus (ie, rounding off of the tuberosities so that the proximal humerus is spherical) as well as other changes in humeral anatomy (**FIG 2A,B**)
  - "Acetabularization" of the acromion-coracoid-glenoid socket (ie, sculpting of a concavity matching the femoralized proximal humerus)
  - The amount of superior and medial erosion of the acromion and upper glenoid
- A true axillary view (**FIG 2C,D**) may reveal:
  - The degree of medial glenoid erosion, ie, the amount of glenoid bone stock available for reconstruction
  - The presence of anterior or posterior glenoid erosion and humeral subluxation, indicating a more complex pattern of instability
- An anteroposterior (AP) view of the proximal humerus with the arm in 30 degrees of external rotation with respect to the x-ray beam may reveal:
  - The approximate size of the humeral medullary cavity that may be used in prosthetic reconstruction

- Any humeral deformities that may affect prosthetic reconstruction
- We do not routinely use either CT or MRI scans, but they may be useful in clarifying the pathology.
  - CT scans may help with:
    - Defining glenoid bone volume and deformities
    - Defining the glenohumeral relationships
  - MRI scans may help with:
    - Determining the condition of the different rotator cuff tendons
    - Determining the condition of the different rotator cuff muscles
    - The volume and location of fluid in the joint
    - Other pathology, such as tumor or avascular necrosis
- Factors suggesting that the cuff defect is likely to be irreparable include:
  - Insidious, atraumatic onset of cuff deficiency
  - Advanced age of the patient
  - History of repeated corticosteroid injections
  - Systemic illness
  - History of smoking
  - Previous unsuccessful attempts at rotator cuff repair
  - Muscle atrophy
  - Superior displacement or superior instability of the glenohumeral joint
  - Anterosuperior escape
  - Pseudoparalysis

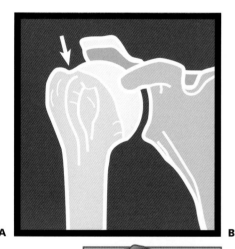
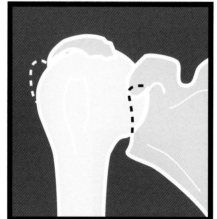
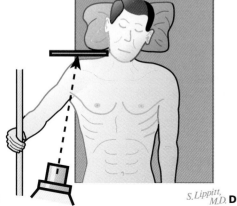
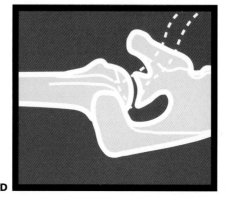

A　**B**　**C**　*S. Lippitt, M.D.* **D**

FIG 2 • **A.** Normal glenoid and normal head–glenoid relationship are seen on this AP radiograph in the plane of the scapula. **B.** Superior glenoid erosion and upward displacement of the head are seen on this AP radiograph in the plane of the scapula. This demonstrates "femoralization" of the proximal humerus and "acetabularization" of the coracoacromial arch. **C,D.** A proper axillary view will reveal anterior, posterior, or medial glenoid erosion. (Copyright Steven B. Lippitt, MD.)

DIFFERENTIAL DIAGNOSIS

- Milwaukee shoulder
- Neurotrophic (Charcot) arthropathy
- Septic arthritis
- Nonseptic inflammatory arthropathy

NONOPERATIVE MANAGEMENT

- An acute rotator cuff tear is a matter of relative urgency, but a chronic cuff defect coupled with glenohumeral arthritis provides the opportunity for nonoperative management, including:
  - Range-of-motion exercises in an attempt to resolve the stiffness that may accompany this condition (eg, the four-quadrant stretching program)
  - Gentle progressive strengthening exercises for the deltoid and the rotator cuff musculotendinous units that remain intact (eg, the two-hand progressive supine press)
- Mild nonnarcotic analgesics may be useful in symptom control.
- However, injections of corticosteroids into the shoulder may compromise the integrity of the remaining tendons and increase the risk of infection.

SURGICAL MANAGEMENT

Preoperative Planning

- Consideration of surgical management is based on the type of involvement (Table 1), the patient's overall health and well-being, and the risk–benefit ratio in trying to meet the patient's goals for treatment.
- With each of the procedures, the patient must be well-informed and give informed consent to the risk of infection, neurovascular injury, pain, stiffness, weakness, fracture, instability, loosening of components, anesthetic complications, and the possible need for revision surgery.

Conventional Hemiarthroplasty, Total Shoulder Arthroplasty, and Special Hemiarthroplasty

- Use AP radiograph in the plane of the scapula and axillary view to identify medial, superior, anterior, posterior, or inferior glenoid erosion.
- Use AP humeral radiograph to estimate the size and fit of the humeral component (**FIG 3**).
- Give prophylactic antibiotics.

Delta or Reverse Arthroplasty:

- Use AP radiograph in the plane of the scapula and transparent glenoid template to estimate the most inferior position of the glenoid that will result in the inferior screw being contained in the thick bone of the scapular axillary border.
- Use AP humeral radiograph to estimate the size and fit of the diaphyseal and metaphyseal humeral components.

Positioning

- All procedures can be performed in the beach chair position. This position is comfortable and safe for the patient, and allows good access for the anesthesiologist and the surgeon.
- The patient is positioned and secured with the glenohumeral joint at the edge of the operating table.
- The forequarter is doubly prepped, and the arm is draped so it can be moved freely.

Approach

- Although some surgeons advocate a deltoid-incising lateral approach, we prefer the deltopectoral approach, because it is effective, familiar, versatile, safe, and extensile.
- Each procedure strives to completely preserve and protect the deltoid and the axillary nerve.
- Each procedure includes a complete mobilization of the humeroscapular motion interface with resection of all scar,

Table 1	Types of Arthritis and Irreparable Rotator Cuff Defects and Their Characteristic Features						
Glenohumeral Joint Surface	**Rotator Cuff**	**Register (Glenohumeral Joint Alignment)**	**Active Elevation**	**Coracoacromial Arch**	**Anterior Superior Escape**	**Deltoid**	**Surgical Significance**
Arthritic	Irreparable supraspinatus	Glenohumeral joint aligned	>90 degrees, but weak	Intact	Absent	Intact	Consider conventional hemi- or total shoulder arthroplasty
Arthritic	Irreparable supraspinatus	Superior displacement with acromiohumeral stability	>90 degrees, but weak	Intact	Absent	Intact	Consider conventional or special (eg, CTA) hemi-arthroplasty
Arthritic	Irreparable supraspinatus and infra-spinatus	Superior displacement without acromiohumeral stability	<45 degrees	Compromised	Present	Intact	Consider Delta or reverse arthroplasty
Arthritic	Irreparable supraspinatus and infra-spinatus	Superior displacement without acromiohumeral stability	<45 degrees	Compromised	Present	Severe compromise	No good surgical options
Failed prosthetic	Irreparable supraspinatus and infra-spinatus	Superior displacement without acromiohumeral stability	<45 degrees	Compromised	Present	Intact	Consider Delta or reverse arthroplasty

CTA, cuff tear arthropathy.

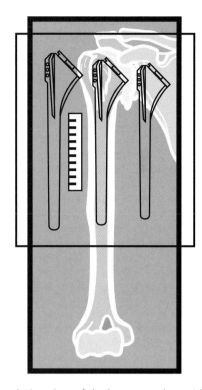

FIG 3 • Templating view of the humerus taken with the arm in 30 degrees of external rotation with respect to the x-ray beam and with a magnification marker. (Copyright Steven B. Lippitt, MD.)

suture, and suture anchors from previous surgical procedures, and hypertrophic bursa.

- This débridement permits complete assessment of the surgical anatomy.
- The integrity of the acromion and coracoacromial ligament is assessed and preserved.
- The subscapularis and subjacent capsule are incised from their attachment to the humerus at the lesser tuberosity.
- A 360-degree subscapularis release is carried out while the axillary nerve is protected.
- One of two types of reconstruction is selected:
  - Anatomic arthroplasty, with one of the following:
    - Hemiarthoplasty using a conventional prosthesis
    - Total glenohumeral arthroplasty
    - Hemiarthroplasty with a special head (eg, Delta CTA [cuff tear arthropathy; DePuy, Inc., Warsaw, IN])
  - Delta or reverse arthroplasty
- At the conclusion of the arthroplasty, the subscapularis is repaired to the bone of the cut humeral surface adjacent to the lesser tuberosity using six sutures of no. 2 nonabsorbable suture passed through drill holes.
- A suction drain is placed just anterior to the subscapularis and led out through a long subcutaneous track to exit the skin of the lateral arm.
- Dry sterile dressings are applied.
- Continuous passive motion is used for 36 hours for all reconstructions except for the Delta or reverse arthroplasty.
- After the Delta arthroplasty, the arm is immobilized for 36 hours.

<hr>

TECHNIQUES

CONVENTIONAL HEMIARTHROPLASTY, TOTAL SHOULDER ARTHROPLASTY, AND SPECIAL HEMIARTHROPLASTY

Incision and Approach

- Create a deltopectoral incision.
- Lyse adhesions and remove bursa from the humeroscapular motion interface.
- Verify irreparability of the rotator cuff tear and resect useless tendon tissue. If useful cuff elements remain, tag for later reattachment.
- Incise susbscapularis and capsule from insertion to lesser tuberosity, preserving maximal length of tendon.
- Release inferior capsule from humerus.
- Identify axillary nerve.
- Perform a 360-degree subscapularis release.

Humeral Preparation and Implant Sizing

- Insert progressively larger reamers into the canal, stopping at the first endocortical bite (**TECH FIG 1A**).
- Resect the humeral head in 30 degrees of retroversion and 45 degrees with the long axis of the shaft (**TECH FIG 1B**).
- Measure height and diameter of the curvature of the resected head (**TECH FIG 1C**).
- Mince bone of the humeral head to make autogenous graft.
- If the glenoid is rough and eroded medially, but not superiorly, and if the infraspinatus and subscapularis are intact or robustly reconstructable, and if the patient has soft glenoid bone (as in rheumatoid arthritis), consider inserting a prosthetic glenoid component.
- Using minced autogenous bone from the humeral head, perform impaction autografting of the humeral canal so that the prosthetic stem will achieve a snug press-fit (**TECH FIG 1D**).
- If a partial rotator cuff repair can be carried out, perform that before definitive sizing of component, because repair may diminish the room available for the prosthesis (**TECH FIG 1E**).
- If glenoid arthroplasty has been performed, select the humeral head prosthesis with the appropriate diameter of curvature for the glenoid.
  - If glenoid arthroplasty has not been performed, select the humeral head prosthesis with the diameter equal to that of the resected head.

Component Placement

- With the trial component in position, resect any prominent tuberosity that may abut against the coracoacromial arch on elevation of the arm (**TECH FIG 2A,B**).
- Consider a special humeral head (eg, CTA head) to cover the area of the greater tuberosity (**TECH FIG 2C**).

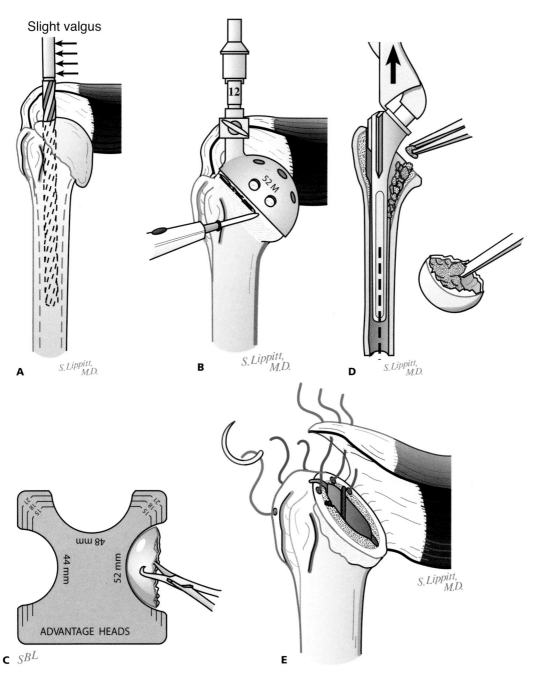

TECH FIG 1 • A. Reaming the humerus until the first endocortical bite is achieved. **B.** Marking the humeral osteotomy at 45 degrees with the reamed axis of the shaft and in 30 degrees of retroversion. Care must be taken to protect the rotator cuff in making the osteotomy. **C.** Measuring the resected head to determine the diameter of curvature and the height. **D.** Impaction grafting of the medullary canal to achieve a secure press-fit without jeopardizing the strength of the diaphyseal cortex. **E.** Partial repair of the rotator cuff to the edge of the resected humerus. (Copyright Steven B. Lippitt, MD.)

- Select the humeral head height that, on trial reduction, allows 40 degrees of external rotation with the subscapularis approximated, 50% posterior translation on the posterior drawer test, and 60 degrees of internal rotation when the arm is abducted to 90 degrees (**TECH FIG 2D–G**).
- Place six no. 2 nonabsorbable sutures in the anterior humeral neck cut for reattachment of the subscapularis (**TECH FIG 2H**).
- Assemble the definitive humeral prosthesis.
- Insert the prosthesis in the impaction-grafted medullary canal.

Final Contouring and Wound Closure

- Ensure smooth passage of the proximal humerus beneath the coracoacromial arch. If abutment occurs, perform smoothing on the humeral side, preserving the integrity of the arch.
- Repair the subscapularis.
- Insert drain.
- Close the deltopectoral interval.
- Perform subcutaneous and skin closure.
- Apply sterile dressings.

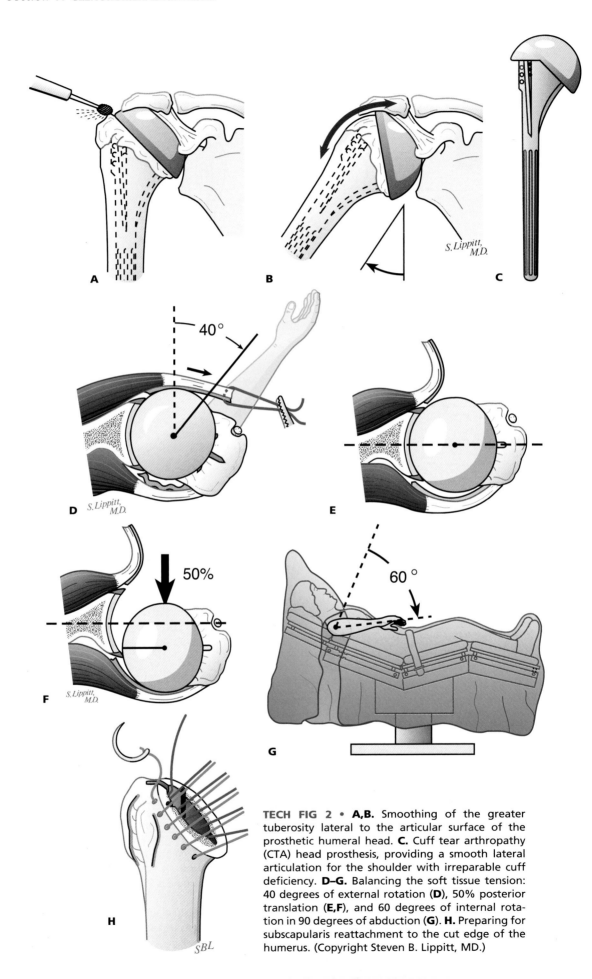

TECH FIG 2 • **A,B.** Smoothing of the greater tuberosity lateral to the articular surface of the prosthetic humeral head. **C.** Cuff tear arthropathy (CTA) head prosthesis, providing a smooth lateral articulation for the shoulder with irreparable cuff deficiency. **D–G.** Balancing the soft tissue tension: 40 degrees of external rotation (**D**), 50% posterior translation (**E,F**), and 60 degrees of internal rotation in 90 degrees of abduction (**G**). **H.** Preparing for subscapularis reattachment to the cut edge of the humerus. (Copyright Steven B. Lippitt, MD.)

DELTA OR REVERSE ARTHROPLASTY

Incision and Approach

- Make a deltopectoral incision.
- Lyse adhesions and remove bursa from the humeroscapular motion interface, protecting deltoid, acromion, and residual cuff tissue.
- Verify irreparability of the rotator cuff tear and resect useless tendon tissue.
- Tag any potentially reparable elements of the cuff that are identified, for later use.
- Incise the subscapularis and capsule from insertion to lesser tuberosity, preserving maximal length of the tendon.
- Release the inferior capsule from the humerus.
- Identify the axillary nerve.
- Perform a 360-degree subscapularis release.

Humeral Preparation

- Insert humeral resection guide stem into medullary canal (**TECH FIG 3A**).
- Resect humeral head in zero degrees of retroversion (**TECH FIG 3B**).
- When the arm is pulled distally, the plane of the humeral cut should pass just below the inferior glenoid.

Glenoid Preparation

- Dissect the capsule from the anterior glenoid down to and around the inferior pole so that the upper axillary border of the scapula can be palpated and seen, releasing the origin of the long head of the triceps as necessary.
- Check radiographs and exposed glenoid to identify abnormal glenoid anatomy (eg, superior, inferior, anterior, posterior, inferior or medial erosion, as well as defects from previous surgery [such as earlier arthroplasty]).
  - Note the relation of the inferior glenoid lip to the axillary border of the scapula.
- Remove the labrum and cartilage from the glenoid.
- Mark a point 13 mm anterior to the posterior rim of the glenoid and 19 mm superior to the inferior glenoid rim.

- Drill the guidewire into the glenoid at this point (**TECH FIG 4A**).
- Place the metaglene of the Delta prosthesis (**TECH FIG 4B**) over this guidewire, with the peg laterally, to verify the appropriateness of this center point.
  - The inferior aspect of the metaglene should align with a line extended from the axillary border of the scapula.
- When the rim of the metaglene is flush with the extrapolated axillary border, remove the metaglene and drill a central hole with the step drill (**TECH FIG 4C**).
- Ream the glenoid conservatively, removing only enough bone to make the surface relatively flat and making sure the reamer handle remains perpendicular to the face of the glenoid (**TECH FIG 4D**).

Metaglene Placement

- Insert the metaglene peg into the central hole (**TECH FIG 5A**).
- Palpate the anterior and posterior aspects of the axillary border of the scapula and rotate the metaglene so the inferior screw hole is centered over the axillary border.
  - Recall that the inferior locking screw makes a 16-degree angle with the central peg.
  - Using a drill guide, drill a hole for the inferior locking screw, checking frequently to ensure that the drill is in bone by pushing on the drill while it is not rotating.
  - Use a 2-mm drill bit unless the bone is hard (**TECH FIG 5B**).
- At least 36 mm of intraosseous drilling should be achieved.
  - If not, re-examine rotation of the metaglene with respect to the axillary border (**TECH FIG 5C**).

Screw Fixation

- Insert the inferior locking screw (**TECH FIG 6A**).
- Drill and insert the superior locking screw using similar technique (**TECH FIG 6B,C**).

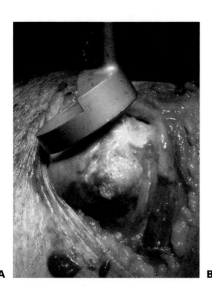
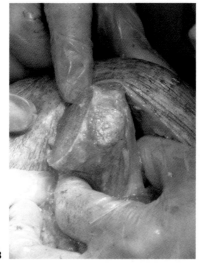

TECH FIG 3 • A. Humeral resection guide inserted for cut at 0 degree of retroversion. **B.** Resected humerus after removal of osteophytes. (Copyright Frederick A. Matsen, MD.)

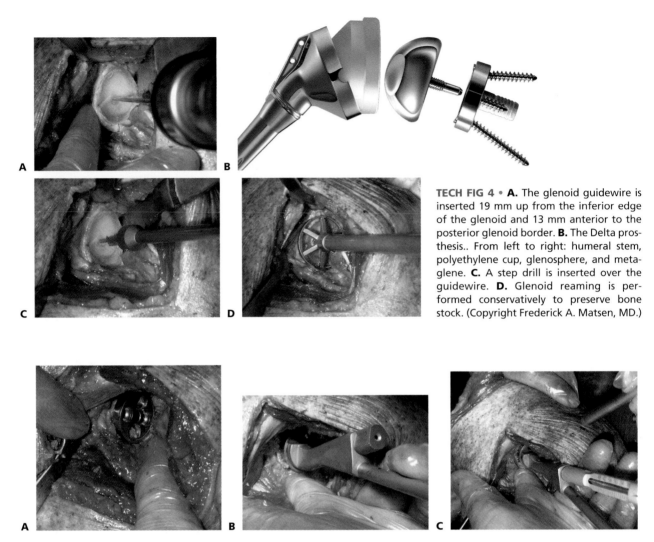

TECH FIG 4 • A. The glenoid guidewire is inserted 19 mm up from the inferior edge of the glenoid and 13 mm anterior to the posterior glenoid border. **B.** The Delta prosthesis.. From left to right: humeral stem, polyethylene cup, glenosphere, and metaglene. **C.** A step drill is inserted over the guidewire. **D.** Glenoid reaming is performed conservatively to preserve bone stock. (Copyright Frederick A. Matsen, MD.)

TECH FIG 5 • A. Inserting the metaglene, noting its flush position with the inferior glenoid. **B.** Drill guide aligned with the axillary border of the scapula. **C.** Verifying the intraosseous position of the inferior drill hole by direct palpation. (Copyright Frederick A. Matsen, MD.)

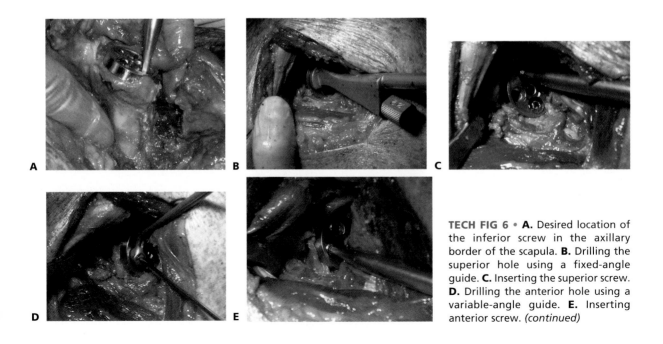

TECH FIG 6 • A. Desired location of the inferior screw in the axillary border of the scapula. **B.** Drilling the superior hole using a fixed-angle guide. **C.** Inserting the superior screw. **D.** Drilling the anterior hole using a variable-angle guide. **E.** Inserting anterior screw. *(continued)*

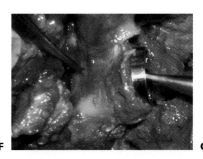

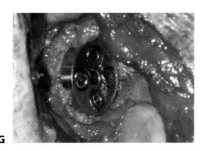

TECH FIG 6 • *(continued)* **F.** The desired position of the anterior screw exiting deep in the subscapularis fossa. **G.** Four screws in place in the metaglene. (Copyright Frederick A. Matsen, MD.)

- Drill and insert the anterior nonlocking screw, guiding orientation by palpating the anterior glenoid neck (**TECH FIG 6D–F**).
- Drill and insert the posterior nonlocking screw (**TECH FIG 6G**).
- Once screws have been placed, check the security of metaglene fixation.
- Insert a trial glenosphere onto the metaglene.
- Inspect the inferior aspect of the glenoid, removing any bone that may abut against the humeral polyethylene component.
  - Adequacy of bone resection can be verified by placing a trial polyethylene humeral component over the glenosphere and making sure it can be adducted fully, recalling that the humeral cup makes a 65-degree angle with the humeral shaft.

Humeral Preparation

- Prepare the humeral canal in a manner that preserves bone stock by insertion of progressively larger reamers until cortical contact is just achieved (**TECH FIG 7A,B**).

- Insert a trial stem with a metaphyseal reamer guide in 0 degrees of rotation (**TECH FIG 7C**).
- Ream the metaphysis until bone purchase is achieved (**TECH FIG 7D**).

Trial Placement

- Perform trial reduction of the prepared humerus (without trial components) to see if the reamed metaphysis can be reduced to the glenosphere, indicating that the humeral resection is adequate (**TECH FIG 8A**).
- Assemble and insert the trial humeral component in 0 degrees of retroversion with a 3-mm trial plastic component (**TECH FIG 8B**).
- Reduce the joint (**TECH FIG 8C,D**) and check for:
  - Medial abutment of plastic against the axillary border of the glenoid
  - Stability
  - Range of motion
  - Minimal (<2 mm) distraction on distal traction
- If the joint cannot be reduced, consider lowering the humeral component position by sequentially resecting small amounts of humeral bone.

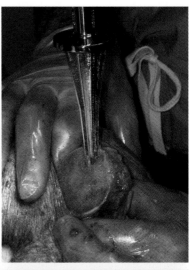

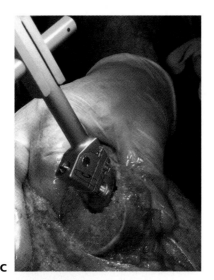

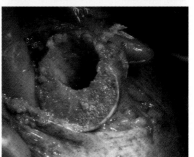

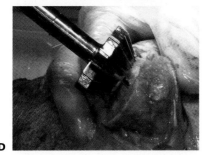

TECH FIG 7 • **A.** Medullary reaming of the humerus using a lateral starting point. **B.** Reamed medullary canal of the humerus. **C.** Inserting the metaphyseal reaming guide in 0 degrees of retroversion to the depth appropriate for the 36-mm prosthesis. **D.** Reaming the metaphysis over the metaphyseal reaming guide. (Copyright Frederick A. Matsen, MD.)

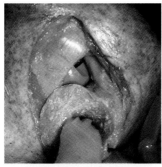
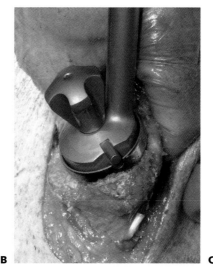
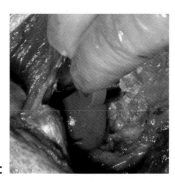
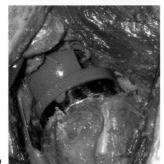

TECH FIG 8 • A. Trial reduction of the humerus. **B.** Insertion of a trial humeral component. **C,D.** Reducing the trial components. (Copyright Frederick A. Matsen, MD.)

Final Component Placement

- Insert the glenosphere into the metaglene, making sure it is aligned to avoid cross-threading and making sure it is fully seated.
- Securely assemble the definitive humeral component with a strong crescent wrench.
- Brush and irrigate the humeral medullary canal.
- Insert a cement restrictor 13 cm distal to the lateral aspect of the humeral cut.
- Place six drill holes and no. 2 nonabsorbable sutures in the anterior neck cut for later reattachment of the subscapularis.
- Repair the posterior cuff, if possible.
- Cement the assembled humeral component in 0 degrees of retroversion without a polyethylene insert.
- Trial different heights of polyethylene liners, starting with 3 mm, reducing shoulder to discover the height that allows for reduction but less than 2 mm of distraction, checking again for abutment of adducted plastic against the lateral glenoid bone inferiorly.
- Insert the definitive polyethylene component, making sure it seats fully.
- Irrigate the wound completely.
- Reduce the joint.

Wound Closure

- Repair the subscapularis to sutures previously placed at the anterior neck cut.
- Place a suction drain.
- Close the deltopectoral interval, close the subcutaneous layer, and close the skin with staples.
- Apply dry sterile dressings and an axillary pad.

PEARLS AND PITFALLS

Glenohumeral arthritis is a chronic condition, so there is no rush to surgical judgment.	▪ Try gentle range-of-motion and deltoid-strengthening exercises.
Individuals with these conditions often are elderly and frail.	▪ Perform a thorough preoperative assessment and minimize surgical risk factors before surgery.
In revision surgery, especially revision arthroplasty, be aware of indolent infection, especially with *Staphylococcus epidermidis* and *Propionibacter acnes*.	▪ Obtain multiple intraoperative cultures for these organisms and hold cultures for 2 weeks.
In "irreparable" cuff tears, the cuff often is partially reparable	▪ At surgery, seek subscapularis and infraspinatus elements that are reparable.
Tissues are fragile in these patients	▪ Treat deltoid, acromion, glenoid, and humeral bone gently.
Patients with irreparable cuff tears and arthritis are prone to effusions and postsurgical hematomas	▪ Drain the surgical site and rehabilitate slowly.

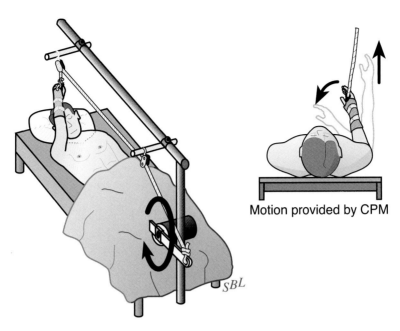

FIG 4 • Continuous passive motion. (Copyright Steven B. Lippitt, MD.)

POSTOPERATIVE CARE

▪ Hemiarthroplasty with a conventional prosthesis, total glenohumeral arthroplasty, or hemiarthroplasty with a special head (eg, CTA)
  ▪ Institute a continuous passive motion (**FIG 4**) and early active assisted motion protocol as soon as possible postoperatively (unless major partial cuff repair has been carried out).
  ▪ Elevation of the arm to 140 degrees is achieved before the patient leaves the medical center.
  ▪ For 6 weeks, external rotation is limited to what was easily achievable on the operating table.
  ▪ Gentle progressive strengthening exercises, including the supine press, usually are started at 6 weeks.
▪ Delta or reverse arthroplasty
  ▪ Institute hand-gripping and active elbow flexion postoperatively.
  ▪ Motion is withheld for 36 hours to minimize the risk of hematoma formation.
  ▪ Gentle activities, such as eating, are started at 36 hours, followed by the slow, progressive addition of other activities, reminding the patient of the need for the shoulder bones and muscles to have time to remodel to their new loading patterns.
  ▪ Avoid lifting anything heavier than 1 pound for 3 months.

OUTCOMES

▪ The highly variable patient characteristics, shoulder pathology, and surgical techniques make general statements about functional and prosthetic survival difficult.
  ▪ For this reason, a conservative approach to surgery is advised.

COMPLICATIONS

▪ Systemic perioperative
  ▪ Anesthetic complications
  ▪ Deep venous thrombosis
  ▪ Atelectasis
  ▪ Cardiac events
▪ Local perioperative
  ▪ Intraoperative fracture of humerus, glenoid, acromion
  ▪ Axillary nerve or plexus injury
  ▪ Deltoid injury
▪ Postoperative
  ▪ Hematoma
  ▪ Infection
  ▪ Dislocation
  ▪ Failure of tissue repair
  ▪ Fracture of humerus, glenoid, acromion
  ▪ Prosthetic loosening
  ▪ Pain
  ▪ Weakness
  ▪ Failure to regain function

REFERENCES

1. Boileau P, Watkinson D, et al. Neer Award 2005. The Grammont reverse shoulder prosthesis: Results in cuff tear arthritis, fracture sequelae, and revision arthroplasty. J Shoulder Elbow Surg 2006;15: 527–540.
2. Boileau P, Watkinson DJ, et al. Grammont reverse prosthesis: Design, rationale, and biomechanics. J Shoulder Elbow Surg 2005;14 (1 Suppl S):147S–161S.
3. Frankle M, Levy JC, et al. The reverse shoulder prosthesis for glenohumeral arthritis associated with severe rotator cuff deficiency: a minimum two-year follow-up study of sixty patients' surgical technique. J Bone Joint Surg Am 2006;88A(Suppl 1 Pt 2):178–190.
4. Frankle M, Siegal S, et al. The reverse shoulder prosthesis for glenohumeral arthritis associated with severe rotator cuff deficiency: a minimum two-year follow-up study of sixty patients. J Bone Joint Surg Am 2005;87A:1697–1705.
5. Guery J, Favard L, et al. Reverse total shoulder arthroplasty. Survivorship analysis of eighty replacements followed for five to ten years. J Bone Joint Surg Am 2006;88A:1742–1747.
6. Harman M, Frankle M, et al. Initial glenoid component fixation in reverse total shoulder arthroplasty: a biomechanical evaluation. J Shoulder Elbow Surg 2005;14(1 Suppl S):162S–167S.

7. Mahfouz M, Nicholson G, et al. In vivo determination of the dynamics of normal, rotator cuff-deficient, total, and reverse replacement shoulders. J Bone Joint Surg Am 2005;87A(Suppl 2):107–113.

8. Matsen FA III, Lippitt SB. Shoulder Surgery: Principles and Procedures. Philadelphia: WB Saunders, 2003.

9. Neyton L, Walch G, et al. Glenoid corticocancellous bone grafting after glenoid component removal in the treatment of glenoid loosening. J Shoulder Elbow Surg 2006;15:173–179.

10. Nyffeler RW, Werner CM, et al. Biomechanical relevance of glenoid component positioning in the reverse Delta III total shoulder prosthesis. J Shoulder Elbow Surg 2005;14:524–528.

11. Nyffeler RW, Werner CM, et al. Analysis of a retrieved Delta III total shoulder prosthesis. J Bone Joint Surg Br 2004;86B:1187–1191.

12. Rockwood CA, Matsen FA III, Wirth MA, et al, eds. The Shoulder, ed 3. Philadelphia: WB Saunders, 2004.

13. Werner CM, Steinmann PA, et al. Treatment of painful pseudoparesis due to irreparable rotator cuff dysfunction with the Delta III reverse-ball-and-socket total shoulder prosthesis. J Bone Joint Surg Am 2005;87A:1476–1486.

Chapter 27

Pectoralis Major Repair

Matthew D. Pepe, Bradford S. Tucker, and Carl Basamania

DEFINITION

▪ Pectoralis major ruptures are injuries to the one of the largest and strongest muscles of the shoulder region.
▪ Injuries can be divided into complete and partial tears.
  ▪ Complete tears typically occur at the tendon-to-bone junction and involve both heads.
  ▪ Partial tears can occur to either the sternocostal or the clavicular head.
  ▪ Both types may also occur at the musculotendinous junction or the muscle itself.

ANATOMY

▪ The pectoralis major is a broad triangular muscle that originates from the medial clavicle, anterior sternum, costal cartilages to the sixth rib, and external obliques.
▪ It inserts into the proximal humerus on the lateral edge of the bicipital groove. It has two distinct heads: the smaller clavicular head and the larger sternocostal head.
▪ The pectoralis major tendon is about 5 cm long. The insertion site has two distinct laminae. The clavicular head is anterior and distal and is about 1 cm long, and the sternocostal head inserts posterior and is 2.5 cm long.[3]
▪ The sternocostal head spirals 180 degrees on itself, inserting posterior to the clavicular head, creating a rolled inferior surface that is the axillary fold (**FIG 1**).
▪ The function of the pectoralis major varies depending on the division. Its primary function is to adduct the humerus and its secondary role is to forward flex and internally rotate. The clavicular head primarily forward flexes and horizontally adducts. The sternocostal head internally rotates and adducts.

PATHOGENESIS

▪ Pectoralis major ruptures typically occur when a powerful eccentric or concentric forward flexion or adduction load to the humerus (such as heavy bench pressing) occurs. The final

30 degrees of humeral extension disproportionally stretches the inferior fibers of the sternocostal head, putting it at a mechanical disadvantage and predisposing it to injury. The inferior fibers fail first, followed by progression toward the clavicular head.
▪ Ruptures may also occur when a traction injury such as rapid extension, abduction, or external rotation force is applied to the extremity (such as catching oneself during a fall).
▪ Injuries to the muscle belly can also be caused by a direct blow, which can result in hematoma formation.
▪ Patients often hear or feel a rip or tear in the shoulder region, feel a burning pain, and occasionally hear a pop.
▪ Younger patients (under 30 years) tear at the tendon–bone insertion, whereas patients over 30 tend to tear at the musculotendinous junction.
▪ Swelling and ecchymosis occur from several hours to days after the injury in the lateral chest wall, upper arm, or axilla.
▪ Medial muscle retraction along with loss of the axillary fold may not be evident for several days until the swelling subsides.
▪ Anabolic steroids weaken the muscle–tendon unit, making patients more susceptible to tears.[1]

NATURAL HISTORY

▪ Weakness of the affected shoulder in adduction, forward flexion, and internal rotation can be expected with nonoperative treatment of full-thickness tears of both heads or of partial tears of the sternocostal head.
▪ Isokinetic strength testing has demonstrated 25% to 50% deficits of strength in adduction and internal rotation in preoperative patients and people treated nonoperatively.[3,4,9]
▪ Cosmetic deformity occurs secondary to the loss of the tendon in the axillary fold as well as from the medial retraction that occurs during contraction of the muscle.
▪ Partial tears will elicit a variable degree of weakness and deformity, depending on the amount and location of tendon torn.

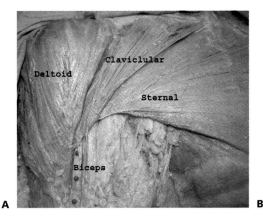
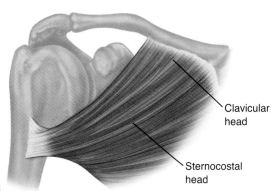

FIG 1 • **A.** Anatomy of the pectoralis major. Two distinct heads are clearly demonstrated. **B.** The clavicular portion of the tendon inserts anterior and distal. The sternocostal lamina inserts posterior and proximal.

■ The initial pain and cramping that occurs during contraction of the pectoralis major usually subsides in 2 to 3 months.
■ Patients treated nonoperatively for full-thickness tears will complain of weakness and fatigue with recreational and occupational activities as well as the cosmetic deformity.

PATIENT HISTORY AND PHYSICAL FINDINGS

■ A previous history of pain is not typical.
■ The patient's occupation and involvement in sports and weight-lifting activities are important in decision making regarding treatment.
■ Physical examination initially will yield painful range of motion of the shoulder and arm. When the swelling subsides, patients typically have full range of motion of the glenohumeral joint.
■ Swelling and ecchymosis are variable depending on the chronicity and the degree of the tear.
■ Isometric or resisted adduction and forward flexion will show the loss of the tendon in the axillary fold and medial retraction of the pectoralis muscle.
■ The examiner should instruct the patient to hold the arm at 90 degrees of abduction, and the anterior head of the deltoid will be accentuated. If the arm is held in forward flexion, the clavicular head will be accentuated (**FIG 2A**).
■ Having patients press their hands together in front of their body for isometric adduction allows inspection of both sides at the same time and simultaneous palpation (**FIG 2B**).
■ Manual strength testing will demonstrate weakness in adduction and forward flexion.

IMAGING AND OTHER DIAGNOSTIC STUDIES

■ A standard shoulder radiographic series is obtained to rule out fractures, avulsions, or signs of instability.

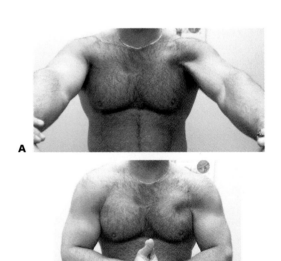

FIG 2 • **A.** Resisted forward flexion demonstrates the intact clavicular head and the defect from the ruptured sternocostal head. The retracted sternocostal head is evident. **B.** Isometric adduction demonstrating the normal contour of the right pectoralis major compared with the medially retracted left sternocostal head.

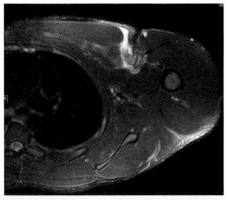
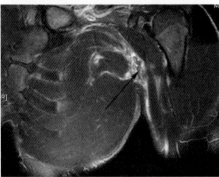

FIG 3 • Axial and coronal T2-weighted MRIs.

■ An MRI of the chest, with attention to the pectoralis major tendon, may be obtained to evaluate the location of the tear or assist in making the diagnosis.[6,11] It has been shown to be beneficial in differentiating musculotendinous junction ruptures from tendinous avulsions and may change the treatment strategy.[11] It is difficult, however, to distinguish between complete and partial ruptures (**FIG 3**).
■ Ultrasound may be used to identify the location and severity of the tear. Results, however, are user-dependent.

DIFFERENTIAL DIAGNOSIS

■ Rotator cuff tears
■ Proximal biceps tear
■ Anterior shoulder instability
■ Deltoid rupture
■ Latissimus dorsi tear
■ Brachial plexus injury

NONOPERATIVE MANAGEMENT

■ Nonoperative treatment is indicated for medial tears, intramuscular tears, or tears at the musculotendinous junction in some people. Also, nonoperative treatment should be considered in low-demand patients with complete or partial distal tendon ruptures.
■ Nonoperative treatment begins with a sling for the first 7 to 10 days. Ice should be applied intermittently for the first 72 hours.
■ Gentle active assisted range of motion is then begun, avoiding aggressive external rotation, abduction, or extension stretching in the initial phases.
■ Strength training is typically initiated at 6 to 8 weeks. Depending on the level of occupational or sporting demands, patients may return between 8 and 12 weeks.

▪ Strength deficits of 25% and 50% can be expected with nonoperative treatment.[5]

SURGICAL MANAGEMENT

▪ Pectoralis major repair is recommended for all complete distal tears, partial distal tears in high-demand patients, and musculotendinous junction tears in high-demand patients with large defects.

▪ A direct tendon-to-bone repair with heavy, nonabsorbable sutures is performed for complete distal tears and sternocostal tears.

▪ A side-to-side repair is used for musculotendinous junction tears.

Preoperative Planning

▪ A standard examination under anesthesia of the glenohumeral joint is performed to evaluate for instability.

Positioning

▪ The patient is placed in the 30-degree modified beach chair position. The shoulder and arm are prepared free. A shoulder positioning device is helpful, but not necessary, to position the arm during surgery (**FIG 4**).

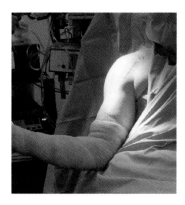

FIG 4 ▪ Operative setup. The patient is placed in the beach chair position with the arm draped free.

Approach

▪ An anterior approach to the shoulder and proximal humerus is used—the internervous plane between the axillary nerve of the deltoid and the superior and inferior pectoral nerves of the pectoralis major.

PECTORALIS MAJOR REPAIR USING DRILL HOLES

▪ Our preferred technique for direct primary repair of the pectoralis major tendon is to attach the tendon directly to the humeral cortex using drill holes.

▪ A limited 4- to 5-cm deltopectoral incision is made (**TECH FIG 1A**). The cephalic vein is identified and retracted laterally with the deltoid.

▪ The biceps tendon is identified, gaining access to the insertion of the pectoralis major just lateral to the biceps tendon in the proximal humerus. In cases of musculotendinous junction tears or partial tears, the entire tendon or a portion of it will be intact.

▪ Medial dissection is then performed to identify the retracted tendon. The sternocostal and clavicular heads are identified as well as the location of the tendon or musculotendinous junction tear.

▪ In cases of complete tears, the tendon is typically retracted medially and folded upon itself, identifiable by palpation.

▪ A traction suture is placed in the tendon, and stepwise gentle blunt mobilization of the muscle and tendon is performed.

▪ The excursion of the tendon is then tested. Even in cases of chronic tears, the tendon can typically be mobilized to reach the humerus without difficulty.

▪ The tendon edge is freshened with a scalpel. A no. 5 braided, nonabsorbable suture is used in a Bunnell or modified Mason-Allen locking stitch in the end of the tendon (**TECH FIG 1B**). Two or three sutures are used, spaced about 1 cm apart, depending on the width of the tendon.

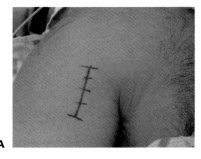

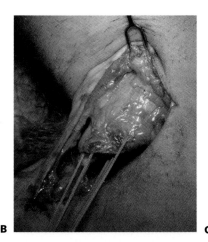

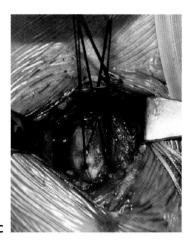

TECH FIG 1 ▪ Drill hole technique. **A.** Limited deltopectoral incision. **B.** Modified Mason-Allen stitch in tendon edge. **C.** Drill hole placement with 2-0 Vicryl sutures placed. (*continued*)

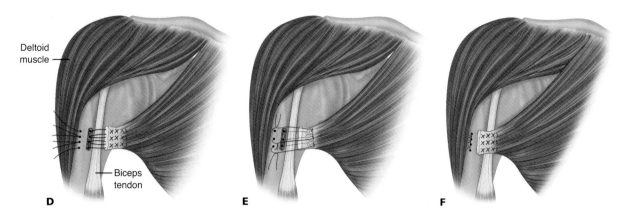

D   **E**   **F**

TECH FIG 1 • (*continued*) **D.** Bunnell technique with sutures passed and ready to tie. The central holes are shared by two sutures. **E.** Suture passage when modified Mason-Allen stitch is used. The deep suture is passed through the drill holes. **F.** Bunnell technique after suture tying.

- The insertion site lateral to the biceps tendon is decorticated with a burr.
- A commercially available drill can be used to drill the proximal and distal sets of holes. A bridge of 8 to 10 mm is adequate secondary to the thickness of the humerus.
  - The holes usually need to be overdrilled with a 2-mm drill bit, as the humeral cortex is extremely strong and thick.
- A needle with a matching radius of curvature is then used to pass a 2-0 looped Vicryl passing suture (**TECH FIG 1C**). Each corresponding suture is passed using the 2-0 Vicryl passing suture.

- The central drill holes are shared by the upper and lower respective sutures in a horizontal mattress configuration for the Bunnell technique (**TECH FIG 1D**).
- If a modified Mason-Allen stitch was used, the deep suture is passed through the drill hole and the knot tied on the upper surface of the tendon (**TECH FIG 1E**).
- The sutures are then tied with the arm in adduction and internal rotation to ensure apposition of the tendon to the humerus (**TECH FIG 1F**).
- Alternatively, the drill holes may be made freehand and the sutures passed with either a free needle or a loop of 24-gauge wire.

PECTORALIS MAJOR REPAIR USING SUTURE ANCHORS

- The musculotendinous unit is mobilized in the same way as described for drill hole repair. The humeral cortex is decorticated with a burr.
- Two or three suture anchors are then placed in the humeral insertion, spaced 1 cm apart. The sutures are passed in a Kessler mattress stitch through the distal pectoralis tendon (**TECH FIG 2**).
- One limb is passed in a simple fashion. This is used as the post during tying so the knot slides and apposes the tendon to the humerus without the knot lying in the repair site.
- Metallic anchors loaded with braided, nonabsorbable no. 5 sutures are used, as the humeral cortex in this region may be too thick to accept an absorbable anchor.

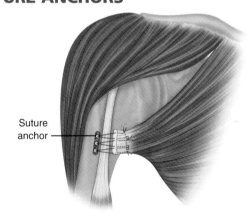

TECH FIG 2 • Suture anchor technique: placement of sutures and passage through the tendon edge.

MUSCULOTENDINOUS JUNCTION REPAIRS

- Multiple figure 8 or modified Kessler sutures of a no. 2 braided, nonabsorbable suture are used on both the superficial and deep layers.

- The quality of the repair depends on the strength and the amount of tendon left on the muscular side.

PEARLS AND PITFALLS

Indications for repair	■ A discussion and risk–benefit analysis is necessary in patients with partial and musculotendinous junction ruptures.
Tendon mobilization	■ Medial dissection is required to free the perimuscular adhesions in chronic ruptures. The neurovascular bundle is rarely at risk.
Suture passing	■ Using a commercially available matched drill and needle facilitates suture passage through the humerus (CurvTek). Because of the thickness of the humerus, overdrilling the holes makes needle passage easier.
Chronic tears	■ Repair of pectoralis major ruptures is feasible up to 5 years after the injury. The outcome of chronic repairs is not as good as that of acute repairs, with residual weakness as the most common complaint.

POSTOPERATIVE CARE

■ The arm is kept in a sling for 6 weeks postoperatively. It is removed from the sling one or two times daily for gentle, progressive passive and active assisted range of motion of the shoulder, elbow, wrist, and hand.

■ The extremes of abduction and external rotation are avoided for the first 6 weeks. At this time, the sling is removed and unrestricted movement is allowed. In addition, strengthening is begun.

■ Return to full activities is generally achieved between 3 and 5 months.

OUTCOMES

■ There are no large prospective or randomized studies in the literature comparing operative and nonoperative treatment. Results are universally good with acute repairs (within 8 weeks).

■ Park and Espiniella[7] in 1970 evaluated 30 patients with pectoralis major ruptures. The results were 90% good to excellent results with operative repair versus 75% with nonoperative treatment.

■ McEntire and colleagues[5] in 1972 compared operative and nonoperative treatment in 11 patients. Again, operative repair had a more favorable outcome at 88% versus 83%, with a higher ratio of excellent to good results.

■ Zenman and coworkers[10] in 1979 reviewed nine athletes with pectoralis major ruptures. Four patients were treated with surgical repair and had excellent results. All five of the patients treated nonoperatively had residual weakness, and two were dissatisfied with their outcome.

■ Kretzler and Richardson[3] in 1989 reported on their results after repair of 16 distal tendon tears. Eighty-one percent regained full motion and strength. Two repairs that occurred 5 years after the injury had persistent weakness.

■ Wolfe and colleagues[9] in 1992 evaluated 14 patients with pectoralis major ruptures, half of whom were treated with operative repair. Cybex strength testing demonstrated normal strength in the repaired patients, with persistent weakness in the unrepaired group.

■ Jones and Matthews[2] in 1988 reviewed the literature and concluded that acute repair within 7 days has 57% excellent and 30% good results. Repair in the setting of a chronic tear yielded 0% excellent and 60% good results. They concluded that although chronic repair is possible even up to 5 years after the injury, the outcome is not as good as an acute repair, with a high likelihood of persistent weakness and cosmetic deformity.

■ Schepsis and colleagues[8] in 2000 found that operatively repaired patients (both acute and chronic) had significantly better outcomes than conservatively treated patients.

■ There are no studies to date documenting rerupture after repair.

COMPLICATIONS

■ Complications are relatively infrequent after pectoralis major repair. One patient experienced loss of abduction.[3] Another patient had ulnar-sided hand paresthesias of unknown etiology that spontaneously resolved.[8]

■ There have been several reports of complications in the elderly after rupture and nonsurgical management. One patient needed a blood transfusion. Two died of sepsis from an infected hematoma. Myositis ossificans developed in one patient 4 months after rupture.

REFERENCES

1. Hunter MB, Shybut GT, Nuber G. The effect of anabolic steroid hormones on the mechanical properties of tendons and ligaments. Trans Orthop Res Soc 1986;11:240.
2. Jones MW, Matthews JP. Rupture of the pectoralis major in weightlifters: a case report and review of the literature. Injury 1988; 19:219.
3. Kretzler HH, Richardson AB. Rupture of the pectoralis major muscle. Am J Sports Med 1989;17:453.
4. Liu J, Wu J, Chang S, Chou Y, et al. Avulsion of the pectoralis major tendon. Am J Sports Med 1992;20:366–368.
5. McEntire JE, Hess WE, Coleman SS. Rupture of the pectoralis major muscle: a report of eleven injuries and review of fifty-six. J Bone Joint Surg Am 1972;54A:1040–1046.
6. Miller MD, Johnson DL, Fu FH, et al. Rupture of the pectoralis major muscle in a collegiate football player: use of magnetic resonance imaging in early diagnosis. Am J Sports Med 1993;21: 475–477.
7. Park JY, Espiniella LJ. Rupture of the pectoralis major muscle: a case report and review of the literature. J Bone Joint Surg Am 1970; 52A:577.
8. Schepsis AA, Grafe MW, Jones HP, et al. Rupture of the pectoralis major muscle: outcome after repair of acute and chronic injuries. Am J Sports Med 2000;28:9–15.
9. Wolfe SW, Wickiewicz TL, Cavanaugh JT. Ruptures of the pectoralis major muscle: an anatomic and clinical analysis. Am J Sports Med 1992;20:587.
10. Zenman SC, Rosenfeld RT, Liscomb PR. Tears of the pectoralis major muscle. Am J Sports Med 1979;7:343.
11. Zvijac JE, Schurhoff MR, Hechtman KS, et al. Pectoralis major tears: correlation of magnetic resonance imaging and treatment strategies. Am J Sports Med 2006;34:289–294.

Jon J. P. Warner and Bassem Elhassan

DEFINITION

▪ The snapping scapula syndrome first was described by Boinet in 1867.[14]

▪ It is characterized by painful scapular motion with associated crepitus during scapulothoracic motion, with or without a clear history of injury or trauma.

▪ It has also been referred to as *scapulothoracic bursitis, retroscapular creaking, superior scapular syndrome,* and *retroscapular pain.*[3,7,11,14]

▪ The associated audible crepitus, which can be tactile in most instances, has been described by Milch and Burman[11] as a tactile-acoustic phenomenon, possibly generated secondary to an abnormality in the scapulothoracic interval.

▪ This crepitus is divided into three classes, based on the volume of the sound produced.[10]

  ▪ The first group is considered physiologic, with what is described as a "gentle friction" sound.

  ▪ The second group, which includes most patients with the snapping scapular syndrome, features a louder grating sound.

  ▪ The third group is defined by a loud snapping noise that is considered pathologic in most cases.

ANATOMY

▪ The scapulothoracic articulation consists of the interface between the anterior aspect of the scapula and the ribs in the posterior aspect of the convex thoracic chest wall (**FIG 1**).

▪ This articulation is cushioned by several muscles, specifically the subscapularis and the serratus anterior.

▪ In addition, two major and four minor bursae have been described in the scapulothoracic articulation[6,7,23] (Fig 1).

  ▪ The two major bursae are the infraserratus bursa, located between the serratus anterior muscle and the chest wall, and the supraserratus bursa, located between the serratus anterior and the subscapularis muscles.

  ▪ The four minor bursae are distributed as follows: two at the superomedial angle of the scapula, one at the inferior angle of the scapula, and one at the medial base of spine of the scapula, underlying the trapezius muscle.

▪ While the major bursae have been found consistently in cadaveric and clinical studies, those of the minor bursae were not.[3,19,20]

PATHOGENESIS

▪ Incongruence of the scapulothoracic articulation has been postulated to be the main cause of the snapping scapular syndrome, which may or may not be associated with bony anomalies of this region.[13,17]

▪ Maltracking or dynamic compression of the scapulothoracic articulation has been postulated as a main etiology of this syndrome, because it leads to irritation of the bursa secondary to pathologic contact between the ribs and the superior angle of the scapula.[4,22]

  ▪ This maltracking is considered to be a soft tissue cause of snapping scapula syndrome, which has been reported in cases of subscapularis atrophy secondary to glenohumeral fusion and long thoracic nerve palsy.[11,24]

  ▪ Clinical studies and histologic findings of muscle intrafascicular fibrosis, bursitis, edema, and shoulder girdle muscle atrophy support this hypothesis.[7,17]

▪ Bony or skeletal causes of snapping scapula syndrome are rare. These include scapular osteochondromas and exostoses (**FIG 2**), anterior angulation of the scapula, scapula fracture, scapular tubercle of Luschka, skeletal abnormalities of the vertebrae (omovertebral bone), and abnormal angulations and tumors of the ribs.[10,11,21]

NATURAL HISTORY

▪ Patients with snapping scapula syndrome usually complain of pain around the shoulder girdle.

▪ This pain most often is secondary to bursitis in the scapulothoracic articulation. Constant motion irritates the soft tissues, leading to inflammation and a cycle of chronic bursitis and scarring.

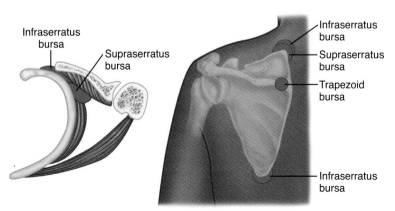

FIG 1 ▪ Four different bursae are shown—two infraserratus, one supraserratus, and one trapezoid bursae.

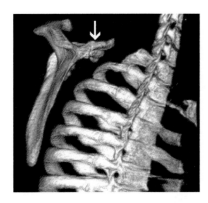

FIG 2 • An osteochondroma (*arrow*) of the superomedial angle of the scapula may, rarely, be the cause of snapping scapula syndrome.

▪ The chronic inflammation of the bursae will lead to fibrotic, scarred, and tough bursal tissues that can lead to mechanical impingement and pain with motion, resulting in further inflammation.

▪ Once the patient reaches this level of chronic bursal inflammation, the symptoms rarely subside by themselves without trial of rest and physical therapy.

▪ In many cases, especially when the cause of snapping is skeletal, surgical intervention becomes essential to manage this problem.

PATIENT HISTORY AND PHYSICAL FINDINGS

▪ Patients with scapulothoracic bursitis report a history of pain in the shoulder or neck with overhead activities for months or years and often have a history of repetitive overuse in work or recreation or a history of trauma.

▪ A history of neck injury, shoulder injury or fracture, or previous shoulder surgery should be ruled out.

▪ Audible or palpable crepitus may accompany the symptoms with scapulothoracic motion; this is another indication for the location of the symptomatic inflamed bursa.

▪ Some patients report a family history of the disorder and have bilateral symptoms.

▪ Localized tenderness is an indication for the site of scapulothoracic bursitis.

▪ Improvement of symptoms by lifting the scapula off the chest wall helps localize the source of pathology to the scapulothoracic articulation.

▪ Diagnosis is confirmed if significant relief or even elimination of the pain occurs when local anesthetic and corticosteroids are injected in the scapulothoracic bursa under the superomedial border of the scapula.

▪ The examiner also must assess soft tissue tightness, muscle strength, and flexibility around the involved shoulder.

▪ Special attention should be directed to rule out tight trapezius, pectoralis minor, or levator scapula muscles, as well as weakness of any of the scapular muscles, specifically the serratus anterior and the trapezius.

▪ In patients with winging of the scapula, a careful neuromuscular examination should be performed to differentiate true winging from compensatory pseudo-winging that might originate from a painful scapulothoracic articulation.

IMAGING AND OTHER DIAGNOSTIC STUDIES

▪ Radiologic studies should include an anterior-posterior (AP) and tangential (Y) views of the shoulder, to identify bony abnormalities in the scapula and ribs (**FIG 3A**).

▪ A CT scan may be needed for more bony definition. Its role, with or without three-dimensional reconstruction, is still debated,[9,13] but in patients with suspected bony skeletal abnormality, the CT scan might be helpful (**FIG 3B**).

▪ Fluoroscopy could be used to visualize the snapping during simulated shoulder motion.

▪ MRI can identify the location and size of the inflamed bursa, but its usefulness is debated. The senior author does not believe that the MRI is necessary and has never ordered it in any of his cases.

▪ Nerve conduction and electromyography studies are useful if a neurologic injury is suspected as the reason for scapula winging.

DIFFERENTIAL DIAGNOSIS

▪ Soft tissue lesions, such as atrophied muscle
▪ Fibrotic muscle
▪ Anomalous muscle insertion
▪ Subscapular elastofibroma. This tumor is nonneoplastic and appears to form in response to repetitive injury or microtrauma. Most patients who have this tumor complain of a palpable mass rather than pain.
▪ Cervical spondylosis and radiculopathy
▪ Periscapular muscle strain
▪ Glenohumeral pathology

NONOPERATIVE MANAGEMENT

▪ The initial management of snapping scapula syndrome, once the diagnosis has been made, is conservative.

▪ Rest, activity modification, and nonsteroidal anti-inflammatory medications should be started.

▪ Next, physical therapy should be initiated to restore the normal kinematics of the shoulder and prevent it from sloping.

▪ Weakness in the serratus anterior, even if subtle, may lead to tilting of the scapula forward, thus increasing the friction and rubbing of the upper medial pole of the scapula on the thoracic ribs. This will cause irritation and inflammation of the scapulothoracic bursae.

▪ Therapy should emphasize periscapular muscle strengthening, particularly the serratus anterior and subscapulari, which can elevate the scapula off the chest wall when they are hypertrophied.[1,17]

▪ Taping, a figure-8 harness, scapulothoracic bracing, or postural training can serve to minimize shoulder sloping and thoracic kyphosis.

▪ Injection of corticosteroid and local anesthetic into the scapulothoracic bursa can be diagnostic and also may be therapeutic and helpful in the rehabilitation program.

▪ There is no consensus on how long the patient should be kept on trial of physical therapy. The underlying diagnosis is important. In general, a 3- to 6-month trial is a good estimate.

▪ If the diagnosis is certain, no structural anatomic lesion is present, and the patient has failed 3 to 6 months of appropriate conservative treatment, then surgical options should be considered.

▪ The threshold to proceed to surgical intervention also should be much lower if the patient has a real structural lesion such as a bony exostosis or an osteochondroma.

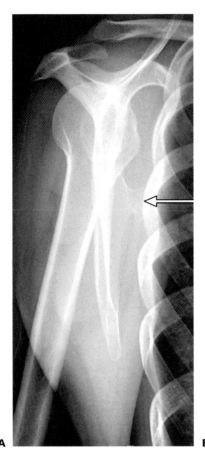
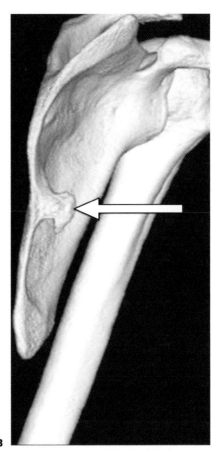

FIG 3 • **A.** A Y-scapular view showing a prominent osteochondroma (*arrow*) of the body of the scapula, causing symptomatic snapping. **B.** A three-dimensional CT scan shows the bony anatomy in more detail. The arrow points to the same osteochondroma.

SURGICAL MANAGEMENT

Preoperative Planning

▪ All radiographs are reviewed before surgery.
▪ The decision to operate is made based on relief of pain with anesthetic injection into the scapulothoracic region in patients who failed conservative management, or in patients who have symptomatic snapping scapula syndrome secondary to structural lesion.
▪ The different surgical approaches, as well as the technique that the surgeon decides to perform, are discussed with the patient before surgery.

Positioning

▪ The patient is positioned in the prone position for both arthroscopic and open techniques (**FIG 4**).
▪ The involved arm is placed in internal rotation against the patient's lower back (chicken-wing position). This will cause the scapula to wing out from the thorax and make the superomedial angle more prominent.
▪ The surgeon stands on the side opposite the scapula to be operated to get the best access to the surgical field.

Approach

▪ Multiple surgical approaches are available that can decompress the impingement in the superomedial region of the scapula.

▪ These include open surgical decompression, arthroscopic surgical decompression, or a combination of the two approaches.
▪ Each of these approaches may include bursectomy alone, bony resection of the superomedial aspect of the scapula alone, or a combination.

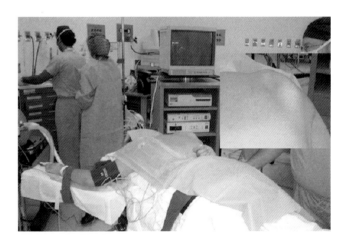

FIG 4 • The operating room setup for arthroscopic scapulothoracic bursectomy. The patient is positioned prone with the hand of the involved shoulder placed behind the back in order to lift the scapula off the chest wall.

OPEN DECOMPRESSION

- A longitudinal incision is made along the medial scapular edge (**TECH FIG 1A**).
- Subcutaneous undermining is performed to expose the superior portion of the scapula, from the level of the scapula spine to the superomedial angle of the scapula.
- Splitting and elevation of the trapezius in line with its fibers is performed at the level of the scapular spine, and

the superomedial edge of the scapula is exposed (**TECH FIG 1B**).

- The levator scapulae and rhomboids are detached from the superior and medial edge of the scapula to expose the upper scapula border (**TECH FIG 1C**).
- Care is taken not to dissect into the rhomboids or fully detach them so as not to injure the dorsal scapular nerve,

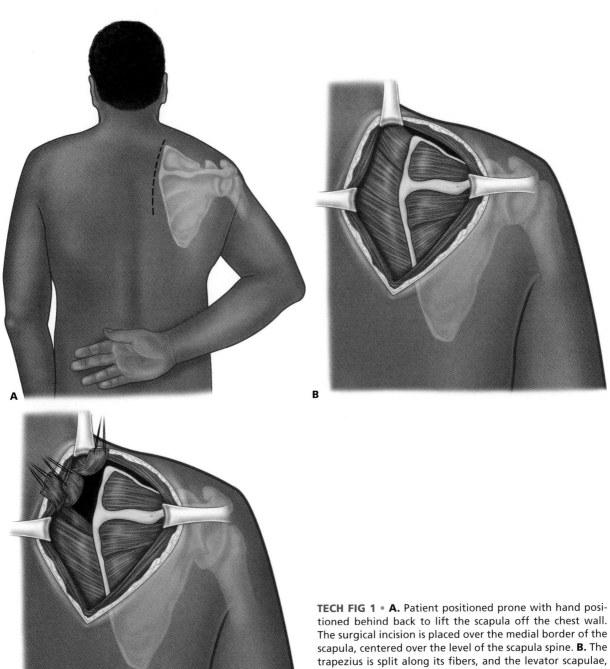

TECH FIG 1 • A. Patient positioned prone with hand positioned behind back to lift the scapula off the chest wall. The surgical incision is placed over the medial border of the scapula, centered over the level of the scapula spine. **B.** The trapezius is split along its fibers, and the levator scapulae, the rhomboids, and the posterior surface of the scapula are exposed. **C.** The levator scapulae, rhomboid major, and rhomboid minor are detached from their insertion on the scapula and tagged with sutures. *(continued)*

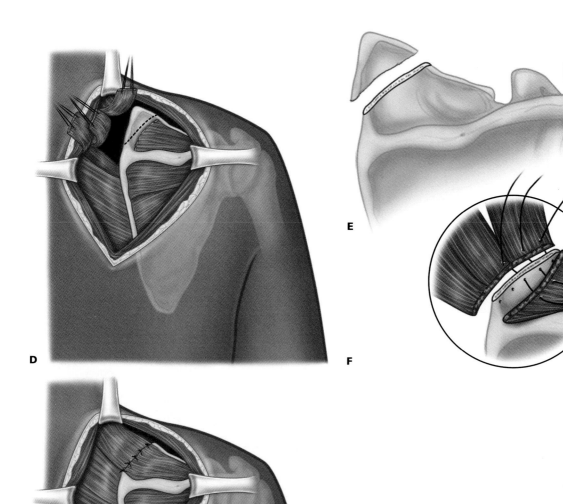

TECH FIG 1 • *(continued)* **D,E.** Resection of the superomedial border of the scapula. **F.** The detached muscles are reattached to the scapula through drill holes. **G.** The final repair of the detached levator scapulae and rhomboids.

which usually is located 2 cm medial to the medial scapular edge.

- The serratus anterior muscle is left intact.
- A retractor is placed underneath the scapula to lift it away from the thoracic ribs.
- The scapulothoracic bursa is identified against the ribs, underneath the serratus anterior muscle.
- A clamp is used to grasp the bursa, and sharp excision of it is performed from superior to inferior.
- Subperiosteal elevation of the muscles around the superomedial border of the scapula, including the supraspinatus, infraspinatus, subscapularis, and serratus

anterior muscles, is performed with the use of electocautery to expose 1 to 2 cm of bone (**TECH FIG 1D**).

- This exposed portion of the superomedial portion of the scapula is resected with use of an oscillating saw (**TECH FIG 1E**).
- Once the bony resection is accomplished, drill holes are placed into the upper-medial border of the scapula in order to reattach the muscles to their anatomic insertion (**TECH FIG 1F**) using a no. 2 nonabsorbable braided suture (**TECH FIG 1G**).
- The skin is closed with absorbable subcuticular suture.

ARTHROSCOPIC BURSECTOMY

- Positioning is the same as in open decompression.
- Placement of the arm in the chicken-wing position results in scapula winging and protraction off the posterior thorax, which facilitates the entry of the arthroscopic instruments in the bursal space.
- Standard arthroscopic portals are used.
- The initial "safe" portal is placed at the level of the scapular spine, 2 cm medial to the scapular edge, to avoid injury to the dorsal scapular nerve and artery (**TECH FIG 2A**).
- The scapulothoracic space is localized with a spinal needle and distended with approximately 30 mL of saline, and the portal is created.
- A blunt obturator is inserted into the scapulothoracic (subserratus) bursa between the posterior thoracic wall and the serratus anterior muscle.
- Care should be taken to avoid overpenetration through the serratus anterior into the subscapular space or through the chest wall.
- A 30-degree arthroscope is inserted into the scapulothoracic space, which was distended with fluid infiltration.
- Use of a fluid pump is optional. Our preference is to use an arthroscopy pump but keep the pressure low, at around 30 mm Hg, to minimize fluid extravasation.
- A spinal needle is used to localize the second portal under direct visualization.
- This portal is inserted, in most instances, in line with and approximately 4 cm distal to the first portal.
- A bipolar radiofrequency device and a motorized shaver are introduced into a 6-mm cannula through the lower portal, and used to resect the bursal tissue. Because the inflamed scapulothoracic bursa is a potential source of bleeding during arthroscopic shaving, the radiofrequency device becomes particularly useful to minimize bleeding in these tissues (**TECH FIG 2B**).
- A methodic approach to resection should be followed, because there are no real landmarks.
- Ablation of tissues should be performed from medial to lateral and then from inferior to superior.
- The surgeon should be ready to switch portals and should have a 70-degree athroscope ready to facilitate visualization. A probe can be used to palpate the scapula and serratus muscle superiorly and the ribs and intercostal muscles inferiorly.
- An additional superior portal may be placed as needed. We prefer not to use this portal, because it may place the accessory spinal nerve, transverse cervical artery, and dorsal scapular neurovascular structures at risk.
- After complete bursectomy is performed, the arthroscopic instruments are withdrawn, and skin closure is performed with absorbable subcuticular sutures.

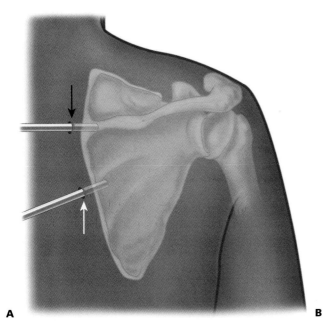
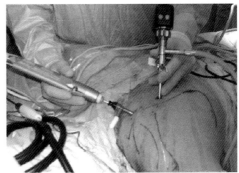

TECH FIG 2 • A. Locations of the arthroscopic portals. A proximal (safe) portal (*black arrow*) is placed 2 cm medial to the spine of the scapula. A distal portal (*white arrow*) is placed in line with and 4 cm distal to the proximal portal. **B.** Sites of portal placement. The shaver and the camera can be placed interchangeably in either portal for viewing and shaving.

ARTHROSCOPIC BURSECTOMY AND PARTIAL SUPEROMEDIAL SCAPULECTOMY

- First, all the steps for arthroscopic bursectomy are followed.
- After the bursa has been completely resected, the superomedial angle of the scapula is localized by palpation through the skin.
- Detachment of the conjoined insertion of the levator scapulae, supraspinatus, and rhomboids is performed with the use of the radiofrequency device.

- A motorized shaver and a burr are used to perform a partial scapulectomy. We do not attempt to repair the periosteal sleeve; it is allowed to heal through scarring.
- The rest of the steps are the same as those for arthroscopic bursectomy.

ARTHROSCOPIC BURSECTOMY AND OPEN PARTIAL SUPEROMEDIAL SCAPULECTOMY

- The decision to perform the superomedial scapular bony resection through a small skin incision rather than through the arthroscope may be made either before surgery or at the time of surgery.
- If full definition of the superomedial border of the scapula becomes difficult because of swelling from the arthroscopic fluid, then bony resection is performed through a small skin incision.
- A 4- to 6-cm incision is performed obliquely over the superomedial border of the scapula (see Tech Fig 1A).

- The trapezius muscle is split, and the levator scapulae and rhomboids are detached from the superomedial angle (see Tech Fig 1B,C).
- The superomedial angle of the scapula is resected. Then the levator scapulae and rhomboids are repaired to the superior scapula through drill holes (see Tech Fig 1D).
- Skin closure is performed with absorbable subcuticular sutures.

PEARLS AND PITFALLS

Indications	▪ Appropriate history, physical examination, and review of radiographs should be done. ▪ Diagnostic injection is very helpful to confirm the diagnosis and predict a good surgical outcome.
Contraindications to arthroscopic decompression	▪ Symptoms that originate from the trapezoid bursa. This bursa is superficial to the scapulothoracic space, and, therefore, removing it will not remove the pathologic tissue.
Positioning	▪ Patient prone, with hand of the affected shoulder behind the back to elevate and protract the scapula. ▪ Surgeon should be standing by the opposite shoulder.
Open decompression	▪ Avoid suprascapular notch during bony resection. ▪ It is essential to reattach the detached muscles to the scapula through bony drill holes.
Arthroscopic decompression	▪ Use a spinal needle for localization of the scapulothoracic space. ▪ Care should be taken to avoid over-penetration through the serratus anterior into the subscapular space or through the chest wall. ▪ Use of a bipolar radiofrequency device is essential to avoid bleeding from the inflamed bursa. ▪ Complete bursectomy should be performed.

POSTOPERATIVE CARE

- After open decompression and a combined arthroscopic and open approach:
  - The patient is kept in a sling, and gentle, passive range of motion is started early after surgery and continued for 4 weeks.
  - After 4 weeks, active range of motion is started.
  - Strengthening is allowed at 8 to 12 weeks.
- After arthroscopic decompression:

- The patient is kept in a sling and allowed passive and active assisted range-of-motion exercises immediately after surgery.
- After 4 weeks, isometric exercises are started.
- Strengthening of the periscapular muscles begins by 8 weeks.

OUTCOMES

- No published reports have compared the outcomes of different surgical techniques of scapulothoracic decompression.

■ The outcome of open decompression, as reported in the literature, has been good.[7,12,17,18]

■ No large series have been published reporting the outcome of arthroscopic scapulothoracic decompression for symptomatic snapping scapular syndrome.

■ Early results from small series of patients who underwent arthroscopic decompression seem promising, with minimal morbidity and early return to work.[2,5,8,15,16]

COMPLICATIONS

■ Recurrence of symptoms secondary to incomplete resection

■ Pneumothorax

■ Iatrogenic injury to the neurovascular structures around the superomedial border of the scapula

■ Aggressive bony resection risking injury to the suprascapular nerve through the notch

■ Insufficiency of the scapular muscles due to detachment after surgery

REFERENCES

1. Carlson HL, Haig AJ, Stewart DC. Snapping scapula syndrome: three case reports and an analysis of the literature. Arch Phys Med Rehabil 1997;78:506–511.
2. Chan BK, Chakrabarti AJ, Bell SN. An alternative portal for scapulothoracic arthroscopy. J Shoulder Elbow Surg 2002;11:235–240.
3. Ciullo JV, Jones E. Subscapular bursitis: conservative treatment of "snapping scapula" or "wash-board syndrome." Orthop Trans 1992–1993;16:740.
4. Glousman R, Jobe F, Tibone J, et al. Dynamic electomyographic analysis of the throwing shoulder with glenohumeral instability. J Bone Joint Surg Am 1988;70A:220.
5. Harper GD, McIlroy S, Bayley JI. Arthroscopic partial resection of the scapula for snapping scapula: a new technique. J Shoulder Elbow Surg 1999;8:53–58.
6. Kolodychuk LB, Reagan WD. Visualization of the scapulothoracique articulation using an arthroscope: A proposed technique. Orthop Trans 1993–1994;17:1142–1148.
7. Kuhn JE, Plancher KD, Hawkins RJ. Symptomatic scapulothoracique crepitus and bursitis. J Am Acad Orthop Surg 1998;6:267–272.
8. Lehtinen JT, Cassinelli E, Warner JJ. The painful scapulothoracic articulation. Clin Orthop Relat Res 2004;423:99–105.
9. Manske RC, Reiman MP, Stovak ML. Nonoperative and operative management of snapping scapula. Am J Sports Med 2004;32:1554–1565.
10. Milch H. Partial scapulectomy for snapping of the scapula. J Bone Joint Surg Am 1950;32A:561–566.
11. Milch H, Burman MS. Snapping scapula and humerus varus: report of six cases. Arch Surg 1933;26:570–588.
12. Morse BJ, Ebraheim NA, Jackson WT. Partial scapulectomy for snapping scapula syndrome. Orthop Rev Relat Res 1993;22:1141–1144.
13. Mozes G, Bickels J, Ovadia D, et al. The use of three-dimensional computed tomography in evaluating snapping scapula syndrome. Orthopedics 1999;22:1029.
14. Parsons TA. The snapping scapula syndrome and subscapular exostoses. J Bone Joint Surg Br 1973;55B:345–349.
15. Pavlik A, Ang K, Coghlan J, et al. Arthroscopic treatment of painful snapping of the scapula by using a new superior portal. Arthroscopy 2003;19:608–611.
16. Pearse EO, Bruguera J, Massoud S, et al. Arthroscopic management of the painful scapula. Arthroscopy 2006;22:755–761.
17. Percy EL, Birbrager D, Pitt MJ. Scapping scapula: a review of the literature and presentation of 14 patients. Can J Surg 1988;31:248.
18. Richards RR, McKee MD. Treatment of painful scapulothoracic crepitus by resection of the superomedial angle of the scapula: a report of three cases. Clin Orthop Relat Res 1989;247:111–116.
19. Ruland LJ III, Ruland CM, Matthews LS. Scapulothoracic anatomy for the arthroscopist. Arthroscopy 1995;11:52.
20. Sisto DJ, Jobe FW. The operative treatment of scapulothoracic bursitis in professional pitchers. Am J Sports Med 1986;14:192.
21. Strizak AM, Cowen MH. The snapping scapula syndrome: a case report. J Bone Joint Surg Am 1982;64A:941–942.
22. Warner JJ, Micheli LJ, Arslanian LE, et al. Scapulothoracic motion in normal shoulder and shoulders with glenohumeral instability and impingement syndrome. A study using Moire topographic analysis. Clin Orthop Relat Res 1992;(285):191.
23. Williams JJ, Micheli LJ, Arslanian LE, et al. Scapulothoracic motion in normal shoulders with glenohumeral instability and impingement syndrome. A study using Moire topographic analysis. Clin Orthop Relat Res 1992;285:191–198.
24. Wood VE, Verska JM. The snapping scapula in association with the thoracic outlet syndrome. Arch Surg 1989;124:1335–1337.

Chapter 29

Eden-Lange Procedure for Trapezius Palsy

Jonathan H. Lee and William N. Levine

DEFINITION

- Trapezius palsy results from a disruption of cranial nerve (CN) XI, also known as the *spinal accessory nerve.*
- Because the trapezius is innervated exclusively by CN XI, any disruption causes trapezius palsy.
- Spinal accessory nerve palsy is a rare but well-described complication of cervical lymph node biopsy.[15,17]
- The trapezius plays an integral part in stabilization of the scapula, and dysfunction leads to painful shoulder disability.
- Nonoperative treatment, including strengthening of the functioning thoracoscapular muscles, does not provide satisfactory clinical results.[2,4]
- Transfer of the levator scapulae, rhomboid major, and rhomboid minor (Eden-Lange procedure, or triple transfer) is an accepted technique for this difficult problem.[16]
- The procedure was first described by Eden[5] in 1924 and then corroborated by Lange[9] in 1951 and Francillon[7] in 1955, all reporting satisfactory short-term results. Further modifications have improved on the initial procedure.[1]
- Lateral transfer of the insertions of the three muscles allows the scapula to be stabilized in a position of abduction and anterior flexion.[15]

ANATOMY

- The trapezius muscle is broad and superficial, taking its origin from the C7–T12 spinous processes and inserting on the acromion, clavicle, and spine of the scapula (**FIG 1A**).
- Its function is to elevate and rotate the scapula; absence of the trapezius leads to lateral winging of the scapula.
- In the posterior cervical triangle, CN XI is located in the subcutaneous tissue; this superficial location renders it susceptible to damage during procedures such as cervical lymph node biopsy.
- Functionally, the trapezius can be divided into three separate parts: upper, middle, and lower.
- The upper portion consists of descending fibers and functions as an aid to suspension of the shoulder girdle, allowing shrugging of the shoulder. The middle portion consists of transverse fibers and contributes to abduction and rotation of the inferior angle of the scapula. The ascending fibers of the lower portion (along with the serratus anterior) anchor the scapula to the chest wall.
- Scapular winging occurs in both spinal accessory and serratus anterior palsy. In serratus palsy, the inferior angle of the scapula is noted to rotate medially (**FIG 1B**), whereas in trapezius palsy, the scapula rotates laterally (**FIG 1C,D**).

PATHOGENESIS

- Paralysis of the trapezius most often results from injury to the spinal accessory nerve during cervical lymph node biopsy.[13]
- Other causes include trauma (including traction injuries) or injuries from other surgical procedures, such as radical neck dissection.[1]

- In one instance, a CN XI palsy was reported to have occurred after a viral infection.[13]
- Idiopathic CN XI paralysis also has been reported.[6]
- Patterson[11] reported trapezius palsy after acromioclavicular and sternoclavicular dissociation.
- Even rarer causes include post-carotid endarterectomy and post-catheterization of the internal jugular vein.[3]
- In most cases, patients report pain and present with visible deformity and dysfunction of the shoulder girdle.

NATURAL HISTORY

- Trapezius palsy most often results from iatrogenic causes, as noted earlier, and, if left untreated, will lead to progressively worsening altered biomechanics and pain of the shoulder girdle.
- Radiating arm pain is thought to be the result of traction on the brachial plexus caused by drooping of the shoulder girdle.[13]

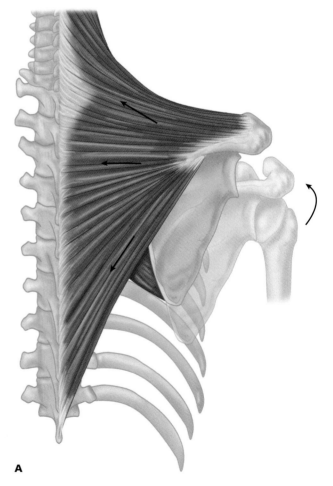

A

FIG 1 • **A.** Schematic of the three parts of the normal trapezius muscle: upper, middle, and lower. *(continued)*

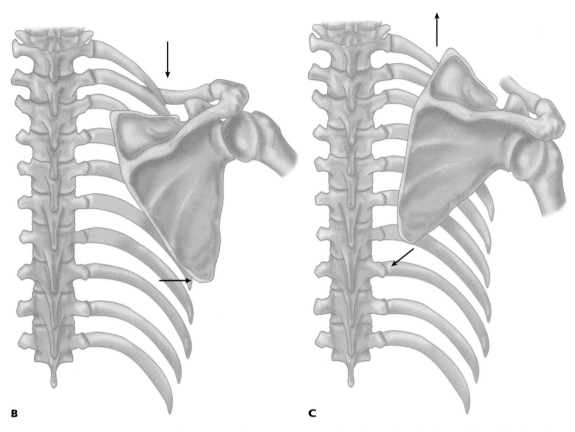

B

C

FIG 1 • *(continued)* **B.** Schematic of trapezius palsy, demonstrating lateral scapular winging and shoulder drooping. **C.** Schematic of serratus anterior palsy, demonstrating medial scapular winging.

■ Although nonoperative management can provide reduction of pain, it does not lead to return of function, and patients treated without surgery usually go on to progressive shoulder dysfunction.

■ Typically, the initial presentation is acute shoulder pain without palsy, with weakness of anterior elevation and abduction appearing after a few days (with slow diminution of pain). Atrophy of the trapezius becomes clinically apparent after a few weeks.[16]

PATIENT HISTORY AND PHYSICAL FINDINGS

■ Altered mechanics of the entire shoulder girdle are possible with trapezius palsy.

■ The classic winging of the scapula seen in CN XI palsy is characterized by downward and lateral translation of the scapula.

■ The patient should be observed from behind so comparison can be made with the contralateral side.

■ Signs unique to CN XI palsy include lateral winging of the scapula (**FIG 2A**), an asymmetric neckline, pain, weakness of shoulder abduction, and forward elevation.[14] Visible atrophy of the trapezius muscle should be noted[16] (**FIG 2B**).

■ Symptoms include weakness made worse by prolonged use of the arm, a feeling of a heavy arm, and a dull pain radiating from the scapula to the forearm (and occasionally with radiation to the hand). The radiation of pain is described as mimicking thoracic outlet syndrome (medial aspect of the upper limb). Pain typically is made worse by abduction of the shoulder as

well as forward elevation.[16] Some patients also reported paresthesias in the distribution of the auricular nerve (posterolateral side of the neck).[16]

■ Patients also often state that the arm feels difficult to control.[13]

■ It should be noted, however, that occasionally patients are pain free and present only with winging and drooping of the scapula.

■ Range of motion is decreased in elevation as well as abduction, and typically is limited to 90 degrees.[13] Teboul et al[16] report average active abduction of 78 degrees (range 30 to 140 degrees), and active forward flexion of 110 degrees (range 50 to 180 degrees). As a result, overhead activities are not possible, nor is shrugging of the shoulder.

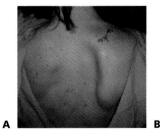
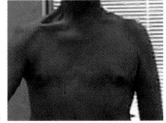

A

B

FIG 2 • **A.** Patient with a trapezius palsy demonstrating characteristic scapular winging. **B.** Anterior sternocleidomastoid muscle wasting due to the spinal accessory nerve palsy.

▪ External rotation of the shoulder and elbow flexion are not affected by CN XI lesions.[16]

▪ Reports of stiffness and passive range of motion are somewhat contradictory in the literature. Romero and Gerber[13] state that patients did not always present with a stiff shoulder but passive range of motion typically was decreased. On the other hand, Teboul et al[16] report that patients often presented with stiffness but with no deficit in passive range of motion.

▪ Often, the diagnosis of CN XI dysfunction is one of exclusion, and it is not until an unsuccessful trial of physical therapy that a patient is referred for an electrodiagnostic study and spinal accessory nerve palsy is confirmed.

▪ The necessity for electrodiagnostic testing is an issue of debate in the literature. Romero and Gerber[13] state that this testing is not necessary to establish the diagnosis of CN XI palsy, but that it can be a valuable tool if other nerve lesions are suspected. Setter et al[14] advocate electrodiagnostic testing as part of the initial workup.

▪ Evaluate the scapula for signs of lateral translation by asking patient to perform a wall push-up.

▪ Spinal accessory nerve (CN XI) palsy also affects the sternocleidomastoid muscle.

IMAGING AND OTHER DIAGNOSTIC STUDIES

▪ A standard five-view shoulder series (including true AP views of the glenohumeral joint in neutral, external, and internal rotation; as well as a scapular Y and axillary view) is required for every patient, although osseous pathology typically is not associated with CN XI palsy.

▪ MRI is not necessary, although it could be useful to assess the degree of fatty atrophy of the trapezius muscle as well as to help rule out any associated pathology such as rotator cuff injury.

▪ Electrodiagnostic testing is recommended in every case, according to Setter et al.[14] Not only will an EMG help confirm the diagnosis of spinal accessory nerve palsy, but it also will serve as confirmation that the muscles to be used in the transfer procedure are functioning normally.

DIFFERENTIAL DIAGNOSIS

▪ Missed diagnosis of spinal accessory nerve palsy is the rule,[13] most likely owing to the rare nature of the condition.

▪ Other possible types of shoulder dysfunction that may confuse the issue include serratus palsy and rotator cuff pathology.

▪ It is crucial to be able to differentiate between spinal accessory nerve (trapezius) palsy and long thoracic nerve (serratus) palsy. In serratus palsy, the inferior angle of the scapula rotates medially, whereas in trapezius palsy, the inferior angle of the scapula rotates laterally.

NONOPERATIVE MANAGEMENT

▪ Typically, if the injury is not detected within 6 months (after which point nerve repair usually is not recommended), a 12-month trial of nonoperative treatment is recommended.[14]

▪ Due to possible compensation by the levator scapulae, the impact of injury to the spinal accessory nerve must be determined individually for each patient.[8]

▪ Maxillofacial surgeons have reported that 30% to 49% of patients do not exhibit any clinical symptoms after radical neck dissection where the spinal accessory nerve is sacrificed.[10]

▪ If the CN XI palsy is symptomatic, pain sometimes can be relieved after a course of nonoperative treatment, but satisfactory return to function cannot be achieved.

▪ Strengthening of the remaining scapulothoracic muscles does not compensate for the trapezius deficit, and, in one study, patients who elected nonoperative management could not elevate their arms above the horizontal.[13]

▪ One study has reported favorable results with nonoperative management in sedentary or elderly persons because discomfort was alleviated.[12]

SURGICAL MANAGEMENT

▪ If trapezius palsy is detected early, microsurgical repair or reconstruction of the nerve can be considered. Timing of the repair attempt is controversial; some authors believe that repair should only be attempted if diagnosis is confirmed within 6 months of injury,[14] whereas other surgeons advocate repair up to 20 months from the time of the nerve insult.[16]

▪ In patients with spontaneous spinal accessory palsy for whom conservative treatment has not been helpful, some authors advocate proceeding directly to muscle transfer reconstruction, because nerve procedures have produced poor results.[15]

▪ Patients who have failed nerve repair attempt or conservative therapy should be considered surgical candidates for the Eden-Lange procedure, the current procedure of choice for stabilization of the scapula after CN XI palsy.

▪ Timing of the Eden-Lange procedure also is controversial. Typically, however, reconstructive surgery is recommended if more than 12 months has elapsed since the injury.[17]

▪ The goal of the Eden-Lange procedure is to reconstruct the three parts of the trapezius muscle. Because the rhomboid major and minor and levator scapulae have medial insertions, they are not capable of stabilizing the scapula unless they are transferred laterally.[16]

Preoperative Planning

▪ It is imperative to have appropriate preoperative discussions with the patient so that he or she understands the procedure, the postoperative rehabilitation program, and the timeframe within which improvement should be expected.

Positioning

▪ The patient is placed in the lateral decubitus position with thoracic, pubic, and sacral supports.[15,16] The entire upper extremity, including the shoulder girdle, should be draped free (**FIG 3**).

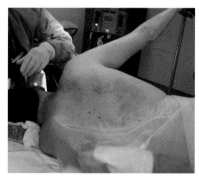

FIG 3 ▪ The patient is placed in the lateral decubitus position with the entire extremity draped free.

EXPOSURE

- Teboul et al[16] describe an incision starting from the spine of the scapula and progressing along its medial angle up to a point 2 cm above the inferior angle of the scapula (**TECH FIG 1A**).
- The trapezius is then divided and retracted, and the three muscles of interest (the levator scapulae,

rhomboid major, and rhomboid minor) are identified and dissected and marked with vessel loops (**TECH FIG 1B**).

- The supraspinatus and infraspinatus must be elevated 3 to 5 cm to expose their respective fossae for transfer of the rhomboids[16] (**TECH FIG 1C**).

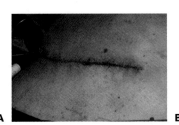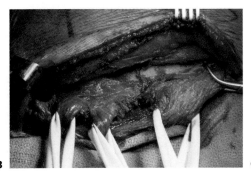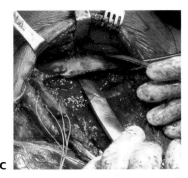

TECH FIG 1 • A. The major incision is made along the medial border of the scapula, extending superiorly to allow exposure to the levator scapula, rhomboid minor, and rhomboid major for their planned transfers. **B.** The levator scapula, rhomboid minor, and rhomboid major are identified and individually released from their scapular attachment sites for lateral transfer. **C.** The supraspinatus and infraspinatus are elevated at least 5 cm medially to allow appropriate exposure of the scapula.

RHOMBOID TRANSFER

- A series of transosseous mattress sutures are placed in anticipation of transferring the rhomboids. At least four mattress sutures are used in the infraspinous fossa (**TECH FIG 2A**) and two in the supraspinous fossa.
- The rhomboids are advanced about 3 cm laterally and attached to the scapula with heavy, nonabsorbable transosseous sutures (**TECH FIG 2B**).

Modification

- Bigliani et al[1] proposed a modification of the procedure in which the rhomboid minor is transferred cephalad to the scapular spine, thereby closing the gap between the rhomboid minor and the levator scapulae (**TECH FIG 3**).
- In this modification, the new position of the rhomboid minor more efficiently substitutes for the middle part of the trapezius.

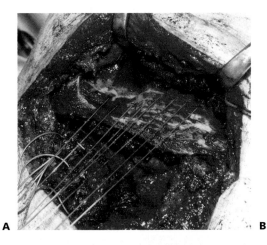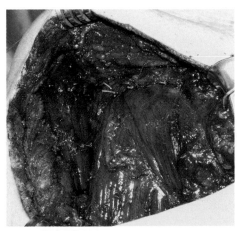

TECH FIG 2 • A. A series of drill holes are made, and transosseous sutures are placed in preparation for securing the transferred muscles. **B.** The rhomboid minor and major are transferred to the supra- and infraspinous fossae, respectively.

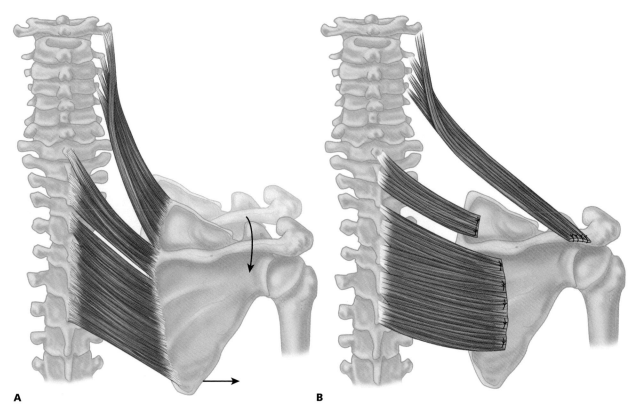

TECH FIG 3 • **A.** Normal position of the levator scapula, rhomboid minor, and rhomboid major on the medial border of the scapula. **B.** Lateral transfer of the levator scapula, rhomboid minor, and rhomboid major. This modification includes transfer of the rhomboid minor to the supraspinatus fossa.

LEVATOR TRANSFER AND WOUND CLOSURE

- A second incision is made about 5 to 7 cm from the posterolateral corner of the acromion for transfer of the levator scapulae (**TECH FIG 4A**).
- Care must be taken to ensure that the levator has been dissected laterally enough to allow tension-free excursion to the scapular spine (**TECH FIG 4B**). The levator is

then transferred subcutaneously and affixed with a series of heavy nonabsorbable sutures.
- The infraspinatus muscle is then sutured over the new rhomboid muscle insertions and, finally, the wounds are closed in layers.

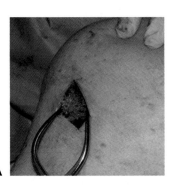

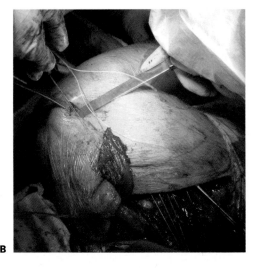

TECH FIG 4 • **A.** The second incision is made 5 to 7 cm medial to the posterolateral corner of the acromion for transfer of the levator scapula muscle. **B.** Excursion of the levator is confirmed before the muscle is subcutaneously tunneled to the planned transfer site.

PEARLS AND PITFALLS

Rhomboid transfer	▪ Separate the rhomboid minor from the rhomboid major so they can be transferred separately. ▪ The infraspinatus and supraspinatus are elevated from their respective fossae for approximately 5 cm. This modification of the original procedure permits the rhomboid minor to be transferred to a position that better substitutes for the action of the middle trapezius. ▪ Care should be taken to prevent injury to the suprascapular nerve, which lies on the deep surface of the supraspinatus muscle.
Levator transfer	▪ Dissect the levator scapula far enough laterally to allow tension-free transfer to the scapular spine. ▪ Avoid iatrogenic injury to the transverse cervical artery and the dorsal scapular nerve, which run superficial and deep, respectively, to the levator scapulae and then terminate into the deep surface of the rhomboids near their insertion onto the scapula. ▪ A tunnel is created through the atrophied trapezius, in line with its upper fibers, for passage of the tagged levator scapulae. ▪ The levator should not be transferred too far laterally, because this can cause a web-like deformity in the neck. A good position is 5 to 7 cm from the posterior lateral corner of the acromion.

POSTOPERATIVE CARE

▪ Most authors advocate immobilization for 6 weeks postoperatively, followed by initiation of physical therapy (passive and active).[13,14,16]

▪ Romero and Gerber[13] prefer an abduction splint, whereas Teboul et al[16] suggest securing the arm to the chest with an elastic bandage.

▪ Our routine postoperative protocol is to use a foam wedge or orthosis for the first 4 weeks, keeping the arm in 60 to 70 degrees of abduction. We encourage early passive range of motion above the wedge or orthosis to prevent stiffness (forward elevation to 130 degrees and external rotation to 40 degrees in the first 4 weeks).

▪ At 4 weeks, the wedge is discontinued, and gentle strengthening exercises are added. We have designed a progressive strengthening program that uses rubber tubing, free weights, and medicine ball throws to achieve dynamic scapular stability. All of the exercises in the protocol are designed to strengthen the transferred levator scapula and rhomboids.

OUTCOMES

▪ The Eden-Lange procedure produces satisfactory results for the difficult problem of trapezius palsy.

▪ In a study in which 16 patients were reviewed at a mean follow-up of 32 years, clinical outcomes were noted to be excellent in 9 patients, fair in 2 patients, and poor in 1 patient (as determined by Constant score).[13] Some patients with outcomes that were less than satisfactory also had dorsal scapular and long thoracic lesions.

▪ Romero and Gerber[13] describe a radiographic outcomes measure that uses an AP radiograph to measure the angle between a line drawn between the cranial and caudal ends of the glenoid with a vertical axial line. This measurement was compared to the contralateral side, and no statistical differences were found.

▪ Another recent study[16] concluded that muscle transfer should be performed only after previous nerve repair surgery had failed or when more than 20 months has elapsed since the injury was incurred. In this series of 7 patients treated with the Eden-Lange procedure (the other 20 patients were treated with nerve surgery), results were excellent in 3 patients, good in 1 patient, and poor in 3 patients. Teboul et al[16] state that two factors are most predictive of a poor result following reconstructive surgery: if the patient is older than 50 years or the lesion is caused by radical neck dissection, penetrating injury, or spontaneous palsy.

COMPLICATIONS

▪ Complications associated with the Eden-Lange procedure, in addition to the usual surgical risks, include failed integration of the transferred muscles with resultant continued dysfunction. Such a complication is discussed rarely, and we were only able to find one report of a failure of muscle integration.[16]

▪ Patient compliance with strict immobilization for the first 6 weeks after surgery is important to avoid pull-out of the transferred muscles, especially the rhomboids, which, unlike the levator scapulae, are not attached to their new scapular insertion with the tendo-osseous interface intact.

▪ Initial complications do not seem to be the problem with the Eden-Lange procedure; rather, the primary complication appears to be later effects of functional outcome falling short of expectations.

▪ Iatrogenic dysfunction resulting from no longer having a physiologic levator scapula or rhomboids is not, to our knowledge, discussed in the literature. However, because the origin of these muscles is merely being transposed more laterally, it does not appear that the Eden-Lange procedure creates a new problem while fixing the old one.

▪ In cases of failure of the procedure, where pain and dysfunction continue, scapulothoracic arthrodesis can be performed as a salvage procedure.

REFERENCES

1. Bigliani LU, Compito CA, Duralde XA, et al. Transfer of the levator scapulae, rhomboid major, and rhomboid minor for paralysis of the trapezius. J Bone Joint Surg Am 1996;78:1534–1540.
2. Bigliani LU, Perez-Sanz JR, Wolfe IN. Treatment of trapezius paralysis. J Bone Joint Surg Am 1985;67:871–877.
3. Burns S, Herbison GJ. Spinal accessory nerve injury as a complication of internal jugular vein cannulation. Ann Intern Med 1996;125:700.
4. Dunn AW. Trapezius paralysis after minor surgical procedures in the posterior cervical triangle. South Med J 1974;67:312–315.
5. Eden R. Zur behandlung der trapeziuslahmung mittels muselplastik. Deutsche Zeitschr Chir 1924;184:387–397.
6. Eisen A, Bertrand G. Isolated accessory nerve palsy of spontaneous origin. A clinical and electromyographic study. Arch Neurol 1972;27:496–502.
7. Francillon MR. Zur Behandlung de Accesoriuslahmung. Schweiz Med Wochenschr 1955;33:787–788.

8. Kondo M, Shiro T, Yamada M. Changes of the tilting angle of the scapula following elevation of the arm. In Bateman JE, Walsh RP, eds. Surgery of the Shoulder. Philadelphia: BC Decker, 1984:136–138.

9. Lange M. Die Behandlung der irreparablen Trapeziuslahmung. Langenbecks Arch Klin Chir 1951;270:437–439.

10. Leipzig B, Suen JY, English JL, et al. Functional evaluation of the spinal accessory nerve after neck dissection. Am J Surg 1983;146:526–530.

11. Patterson WR. Inferior dislocation of the distal end of the clavicle: a case report. J Bone Joint Surg Am 1967;49A:1184–1186.

12. Pelissier J, Lopez S, Herisson C, et al. [Shoulder pain and trapezius paralysis: Evaluation of a rehabilitation protocol.] Rev Rhum Mal Osteoartic 1990;57:319–321. In French.

13. Romero J, Gerber C. Levator scapulae and rhomboid transfer for paralysis of trapezius: The Eden-Lange procedure. J Bone Joint Surg Br 2003;85B:1141–1145.

14. Setter KJ, Voloshin I, Bigliani LU. Operative treatment of spinal accessory nerve palsy. Techniques in Shoulder and Elbow Surgery 2004;5:25–36.

15. Teboul F, Bizot P, Kakkar R, et al. Surgical management of trapezius palsy. J Bone Joint Surg Am 2005;87(Suppl 1):285–291.

16. Teboul F, Bizot P, Kakkar R, et al. Surgical management of trapezius palsy. J Bone Joint Surg Am 2004;86A:1884–1890.

17. Wiater JM, Bigliani LU. Spinal accessory nerve injury. Clin Orthop Relat Res 1999;368:5–16.

Chapter 30

Pectoralis Major Transfer for Long Thoracic Nerve Palsy

Raymond A. Klug, Bradford O. Parsons, and Evan L. Flatow

DEFINITION

- Long thoracic nerve palsy leads to classical scapular winging because of weakness of the serratus anterior muscle (**FIG 1**).
  - Other types of winging include trapezius winging and rhomboid winging.
- Lesions of the long thoracic nerve can range from paresis to complete paralysis, leading to varying degrees of shoulder dysfunction.
- The serratus anterior muscle functions to stabilize the scapula against the chest wall, thus providing a fulcrum for the humerus to push against while moving the arm in space.[3,4]
  - Without this fulcrum, shoulder elevation is weakened, which leads to inability to use the arm in forward activities.
  - Forward elevation of the shoulder is most severely affected, followed by shoulder abduction.

ANATOMY

- The serratus anterior is a large broad muscle that covers the lateral aspect of the thorax. It has digitations that take origin from the upper nine ribs, pass deep to the scapula, and insert on the medial aspect of the scapula.[15]
- The muscle has three divisions.[5]
  - The first division consists of one slip and takes origin from the first two ribs. This division runs slightly upward and inserts on the superior angle of the scapula.
  - The second division is made up of three slips from the second, third, and fourth ribs, and inserts on the anterior surface of the medial border of the scapula.
  - The third division, which consists of the inferior five slips from ribs five through nine, inserts on the inferior angle of the scapula. Because this division has the longest course it has the longest lever-arm and the most power for scapular rotation.
- The serratus anterior muscle stabilizes the scapula against the chest wall, creating a fulcrum for the proximal humerus to lever against while moving the arm in space.
  - The serratus anterior protracts and upwardly rotates the glenoid.
  - Its direction of pull brings the inferomedial border of the scapula anteriorly. The inferior border of the scapula is pulled forward with forward elevation of the arm. This causes the glenoid to tip posteriorly and allow full forward elevation without impingement.
  - With weakness of the serratus anterior muscle, the scapula translates superiorly and medially, and the inferior border rotates medially and dorsally (**FIG 2A**).
- The serratus anterior muscle is innervated by the long thoracic nerve, which arises from the ventral rami of cervical roots C5–7.
  - The C5 and C6 roots pass through the scalenus medius muscle and merge before they receive a branch from C7.
  - The nerve enters the axillary sheath at the level of the first rib and travels posteriorly in the axilla.
  - It then passes over a prominence in the second rib and descends along the lateral chest wall, where it enters the serratus anterior fascia and then the muscle itself (**FIG 2C**).[5,15]
- The total length of the nerve is about 24 cm, and there are several possible points of injury.
  - Proximally, as well as distally along the chest wall, the nerve is susceptible to injury because of its superficial location.
  - The nerve is tethered in the axillary sheath, which places it on stretch with forward elevation of the arm.

PATHOGENESIS

Scapular Winging

- Scapular winging may be due to primary, secondary, or voluntary causes.[8]
- Primary scapular winging can be divided into neurologic, bony, and soft tissue types.
  - Neurologic disorders, which are most common, include:
    - Long thoracic nerve palsy (serratus anterior weakness)
    - Spinal accessory nerve palsy (trapezius weakness)
    - Dorsal scapular nerve palsy (rhomboid weakness)
    - Trapezius weakness winging may be distinguished from serratus winging by the position and direction of scapular laxity (see Fig 2A,B).
  - Bony abnormalities include osteochondromas of the scapula or fracture malunion.
  - Soft tissue disorders include:
    - Soft tissue contractures, causing winging
    - Muscular disorders such as fascioscapulohumeral dystrophy

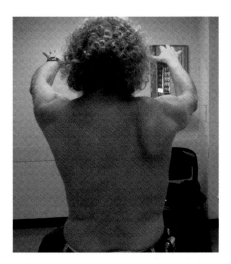

FIG 1 • Clinical photograph of serratus winging.

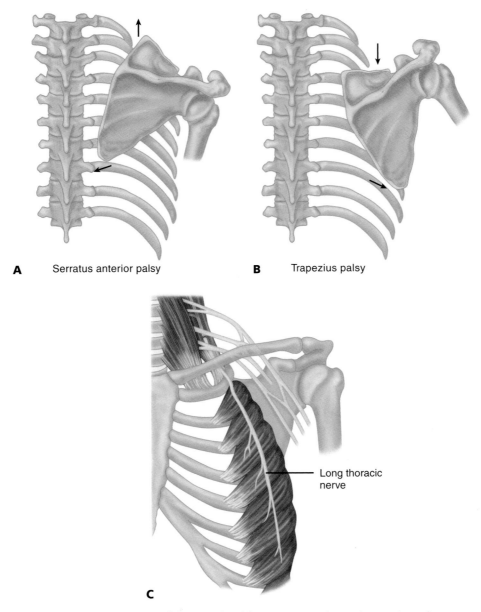

A Serratus anterior palsy

B Trapezius palsy

C

FIG 2 • A,B. Resting position of the scapula with serratus anterior and trapezius palsy. **C.** Superficial location of the long thoracic nerve.

■ Congenital absence or traumatic rupture of the parascapular muscles

■ Scapulothoracic bursitis

■ Secondary winging may occur following disorders of the glenohumeral joint. The most common causes are multidirectional and posterior instability.

■ The sequence of events leading to secondary scapular winging due to primary shoulder pathology is as follows:

■ Primary glenulohumeral or subacromial pathology, *leading to*

■ Limited glenulohumeral motion, *leading to*

■ Increased compensatory scapulothoracic motion, *leading to*

■ Increased demand on periscapular muscles, *leading to*

■ Fatigue of periscapular muscles—serratus, trapezius, and rhomboids—*leading to*

■ Secondary scapular winging

■ Voluntary winging may occur in psychiatric patients or for secondary gain.

Long Thoracic Nerve Palsy

■ Long thoracic nerve palsy is the most common cause of serratus dysfunction resulting in symptomatic scapular winging, especially in those patients who fail nonoperative management and are being considered for pectoralis tendon transfer.[1]

■ Long thoracic nerve palsy has been reported to result from idiopathic, iatrogenic, viral, compressive, or traumatic (blunt or penetrating) causes.[15]

■ Most injuries are neurapraxic, due to blunt trauma.

■ Lesions also may occur through entrapment of the fifth or sixth cervical roots at the level of the scalenus medius, during traction over the second rib, or with traction and compression at the inferior angle of the scapula with general anesthesia or prolonged abduction of the arm.

■ Iatrogenic injuries may occur during radical mastectomy, first rib resection, or transaxillary sympathectomy, or during surgical positioning.[6]

■ Other less common causes include viral illnesses, Parsonage-Turner syndrome, isolated long thoracic neuritis, immunizations, or C7 nerve root lesions.

  ■ Often, the cause is idiopathic, with a questionable history of trauma or viral illness.

Pathoanatomy

■ A mechanical advantage is gained by stabilization of the scapula against the chest wall.

  ■ With loss of this mechanical advantage, forward elevation against resistance is decreased owing to scapulothoracic motion.

■ Additional types of shoulder pathology can result secondary to stabilization of the scapula:

  ■ Impingement due to relative anterior rotation of the acromion (**FIG 3**)

  ■ Weakness due to loss of mechanical advantage in forward elevation

  ■ Adhesive capsulitis from disuse

■ With complete paralysis of the serratus anterior, complete forward elevation and abduction greater than 110 degrees are not possible.[3,15]

NATURAL HISTORY

■ As mentioned previously, most injuries to the long thoracic nerve are neurapraxic from stretch of the nerve or blunt trauma.

■ Most cases resolve spontaneously without operative intervention within 12 months, although maximal recovery may take up to 24 months.[2,7,9]

■ The exception to this rule is injury due to nerve laceration from penetrating trauma or iatrogenic injury.

PATIENT HISTORY AND PHYSICAL FINDINGS

■ A thorough history (including previous illnesses, procedures and interventions, hand dominance, and activity level) and complete examination of the shoulder and back are essential.

■ Treatment often is delayed, and diagnosis may become apparent only after failed treatment for other disorders.

  ■ Furthermore, patients may develop secondary stiffness from disuse, and this may be the primary complaint.

■ Patients often present with vague complaints of shoulder pain or weakness with overhead activities.

  ■ Because winging may be subtle, the patient must be undressed from the waist up, viewed from the back, and tested with provocative maneuvers such as resisted forward elevation and pushups against a wall.

■ Pain may come from several sources, making diagnosis of long thoracic nerve palsy based on pain distribution difficult.

  ■ Compensatory overuse of the remaining scapulothoracic musculature may cause pain localized posteriorly about the scapula.

  ■ Patients may present with impingement-type pain with forward elevation.

  ■ In secondary winging, pain may result from an underlying diagnosis such as glenohumeral instability.

  ■ With severe pain, long thoracic neuritis or Parsonage-Turner syndrome should be considered.

■ Physical examination usually reveals classic winging, with the scapula translated medially and the inferior border rotated toward the midline (see Fig 1).

■ Patients may present with varying degrees of weakness of forward elevation of the arm.

  ■ Resisted testing may accentuate winging, as will having the patient do a pushup against a wall.

  ■ Weakness of forward elevation may be decreased by manual scapular stabilization against the chest wall by an examiner, the so-called "scapular stabilization test."[13]

IMAGING AND OTHER DIAGNOSTIC STUDIES

■ Plain radiographs of the shoulder, cervical spine, and chest should be part of the workup.

  ■ Although radiographs rarely are diagnostic, bony abnormalities such as osteochondromas, cervical spondylosis, or scoliosis may be evident.

  ■ CT or MRI scans may be helpful in these situations, but are often not necessary.

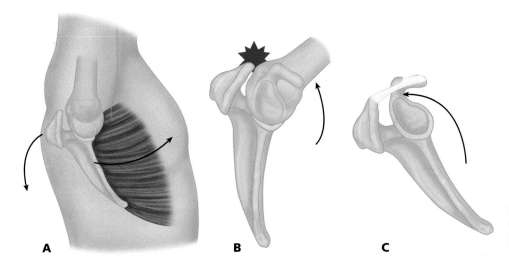

FIG 3 • Normal and abnormal scapular kinematics and its relationship to subacromial impingement syndrome.

A   **B**   **C**

■ Electromyographic and nerve conduction velocity studies are useful in confirming the diagnosis as well as following patients clinically.

   ■ Additionally, in idiopathic cases or where dystrophy is suspected, these tests may be helpful in ruling out other neuromuscular disorders (such as fascioscapulohumeral dystrophy) that may preclude muscle transfer as an option for scapular stabilization.

   ■ Serial studies every 3 months are recommended.

   ■ Studies should include cervical roots, brachial plexus, and the spinal accessory nerve.

DIFFERENTIAL DIAGNOSIS

■ Rotator cuff tear
■ Fracture malunion
■ Glenohumeral instability
■ Impingement
■ Acromioclavicular joint disease
■ Biceps tendinitis
■ Neurologic disorders
■ Suprascapular nerve entrapment
■ Scoliosis
■ Scapular osteochondroma

NONOPERATIVE MANAGEMENT

■ Whether idiopathic, viral, or compressive, almost all cases of serratus winging from long thoracic palsy resolve spontaneously within 1 to 2 years.[2,7,9]

   ■ Without a clear history of penetrating trauma, all patients initially should be treated conservatively (**FIG 4**).

   ■ Physical therapy should consist of range-of-motion exercises to avoid secondary glenohumeral stiffness.

   ■ Braces and orthotics that have been designed to stabilize the scapula to the chest wall may provide symptomatic

relief. Their use is controversial, however, and many patients find them cumbersome.

   ■ Some authors have recommended bracing to decrease continued traction on the nerve.[14]

SURGICAL MANAGEMENT

■ Patients for whom nonoperative treatment has failed and who have persistent symptomatic scapular winging are candidates for surgical stabilization.

■ Patients often are given up to 24 months to recover nerve and muscle function before surgical repair is considered.

   ■ However, Fery[2] has reported that up to 25% of patients with serratus anterior paralysis may fail nonoperative treatment.

   ■ Patients who have penetrating trauma or iatrogenic injury, where a long thoracic nerve transection is suspected, may be indicated for acute nerve exploration and repair.

■ Historically, three different procedures have been used to treat patients with symptomatic serratus anterior dysfunction: scapulothoracic fusion, static stabilization procedures, and dynamic muscle transfers.

   ■ Scapulothoracic fusion is mainly a salvage procedure, sometimes used in patients with previous failures or in patients with dystrophies, such as fascioscapulohumeral dystrophy, where multiple muscles may be affected.

   ■ Static stabilization uses fascial slings or tethers to help stabilize the scapula.

   ■ These procedures have fallen out of favor because the slings may gradually stretch out, with subsequent loss of scapular stability.

■ Dynamic muscle transfers, first described by Tubby[12] in 1904, have been found to offer the optimal recovery and result in nearly normal scapulothoracic motion.

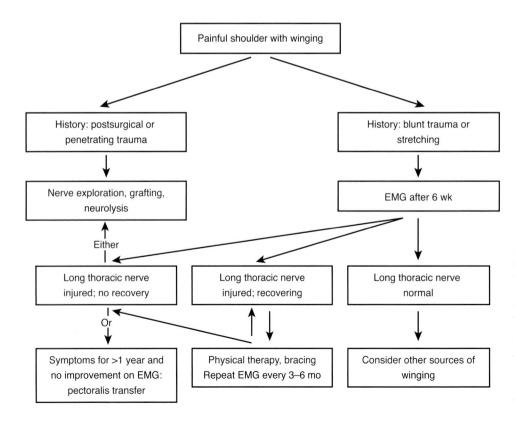

FIG 4 • Algorithm for treatment of serratus palsy. EMG, electromyography. (Adapted from Kuhn JE. The scapulothoracic articulation: anatomy, biomechanics, pathophysiology, and management. In: Iannotti JP, Williams GR Jr., eds. Disorders of the Shoulder: Diagnosis and Management, ed 2. Philadelphia: Lippincott Williams & Wilkins, 2007:1058–1086.)

Numerous different transfers have been described, but most surgeons currently perform a transfer of the sternal head of the pectoralis major to the inferior angle of the scapula to reconstruct the function of the deficient serratus anterior.

■ The sternal head of the pectoralis is preferred because it has good excursion and similar power to the serratus, and its fiber orientation is similar to that of the serratus.[1,2]

Preoperative Planning

■ Preoperative planning should include a discussion with the patient regarding allograft versus autograft augmentation of the pectoralis transfer.

■ Typical options include contralateral fascia lata or semitendinosus autograft, or semitendinosus allograft.

■ A tendon stripper is needed for autograft harvest if desired.

■ A 5-mm round trip burr or drill bit is needed to fashion a tunnel through the inferior angle of the scapula.

■ Heavy nonabsorbable suture (no. 2 or no. 5) is needed to attach the pectoralis transfer and prepare the graft augmentation.

Patient Positioning

■ The patient is placed supine in the beach chair position, with care taken to leave access to the midline posteriorly and anteriorly.

■ A pad is placed behind the midline of the thorax to improve posterior exposure.

■ The forequarter is draped free with the entire scapula in the surgical field.

■ A pneumatic arm positioner (Spider Limb Positioner, Tenet Medical Engineering, distributed by Smith & Nephew Endoscopy, Andover, MA) is helpful during the procedure to maintain position of the extremity.

■ If fascia lata or semitendinosus autograft is to be harvested, the lower extremity must be prepped and draped free as well.

Approach

■ The following section describes our preferred technique for transfer of the sternal head of the pectoralis major to the inferior angle of the scapula for serratus anterior dysfunction.

EXPOSURE

■ A 10- to 15-cm incision is made in the axillary crease posterior to the lateral border of the scapula (**TECH FIG 1A**).

■ The deltopectoral interval is developed, and the cephalic vein is retracted laterally.

■ The pectoralis tendon is identified at its humeral insertion.

■ The sternal head, which lies deep to the clavicular head, is identified and isolated bluntly (**TECH FIG 1B,C**).

■ Often, abduction and external rotation of the extremity is helpful in exposing the sternal head.

■ The sternal head insertion is released sharply from the humerus, taking care not to damage the underlying long head of the biceps tendon or the clavicular head of the pectoralis major (**TECH FIG 1D,E**).

■ Traction sutures are placed into the sternal head tendon, and the muscle belly is freed of adhesions medially.

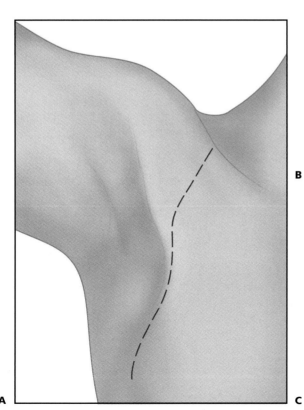
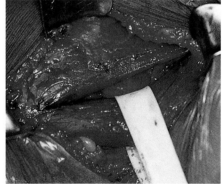
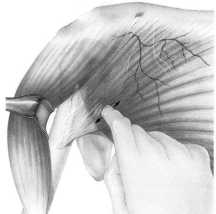

TECH FIG 1 • A. Axillary incision used for pectoralis major transfer. **B,C.** The sternal head, which lies deep to the clavicular head, is identified and isolated bluntly. *(continued)*

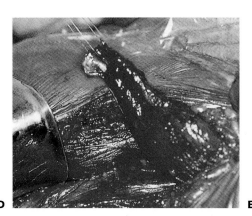
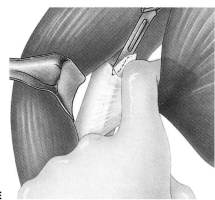

TECH FIG 1 • *(continued)* **D,E.** The sternal head insertion is released sharply from the humerus, taking care not to damage the underlying long head of the biceps tendon or the clavicular head of the pectoralis major. (**B–E:** from Post M. Orthopaedic management of neuromuscular disorders. In: Post M, Flatow EL, Bigliani LU, Pollack RG, eds. The Shoulder: Operative Technique. Philadelphia: Lippincott Williams & Wilkins, 1998:201–234.)

GRAFT HARVESTING

- At this point, attention is turned to the fascia lata harvest, or preparation of the allograft tendon.
  - For fascia lata harvest, two small incisions (2 to 3 cm) are made on the lateral aspect of the thigh, about 20 cm apart.
  - After incision, the fascia lata is exposed and cleaned with an elevator between the two incisions.
  - Once the fascia lata is identified and isolated, a tendon stripper is used to harvest a graft approximately 6 cm × 20 cm.

- The graft is then folded over itself and tubularized using heavy, nonabsorbable suture.
- Once prepared, the graft is woven into the sternal head tendinous origin and secured with heavy, nonabsorbable suture (**TECH FIG 2**).

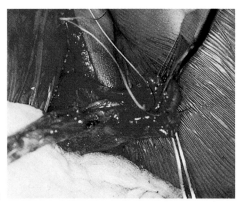
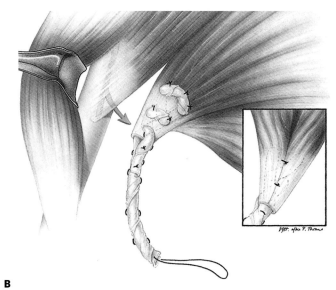

TECH FIG 2 • Once prepared, the graft is woven into the sternal head tendinous origin and secured with heavy, nonabsorbable suture. (From Post M. Orthopaedic management of neuromuscular disorders. In: Post M, Flatow EL, Bigliani LU, et al, eds. The Shoulder: Operative Technique. Philadelphia: Lippincott Williams & Wilkins, 1998:210–234.)

SCAPULAR EXPOSURE, PREPARATION, AND TENDON ATTACHMENT

- After the pectoralis tendon and graft are ready, the scapula is exposed.
- The inferior angle of the scapula is identified and exposed by blunt dissection along the chest wall.
- The latissimus dorsi and teres major tendons are retracted distally, and the lateral neurovascular structures are avoided by staying medial.
- Once the inferior angle of the scapula is identified, it is exposed subperiosteally, and a 6- to 8-mm burr hole is made 2 cm from the lateral and inferior border of the scapula.
- The graft is then passed through the bone hole from anterior to posterior, tensioning the graft while reducing the scapula on the chest wall, so that the native pectoralis tendon is flush with the bone tunnel.
- The graft is then looped through the hole in the inferior scapula and sutured to itself using heavy, nonabsorbable suture (**TECH FIG 3**).
    - It is necessary to ensure that native pectoralis tendon is brought to the scapula, because the tendon graft may stretch over time.

TECH FIG 3 • The graft is looped through the hole in the inferior scapula and sutured to itself using heavy, nonabsorbable suture. (From Post M. Orthopaedic management of neuromuscular disorders. In: Post M, Flatow EL, Bigliani LU, et al, eds. The Shoulder: Operative Technique. Philadelphia: Lippincott Williams & Wilkins, 1998:210–234.)

- The wound is then closed in layers over a drain.
- The extremity is placed in a sling and a scapulothoracic orthosis, which maintains pressure on the scapula against the chest wall.

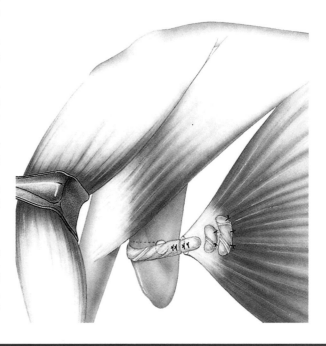

PEARLS AND PITFALLS

- Electromyography is helpful in identifying patients with dystrophy or other palsies, which may preclude the possibility of a sternal head transfer for serratus anterior dysfunction.
- Patients with blunt trauma or idiopathic etiologies initially should be managed nonoperatively, because most will recover serratus anterior function.
- The sternal head lies deep to the clavicular head, and positioning the arm in abduction and external rotation can help identify the insertion of the tendon.
- When approaching the inferior scapula, care is taken to stay medial while retracting the latissimus and teres major distally, because the neurovascular structures are lateral.
- The scapula should be reduced to the chest wall by an assistant before tensioning the pectoralis transfer.
- Avoid scapular fracture by keeping the osseous tunnel a minimum of 1 cm away from the scapular borders.
- The sternal head is lengthened by autograft or allograft, but it is critical to have native, living pectoralis tendon attached directly to the inferior scapula. The auto- or allograft is meant for augmentation.

POSTOPERATIVE CARE

- Patients are kept immobilized in the sling and orthosis for 6 weeks.
- After 6 weeks, range-of-motion exercises are begun, and the brace is discontinued.
- Strengthening exercises are begun as motion returns.
- Patients are restricted from heavy lifting or manual labor for 6 months.

OUTCOMES

- Most series of sternal head transfer for serratus anterior dysfunction and scapular winging report good to excellent results with improvement in function, relief of pain, and correction of winging.
    - Post[11] reported on eight patients treated with sternal head transfer with excellent results.
    - Connor et al[1] reported on 11 patients, 10 of whom (91%) had significant improvement in pain and function and relief of winging.
    - Warner and Navarro[13] reported that seven of eight patients had excellent results, with the only unsatisfactory outcome following a deep infection.
    - Conversely, Noerdlinger et al[10] reported that of 15 patients treated, only 7 (47%) had good to excellent results. They found that those patients who lacked external rotation at follow-up

had poorer results, and that more aggressive therapy regarding rotation may be needed.

COMPLICATIONS

- Seroma and infection[13]
- Neurovascular injury
- Scapular fracture through bone tunnel
- Shoulder stiffness[10]
- Graft loosening and loss of tension[11]

REFERENCES

1. Connor PM, Yamaguchi K, Manifold SG, et al. Split pectoralis major transfer for serratus anterior palsy. Clin Orthop Relat Res 1997; 341:134–142.
2. Fery A. Results of treatment of anterior serratus paralysis. In Post M, Morrey BF, Hawkins R, eds. Surgery of the Shoulder. St. Louis: Mosby-Year Book, 1990:325–329.
3. Gregg JR, Labosky D, Harty M, et al. Serratus anterior paralysis in the young athlete. J Bone Joint Surg Am 1979;61A:825–832.
4. Inman VT, Saunders JB, Abbott LC. Observations on the function of the shoulder joint. J Bone Joint Surg 1944;26:1–30.
5. Jobe CM. Gross anatomy of the shoulder. In Rockwood CA Jr, Matsen FA III, eds. The Shoulder. Philadelphia: WB Saunders, 1998:34–94.
6. Kauppila LI, Vastamaki M. Iatrogenic serratus anterior paralysis. Long-term outcome in 26 patients. Chest 1996;109:31–34.
7. Kuhn JE, Hawkins RJ. Evaluation and treatment of scapular disorders. In Warner JJ, Iannotti JP, Gerber C. Complex and Revision Problems in Shoulder Surgery. Philadelphia: Lippincott-Raven, 1997:357–376.
8. Kuhn JE, Plancher KD, Hawkins RJ. Scapular winging. J Am Acad Orthop Surg 1995;3:319–325.
9. Leffert RD. Neurologic problems. In Rockwood CA Jr, Matsen FA III, eds. The Shoulder. Philadelphia: WB Saunders, 1998:965–988.
10. Noerdlinger MA, Cole BJ, Stewart M, et al. Results of pectoralis major transfer with fascia lata autograft augmentation for scapula winging. J Shoulder Elbow Surg 2002;11:345–350.
11. Post M. Pectoralis major transfer for winging of the scapula. J Shoulder Elbow Surg 1995;4:1–9.
12. Tubby AH. A case illustrating the operative treatment of paralysis of the serratus magnus by muscle grafting. Br Med J 1904;2:1159–1160.
13. Warner JJ, Navarro RA. Serratus anterior dysfunction. Recognition and treatment. Clin Orthop Relat Res 1998;349:139–148.
14. Watson CJ, Schenkman M. Physical therapy management of isolated serratus anterior muscle paralysis. Phys Ther 1995;75:194–202.
15. Wiater JM, Flatow EL. Long thoracic nerve injury. Clin Orthop Relat Res 1999;368:17–27.

Shadley C. Schiffern and Sumant G. Krishnan

DEFINITION

▪ Refractory disorders of the scapulothoracic articulation have been reported to result in debilitating pain and dysfunction that may require surgical management.

▪ The most common clinical presentation, scapular winging,[12] was first reported in the published literature in 1723, and several etiologies for scapular winging have been documented since then.

▪ Soft tissue operations (eg, pectoralis major tendon transfer) have had reported success in stabilizing the dyskinetic scapula in appropriate patients.

▪ Despite successful clinical outcomes, a population of patients experience recurrent symptomatic scapular winging even after pectoralis major transfer.[6,10,12]

 ▪ Several authors[5,7,10,12] report that arthrodesis is the treatment of choice for these failed muscle transfers. For failed pectoralis transfer or significant (ie, irreducible) fixed winging, scapulothoracic arthrodesis can be a successful salvage operation for these patients.[14]

ANATOMY

▪ The scapula is positioned over the posterolateral aspect of the rib cage, overlying ribs 1 to 7. It is suspended from the sternum by the clavicle anteriorly and plays an important role in positioning the upper extremity for proper function.

▪ The lateral scapula includes the glenoid fossa for articulation with the humeral head.

▪ The scapula provides an attachment for 16 muscles, which help maintain it in functional positions. It articulates on the thoracic cavity, allowing rotation, protraction, and retraction.

▪ A thin bursal layer separates the scapula from the underlying ribs.

PATHOGENESIS

▪ Dysfunction of the scapulothoracic articulation has been well documented in the peer-reviewed literature.

▪ The most common manifestation of scapulothoracic dysfunction is symptomatic scapular winging[7,12] (**FIG 1**).

 ▪ Traumatic injuries to the serratus anterior muscle or the long thoracic nerve have been reported to cause symptomatic winging.[7,8,11,12,19,20]

 ▪ Atraumatic etiologies, such as neuralgic amyotrophy, polio, and the muscular dystrophies, also may produce disabling scapular winging.[1,2,4,5,8,10,15,16]

 ▪ Intolerable winging also has been demonstrated in association with other bony abnormalities (eg, rib or scapular osteochondromas and malunited scapular fractures) or soft tissue lesions (eg, scapular-stabilizing muscle contractures, muscle avulsions, and scapulothoracic bursitis).[3,11,12]

 ▪ Recent authors[18] have reported a significant incidence of scapular winging secondary to glenohumeral joint lesions such as rotator cuff tears and glenohumeral instability (especially posterior and multidirectional instability).

▪ The scapulothoracic articulation also is a potential source of debilitating pain in the shoulder girdle.

 ▪ Several authors[9,13,17,18] have documented the incidence of painful scapulothoracic crepitus ("snapping scapula" syndrome) and scapulothoracic bursitis.

 ▪ Painful crepitus can be due to interposed muscle, fibrous and granulomatous lesions, or bony incongruity associated with osteochondromata, fractures, scoliosis, or kyphosis.[13]

NATURAL HISTORY

▪ Most patients who present with symptomatic scapular winging, scapulothoracic pain, or crepitus respond to nonoperative measures.

▪ A subset of this patient population, however, experiences complex scapulothoracic dysfunction or pain refractory to conservative measures.

PATIENT HISTORY AND PHYSICAL FINDINGS

▪ Patients presenting with scapulothoracic disorders typically complain of debilitating pain, shoulder dysfunction, or scapulothoracic crepitus.

▪ Physical findings commonly include scapular winging, crepitus, alterations in normal scapulohumeral rhythm, or neurologic deficits.

▪ Physical examination should focus on the resting posture of the scapula, as well as its dynamic position.

 ▪ Both scapulae should be observed and palpated while the arms are elevated or while the patient performs a wall push-up. These dynamic tests may make subtle winging more obvious.

 ▪ The pattern of winging distinguishes between serratus anterior dysfunction (long thoracic nerve) or trapezius palsy (spinal accessory nerve).

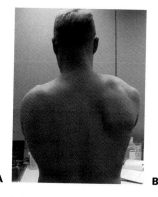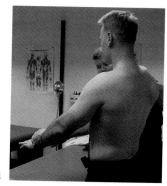

FIG 1 • A. Moderate dynamic scapular winging demonstrated with slow forward elevation of the arms in the frontal plane. **B.** The same patient demonstrating marked medial winging with the resisted elevation at 30 degrees.

▪ The more common medial winging is consistent with serratus anterior dysfunction, whereas lateral winging is observed in trapezius palsy.

▪ Further assessment includes the scapula stabilization test to assess for fixed or correctable winging. This test is crucial in determining fixed versus reducible winging. It demonstrates the amount of discomfort the patient has and indicates the extent to which reduction of the scapula will relieve that discomfort.

▪ Painful crepitus localized to the scapulothoracic region is verified by diagnostic injection, in which 1% lidocaine is injected beneath the medial border of the scapula into the scapulothoracic bursa. Improvement in pain may be noted in the examination room, further supporting the diagnosis.

IMAGING AND OTHER DIAGNOSTIC STUDIES

▪ Standard plain radiographs of the shoulder, including anteroposterior views in internal and external rotation, axillary lateral views, and scapula Y views are obtained to evaluate the status of the clavicle, acromioclavicular joint, glenohumeral joint, and bony contour of the scapula.

▪ CT scans, including axial images and reformatted coronal and sagittal images, provide further detail, and may be required to assess scapula morphology and the presence of exostoses or deformity.

▪ Electromyography and nerve conduction velocity are important to verify neurologic dysfunction of the long thoracic or spinal accessory nerves.

DIFFERENTIAL DIAGNOSIS

▪ Long thoracic nerve palsy
▪ Spinal accessory nerve palsy
▪ Glenohumeral joint derangement with secondary scapular winging
▪ Scapulothoracic bursitis
▪ Snapping scapula
▪ Scapular exostosis or osteochondroma

NONOPERATIVE MANAGEMENT

▪ Nonoperative treatment is the cornerstone of management of scapulothoracic dysfunction.

▪ Therapeutic modalities involve supervised scapular–stabilizer and glenohumeral stretching and strengthening, the judicious use of oral anti-inflammatory medications, and selective cortisone injections.

SURGICAL MANAGEMENT

▪ Patients who have failed an extensive nonoperative course are candidates for surgical treatment.

▪ Surgical options for scapulothoracic dysfunction include:
  ▪ Arthroscopic or open decompression and bursectomy or medial border scapulectomy for painful crepitus
  ▪ Split pectoralis major tendon transfer for dynamic winging
  ▪ Scapulothoracic arthrodesis

▪ Surgical indications for scapulothoracic arthrodesis include the following clinical situations:
  ▪ For patients with disabling pain associated with crepitus, failure of previous resection of the superomedial border of the scapula is an indication for fusion.

▪ For patients with disabling pain associated with fixed scapular winging or failed pectoralis transfer, indications for fusion include:
  ▪ Significant winging
  ▪ Difficulty in reducing the scapula with the "scapular stabilization test"
  ▪ Significant pain relief (>75%) that substantially improved function during a scapular stabilization test

Preoperative Planning

▪ Preoperative anesthesia consultation is recommended. We use general anesthesia with a double-lumen endotracheal tube to allow for selective deflation of the ipsilateral lung during wire passage.

Positioning

▪ Patients are placed in the prone position.
▪ Care is taken to pad all bony prominences.
▪ The entire involved arm, scapula, and ipsilateral posterior iliac crest are prepped and draped to the midline of the spine (**FIG 2**).
  ▪ It is essential that the entire arm be prepped and draped in the surgical field to allow for appropriate manipulation of the scapula and accurate placement of the scapula on the rib cage for fusion.

Approach

▪ A direct approach to the scapulothoracic articulation along the medial border of the scapula is used. This approach allows excellent exposure of the underlying ribs and undersurface of the scapula. The superficial location of the scapula makes this approach relatively straightforward.

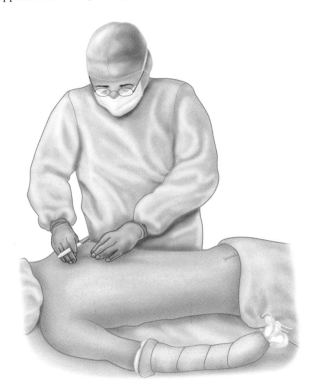

FIG 2 • Patient in the prone position. The surgical preparation must include the entire arm and the back, extending medially past the midline of the spine and inferiorly to include the posterior superior iliac crest.

EXPOSURE

- The incision is placed along the medial border of the scapula from just superior to the scapular spine to the inferior angle.
- The superficial fascia is incised, and the trapezius muscle is identified and retracted medially (**TECH FIG 1A**). The rhomboid muscles are incised off the medial edge of the scapula and are tagged for reattachment before closure (**TECH FIG 1B**).
- With the rhomboid muscles elevated, a rake retractor can be placed on the anterior surface of the medial

scapular border to retract the medial scapula away from the rib cage (**TECH FIG 1C**).

- About one third of the musculature of the serratus anterior and the subscapularis is resected from medial to lateral off the anterior surface of the scapula to allow for a wide fusion surface (**TECH FIG 1D**).
- Care must be taken to avoid resecting the subscapularis beyond the midline of the scapula to prevent denervation.

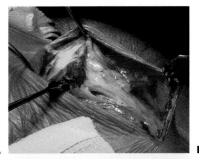
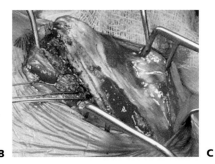
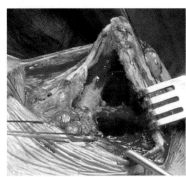
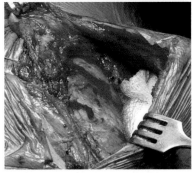

TECH FIG 1 • **A.** Superficial dissection proceeds down to the trapezial fascia, and the trapezius is retracted medially. **B.** The rhomboids are released from the medial border of the scapula and tagged for later repair. **C.** A retractor is positioned on the medial border of the scapula, and the scapula is elevated, allowing for dissection of the scapulothoracic articulation and underlying ribs. **D.** Following dissection of one third of the serratus anterior and subscapularis musculature, a wide fusion bed is visualized overlying the ribs.

BONY PREPARATION

- The anterior surface of the scapula is now roughened slightly with a burr (**TECH FIG 2A**). Care must be taken during this maneuver to avoid thinning the medial border excessively, because that could lead to fracture during hardware fixation.
- Next, the scapula is reduced to the rib cage in approximately 20 to 25 degrees of external rotation from the midline to maximize subsequent shoulder range of motion (most notably elevation and external rotation).
- If patients demonstrated concomitant multidirectional glenohumeral instability with a symptomatic inferior component, the scapula is rotated externally 35 to 40 degrees from the midline to use the inferior glenoid rim to buttress against inferior translation.

- The ribs corresponding to the decorticated anterior surface of the scapula are identified, and the scapula is again retracted to allow for rib preparation.
  - Depending on the size and configuration of the scapula, three or four ribs typically will be used in the fusion (usually the third to sixth ribs).
- The periosteum is incised carefully in a longitudinal direction and stripped off each rib (**TECH FIG 2B,C**).
- The ribs are minimally roughened with a burr down to bleeding bone.
- It is essential to remove all areas of soft tissue between the scapula and rib cage to permit maximum bony contact between the anterior surface of the scapula and the ribs (**TECH FIG 2D**).

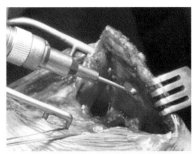
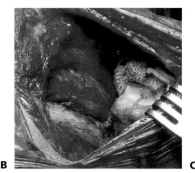
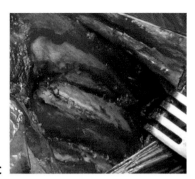

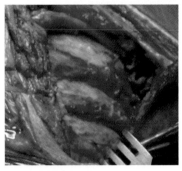

TECH FIG 2 • A. The anterior surface of the scapula is lightly decorticated with a motorized oval burr. **B.** The first rib has been prepared with the periosteum incised and stripped off of the rib, ready for light decortication. **C.** Rib preparation continues, exposing the bony surface of the ribs corresponding to the undersurface of the scapula. This typically involves three to four ribs. **D.** Appearance of the rib surface after light decortication to a bleeding bony surface. Note that in this case, three ribs were prepared for the fusion surface.

WIRE PASSAGE AND PLACEMENT OF SEMITUBULAR PLATE

- At this time, the involved lung is deflated before cerclage wires are passed around the ribs, to minimize trauma to the lung fields.
- Using rib and periosteal dissectors, a cerclage wire with a minimum diameter of 1.5 mm is passed carefully around each of the exposed ribs at the level where the medial border of the scapula will be placed on the rib cage (**TECH FIG 3A,B**).

- After passage of the cerclage wires, a one-third semitubular large fragment plate (usually with 5 or 6 holes, depending on the size of the scapula) is lined up on the posterior aspect of the medial border of the scapula (the thickest part of the scapula; **TECH FIG 3C**).
- A 3-mm burr is used to make holes through the scapula corresponding to the holes in the semitubular plate (**TECH FIG 3D**).

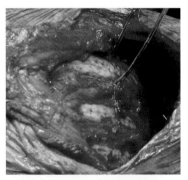
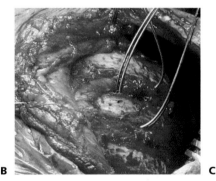
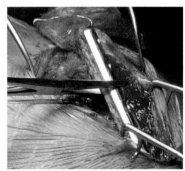

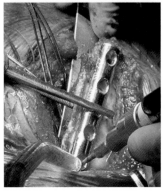

TECH FIG 3 • A. A 1.5-mm wire is passed around the rib using rib and periosteal elevators. The lung is deflated by the anesthesia team before the wire is passed to minimize damage to the underlying pleura. **B.** Wires are passed around each of the ribs to be involved in the fusion construct. **C.** A one-third semitubular plate (typically with 5 or 6 holes) is positioned over the medial border of the scapula. **D.** Holes are drilled in the scapula, corresponding to the plate, with a 3-mm motorized burr. A skid retractor is placed beneath the scapula to protect the underlying thoracic cavity.

REDUCTION AND PLATE FIXATION

- Cancellous bone is now harvested from the posterior iliac crest in routine fashion through a separate incision paralleling the path of the cluneal nerves.
  - If more bone graft is desired, either allograft cancellous chips or a synthetic bone graft substitute can be added.
- The wires are now passed through the scapula and semitubular plate (**TECH FIG 4A**), and the bone graft is placed between the scapula and ribs.

- The scapula is reduced to the underlying ribs (**TECH FIG 4B**), and the wires are sequentially tightened with the scapula held in 20 to 25 degrees of external rotation from the midline (**TECH FIG 4C,D**).
  - The semitubular plate allows uniform stress distribution once the wires are tightened (**TECH FIG 4E,F**).
- The wires are cut, and attention is turned to closure of the wound (**TECH FIG 4G**).

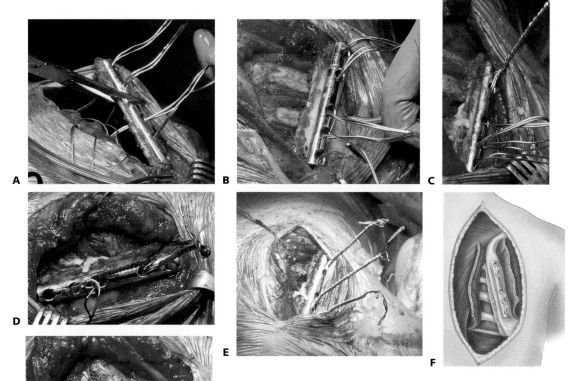

TECH FIG 4 • A. The previously placed wires are then passed through the scapula and plate in the appropriate position. **B.** The scapula is reduced into the predetermined position overlying the ribs and held in place before wire tightening. **C,D.** The wires are tightened sequentially, applying uniform tension on the plate and compressing the scapula against the ribs. **E.** The final position of the scapula after fixation with the wires. Note the autologous bone graft seen along the medial border. **F.** Illustration of the final construct. **G.** The wires are then cut, and attention is turned to wound closure.

WOUND CLOSURE AND CHEST TUBE PLACEMENT

- The lung is reinflated, and irrigation is used to assess for a pneumothorax, which may be present.
- The rhomboids are then reattached to the medial aspect of the scapula (**TECH FIG 5**), and the subcutaneous tissue and skin are closed in the usual fashion.
- A thoracotomy tube is inserted if necessary, both to treat any associated pneumothorax and to drain any reactive pleural effusion that may develop postoperatively.

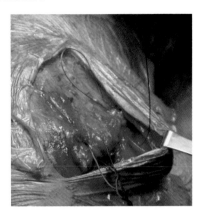

TECH FIG 5 • The rhomboids are repaired securely to the medial border of the scapula. This provides adequate coverage of the hardware.

PEARLS AND PITFALLS

Avoiding pulmonary complications	▪ Use double-lumen tube and deflate lung ▪ Meticulous subperiosteal passage of rib cerclage wires ▪ Thoracotomy tube when necessary
Avoiding hardware complications and nonunion	▪ Minimum size for wire is 1.50 mm ▪ Use posterior iliac crest autograft ▪ Use cancellous autograft ▪ Immobilize in "gunslinger" or similar brace
Avoiding neurologic complications	▪ Prevention of intercostal neuralgia by minimizing trauma to intercostal nerves is the best method to reduce neurologic complications.
Avoiding wound complications	▪ Infection is rare, but surgeons must maintain vigilance.

POSTOPERATIVE CARE

▪ The patient is placed in a "gunslinger" brace, immobilizing the arm in neutral rotation (**FIG 3**), and a postoperative chest radiograph is obtained to document any hemo- or pneumothorax.

▪ If a chest tube has been placed, it is removed 1 or 2 days postoperatively, depending on chest tube outputs and pulmonary status.

▪ Patients are immobilized in the brace for 12 weeks.

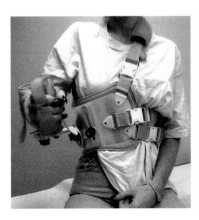

FIG 3 • "Gunslinger" brace with the arm positioned in neutral rotation.

▪ Rehabilitation is commenced at 12 weeks with a gentle passive range-of-motion program that emphasizes forward elevation and external rotation.

▪ Three weeks later, the patient is progressed to an active range-of-motion program.

▪ A strengthening program involving resisted exercises is begun 6 weeks after the gunslinger brace is removed.

OUTCOMES

▪ Despite the significant complication rate (nearly 50%) that accompanies scapulothoracic arthrodesis, this operation has been documented to provide improvements in both pain and functional disability.

▪ A high level of patient satisfaction when patients are chosen appropriately and expert surgical technique is used can make this operation rewarding for both patient and surgeon.

▪ In one series of 23 patients undergoing scapulothoracic fusion, mean ASES scores improved from 35.8 to 40.1. Postoperative pain scores decreased from mean 5.5 to 4.7. Mean patient satisfaction was 9.5 out of 10 for the surgical procedure, and 91% of patients reported that they would undergo the procedure again.[14]

COMPLICATIONS

▪ Complications are not uncommon with this procedure and have been reported to be as high as 50% in some series.[14]

■ The most commonly cited complications associated with this procedure include:
  ■ Pneumothorax
  ■ Hemothorax
  ■ Hardware complications, including wire breakage, nonunion, and pseudoarthrosis
  ■ Neurologic complications, including intercostal neuralgia
  ■ Wound complications, including infection or wound dehiscence

REFERENCES

1. Bunch WH, Siegel IM. Scapulothoracic arthrodesis in fascioscapulohumeral muscular dystrophy. J Bone Joint Surg Am 1993;75A: 372–376.
2. Connor PM, Yamaguchi K, Manifold SG, et al. Split pectoralis major for serratus anterior palsy. Clin Orthop Relat Res 1997;341: 134–142.
3. Cooley LH, Torg JS. "Pseudowinging" of the scapula secondary to subscapular osteochondroma. Clin Orthop Relat Res 1982;162: 119–124.
4. Fery A. Results of treatment of anterior serratus paralysis. In: Post M, Morrey BF, Hawkins RJ, eds. Surgery of the Shoulder. Philadelphia: Mosby, 1990:325–329.
5. Foo CL, Swann M. Isolated paralysis of the serratus anterior. A report of 20 cases. J Bone Joint Surg Br 1983;65B:552–556.
6. Freedman L, Munro RR. Abduction of the arm in the scapular plane: scapular and glenohumeral movements. J Bone Joint Surg Am 1966; 48A:1503–1510.
7. Gozna ER, Harris WR. Traumatic winging of the scapula. J Bone Joint Surg Am 1979;61A:1230–1233.
8. Gregg JR, LaBosky D, Harty M, et al. Serratus anterior paralysis in the young athlete. J Bone Joint Surg Am 1979;61A:825–832.
9. Harper GD, McIlroy S, Bayley JIL, et al. Arthroscopic partial resection of the scapula for snapping scapula: a new technique. J Shoulder Elbow Surg 1999;8:53–57.
10. Hawkins RJ, Willis RB, Litchfield RB. Scapulothoracic arthrodesis for scapular winging. In Post M, Morrey BF, Hawkins RJ, eds. Surgery of the Shoulder. Philadelphia: Mosby, 1990:340–349.
11. Hays JM, Zehr DJ. Traumatic muscle avulsion causing winging of the scapula. J Bone Joint Surg Am 1981;63A:495–497.
12. Kuhn JE, Plancher KD, Hawkins RJ. Scapular winging. J Am Acad Orthop Surg 1995;3:319–325.
13. Kuhn JE, Plancher KD, Hawkins RJ. Symptomatic scapulothoracic crepitus and bursitis. J Am Acad Orthop Surg 1998;6:267–273.
14. Krishnan SG, Hawkins RJ, Michelotti JD, et al. Scapulothoracic arthrodesis: indications, technique, and results. Clin Orthop Relat Res 2005;435:126–133.
15. Marmor L, Bechtol CO. Paralysis of the serratus anterior due to electric shock relieved by transplantation of the pectoralis major muscle: A case report. J Bone Joint Surg Am 1963;45:156–160.
16. Perlmutter GS, Leffert RD. Results of transfer of the pectoralis major tendon to treat paralysis of the serratus anterior muscle. J Bone Joint Surg Am 1999;81A:377–384.
17. Richards RR, McKee MD. Treatment of painful scapulothoracic crepitus by resection of the superomedial angle of the scapula. Clin Orthop Relat Res 1989;247:111–116.
18. Strizak AM, Cowen MH. The snapping scapula syndrome. J Bone Joint Surg Am 1982;64A:941–942.
19. Warner JJP, Navarro RA. Serratus anterior dysfunction. Clin Orthop Relat Res 1998;349:139–148.
20. Wiater JM, Flatow EL. Long thoracic nerve injury. Clin Orthop Relat Res 1999;368:17–27.

Chapter 32

Suprascapular Nerve Decompression

Andreas H. Gomoll and Anthony A. Romeo

DEFINITION

▪ Suprascapular nerve (SSN) entrapment is an uncommon cause for shoulder pain and weakness. It was initially described by Koppel and Thompson.[11]

▪ SSN entrapment typically occurs at the suprascapular or spinoglenoid notch and presents with symptoms ranging from diffuse shoulder pain to weakness and atrophy of the supraspinatus and infraspinatus muscles.

ANATOMY

▪ The SSN arises from the upper trunk of the brachial plexus, with contributions from C5 and C6 (rarely also C4), and provides branches to the supraspinatus and infraspinatus muscles. It also carries afferent fibers from the glenohumeral joint and rarely also cutaneous fibers from the lateral aspect of the shoulder.

▪ The nerve traverses two potential compression points, at the suprascapular notch and spinoglenoid notch (**FIG 1**), and is accompanied by the suprascapular artery and vein.

▪ At the suprascapular notch, the nerve runs in a fibro-osseous canal formed by the scapular notch and the transverse scapular ligament. Generally, the nerve runs under the ligament, but it is occasionally accompanied by a branch of the main vessels, which course over the ligament.

▪ The suprascapular notch is approximately 4.5 cm medial to the posterolateral corner of the acromion and 3 cm medial to the glenoid rim (supraglenoid tubercle). The spinoglenoid notch is approximately 1.8 cm medial to the glenoid rim and 2.5 cm inferomedial to the supraglenoid tubercle.[3]

▪ Several anatomic studies have described the presence of a spinoglenoid ligament (inferior transverse scapular ligament) at the spinoglenoid notch in 3% to 60% of specimens,[5,6] but its role in nerve entrapment at this level is controversial.

PATHOGENESIS

▪ The most common site of entrapment is at the suprascapular notch, where it can be compressed by a thickened or ossified transverse scapular ligament.

▪ The relative confinement of the nerve at the suprascapular notch also places it at risk for injury due to traction, such as seen either in acute trauma or repetitive overhead activities such as volleyball, tennis, or weightlifting.

▪ Compression from labral ganglions can also occur, typically at the spinoglenoid notch.[1] These cysts can develop as the result of labral tears that allow fluid extravasation but block backflow, similar to a one-way valve.

▪ More recently, traction injury to the nerve has been described as the result of massive, retracted tears of the posterosuperior cuff.[2]

▪ Direct or indirect trauma leading to SSN neuropathy has been described as the result of shoulder dislocation, proximal humerus fracture, or scapular fracture.

▪ Iatrogenic injury to the SSN can occur during distal clavicle resection, positioning during spine surgery, transglenoid drilling for instability repair, shoulder arthrodesis, or the posterior approach to the glenohumeral joint.

NATURAL HISTORY

▪ The natural history depends on the presence or absence of a space-occupying lesion as the cause of SSN neuropathy.

▪ Without compression by a mass, most patients will improve with time and supervised physical therapy.[8]

▪ Conversely, the presence of a mass, such as a cyst or ganglion, usually results in failure of conservative management and will require decompressive surgery.

▪ The natural history of periarticular ganglion cysts in the shoulder is controversial, but they are thought to persist and enlarge with time.[9] In rare instances, spontaneous resolution of ganglion cysts has been documented.

PATIENT HISTORY AND PHYSICAL FINDINGS

▪ SSN neuropathy secondary to compression at the suprascapular notch typically presents as a dull pain in the posterior

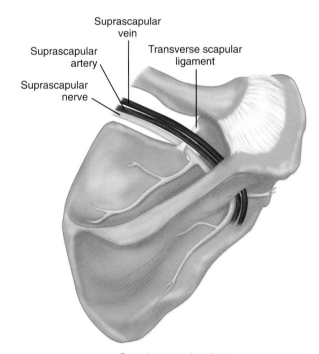

FIG 1 • Anatomy of the suprascapular nerve (SSN). The SSN is accompanied by the suprascapular artery and vein, which course over the transverse scapular ligament (TSL), while the nerve passes underneath. All three then traverse the spinoglenoid notch.

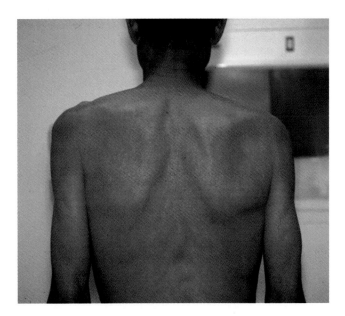

FIG 2 • Posterior photograph of a patient with right infraspinatus muscle wasting secondary to suprascapular nerve entrapment at the spinoglenoid notch.

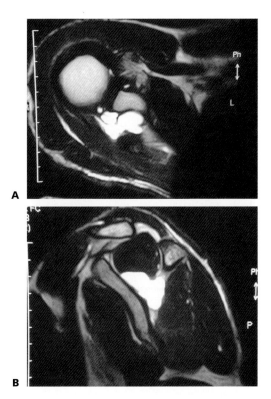

FIG 3 • T2-weighted MR images depicting axial (**A**) and oblique (**B**) sagittal views showing a cyst in the area of the spinoglenoid notch.

and lateral shoulder, but the pain can also be referred to the anterior chest wall, lateral arm, and ipsilateral neck. Compression at the spinoglenoid notch is often comparatively pain-free and presents with isolated infraspinatus atrophy (**FIG 2**).

▪ The patient often provides a history of acute or repetitive trauma to the shoulder, such as a fall on the outstretched hand, or activities such as volleyball, tennis, or weightlifting.

▪ There appears to be an increased incidence of isolated infraspinatus atrophy in asymptomatic volleyball players. This typically responds well to conservative measures.

▪ Depending on the chronicity and degree of compression, varying amounts of weakness in abduction and external rotation can be detected on physical examination.

▪ In longstanding compression, atrophy of the supraspinatus and infraspinatus can be observed.

▪ Atrophy, if present, may assist in differentiating compression at the suprascapular notch from that at the spinoglenoid level, since supraspinatus atrophy occurs only with the former.

▪ Palpation of the spinoglenoid notch and cross-body adduction may reproduce the patient's symptoms.

▪ It is important to exclude other potential sources of pain, such as the cervical spine, acromioclavicular joint, or rotator cuff.

IMAGING AND OTHER DIAGNOSTIC STUDIES

▪ An anesthetic injection into the suprascapular notch can be diagnostic if it results in complete but transient pain relief.

▪ Stryker notch views, or anteroposterior radiographs of the scapula, with a 15- to 30-degrees caudally directed beam, provide visualization of the suprascapular notch. Alternatively, a CT scan can provide good osseous detail in cases of posttraumatic deformity or ossification of the transverse scapular ligament.

▪ MRI can reveal a superior or posterior labral tear and the presence of a ganglion in the area of the suprascapular or

spinoglenoid notch (**FIG 3**). Ganglion cysts present as homogeneous masses with low signal intensity on T1-weighted images and high signal intensity on T2-weighted images.

▪ Electromyography and nerve conduction studies can often provide a conclusive diagnosis by showing denervation potentials, fibrillations, spontaneous activity, and prolonged motor latencies in the supraspinatus or infraspinatus, depending on the level of entrapment.

DIFFERENTIAL DIAGNOSIS

▪ Cervical radiculopathy
▪ Glenohumeral instability
▪ Rotator cuff pathology
▪ Acromioclavicular joint arthrosis

NONOPERATIVE MANAGEMENT

▪ Initial treatment for SSN neuropathy in the absence of a space-occupying lesion is conservative and will lead to near-complete resolution of symptoms in most cases.

▪ Complete resolution of pain and weakness can take more than 1 year.

▪ Supervised physical therapy, followed by a self-directed home exercise program, should consist of range-of-motion exercises, as well as strengthening of the rotator cuff muscles, the deltoid, and the periscapular musculature, including the trapezius, rhomboids, and serratus musculature. Restoring proper scapular function is beneficial in recovery and may prevent recurrence of the injury.

▪ Image-guided cyst aspiration has shown success in about half of patients, with persistence or recurrence in the other half.[9,12]

SURGICAL MANAGEMENT

- Surgical treatment is indicated in patients who have failed to respond to 6 to 12 months of nonoperative measures and continue to have significant pain and dysfunction. SSN neuropathy secondary to a mass is best treated with decompression, and evaluation and potential repair of the glenoid labrum.
- Other sources for shoulder pain and dysfunction should be ruled out if the mass is smaller than 1 cm in diameter or is not directly compressing the neurovascular bundle.

Preoperative Planning

- Oblique sagittal MR imaging allows visualization of the SSN in the supraspinatus fossa, the spinoglenoid notch, and the infraspinatus fossa.
  - If a space-occupying lesion is present, this imaging will assist in preoperative planning by delineating the exact position of the mass and determining whether it is confined to the supraspinatus or the infraspinatus fossa or involves both areas.
- A paralabral ganglion or cyst that is confined to one area, especially when associated with a labral tear or other intra-articular pathology, is often amenable to arthroscopic decompression.
- We have found it useful first to perform a diagnostic shoulder arthroscopy and potential treatment of intra-articular pathology, followed by arthroscopic or open decompression of the SSN.
- Arthroscopic decompression has the potential advantages of treating associated intra-articular lesions, such as labral tears and avoiding the morbidity associated with open procedures.

Positioning

- Either the beach chair or the lateral decubitus position can be used.

OPEN DECOMPRESSION

Approach to the Suprascapular Notch

- Decompression of the suprascapular nerve at the suprascapular notch is best achieved through a trapezius-splitting approach.
  - The anterior approach requires a more complex dissection and therefore carries a higher risk of neurovascular complications. It also offers incomplete visualization of the SSN posterior to the notch and is generally not recommended.
- A saber-type skin incision following the Langer lines is performed over the top of the shoulder. The incision begins posteriorly at the distal third of the scapular spine and extends anteriorly to a point 2 cm medially off the acromioclavicular joint (**TECH FIG 1A**).
- A transverse skin incision parallel to the scapular spine can be chosen instead but produces a less cosmetic scar.
- The trapezius fascia and muscle is divided in line with its fibers for a distance of 5 cm.
- Abduction of the arm decreases tension on the muscle, which if necessary can be elevated off the scapular spine for an extensile exposure.
- The supraspinatus muscle is bluntly dissected off the anterior aspect of the suprascapular fossa and retracted posteriorly to provide access to the suprascapular notch (**TECH FIG 1B**).

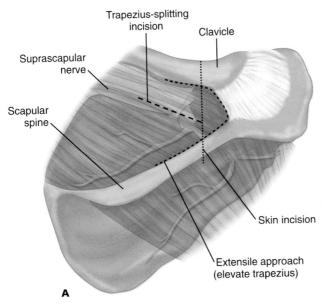
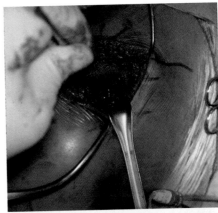
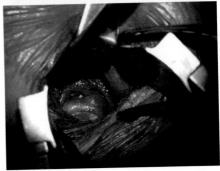

TECH FIG 1 • Schematic and intraoperative photograph demonstrating suprascapular nerve release at the suprascapular notch. **A.** The trapezius muscle is split in line with its fibers. **B.** The suprascapular muscle is bluntly dissected off the suprascapular fossa and retracted to expose the suprascapular notch. **C.** The transverse scapular ligament has been released.

- The overlying suprascapular artery and vein are gently retracted to expose the transverse scapular ligament.
- A small right-angle clamp can be used to bluntly dissect under the ligament and protect the underlying nerve while the ligament is transected with a scalpel.
- Occasionally the nerve is still tethered after release of the transverse ligament, requiring careful resection of the medial aspect of the suprascapular notch. The resected edge of the bone must be smooth at the completion of the procedure.
- If the trapezius was detached during the approach, it should be sutured back to the bone of the scapular spine. If the muscle was only split in line with its fibers, it is reapproximated with interrupted, absorbable sutures.

Approach to the Spinoglenoid Notch

- The posterior approach provides direct visualization of the suprascapular nerve at the spinoglenoid notch.
- A longitudinal skin incision is centered approximately 4 cm medial to the posterolateral corner of the acromion, approximately 5 cm in length. Following Langer lines provides a cosmetically acceptable scar.

- The underlying fascia and deltoid muscle is split in line with its fibers beginning at the level of the scapular spine and extending 5 cm distal from the posterior acromion (**TECH FIG 2A**). A stay suture placed at the distalmost extent of the incision protects against propagation of the split, which carries a risk of injury to the axillary nerve.
- The infraspinatus is identified, dissected off the scapular spine, and retracted inferiorly (**TECH FIG 2B**).
- Commonly, a small area of vascular fibrous tissue is encountered posterior to the site of the spinoglenoid notch, covering the suprascapular neurovascular structures.
- If a ganglion is present, the contents of the cyst should be removed along with the wall (**TECH FIG 2C**).
- A spinoglenoid ligament, if present, should be excised.
- Decompression is complete when the SSN can be followed along its entire length from the spinoglenoid notch until it arborizes into its infraspinatus branches (**TECH FIG 2D**).
- The infraspinatus muscle is allowed to return to its anatomic position.
- The deltoid muscle and fascia is reapproximated with interrupted, absorbable sutures.

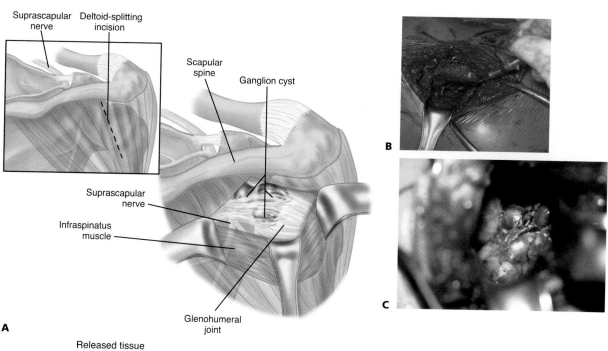

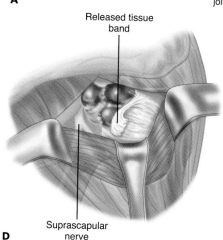

TECH FIG 2 • Schematics and intraoperative photographs showing suprascapular nerve release at the spinoglenoid notch. **A.** The deltoid muscle is split in line with its fibers, beginning about 4 cm medial to the posterolateral corner of the acromion. **B.** The spinoglenoid notch has been exposed. The retractors displace the infraspinatus muscles posteriorly and inferiorly. **C.** A multilobulated ganglion cyst. **D.** The suprascapular nerve is now visible after the soft tissue band has been divided.

ARTHROSCOPIC DECOMPRESSION

Approach to the Suprascapular Notch

- Routine glenohumeral arthroscopy is performed to assess concomitant pathology, especially tears of the superior-posterior labrum.
- The subacromial bursa is resected, extending more medially than what is usual for subacromial decompression.
  - The bursectomy should allow adequate visualization from the acromioclavicular (AC) joint and coracoid anteriorly to the scapular spine posteriorly.
- The coracoid is palpated with a probe or switching stick, which can also be used to bluntly dissect the surrounding soft tissues to expose the coracoclavicular ligaments.
  - Alternatively, the ligaments can be found approximately 15 mm medial to the AC joint and then followed inferiorly to their insertion on the coracoid.
- The conoid ligament attaches to the coracoid just laterally to the suprascapular notch. Fibers of the conoid ligament are in continuity with the transverse scapular ligament.

- The suprascapular notch is typically covered by the supraspinatus muscle and fat, complicating visualization of the neurovascular bundle (**TECH FIG 3A**).
- An accessory portal is created approximately 2 cm medial to the standard Neviaser portal along a line that bisects the angle formed between the clavicle and spine of the scapula. An 18-gauge spinal needle helps with correct positioning of the portal (**TECH FIG 3B**).
- Use of a switching stick or smooth trocar through this accessory portal allows careful, blunt dissection of the fat to expose the suprascapular vessels coursing over the transverse scapular ligament, which presents as glistening white fibers.
- Once adequate visualization has been achieved, the nerve is protected with a probe or small trocar while the overlying ligament is cut with the arthroscopic scissors as far lateral as possible (**TECH FIG 3C–E**).
- The SSN is probed to ensure adequate decompression; any residual compression from the bony structures can be removed with the arthroscopic burr.

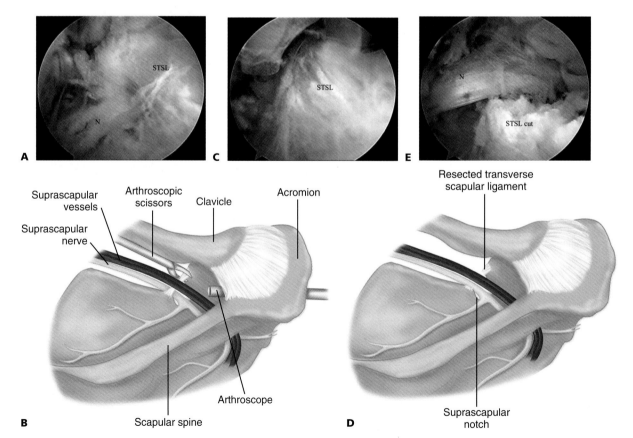

TECH FIG 3 • Schematic and arthroscopic images showing arthroscopic suprascapular nerve release at the suprascapular notch. **A.** After soft tissue removal, the nerve (N) can be visualized underneath the superior transverse scapular ligament (STSL). A blunt trocar is retracting the overlying vessel. **B.** The arthroscope is positioned in the lateral portal and the instruments are introduced through a superior portal, medial to the standard Neviaser portal. **C.** Arthroscopic scissors positioned to cut the STSL. **D,E.** The ligament has been released. *A*, artery. (**A,C,E**: Courtesy of Dr Laurence Higgins.)

Approach to the Spinoglenoid Notch

- Ganglion cysts associated with labral tears are most commonly located at the spinoglenoid notch. They often extend into the infraspinatus fossa.
- With an intact labrum, the joint capsule above the superior-posterior labrum is incised, beginning posterior to the biceps root and extending posteriorly for 2 to 3 cm.
- After incision of the capsule, the fibrous raphe between the supraspinatus and infraspinatus seen lateral to the spinoglenoid notch provides a useful landmark.
- The spinoglenoid notch can be palpated with an arthroscopic instrument, providing a bony landmark that can be correlated with the cyst position as seen on preoperative MR imaging.

- An accessory posterolateral portal is placed after first establishing correct orientation with an 18-gauge spinal needle.
- Similar to open decompression, fibrovascular tissue covers the neurovascular bundle and has to be bluntly dissected with a switching stick or similar tool through the accessory portal before the nerve can be visualized.
- The SSN is positioned medially, in direct contact with the bone of the spinoglenoid notch; the vascular structures are positioned laterally and closer to the glenoid.
- Ganglion cysts are typically located posterior to the nerve and should be removed completely, including the lining.
- After cyst removal, the nerve should be inspected for any additional sites of compression.

POSTOPERATIVE CARE

- The arm is immobilized in a sling for 2 or 3 days for comfort.
- Pendulum exercises commence on postoperative day 1, and active motion is increased as tolerated.

OUTCOMES

- Nonoperative treatment is successful in 80% of patients without space-occupying lesions.[8]
- Open decompression with release of the transverse scapular ligament improved pain and weakness in 73% to 87% of patients.[4,13]

- Reports on the outcomes of arthroscopic decompression are rare, but outcomes seem to approach the success rate of open approaches.

COMPLICATIONS

- Damage to the suprascapular nerve and vessels
- Damage to the spinal accessory nerve if mobilization of the trapezius muscle is carried out far medially
- Incomplete decompression, especially in rare cases of compression at both suprascapular and spinoglenoid notch

PEARLS AND PITFALLS

Arthroscopic decompression	<ul><li>Hemostasis and visualization can be improved by increasing the fluid pressure to 50 mm Hg and using an electrothermal device to cauterize bleeders.</li><li>The decompression should be performed before treatment of any concomitant pathology to avoid further complicating this procedure owing to fluid extravasation and swelling.</li><li>A 70-degree scope is sometimes helpful to visualize the notch.</li><li>Visualization should be performed through the lateral portal, with posterior and accessory medial working portals.</li></ul>

REFERENCES

1. Aiello I, Serra G, Traina GC, et al. Entrapment of the suprascapular nerve at the spinoglenoid notch. Ann Neurol 1982;12:314–316.
2. Albritton MJ, Graham RD, Richards RS II, et al. An anatomic study of the effects on the suprascapular nerve due to retraction of the supraspinatus muscle after a rotator cuff tear. J Shoulder Elbow Surg 2003;12:497–500.
3. Bigliani LU, Dalsey RM, McCann PD, et al. An anatomical study of the suprascapular nerve. Arthroscopy 1990;6:301–305.
4. Callahan JD, Scully TB, Shapiro SA, et al. Suprascapular nerve entrapment: a series of 27 cases. J Neurosurg 1991;74:893–896.
5. Cummins CA, Anderson K, Bowen M, et al. Anatomy and histological characteristics of the spinoglenoid ligament. J Bone Joint Surg Am 1998;80:1622–1625.
6. Demaio M, Drez D Jr, Mullins RC. The inferior transverse scapular ligament as a possible cause of entrapment neuropathy of the nerve to the infraspinatus: a brief note. J Bone Joint Surg Am 1991;73A:1061–1063.
7. Lafosse L, Tomasi A. Technique for endoscopic release of suprascapular nerve entrapment at the suprascapular notch. Tech Shoulder Elbow 2006;7:1–6.
8. Martin SD, Warren RF, Martin TL, et al. Suprascapular neuropathy: results of non-operative treatment. J Bone Joint Surg Am 1997;79A:1159–1165.
9. Piatt BE, Hawkins RJ, Fritz RC, et al. Clinical evaluation and treatment of spinoglenoid notch ganglion cysts. J Shoulder Elbow Surg 2002;11:600–604.
10. Romeo AA, Rotenberg DD, Bach BR Jr. Suprascapular neuropathy. J Am Acad Orthop Surg 1999;7:358–367.
11. Thompson W, Kopell H. Peripheral entrapment neuropathies of the upper extremity. N Engl J Med 1959;260:1261–1265.
12. Tirman PF, Feller JF, Janzen DL, et al. Association of glenoid labral cysts with labral tears and glenohumeral instability: radiologic findings and clinical significance. Radiology 1994;190:653–658.
13. Vastamaki M, Goransson H. Suprascapular nerve entrapment. Clin Orthop Relat Res 1993;297:135–143.

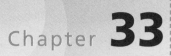

Chapter 33

Open Reduction and Internal Fixation of Supracondylar and Intercondylar Fractures

Joaquin Sanchez-Sotelo

PATIENT HISTORY AND PHYSICAL FINDINGS

- Distal humerus fractures occur in two age groups:
  - Younger patients who sustain high-energy trauma
  - Older patients with underlying osteopenia
- Comminution is the dominant feature of supracondylar and intercondylar fractures and complicates internal fixation.
- The goals of the initial evaluation are to:
  - Understand the fracture pattern.
  - Determine the existence of previous symptomatic elbow pathology.
  - Determine the extent of associated soft tissue (open fractures).
  - Identify associated musculoskeletal or neurovascular injuries.

IMAGING AND OTHER DIAGNOSTIC STUDIES

- Elbow radiographs in the anteroposterior and lateral planes are the first imaging studies obtained and should be carefully scrutinized to identify the fracture lines and fragments as well as the extent of comminution.
  - A complete understanding of the fracture pattern is difficult to obtain based only on simple radiographs because of the complex geometry of the distal humerus and fragment overlapping (**FIG 1A,B**).
- CT with three-dimensional reconstruction is extremely helpful, especially in the more complex cases. It allows the surgeon to look for specific fractured fragments at the time of fixation, facilitating accurate fracture reduction (**FIG 1C,D**).

- Traction radiographs obtained in the operating room with the patient under anesthesia just before surgery also can be helpful, especially if a CT scan is not available.

SURGICAL MANAGEMENT

- Internal fixation is the treatment of choice for most fractures of the distal humerus.
- Modern fixation techniques seem to benefit from:
  - Fixation strategies designed to improve the mechanical stability of the construct
  - Use of precontoured periarticular plates
  - Use of screws locked to the plates
- Elbow arthroplasty should be considered in elderly patients with previous elbow pathology or in very low, comminuted fractures in patients with osteopenia.
- The goal of the internal fixation technique is to achieve a construct stable enough to allow immediate unprotected motion without fear of redisplacement.[12] This can be attained in most distal humerus fractures—even the most complex—provided the following principles are adhered to (**FIG 2**):
  - Plates used for internal fixation are applied so that fixation in the distal fragments is maximized.
  - Distal screw fixation contributes to stability at the supracondylar level, where true interfragmentary compression is achieved.

Approaches

- Adequate exposure is necessary to achieve satisfactory reduction and fixation.
- Subcutaneous transposition of the ulnar nerve is associated with a decreased incidence of postoperative ulnar neuropathy.

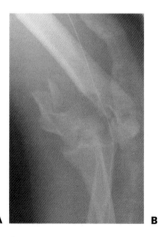
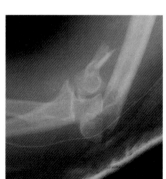
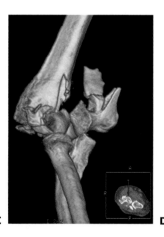
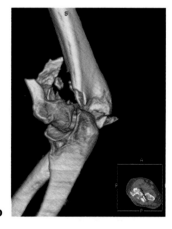

FIG 1 • A,B. AP and lateral radiographs showing a comminuted intra-articular supraintercondylar fracture of the distal humerus. The complexity of the fracture is difficult to appreciate fully because of the geometry of the distal humerus, fracture comminution, and fragment overlapping. **C,D.** The use of CT with three-dimensional reconstruction and surface rendering helps understand the fracture configuration and anticipate the surgical findings.

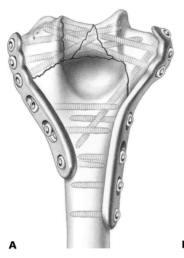 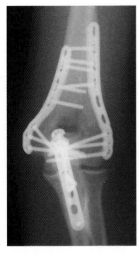

FIG 2 • **A.** Internal fixation using two parallel medial and lateral plates allows maximal fixation of the plates in the distal fragments and increased stability at the supracondylar level. **B.** This postoperative AP radiograph shows anatomic reduction of a complex distal humerus fracture and stable fixation using the principles and technique described in this chapter. The olecranon osteotomy was fixed with a plate. (**A:** Copyright Mayo.)

■ Most fractures require mobilization of the extensor mechanism of the elbow through an olecranon osteotomy, triceps reflection, or triceps split.

■ Simple fractures occasionally may be addressed working on both sides of the triceps without mobilization of the extensor mechanism.

■ Olecranon osteotomy is the preferred surgical approach for internal fixation for most distal humerus fractures.[11]
   ■ Advantages
      ■ Provides excellent exposure

■ Offers the potential of bone-to-bone healing, thereby limiting the risk of triceps dysfunction
   ■ Disadvantages
      ■ Complications: nonunion, intra-articular adhesions
      ■ Hardware removal may be needed.
      ■ Limits the ability for intraoperative conversion to elbow arthroplasty
      ■ May devitalize the anconeus muscle
      ■ The proximal ulna cannot be used as a template to judge reduction and motion.
■ Triceps reflection and triceps split[8] allow preservation of the intact ulna.
   ■ Avoids complications related to olecranon osteotomy
   ■ Facilitates intraoperative conversion to total elbow arthroplasty
   ■ Allows use of the proximal ulna as a template for reduction of the distal humerus articular surface
   ■ Allows assessment of extension deficit after fracture fixation, which is especially useful in fractures requiring metaphyseal shortening
■ Bilaterotricipital approach[1]
   ■ Goals and indications
      ■ The goal is to provide adequate exposure for fracture fixation without violating the extensor mechanism.
      ■ This approach is used only for the more simple fracture patterns (eg, extra-articular or simple intra-articular distal humerus fractures [AO/OTA A, C1, C2]) or when elbow arthroplasty is being considered.
   ■ Advantages
      ■ This approach avoids complications related to the extensor mechanism.
      ■ No postoperative protection is needed.
      ■ Surgical time is decreased.
   ■ Disadvantage
      ■ The procedure provides limited exposure of the articular surface.

SURGICAL APPROACH

Olecranon Osteotomy

■ Chevron osteotomy provides increased stability (**TECH FIG 1A**).

■ The distal apex of the chevron osteotomy is centered with the bare area of the olecranon articular surface.

■ The anconeus is divided with electrocautery in line with the lateral limb of the osteotomy.
   ■ Alternatively, the anconeus may be preserved by dissecting it free on its distal aspect and reflecting it proximally attached to the proximal ulnar fragment.[2]

■ Start the osteotomy with a thin oscillating saw.

■ Complete the osteotomy with an osteotome.
   ■ Decreases risk of damage to the articular cartilage on ulna and humerus
   ■ Creates irregularities at the opposing cut surfaces, which may increase interdigitation

■ Mobilize the fragment to facilitate exposure (**TECH FIG 1B**).

■ Fixation (**TECH FIG 1C**)

■ Some biomechanical studies support the combination of a 7.3-mm cancellous screw and tension band over either a screw alone or K-wires plus tension band; others have found no differences.

■ The author's preferred method uses K-wires plus a tension band.

■ If screw fixation is planned, drill and tap the ulna before performing the osteotomy.

■ Plate fixation is preferred by some.
   ■ It provides improved fixation, but the risk of wound complications is increased.

Triceps Reflection and Triceps Split

■ Bryan-Morrey triceps-sparing approach (**TECH FIG 2**)
   ■ The triceps is elevated from the medial intermuscular septum.
   ■ The forearm fascia and periosteum are incised just lateral to the flexor carpi ulnaris.
   ■ The triceps, forearm fascia, and anconeus are elevated in continuity from medial to lateral.

TECHNIQUES

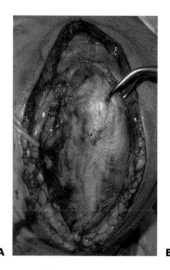
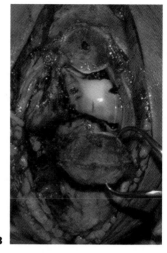
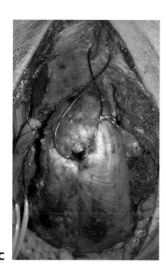

TECH FIG 1 • Olecranon osteotomy provides an excellent exposure for distal humerus fracture fixation. **A.** A chevron osteotomy is initiated with a microsagittal saw and completed with an osteotome. Drilling and tapping before performing the osteotomy facilitates fixation of the osteotomy if screw fixation is selected. **B.** Proximal mobilization of the osteotomized fragment and triceps allows ample exposure of the articular surface and columns. **C.** Fixation may be performed with a cancellous screw and tension band, wires and a tension band, or a plate.

- The anterior bundle of the medial collateral ligament and the lateral ulnar collateral ligament must be preserved to avoid postoperative instability.
- Mayo-modified extensile Köcher approach
  - The triceps is elevated from the lateral intermuscular septum.
  - The triceps and anconeus are elevated in continuity from lateral to medial.

- As noted earlier, the anterior bundle of the medial collateral ligament and the lateral ulnar collateral ligament must be preserved to avoid postoperative instability.

Bilaterotricipital Approach

- The triceps is elevated from the medial and lateral intermuscular septae.
- Lateral dissection can be extended anterior to the anconeus muscle (**TECH FIG 3**).
- Arthrotomy is performed posterior to the medial collateral ligament and lateral collateral ligament complex.

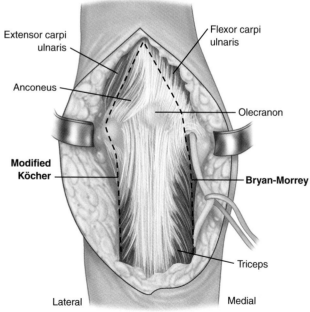

Extensor carpi ulnaris

Anconeus

Modified Köcher

Lateral

Flexor carpi ulnaris

Olecranon

Bryan-Morrey

Triceps

Medial

TECH FIG 2 • The extensor mechanism (ie, triceps, anconeus, and forearm fascia) may be elevated off the ulna subperiosteally in continuity from medial to lateral (Bryan-Morrey approach) or from lateral to medial (Mayo-modified extensile Köcher approach).

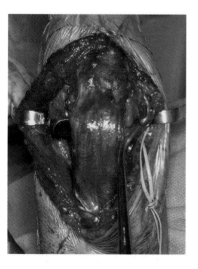

TECH FIG 3 • Fractures with no or limited articular involvement may be fixed working on both sides of the triceps. As shown in this image, the extensor mechanism is left mostly undisturbed.

INTERNAL FIXATION

Technical Objectives

- Screws in the distal fragments (articular segment) should be placed according to the following principles:
  - Every screw should pass through a plate.
  - Each screw should engage a fragment on the opposite side that also is fixed to a plate.
  - As many screws as possible should be placed in the distal fragments.
  - Each screw should be as long as possible.
  - Each screw should engage as many articular fragments as possible.
  - The screws should lock together by interdigitation within the distal segment, thereby rigidly linking the medial and lateral columns together, creating an architectural structure similar to that of an arch or dome.
- Plates are used for fixation.
  - Plates should be applied such that compression is achieved at the supracondylar level for both columns.
  - Plates must be strong enough and stiff enough to resist breaking or bending before union occurs at the supracondylar level.

Provisional Assembly of the Articular Surface and Plate Placement

- Reduce the articular surface fragments anatomically.
  - The proximal ulna and radial head may be used as templates.
- Rotational alignment should be carefully assessed.
- Use smooth K-wires to maintain the reduction provisionally (**TECH FIG 4A**).
  - Two 2.0-mm smooth wires introduced at the medial and lateral epicondyles facilitate provisional placement of the plates and can be replaced by screws later.

- Fine-threaded wires or absorbable pins may be used for definitive fixation of small fracture fragments.
- Medial and lateral plates are placed so that one of the distal holes of each plate slides over the medial and lateral 2.0-mm smooth wires introduced at the medial and lateral epicondyles (**TECH FIG 4B**).
- One cortical screw is loosely introduced into a slotted hole of each plate to hold the plates in place; use of slotted holes for these screws facilitates later adjustments in plate positioning.

Articular and Distal Fixation

- Two or more distal screws are inserted through the plates medially and laterally. As noted, the screws should be as long as possible and engage the opposite column.
  - Before screw application, a large bone clamp is used to compress the articular fracture lines, unless there is comminution of the articular surface.
- The two 2.0-mm smooth pins may be replaced with distal screws without previous drilling, to avoid accidental breakage of the drill when contacting the other screws. Usually, these last screws will interdigitate with the previously applied distal screws, thereby increasing the stability of the construct (**TECH FIG 5**).

Supracondylar Compression and Proximal Plate Fixation

- The proximal screw on one side is backed out, and a large bone clamp is applied distally on that side and proximally on the opposite side to apply maximum compression at the supracondylar level. Compression is maintained by application of one proximal screw in the compression mode (**TECH FIG 6A,B**).
- The same steps are followed on the opposite side.

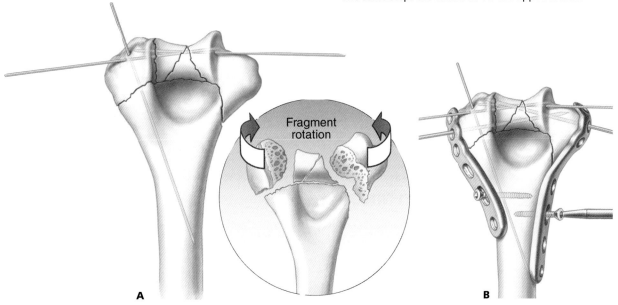

A   B

TECH FIG 4 • A. Anatomic reduction of the articular surface is maintained provisionally with fine wires placed so that they will not interfere with plate and screw application. **B.** The medial and lateral plates are held in place provisionally with two distal 2.0-mm pins (which later will be replaced by screws) and two proximal screws through an oval hole to allow small adjustments in plate positioning. (Copyright Mayo.)

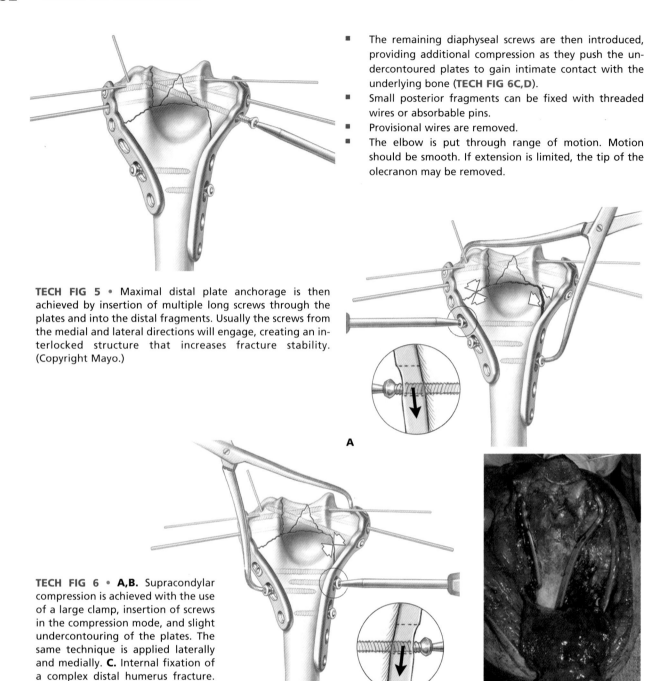

- The remaining diaphyseal screws are then introduced, providing additional compression as they push the undercontoured plates to gain intimate contact with the underlying bone (**TECH FIG 6C,D**).
- Small posterior fragments can be fixed with threaded wires or absorbable pins.
- Provisional wires are removed.
- The elbow is put through range of motion. Motion should be smooth. If extension is limited, the tip of the olecranon may be removed.

TECH FIG 5 • Maximal distal plate anchorage is then achieved by insertion of multiple long screws through the plates and into the distal fragments. Usually the screws from the medial and lateral directions will engage, creating an interlocked structure that increases fracture stability. (Copyright Mayo.)

A

TECH FIG 6 • **A,B.** Supracondylar compression is achieved with the use of a large clamp, insertion of screws in the compression mode, and slight undercontouring of the plates. The same technique is applied laterally and medially. **C.** Internal fixation of a complex distal humerus fracture. (**A,B:** Copyright Mayo.)

B

C

SUPRACONDYLAR SHORTENING

- In cases with supracondylar comminution (ie, bone loss), compression at the supracondylar level cannot be achieved unless the humerus is shortened into a non-anatomic reduction that will provide adequate bone contact (**TECH FIG 7A,B**).
  - The humerus may be shortened between a few millimeters and 2 cm with only minor losses in extension strength.[9]
- Bone is trimmed from the diaphysis to ensure adequate bone contact with the distal fragments.

- The distal fragments are translated proximally and anteriorly. Anterior translation is necessary to create room for the radial head and the coronoid in flexion.
- The fracture is fixed in the desired position using the technique described previously.
- A new deep and wide olecranon fossa is created by removing bone from the distal and posterior aspect of the diaphysis (**TECH FIG 7C**). Otherwise, extension will be restricted.

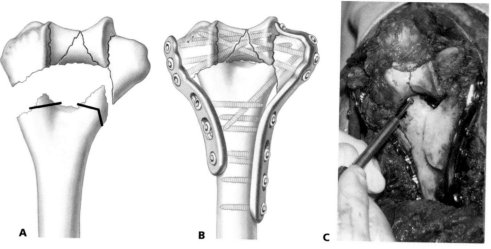

TECH FIG 7 • In cases of severe supracondylar comminution, adequate interfragmentary contact and compression takes priority over anatomic reduction. The humerus may be shortened anywhere from a few millimeters to 2 cm by trimming the bony spikes of the diaphysis (**A**), advancing the distal segment proximally and anteriorly, and fixing it in a nonanatomic fashion (**B**). **C.** The olecranon fossa is recreated in this case by removing bone from the posterior aspect of the diaphysis with a burr. (**A,B:** Copyright Mayo.)

PEARLS AND PITFALLS

Olecranon osteotomy	▪ Position the apex of the osteotomy distally. ▪ Use a thin oscillating saw to minimize bone loss. ▪ If plate fixation is preferred, consider drilling the holes for the plate before beginning the osteotomy. This facilitates plate fixation of the osteotomy at the conclusion of the surgery. ▪ Similarly, if tension band fixation with an intramedullary screw is preferred, predrill the screw hole.
Triceps reflection and triceps split	▪ Subperiosteal detachment of the extensor mechanism is critical to preserve its thickness and facilitate a strong reattachment. ▪ Reproduce anatomic reattachment of the extensor mechanism. ▪ Use heavy nonabsorbable suture (no. 5 Ethibond [Ethicon, Inc., Somerville, NJ] or no. FiberWire [Arthrex, Inc., Naples, FL]) through bone. ▪ Protect extension against resistance for 6 weeks.
Bilaterotricipital approach	▪ Separate the triceps from the underlying medial and lateral joint capsules. ▪ Resect the posterior capsule and fat pad to improve visualization.

POSTOPERATIVE MANAGEMENT

▪ After closure, the elbow is placed in a bulky noncompressive dressing with an anterior plaster splint to maintain the elbow in extension, and the upper extremity is kept elevated.

▪ Motion is initiated according to the extent of soft tissue damage. Motion usually can be initiated on the first or second postoperative day, but it may be necessary to wait for several days in the case of open fractures or severe soft tissue damage.

▪ Most patients benefit from a program of continuous passive motion for the first week or two after fixation; some may benefit from a longer period of passive motion.

▪ When postoperative motion fails to progress as expected, a program of patient-adjusted static flexion and extension splints is implemented.

▪ Treatment with indomethacin or single-dose radiation to the soft tissues shielding the fracture site may be considered for patients with high risk of heterotopic ossification, such as those with associated head or spinal trauma as well as those who require several surgeries in a short period of time.

OUTCOMES

▪ The results of internal fixation for fractures of the distal humerus using modern techniques are summarized in Table 1.

  ▪ The results of the different studies are difficult to interpret, because the severity of the injuries included cannot be compared, and there may be variations in the accuracy of range-of-motion measurements.

▪ Improvements in fixation techniques have resulted in a decreased rate of hardware failure and nonunion, but range of motion is not reliably restored in every patient.

COMPLICATIONS

▪ Infection
▪ Nonunion
▪ Stiffness, with or without heterotopic ossification
▪ Need for removal of the hardware used for fixation of the olecranon osteotomy
▪ Posttraumatic osteoarthritis or avascular necrosis requiring interposition arthroplasty or elbow replacement

Table 1   Results of Internal Fixation for Distal Humerus Fractures Affecting the Humeral Columns

Study	No.	Mean Age (Range) (y)	Follow-up (mo)	Fracture Type (no.) (AO Classification)	Open	Mean Degrees ROM (range)	Overall results*	Complications (no.)	Reoperations (no.)
Jupiter et al[5]	34	57 (17–79)	70 (25–139)	C1 (13) C2 (2) C3 (19)	14 (41%)	76% achieved at least 30–120	79% satisfactory*	Nonunion (2) Refracture (1) Olecranon osteotomy nonunion (2) Class II HO (1) Ulnar neuropathy (4) Median neuropathy (1)	Hardware removal (24) Capsulectomy (3) HO removal (1) Nerve decompression (4)
Henley et al[4]	33	32 (15–61)	18.3	C1 (23) C2 (8) C3 (2)	14 (42%)	Mean extension, 19; mean flexion 126	92% satisfactory* (only 25 patients evaluated)	Hardware failure (5) Infection (2) Olecranon osteotomy nonunion (2) Class II HO (2)	Repeat ORIF (2) TBW removal (6) Olecranon osteotomy repeat ORIF (2)
Sanders et al[14]	17	51 (12–85)	>24	C1 (4) C2 (3) C3 (10)	7 (41%)	108 (55–140)	76% satisfactory*	Delayed union (2) Infection (2) Pulmonary embolism (1) Ulnar neuropathy (1)	Hardware removal (3) Ulnar nerve decompression (1)
McKee et al (closed fractures)[7]	25	47 (19–85)	37 (18–75)	C (25)	None	108 (55–140)	Mean DASH: 20 (0–55)	Ulnar neuritis (3) Transient radial nerve palsy (1) Nonunion (1) Malunion (1)	TBW removal (3) Repeat ORIF (1) Elbow release (2)
McKee et al (open fractures)[6]	26	44 (17–78)	51 (10–141)	C1 (5) C2 (13) C3 (8)	100%	97 (55–140)	Mean DASH 23.7 (0–57.5) 60% satisfactory MEPS	Septic nonunion (1) Delayed union (4) Transient radial nerve palsy (1)	Repeat ORIF (3)
Pajarinen et al[10]	21	44 (16–81)	24 (10–41)	C1 (6) C2 (12) C3 (3)	5 (24%)	107 (98–116)	56% satisfactory OTA	Deep infection (1) Nonunion (2) Traumatic nerve injuries (3) Olecranon osteotomy nonunion (1)	Repeat ORIF (2)
Gofton et al[3]	23	53 (16–80)	45 (14–89)	C1 (3) C2 (11) C3 (9)	7 (30%)	122 (extension loss 19 ±12, flexion 142 ± 6)	Mean DASH: 12 (0–38) Subjective satisfaction: 93% 87% satisfactory MEPS	Deep infection (1) Olecranon osteotomy nonunion (2) Class II HO (3) Avascular necrosis (1) Reflex sympathetic dystrophy (1) Capitellar nonunion (1)	Olecranon osteotomy repeat ORIF (2) Elbow release (3) Capitellar ORIF (1)
Soon et al[15]	15	43 (21–80)	12 (2–27)	B (3) C1 (4) C2 (4) C3 (4)	None	109 (45–145)	86% satisfactory MEPS	Transient ulnar neuritis (2) Hardware failure (3) Nonunion (1)	Total elbow arthroplasty (1) Repeat ORIF (3) Elbow manipulation or release (4)
Sanchez-Sotelo et al[13]	32	58 (16–99)	24 (12–60)	A3 (3) C2 (4) C3 (25)	13 (44%)	Mean extension: 26 (0–55) Mean flexion: 124 (80–150)	83% satisfactory MEPS	Delayed union (1) Ulnar neuropathy (6) Class II HO (5) Infection (1)	Wound debridement or coverage (4) Bone grafting (1) HO removal (4) HO removal and distraction arthroplasty (1) Triceps reconstruction (1)

Class II HO, heterotopic ossification restricting motion; DASH, Disabilities of the Arm, Shoulder and Hand questionnaire; MEPS, Mayo Elbow Performance Score; ORIF, open reduction and internal fixation; OTA, Orthopedic Trauma Association rating; ROM, range of motion; TBW, tension band wiring.
* According to the Jupiter rating system.

REFERENCES

1. Alonso-Llames M. Bilaterotricipital approach to the elbow. Its application in the osteosynthesis of supracondylar fractures of the humerus in children. Acta Orthop Scand 1972;43:479–490.
2. Athwal GS, Rispoli DM, Steinmann SP. The anconeus flap transolecranon approach to the distal humerus. J Orthop Trauma 2006;20: 282–285.
3. Gofton WT, Macdermid JC, Patterson SD, et al. Functional outcome of AO type C distal humeral fractures. J Hand Surg Am 2003;28: 294–308.
4. Henley MB, Bone LB, Parker B. Operative management of intra-articular fractures of the distal humerus. J Orthop Trauma 1987; 1:24–35.
5. Jupiter JB, Neff U, Holzach P, et al. Intercondylar fractures of the humerus. An operative approach. J Bone Joint Surg Am 1985;67: 226–239.
6. McKee MD, Kim J, Kebaish K, et al. Functional outcome after open supracondylar fractures of the humerus. The effect of the surgical approach. J Bone Joint Surg Br 2000;82B:646–651.
7. McKee MD, Wilson TL, Winston L, et al. Functional outcome following surgical treatment of intra-articular distal humeral fractures through a posterior approach. J Bone Joint Surg Am 2000;82A:1701–1707.
8. Morrey BF. Anatomy and surgical approaches. In: Morrey BF, ed. Joint Replacement Arthroplasty. Philadelphia: Churchill-Livingstone, 2003:269–285.
9. O'Driscoll SW, Sanchez-Sotelo J, Torchia ME. Management of the smashed distal humerus. Orthop Clin North Am 2002;33:19–33.
10. Pajarinen J, Bjorkenheim JM. Operative treatment of type C intercondylar fractures of the distal humerus: Results after a mean follow-up of 2 years in a series of 18 patients. J Shoulder Elbow Surg 2002;11:48–52.
11. Ring D, Gulotta L, Chin K, et al. Olecranon osteotomy for exposure of fractures and nonunions of the distal humerus. J Orthop Trauma 2004;18:446–449.
12. Sanchez-Sotelo J, Torchia ME, O'Driscoll SW. Principle-based internal fixation of distal humerus fractures. Tech Hand Upper Extremity Surg 2001;5:179–187.
13. Sanchez-Sotelo J, Torchia ME, O'Driscoll SW. Complex distal humeral fractures: internal fixation with a principle-based parallel-plate technique. J Bone Joint Surg Am 2007;89A:961–969.
14. Sanders RA, Raney EM, Pipkin S. Operative treatment of bicondylar intraarticular fractures of the distal humerus. Orthopedics 1992;15: 159–163.
15. Soon JL, Chan BK, Low CO. Surgical fixation of intra-articular fractures of the distal humerus in adults. Injury 2004;35:44–54.

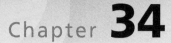

Chapter 34

Open Reduction and Internal Fixation of Capitellum and Capitellar–Trochlear Shear Fractures

Asif M. Ilyas and Jesse B. Jupiter

DEFINITION

▪ Capitellar fractures are uncommon, accounting for less than 1% of all elbow fractures and 6% of all distal humerus fractures.[3]

▪ They often are associated with radial head fractures and posterior elbow dislocations.

▪ A classification system for capitellar fractures has been proposed by Bryan and Morrey[3] and modified by McKee:

▪ Type 1: complete fractures of the capitellum[11]

▪ Type 2: superficial subchondral fractures of the capitellar articular surface[22]

▪ Type 3: comminuted fractures[2]

▪ Type 4: coronal shear fractures that include a portion of the trochlea as well as the capitellum as one piece[17] (**FIG 1**)

▪ Ring and Jupiter[21] have proposed a new classification, expanding on the growing understanding that isolated capitellum fractures are rare and often are involved as part of articular shear fractures of the distal humerus. The classification includes five anatomic components:

▪ The capitellum and lateral aspect of the trochlea

▪ The lateral epicondyle

▪ The posterior aspect of the lateral column

▪ The posterior aspect of the trochlea

▪ The medial epicondyle

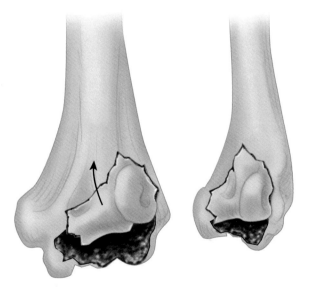

FIG 1 ▪ Type 4 coronal shear fractures of the distal humerus. (Adapted from McKee MD, Jupiter JB, Bosse G, et al. Coronal shear fractures of the distal end of the humerus. J Bone Joint Surg Am 1996;78A:49–54.)

ANATOMY

▪ The two condyles of the distal humerus diverge from the humeral shaft to form the lateral and medial columns, which support the trochlea between them. The anterior aspect of the lateral column is covered with articular cartilage, forming the capitellum. Distally, these two condyles can be visualized as forming a triangle at the end of the humerus.

▪ The capitellum is the first epiphyseal center of the elbow to ossify.

▪ It is covered by articular surface anteriorly but devoid of it posteriorly.

▪ The capitellum is directed distally and anteriorly at an angle of 30 degrees to the long axis of the humerus.

▪ The radial head rotates on the anterior surface of the capitellum in elbow flexion and articulates with its inferior surface in elbow extension.

▪ The lateral collateral ligament inserts next to the lateral margin of the capitellum.

▪ The blood supply of the capitellum is derived posteriorly. It arises from the lateral arcade, which is the anastomosis of the radial collateral arteries of the profunda brachii and the radial recurrent artery.[23]

PATHOGENESIS

▪ Capitellar fractures usually result from a fall on an outstretched hand or forearm as the radial head impacts the capitellum on impact.

▪ Capitellar–trochlear shear fractures involve impaction of the radial head against the lateral column of the distal humerus in a semi-extended position, resulting in a shearing mechanism of the distal humerus.

▪ Fracture fragments vary in size and displace superiorly and anteriorly into the radial fossa, resulting in impingement with elbow flexion.

NATURAL HISTORY

▪ Capitellar fractures occur almost exclusively in adults. These fractures do not occur in children, because in that age group the capitellum is largely cartilaginous, and a similar mechanism of injury would instead cause a supracondylar or lateral condyle fracture.

▪ Capitellar fractures are more common in females, a finding that has been attributed to the higher carrying angle of the elbow.

▪ Elderly patients of both genders are more susceptible to capitellum and complex capitellar–trochlear shear fractures because of the metabolic susceptibilities of osteoporosis.

▪ Displaced fractures that go untreated can have a poor outcome owing to progressive loss of motion and posttraumatic arthrosis.

PATIENT HISTORY AND PHYSICAL FINDINGS

▪ Symptoms of capitellar fractures are similar to those of radial head fractures, including pain and swelling along the lateral elbow and pain with elbow motion.

▪ Although there may be variable loss of forearm rotation, loss of flexion and extension is common, often accompanied by crepitus and pain.

▪ The association of concomitant radial head fractures and ligamentous injuries with capitellar fractures is high.[18]

▪ The shoulder and wrist should be examined for concomitant injury.

IMAGING AND OTHER DIAGNOSTIC STUDIES

▪ Standard radiography is inadequate for accurate assessment of capitellar fractures.

▪ Lateral radiographs are best for obtaining an initial evaluation of capitellar fractures.

▪ Anteroposterior views do not reliably show the fracture, because the outline of the distal humerus is not consistently affected.

▪ The radial head–capitellum view can help identify fractures of the capitellum. This view is a lateral oblique projection taken with the x-ray beam pointing 45 degrees dorsoventrally, thereby eliminating the ulno- and radiohumeral articulation shadows.[10]

  ▪ A type 1 fracture appears as a semilunar fragment sitting superiorly with its articular surface pointing up and away from the radial head in most cases.

  ▪ Type 2 fractures are more difficult to diagnose, depending on the amount of subchondral bone accompanying the articular fragment. They may appear as a loose body lying in the superior part of the joint.

  ▪ Type 3 fractures display variable amounts of comminution.

  ▪ Coronal shear fractures show a characteristic "double arc" sign on lateral radiographic views (**FIG 2A**).

▪ CT scans are necessary for delineating the fracture pattern and should be performed in all cases.

  ▪ CT scanning of the elbow should be done at 1- to 2-mm intervals using axial or transverse cuts.

▪ Three-dimensional (3D) CT reconstructions provide the best detail and ability to appreciate the anatomic orientation of the fracture patterns and should be ordered if 3D imaging is available (**FIG 2B,C**).

DIFFERENTIAL DIAGNOSIS

▪ Radial head fracture
▪ Distal humeral lateral condyle fracture
▪ Elbow dislocation

NONOPERATIVE MANAGEMENT

▪ Truly nondisplaced and isolated capitellum fractures can be splinted for 3 weeks, followed by protected motion. We do not advocate nonoperative management for any other type of capitellum fracture.

▪ Closed reduction techniques, which have been described in the literature, should be performed with caution, and only complete anatomic reduction should be accepted.[4,19]

▪ Capitellar–trochlear shear fractures should not be treated nonoperatively because of their inherent instability and articular incongruity.

SURGICAL MANAGEMENT

▪ The goal of surgery is anatomic reduction and fixation of the fracture to allow for early motion without mechanical block.

  ▪ Long-term goals are pain-free and maximal motion with minimal stiffness.

▪ Capitellar fractures are uncommon, and the wide array of treatment options presented in the literature is based on relatively small series.

  ▪ Treatment options include closed reduction,[4,19] open excision,[1,8,16] open reduction and internal fixation (ORIF), and arthroplasty.[5,9]

▪ With the improvement in techniques for fixation of small fragments and management of articular surfaces, ORIF has become the mainstay of treatment.

  ▪ Advantages of ORIF include restoration of anatomy and stability.

  ▪ Disadvantages include stiffness and failed fixation.

▪ In elderly patients, we do consider total elbow arthroplasty for complex intra-articular distal humerus fractures.

  ▪ Advantages include early return to function and motion.

  ▪ Disadvantages include functional limitations.

Preoperative Planning

▪ Before proceeding with surgery, a thorough understanding of the fracture and its orientation should be obtained with the help of a CT scan, and, if possible, 3D reconstructions.

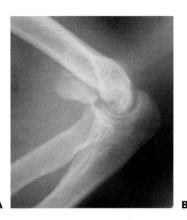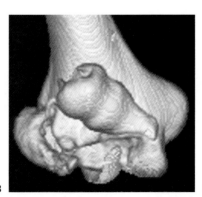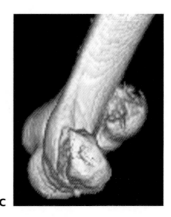

FIG 2 • **A.** Characteristic "double arc" sign on lateral radiographs of coronal shear fractures. **B,C.** 3D CT reconstructions of a coronal shear fracture of the distal humerus.

■ The timing of surgery is important. Fractures preferably should be approached within 2 weeks, before osseous healing sets in, but after swelling has gone down.

■ Ensure that the necessary implants and hardware are available.

■ Reduction and fixation of the fracture will require K-wires, articular or headless screws, and small-fragment AO screws.

■ An image intensifier should be used during surgery to confirm reduction of the fracture and proper positioning of implanted hardware.

Positioning

■ General anesthesia is recommended.

■ The patient usually is positioned supine on the operating table, with a radiolucent hand table.

■ Alternatively, a lateral or prone position can be considered, with the anterior surface of the elbow supported by a padded bolster to use the universal posterior approach.

Approach

■ Either a lateral or posterior midline incision should be used, depending on the nature of the fracture, followed by a lateral approach into the elbow joint.

■ Multiple intervals that can be exploited in the lateral approach to the elbow.

　■ We advocate the Köcher approach, which uses the interval between the extensor carpi ulnaris and the anconeus and affords greater protection of the posterior interosseous nerve.

　■ To increase exposure, the origin of the extensor carpi ulnaris (ECU), extensor digitorum communis, and extensor carpi radialis longus can be raised off of the lateral epicondyle anterior to its interval with the triceps.

■ In many cases, a capsular violation has occurred. This can be exploited and used as the interval to expose the fracture, thereby avoiding the need to cause an additional soft tissue defect.

CAPITELLAR FRACTURES

Exposure

■ The incision should begin 2 cm proximal to the lateral epicondyle and extend 3 to 4 cm distal toward the radial neck.

■ If no large soft tissue or capsular defect is present, a direct lateral Köcher approach between the anconeus and ECU interval is recommended.

■ The common extensor origin is sharply raised off the lateral epicondyle and reflected anteriorly to expose the lateral elbow joint.

　■ Care must be taken to avoid damage to the radial nerve traveling between the brachialis and brachioradialis.

■ Often the lateral ligamentous complex will be avulsed from the distal aspect of the humerus, with or without some aspect of the lateral epicondyle.

　■ This ligamentous violation can be exploited to improve exposure by hinging open the joint on the medial collateral ligament with a varus stress.

■ The capitellar fracture usually is displaced proximally and rotated and has no soft tissue attachments.

Reduction and Fixation

■ The fragment is reduced under direct visualization, held with reduction tenaculums, and provisionally fixed with 0.045-inch K-wires from an anterior-to-posterior direction.

■ Internal fixation options include fixation from posterior to anterior with AO cancellous screws or from either direction with headless compression screws.

■ Cancellous screws are best for fracture fragments with a large subchondral component, as in type 1 fracture fragments. However, extending the dissection posteriorly around the lateral column theoretically increases the risk of osteonecrosis (**TECH FIG 1**).

■ Headless compression screws, such as the Herbert screw, are best for fragments with less subchondral

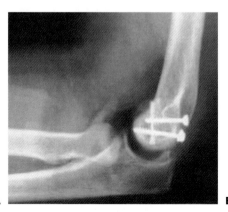
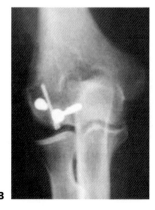

TECH FIG 1 • Fixation of a type 1 capitellum fracture with a headless screw anteriorly and AO screws from posterior to anterior.

A　　　　**B**

bone, such as type 2 and small type 1 fracture fragments. The head of the screw must be buried below the articular surface.

- Excision of fracture fragments is recommended in type 2 fractures with small, thin articular pieces and type 3 comminuted fractures where the fragments are not amenable to internal fixation.
- Fragment reduction and hardware position should be confirmed by image intensifier.

- Unrestricted forearm rotation and elbow flexion–extension without mechanical block or catching should be confirmed intraoperatively.
- If the lateral collateral ligament is found to be avulsed, it should be repaired back to the lateral epicondyle with drill holes and nonabsorbable no. 2 suture or suture anchors.
- The capsule should be closed.
- The retracted extensor origin should be relaxed and closed to the surrounding soft tissue.

CAPITELLAR–TROCHLEAR SHEAR FRACTURES

Exposure

- A posterior midline incision should be made, and full-thickness flaps should be raised medially and laterally off of the extensor mechanism.
  - This incision provides extensile exposure, access to both sides, and ease of osteotomy if necessary (**TECH FIG 2A**).
- Beginning medially, the ulnar nerve should be decompressed in situ behind the medial epicondyle (**TECH FIG 2B**).
- Returning laterally, the interval between the anconeus and the ECU should be developed. In many cases, a capsular violation can be exploited (**TECH FIG 2C**).
- The common extensor origin, including the ECU, extensor digitorum communis, and extensor carpi radialis longus, is then sharply raised off the lateral epicondyle and reflected anteriorly to expose the lateral elbow joint and improve visualization medially.

- Care must be taken to avoid injury to the radial nerve proximally as it travels between the brachialis and brachioradialis, and to the posterior interosseous nerve distally when raising the ECU anteriorly. This may be done by keeping the forearm pronated.
- In many cases, the lateral epicondyle will have avulsed off of the distal humerus, and this traumatic osteotomy can be exploited.
  - Otherwise, a formal lateral epicondyle osteotomy can be performed to enhance visualization while maintaining the integrity of the lateral ligamentous complex.
- Additionally, an olecranon osteotomy may be performed to improve visualization and fixation of fractures extending medially and posteriorly.
- The fracture fragments should now be visualized and accounted for. They are most commonly displaced proximally and internally rotated (**TECH FIG 2D**).

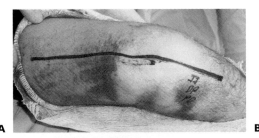
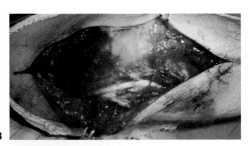
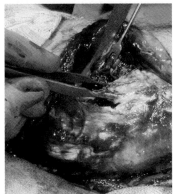
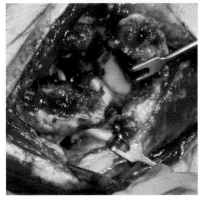

TECH FIG 2 • A. Posterior midline incision used to for capitellar–trochlear shear fractures. **B.** Ulnar nerve compression medially. **C.** Lateral approach to elbow taking advantage of violation of the capsule and extensor muscles at the level of the extensor carpi ulnaris (ECU) and anconeus. **D.** The fracture fragments tend to displace proximally and become internally rotated.

Reduction and Fixation

- The fragment is reduced under direct visualization, held with reduction tenaculums, and provisionally fixed with 0.045-inch K-wires from anterior to posterior (**TECH FIG 3A**).
- Inability to reduce the fracture anatomically may represent fracture impaction, requiring either disimpaction or bone grafting, or both.
- Options for internal fixation include fixation from posterior-to-anterior with AO screws or from either direction with headless compression screws.
- Cancellous screws are best when the fracture fragment has a large subchondral component, but they make it necessary to extend the dissection posteriorly around the lateral column, theoretically increasing the risk of osteonecrosis.

- Headless compression screws, such as the Herbert screw, are best for fragments with less subchondral bone and provide the added benefit that they can be used in either direction, anteriorly or posteriorly. Diligence must be maintained to confirm that the head of the screw is buried below the articular surface when placed anteriorly.
- Fragment reduction and hardware position should be confirmed by image intensifier.
- Unrestricted forearm rotation and elbow flexion–extension without mechanical block or catching should be confirmed intraoperatively.
- The lateral epicondyle, if avulsed or osteotomized, should be repaired with a tension band technique or plate and screws (**TECH FIG 3A,B**).
- The capsule should be closed.
- The interval and released extensor origin should be relaxed and closed to the surrounding soft tissue.

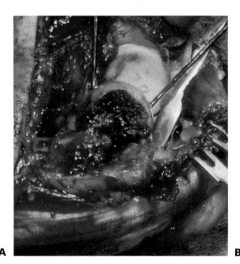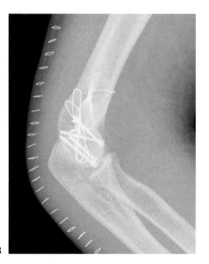

TECH FIG 3 • A. The fracture is reduced and pinned with 0.045-inch K-wires. **B.** Postoperative radiographs illustrate repair of the lateral epicondyle and fracture fixation.

PEARLS AND PITFALLS

Diagnosis	• Diligence should be paid to identifying concomitant injuries such as dislocations, radial head fractures, and ligamentous instability.
Imaging	• Plain radiographs are insufficient, and a CT scan should be performed routinely. • Order 3D reconstructions if possible.
Nonoperative management	• Nonoperative management should be chosen cautiously. Anatomic and stable reduction of the fracture is necessary. Otherwise, a painful elbow with restricted motion may result. • We do not recommend nonoperative management of any capitellar–trochlear shear fractures.
Surgical management	• A straight posterior skin incision will allow ulnar nerve decompression and fracture fixation. • Lateral epicondyle osteotomy can enhance exposure. • Inability to reduce the fracture anatomically may represent impaction of the lateral column and require disimpaction or bone grafting. • Excision of comminuted fragments that cannot be fixed internally is preferred over nonanatomic reduction and malunion. • Concomitant fractures and ligamentous injuries should be treated simultaneously to optimize outcomes.
Postoperative management	• Stable fixation should be sought to allow for early motion. • Heterotopic ossification is common after elbow fractures, and prophylaxis with nonsteroidal anti-inflammatory drugs should be considered.

POSTOPERATIVE CARE

■ If secure fixation has been obtained, immediate mobilization can be initiated postoperatively.
■ If fixation is tenuous, splint or cast the elbow for 3 to 4 weeks, followed by active and assisted range-of-motion exercises.

OUTCOMES

■ Focusing initially on outcomes after ORIF of types 1 and 2 capitellar fractures, multiple small series have shown good results using Herbert screws in an anterior to posterior direction.[6,13,14,20]
■ More recently, Mahirogullari et al[15] reported on 11 cases of type 1 capitellum fractures treated with Herbert screws, which yielded 8 excellent and 3 good results. They recommended fixation in a posterior-to-anterior direction with at least two Herbert screws.
■ Reported outcomes on type 4 capitellar–trochlear shear fractures are limited. McKee et al[17] originally described this pattern and reported on 6 cases.
  ■ Each case involved an extended lateral Köcher approach and fixation with Herbert screws from an anterior to posterior direction. Good or excellent results were achieved in all cases, with average elbow motion of 15 to 141 degrees, and forearm rotation of 83 degrees pronation and 84 degrees supination.
■ Ring and Jupiter examined 21 cases of articular fractures of the distal humerus treated with Herbert screw fixation and found 4 excellent results, 12 good results, and 5 fair results.
  ■ All of the fractures healed and had an average range of motion of 96 degrees. No ulnohumeral instability, arthrosis, or osteonecrosis was reported.
  ■ The authors stressed the importance of proper evaluation of these fractures and awareness that apparent capitellum fractures often are complex articular fractures of the distal humerus.[21]
■ Dubberley et al[7] further subclassified type 4 fractures in their series of 28 cases. They achieved an average range of motion of flexion–extension of 25 degrees less than the contralateral elbow and 4 degrees of supination–pronation less than the contralateral elbow.
  ■ Two comminuted cases required conversion to a total elbow arthroplasty.
  ■ Varied fixation methods were used, including Herbert screws, cancellous screws, absorbable pins, and supplementation with K-wires.

COMPLICATIONS

■ The most common complication of capitellar fractures is loss of elbow motion and residual pain. The compromised motion most commonly is manifested in loss of flexion and extension.
■ Ulnar neuropathy has been noted after ORIF, and some recommend routine ulnar nerve decompression.[21]
■ Osteonecrosis may occur from the initial fracture displacement or surgical exposure. Blood is supplied to the capitellum from a posterior to anterior direction and may be compromised by surgical dissection.
  ■ In symptomatic cases in which revascularization after fixation has not occurred, delayed excision is indicated.

■ Malunions may occur when the patient has delayed seeking treatment, when inadequate reduction or loss of closed reduction occurs, or after ORIF. Malunions result in loss of motion and may require excision of the fragment and soft tissue releases.
■ Nonunions may occur, although this is uncommon. They most likely result secondary to inadequate reduction or lack of revascularization of the fragment.

REFERENCES

 1. Alvarez E, Patel M, Nimberg P, et al. Fractures of the capitellum humeri. J Bone Joint Surg Am 1975;57A:1093–1096.
 2. Broberg MA, Morrey BF. Results of delayed excision of the radial head after fracture. J Bone Joint Surg Am 1986;68A:669–674.
 3. Bryan RS, Morrey BF. Fractures of the distal humerus. In: Morrey BF, ed. The Elbow and Its Disorders. Philadelphia: WB Saunders, 1985:302–399.
 4. Christopher F, Bushnell L. Conservative treatment of fractures of the capitellum. J Bone Joint Surg 1935;17:489–492.
 5. Cobb TK, Morrey BF. Total elbow arthroplasty as primary treatment for distal humerus fractures in elderly patients. J Bone Joint Surg Am 1997;79A:826–832.
 6. Collert S. Surgical management of fracture of the capitulum humeri. Acta Orthop Scand 1977;48:603–606.
 7. Dubberley JH, Faber KJ, Macdermid JC, et al. Outcome after open reduction and internal fixation of capitellar and trochlear fractures. J Bone Joint Surg Am 2006;88A:46–54.
 8. Fowles JV, Kassab MT. Fracture of the capitulum humeri: treatment by excision. J Bone Joint Surg Am 1975;56A:794–798.
 9. Garcia JA, Myulka R, Stanley D. Complex fractures of the distal humerus in the elderly: the role of total elbow replacement as primary treatment. J Bone Joint Surg Br 2002;84B:812–816.
10. Greenspan A, Norman A. The radial head, capitellum view: useful technique in elbow trauma. AJR Am J Roentgenol 1982;138:1186–1188.
11. Hahn NF. Fall von einer besonderes Varietat der Frakturen des Ellenbogens. Z Wund Geburt 1853;6:185.
12. Jupiter JB, Neff U, Ragazzoni P, et al. Unicondylar fractures of the distal humerus: an operative approach. J Orthop Trauma 1988;2:102–109.
13. Lansinger O, Mare K. Fracture of the capitulum humeri. Acta Orthop Scand 1981;52:39–44.
14. Liberman N, Katz T, Howard CV, et al. Fixation of capitellar fractures with Herbert screws. Arch Orthop Trauma Surg 1991;110:155–157.
15. Mahirogullari M, Kiral A, Solakoglu C, et al. Treatment of fractures of the humeral capitellum using Herbert screws. J Hand Surg Eur Vol 2006;31:320–325.
16. Mazel MS. Fracture of the capitellum. J Bone Joint Surg 1935;17:483–488.
17. McKee MD, Jupiter JB, Bosse G, et al. Coronal shear fractures of the distal end of the humerus. J Bone Joint Surg Am 1996;78A:49–54.
18. Milch H. Fractures and fracture-dislocations of the humeral condyles. J Trauma 1964;13:882–886.
19. Ochner RS, Bloom H, Palumbo RC, et al. Closed reduction of coronal fractures of the capitellum. J Trauma 1996;40:199–203.
20. Richards RR, Khoury GW, Burke FD, et al. Internal fixation of capitellar fractures using Herbert screw: a report of four cases. Can J Surg 1987;30:188–191.
21. Ring D, Jupiter JB, Gulotta L. Articular fractures of the distal part of the humerus. J Bone Joint Surg Am 2003;85A:232–238.
22. Steinthal D. Die isolirte Fraktur der eminentia Capetala in Ellengogelenk. Zentralk Chir 1898;15:17.
23. Yamaguchi K, Sweet FA, Bindra R, et al. The extraosseous and intraosseous arterial anatomy of the adult elbow. J Bone Joint Surg Am 1997;79A:1653–1662.

Chapter 35

Open Reduction and Internal Fixation of Radial Head and Neck Fractures

Anshu Singh, George Frederick Hatch III, and John M. Itamura

DEFINITION

- The radial head is distinctive in anatomy and function with unique considerations regarding the diagnostic and treatment options available to the surgeon.
- Radial head and neck fractures are the most common elbow fractures in adults, representing 33% of elbow fractures.
- The original Mason classification was modified by Johnson, then Morrey. Hotchkiss proposed that the classification system be used to provide guidance for treatment. It has poor intraobserver and interobserver reliability (**FIG 1**).[9]
  - Type I fractures are nondisplaced and offer no block to pronation and supination on examination.
  - Type II fractures have displaced marginal segments that block normal forearm rotation. We only include fractures with three or fewer articular fragments, which meet criteria for fractures that can be operatively reduced and fixed with reproducibly good results.
  - Type III fractures are comminuted or impacted articular fractures that are optimally managed with prosthetic replacement.
  - Type IV fractures are associated with elbow instability and should never be resected in the acute setting.

ANATOMY

- The radial head is entirely intra-articular. It has two articulations, one with the humerus, via the radiocapitellar joint, and another with the ulna, via the proximal radioulnar joint (PRUJ).
  - The radiocapitellar joint has a saddle-shaped articulation allowing both flexion and extension as well as rotation.
  - The PRUJ, constrained by the annular ligament, allows rotation of the radial head in the lesser sigmoid notch of the proximal ulna.
    - To avoid creating a mechanical block to pronation and supination, implants must be limited to a 90-degree arc (the "safe zone") outside the PRUJ (**FIG 2**).[4]

- Blood supply to the radial head is tenuous, with a major contribution from a single branch of the radial recurrent artery in the safe zone and minor contributions from both the radial and interosseous recurrent arteries, which penetrate the capsule at its insertion into the neck (**FIG 3**).[13]
- There is considerable variability in the shape of the radial head, from nearly round to elliptical, as well as variability in the offset of the head from the neck.
- The anterior band of the medial collateral ligament (MCL) is the primary stabilizer to valgus stress. The radial head, a secondary stabilizer, maintains up to 30% of valgus resistance in the native elbow. Therefore, in cases where the MCL is ruptured:
  - A radial head that is not reparable should be replaced with a prosthesis and not excised given its biomechanical importance.
  - It may be prudent to protect a repaired radial head from high valgus stress during early range of motion by placing a hinged external fixator.
- The radial head also functions in the transmission of axial load, transmitting 60% of the load from the wrist to the elbow.[10] This is a crucial consideration when the interosseous membrane is disrupted in the Essex-Lopresti lesion.[5] Resection of the radial head in this setting results in devastating longitudinal radioulnar instability, proximal migration of the radius, and possible ulnar-carpal impingement.

PATHOGENESIS

- Radial head fractures result from trauma. A fall on an outstretched hand with the elbow in extension and the forearm in pronation produces an axial or valgus load (or both) driving the radial head into the capitellum, fracturing the relatively osteopenic radial head.
  - Loading at 0 to 35 degrees of extension causes coronoid fractures.
  - Loading at 0 to 80 degrees of extension produces radial head fractures.

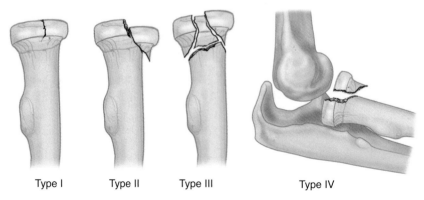

Type I   Type II   Type III   Type IV

FIG 1 • The modified Mason classification for radial head fractures.

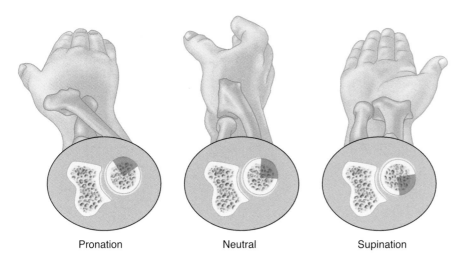

Pronation   Neutral   Supination

FIG 2 • The "safe zone" is a roughly 90-degree arc of the radial head that does not articulate with the ulna in the proximal radioulnar joint with full supination and pronation. With the wrist in neutral rotation, the safe zone is anterolateral.

▪ Associated soft tissue injuries can lead to considerable complications, including pain, arthrosis, stiffness, and disability:
  ▪ MCL injury in 50%
  ▪ Lateral ligament disruption in about 80%
  ▪ Capitellar bone bruises in 90%[8]
  ▪ Capitellar cartilage defects in about 50%

▪ The axial loading may also rupture the interosseous membrane, causing longitudinal radioulnar instability with dislocation of the distal radioulnar joint (DRUJ) (**FIG 4**).

▪ The "terrible triad" injury results from valgus loading of the elbow, disrupting the MCL or lateral ulnar collateral ligament and fracturing the radial head and coronoid process.

NATURAL HISTORY

▪ Results are mixed regarding the efficacy of radial head excision for treatment of radial head fracture. Good or fair results may be possible, with a few caveats:

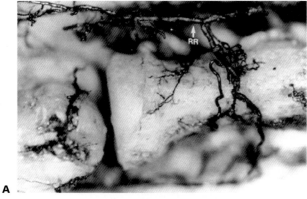

A

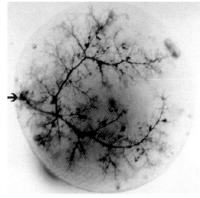

B

FIG 3 • **A.** The radial recurrent artery, a branch of the radial artery, provides the main blood supply to the radial head. **B.** In most cadaveric specimens, a branch of the radial recurrent penetrates the radial head in the safe zone. (From Yamaguchi K, Sweet FA, Bindra R, et al. The extraosseous and intraosseous arterial anatomy of the adult elbow. J Bone Joint Surg Am 1997;79A:1653–1662.)

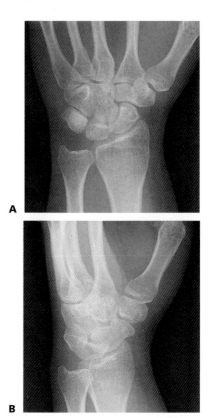

A

B

FIG 4 • **A.** AP radiograph of the wrist in cases of longitudinal radioulnar instability (the Essex-Lopresti lesion). Subtle shortening of the radius is demonstrated. **B.** Lateral radiograph of the wrist may show dorsal subluxation of the distal ulna.

- There is a demonstrable increase in ulnar variance at the wrist and increased carrying angle.
- 10% to 20% loss of strength is expected.
- It is contraindicated in the face of associated soft tissue injuries.
- Radiographic, but usually clinically silent, degenerative changes such as cysts, sclerosis, and osteophytes occur radiographically in about 75% of elbows after radial head excision (**FIG 5**).
- Results of excision are poor in patients with concomitant MCL, coronoid, or interosseous membrane injury.
  - Radial head resection should be reserved for patients with low functional demands or limited life expectancy, and when the surgeon has excluded elbow instability with a fluoroscopic examination.
- Delayed excision of the radial head after failed nonoperative management may be considered with modest increase in function; it has shown 23% fair or poor results at 15 years of follow-up.[3] Other studies suggest that there is no difference between delayed and primary excision.[6]
- Although open reduction and fixation of a comminuted fracture can be attempted, a large series by experienced elbow surgeons found that fixation of a radial head with more than three articular fragments is fraught with poor results.[11]
- Nonanatomic reduction of the shaft or joint may result in limited range of motion due to a cam effect in the PRUJ, but no literature or prospective studies indicate what parameters are "acceptable."

PATIENT HISTORY AND PHYSICAL FINDINGS

- The history typically involves a fall on an outstretched hand followed by pain and edema over the lateral elbow, accompanied by limited range of motion.
- The examiner should note the patient's activity level and profession.
- Physical examination should include neurovascular status and examination of the skin to look for medial ecchymosis, which may suggest injury to the MCL.
  - A detailed examination of the elbow must include bony palpation of the medial and lateral epicondyles, olecranon process, DRUJ, and radial head, as well as the squeeze test

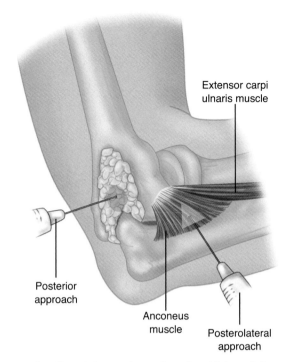

FIG 6 • The elbow joint can be aspirated and injected through the posterior and posterolateral approaches. They are equally effective and should be used based on soft tissue injury.

of the interosseous membrane and DRUJ to screen for potential longitudinal instability.
  - Varus and valgus stress testing, with or without fluoroscopy, can indicate injury to the anterior band of the MCL or to the lateral ulnar collateral ligament, respectively.
- Range-of-motion and stress examinations are vital to proper decision making and may obviate the need for advanced imaging if performed correctly with adequate anesthesia. If omitted, this will lead to undiagnosed associated injuries and may result in flawed decision making.
  - In the emergency department or office, adequate anesthesia may be obtained by aspirating hematoma, then injecting the elbow joint with 5 mL of local anesthetic and examining the elbow under fluoroscopy. This may be performed by the traditional lateral injection in the "soft spot" or posteriorly into the olecranon fossa (**FIG 6**).[12]
  - If operative intervention is clearly indicated, this examination can be performed under a general anesthetic, provided the surgeon and patient are prepared for a change in operative plan as dictated by the examination.
  - Normal values are 0 to 145 degrees of flexion–extension, 85 degrees of supination, and 80 degrees of pronation. The examiner should check for a bony block to motion.

IMAGING AND OTHER DIAGNOSTIC STUDIES

Radiography

- Anteroposterior (AP), lateral, and oblique views are the standard of care, but they underestimate or overestimate joint impaction and degree of comminution (**FIG 7A,B**).
  - A radiocapitellar view with forearm in neutral and at 45 degrees cephalad gives an improved view of the articular surfaces.

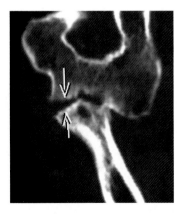

FIG 5 • A CT scan demonstrating symptomatic posttraumatic arthrosis with cyst formation in the ulnohumeral articulation after radial head resection.

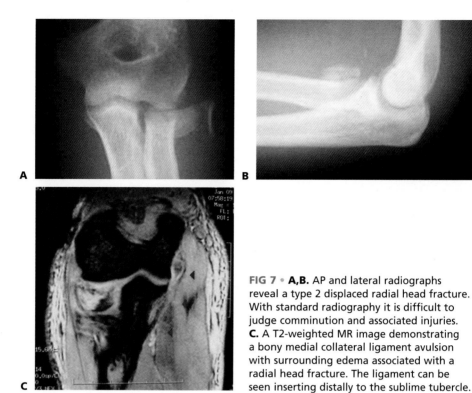

FIG 7 • **A,B.** AP and lateral radiographs reveal a type 2 displaced radial head fracture. With standard radiography it is difficult to judge comminution and associated injuries. **C.** A T2-weighted MR image demonstrating a bony medial collateral ligament avulsion with surrounding edema associated with a radial head fracture. The ligament can be seen inserting distally to the sublime tubercle.

■ If the examination reveals wrist or forearm tenderness, the examiner should have a low threshold for obtaining bilateral wrist posteroanterior (PA) views to rule out an Essex-Lopresti lesion.

Magnetic Resonance Imaging

■ Magnetic resonance imaging (MRI) is a useful adjunct to physical examination for evaluating associated injuries such as collateral ligament tears, chondral defects, and loose bodies,[8] but it is not routinely indicated (**FIG 7C**).

DIFFERENTIAL DIAGNOSIS

■ Simple elbow dislocation
■ Distal humerus fracture
■ Olecranon fracture
■ Septic elbow

NONOPERATIVE MANAGEMENT

■ The standard protocol for treating radial head fractures is shown in FIGURE 8.

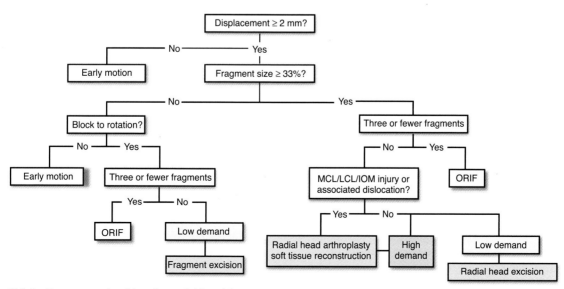

FIG 8 • Treatment algorithm for radial head fractures.

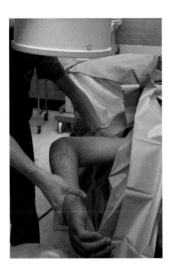

FIG 9 • Intraoperative photograph demonstrating the fluoroscopic examination. This is crucial to proper decision making and may be performed just before operative management.

▪ Conservative management, with a week of sling immobilization followed by range of motion once the acute pain resolves, it is the treatment of choice in nondisplaced radial head fractures, where universally good and excellent results have been reported.

▪ Nonoperative management is also the treatment of choice in fractures with less than 2 mm of displacement, with minor head involvement, and without bony blockage to range of motion.

  ▪ A 7-day period of cast or splint immobilization is followed by aggressive motion after the inflammatory phase.

▪ Our current practice for fractures that are more than 2 mm displaced is to determine whether there is a blockage of motion on fluoroscopic examination.

  ▪ If there is maintenance of at least 50 degrees of both pronation and supination, we recommend conservative treatment.

  ▪ If there is a blockage or instability, excision, fixation, or arthroplasty is recommended based on patient factors and instability.

▪ A recent report regarding the long-term results of nonoperative management (similar to that described) of 49 patients with radial head fractures encompassing over 30% of the joint surface and displaced 2 to 5 mm revealed that 81% of patients had no subjective complaints and minimal loss of motion versus the uninjured extremity. Only one patient had daily pain.[1]

SURGICAL MANAGEMENT

Preoperative Planning

▪ It is essential to review all radiographs and, most importantly, perform thorough history, physical, and fluoroscopic examinations before making an incision.

  ▪ The presence of instability or associated fractures warrants a more extensile approach (**FIG 9**).

Positioning

▪ Positioning depends on the planned approach and the surgeon's preference.

  ▪ We prefer the patient supine with the affected extremity brought across the chest over a bump to allow access to the posterolateral elbow.

  ▪ A tourniquet is placed high on the arm.

Approach

▪ Two approaches, the extensile posterior (Boyd) and posterolateral (Köcher), will be presented (**FIG 10**).

▪ The extensile posterior (Boyd) approach[2] with an interval between the ulna and anconeus allows for excellent visualization compared to traditional approaches. This versatile approach facilitates ORIF or arthroplasty of the radial head if the fracture proves to be more comminuted than preoperative imaging would predict. It can be easily accessed through a universal extensile incision that allows the surgeon to address ligamentous injuries in addition to the radial head fracture.

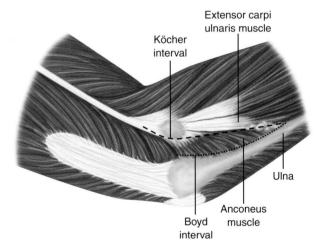

FIG 10 • Surgical intervals for the Boyd approach and the Köcher approach.

BOYD APPROACH

▪ An 8-cm straight longitudinal incision is made just lateral to the olecranon (**TECH FIG 1A**).

▪ Full-thickness skin flaps are developed bluntly over the fascia.

▪ The fascia is longitudinally incised in the interval between the anconeus and ulna (**TECH FIG 1B**).

▪ The anconeus is dissected off the ulna, elevating proximal to distal to preserve the distal vascular pedicle. Great care is taken not to violate the joint capsule or

lateral ulnar collateral ligament by using blunt fashion (**TECH FIG 1C**).

▪ The lateral ulnar collateral ligament and annular ligament complex are sharply divided and tagged from their insertion on the crista supinatorus of the ulna. The radial head and its articulation with the capitellum are now evident (**TECH FIG 1D**).

▪ After repair or replacement, the ligaments are repaired to their insertion with suture anchors.

TECHNIQUES

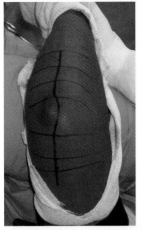
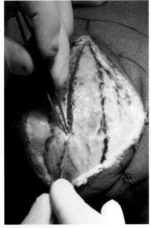
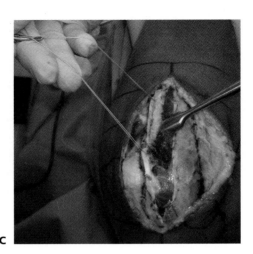

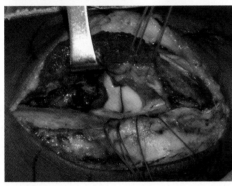

TECH FIG 1 • Boyd approach. **A.** Make an 8-cm longitudinal incision at the junction of the ulna and anconeus starting about four fingerbreadths distal to the olecranon and extending 2 cm proximal to the olecranon. **B.** The interval between the ulna and anconeus is incised sharply, with care taken not to violate the periosteum or muscle to minimize the risk of proximal radioulnar synostosis. **C.** Blunt elevation of the anconeus is crucial to avoid damaging the capsule or lateral ligament complex. **D.** The capsule and lateral ligament complex are tagged during the approach to facilitate final repair with suture anchors.

KÖCHER APPROACH

- The traditional posterolateral (Köcher) approach between the anconeus and extensor carpi ulnaris is cosmetic and spares the lateral ulnar collateral ligament.
  - We recommend not using an Esmarch tourniquet to allow visualization of penetrating veins that help identify the interval.
- A 5-cm oblique incision is made from the posterolateral aspect of the lateral epicondyle obliquely to a point three fingerbreadths below the tip of the olecranon in line with the radial neck (**TECH FIG 2A**).
- The radial head and epicondyle are palpated and the fascia is divided in line with the skin incision.

- The Köcher interval is identified distally by small penetrating veins and bluntly developed, revealing the lateral ligament complex and joint capsule (**TECH FIG 2B**).
- The anconeus is reflected posteriorly and the extensor carpi ulnaris origin anteriorly. The capsule is incised obliquely anterior to the lateral ulnar collateral ligament (**TECH FIG 2C,D**).
- The proximal edge of the annular ligament may also be divided and tagged, with care taken not to proceed distally and damage the posterior interosseous nerve.

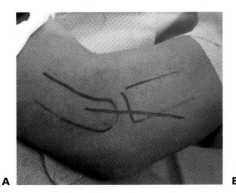
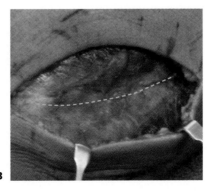

TECH FIG 2 • Köcher approach. **A.** The skin incision proceeds distally from the posterolateral aspect of the lateral epicondyle to the posterior aspect of the proximal radius. **B.** Full-thickness flaps are made and the fascial interval between the extensor carpi ulnaris and anconeus muscles is identified. *(continued)*

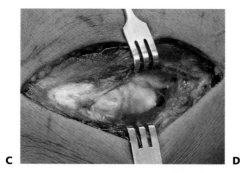

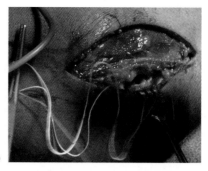

C   D

TECH FIG 2 • *(continued)* **C.** With longitudinal incision of the fascia and blunt division of the muscles, the joint capsule is evident. **D.** The capsule is longitudinally incised and the fascia is tagged with figure 8 stitches for later anatomic repair.

FRACTURE INSPECTION AND PREPARATION

- The fracture is now visible (**TECH FIG 3**).
- The wound is irrigated and loose bodies are removed.
- The forearm is rotated to obtain a circumferential view of the fracture and appreciate the safe zone for hardware placement.
- If comminution (more than three pieces) is evident at this step, we elect to replace the radial head.

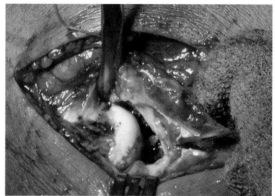

TECH FIG 3 • Here the fractured radial head fragment has violated the lateral capsule, indicating a high-energy injury. The proximal radius is now exposed for fixation or prosthetic replacement.

REDUCTION AND PROVISIONAL FIXATION

- Any joint impaction is elevated and the void filed with local cancellous graft from the lateral epicondyle.
- The fragments are reduced provisionally with a tenaculum and held with small Kirschner wires placed out of the zone where definitive fixation is planned.
- It is acceptable to place this temporary fixation in the safe zone (**TECH FIG 4**).

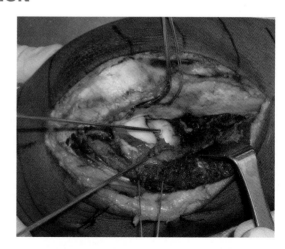

TECH FIG 4 • We prefer to use 0.062-inch Kirschner wires placed outside the zone of planned definitive fixation to provisionally hold the reduction.

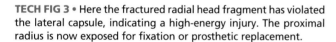

TECHNIQUES

FIXATION

- There are many options for definitive fixation[7]:
  - One or two countersunk 2.0-mm or 2.7-mm AO cortical screws perpendicular to the fracture (**TECH FIG 5A**)
  - Mini-plates (**TECH FIG 5B**)
  - Small headless screws
- Polyglycolide pins
- Small threaded wires
- We prefer to use two small parallel screws for isolated head fractures. For fractures with neck extension, we prefer AO 2.0-mm or 2.7-mm mini-plates along the safe zone.

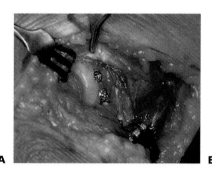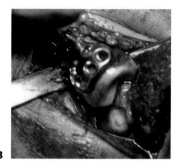

A **B**

TECH FIG 5 • A. Two screws are placed in the safe zone perpendicular to the fracture. **B.** A plate is placed on a radial neck fracture.

CLOSURE

- Any releases or injury to the annular ligament or lateral ulnar collateral ligament must be repaired anatomically. Drill holes with transosseous sutures are a proven method, but most authors now use suture anchors with reproducible results.
- Skin closure is performed in standard fashion with drains at the surgeon's discretion. Small hemovac drains are routinely pulled on postoperative day 1.

PEARLS AND PITFALLS

Protection of the posterior interosseous nerve	■ Pronation of the forearm moves the posterior interosseous nerve away from the operative field during posterior approaches. ■ Dissection should remain subperiosteal.
Comminution	■ We have a low threshold for excision or arthroplasty in the setting of comminution.
Fluoroscopy	■ A fluoroscopy unit should be available for examination under anesthesia before sterile preparation.
Hardware	■ Prosthetic radial head replacement should be discussed with the patient as an option and should be available in the room should the fracture prove to be comminuted. ■ A hinged external fixator should be available if instability may be an issue.
Examination	■ A thorough fluoroscopic examination is the most important factor in deciding what treatment is appropriate. To obtain a true lateral we recommend abducting the arm and externally rotating the shoulder while placing the elbow on the image intensifier.

POSTOPERATIVE CARE

- The elbow is immobilized in a splint for 7 to 10 days.
- Active range of motion is allowed as soon as tolerable. Supervised therapy may be considered if the patient is not making adequate progress.
- Associated injuries may call for more protected range of motion.
- Light activities of daily living are allowed at 2 weeks, with increased weight bearing at 6 weeks.

RESULTS

- The results of open reduction and internal fixation depend both on host factors such as the type of fracture, smoking, compliance, demand, as well as surgical and rehabilitation protocols.
  - In uncomplicated fractures, over 90% satisfactory results can be expected.
  - Complications and resultant secondary procedures will be more likely in cases with undiagnosed instability and associated injury.

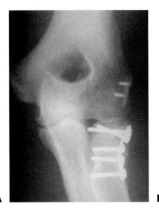 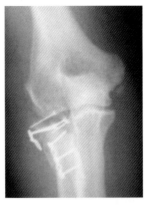 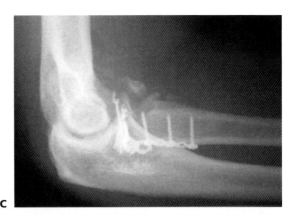

A   B   C

FIG 11 • **A.** AP radiograph demonstrating a screw penetrating the proximal radioulnar joint. **B,C.** Although these low-profile implants were apparently well placed, this patient went on to develop avascular necrosis with fragmentation of the radial head.

COMPLICATIONS

▪ Stiffness is the most common complication, with loss of terminal extension, supination, and pronation being most evident.

▪ Arthritis of the radiocapitellar joint or proximal radioulnar joint

▪ Heterotopic ossification

▪ Symptomatic hardware may require secondary removal (**FIG 11A**).

▪ Infection

▪ Early and late instability from missed or failed treatment of associated injuries

▪ The rate of avascular necrosis is about 10%, significantly higher in displaced fractures. This is expected given that the radial recurrent artery inserts in the safe zone where hardware is placed. This is generally clinically silent.

▪ Loss of reduction

▪ Nonunion (**FIG 11B,C**)

REFERENCES

1. Akesson T, Herbertsson P, Josefsson PO, et al. Primary nonoperative treatment of moderately displaced two-part fractures of the radial head. J Bone Joint Surg Am 2006;88A:1909–1914.
2. Boyd HB. Surgical exposure of the ulna and proximal third of the radius through one incision. Surg Gynecol Obstet 1940;71:86–88.
3. Broberg MA, Morrey BF. Results of delayed excision of the radial head after fracture. J Bone Joint Surg Am 1986;68A:669–674.
4. Caputo AE, Mazzocca AD, Sontoro VM. The nonarticulating portion of the radial head: Anatomic and clinical correlations for internal fixation. J Hand Surg Am 1998;23A:1082–1090.
5. Essex-Lopresti P. Fractures of the radial head with distal radioulnar dislocation. J Bone Joint Surg Br 1951;33B:244–250.
6. Herbertsson P, Josefsson PO, Hasserius R, et al. Fractures of the radial head and neck treated with radial head excision. J Bone Joint Surg Am 2004;86A:1925–1930.
7. Ikeda M, Sugiyama K, Kang C, et al. Comminuted fractures of the radial head: comparison of resection and internal fixation. J Bone Joint Surg Am 2006;88A:11–23.
8. Itamura J, Roidis N, Vaishnav S, et al. MRI evaluation of comminuted radial head fractures. J Shoulder Elbow Surg 2005;14:421–424.
9. Morgan SJ, Groshen SL, Itamura JM, et al. Reliability evaluation of classifying radial head fractures by the system of Mason. Bull Hosp Jt Dis 1997;56:95–98.
10. Morrey BF, An KN, Stormont TJ. Force transmission through the radial head. J Bone Joint Surg Am 1988;70A:250–256.
11. Ring D, Quintero J, Jupiter JB. Open reduction and internal fixation of fractures of the radial head. J Bone Joint Surg Am 2002;84A:1811–1815.
12. Tang CW, Skaggs DL, Kay RM. Elbow aspiration and arthrogram: an alternative method. Am J Orthop 2001;30:256.
13. Yamaguchi K, Sweet FA, Bindra R, et al. The extraosseous and intraosseous arterial anatomy of the adult elbow. J Bone Joint Surg Am 1997;79A:1653–1662.

DEFINITION

- Radial head fractures are the most common fracture of the elbow and usually can be managed either nonoperatively or with open reduction and internal fixation.
- Radial head arthroplasty is indicated for unreconstructable displaced radial head fractures with an associated elbow dislocation or a known or possible disruption of the medial collateral, lateral collateral, or interosseous ligaments.[16]
- Most comminuted radial head fractures have an associated ligament injury, so radial head excision without replacement is uncommonly indicated in the setting of an acute radial head fracture.
- Biomechanical studies have shown that the kinematics and stability of the elbow are altered by radial head excision, even in the setting of intact collateral ligaments,[15] and are improved with a metallic radial head arthroplasty.[19,23]
- Radial head replacement is also indicated to treat posttraumatic conditions such as radial head nonunion and malunion and to manage elbow or forearm instability after radial head excision.

ANATOMY

- The radial head has a circular concave dish that articulates with the spherical capitellum and an articular margin that articulates with the lesser sigmoid notch of the ulna.
- The articular dish has an elliptical shape that varies considerably in size and shape and is variably offset from the axis of the radial neck.
- There is a poor correlation between the size of the radial head and the medullary canal of the radial neck, making a modular implant desirable for an optimal fit.[18]
- Elbow stability is maintained by joint congruity, capsuloligamentous integrity, and an intact balanced musculature.
- The radial head is an important valgus stabilizer of the elbow, particularly in the setting of an incompetent medial collateral ligament, which is the primary stabilizer against valgus force.
- The radial head is also important as an axial stabilizer of the forearm and resists varus and posterolateral rotatory instability by tensioning the lateral collateral ligament.
- The radial head accounts for up to 60% of the load transfer across the elbow.[11]
- The lateral ulnar collateral ligament is an important stabilizer against varus and posterolateral rotational instability of the elbow and should be preserved or repaired after radial head arthroplasty (**FIG 1**).

PATHOGENESIS

- Displaced radial head fractures typically result from a fall on the outstretched arm.
- Axial, valgus, and posterolateral rotational patterns of loading are all thought to be potentially responsible for these fractures.

- Injuries of the medial collateral or lateral collateral ligament or the interosseous ligament are typically associated with comminuted displaced unreconstructable radial head fractures.[6]
- In more severe injuries, dislocations of the elbow and forearm and fractures of the coronoid, olecranon, and capitellum can occur and further impair stability.

NATURAL HISTORY

- Long-term follow-up studies suggest a high incidence of radiographic arthritis with radial head excision, although the incidence of symptomatic arthritis varies widely between series.[4,13,14]
- Biomechanical data have demonstrated an alteration in the kinematics, load transfer, and stability of the elbow after radial head excision[3,15] that may lead to premature cartilage wear of the ulnohumeral joint and secondary pain due to arthritis.
- Metallic radial head replacement in elbows with intact ligaments restores the kinematics and stability similar to that of a native radial head and has been shown to provide good clinical and radiographic outcome in most patients at medium-term follow-up; however, long-term outcome studies are lacking.[3]

PATIENT HISTORY AND PHYSICAL FINDINGS

- The mechanism of injury is typically a fall on the outstretched hand.
- The patient will complain of pain and limitation of elbow or forearm motion.

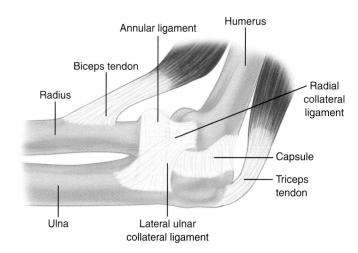

FIG 1 • The ligaments on the lateral aspect of the elbow include the lateral ulnar collateral ligament, the radial collateral ligament, and the annular ligament. The lateral ulnar collateral ligament is an important stabilizer against varus and posterolateral rotational instability of the elbow and should be preserved or repaired after radial head arthroplasty.

- A history of forearm or wrist pain should be sought.
- Inspection may reveal ecchymosis along the forearm or medial aspect of the elbow. Deformity may be evident if there is an associated dislocation.
- Careful palpation of the radial head, the medial and lateral collateral ligaments of the elbow, the interosseous ligament of the forearm, and the distal radioulnar joint should be performed. Local tenderness over one or all of these structures implies a possible derangement of the relevant structure.
- Since associated injuries of the shoulder, forearm, wrist, and hand are common, these areas should be carefully examined.
- Range of motion, including forearm rotation and elbow flexion–extension, should be evaluated. The presence of palpable and auditory crepitus should be noted.
- Loss of terminal elbow flexion and extension is expected as a consequence of a hemarthrosis in acute fractures, while loss of forearm rotation typically is caused by a mechanical impingement.
- A careful neurovascular assessment of all three major nerves that cross the elbow should be performed.
- The examiner should observe for localized or diffuse swelling in the elbow. Effusion represents hemarthrosis due to intra-articular fracture.
- The examiner should compare active and passive range of motion to the uninjured side. Reduced range of motion may be a result of hemarthrosis or mechanical block from a broken fragment. Intra-articular injection of a local anesthetic helps differentiate between reduced range of motion due to a mechanical block versus pain inhibition.
- The examiner should look for varus–valgus instability. Any gapping on the medial or lateral side beneath the examiner's hand is noted. Positive findings suggest mediolateral collateral ligament insufficiency. Typically, this test is positive only when performed under a general anesthetic.
- The lateral pivot shift test is performed. Positive apprehension or a clunk that is seen or felt when the ulna and radius reduce on the humerus suggests posterolateral rotatory instability.

IMAGING AND OTHER DIAGNOSTIC STUDIES

- Anteroposterior (AP), lateral, and oblique elbow radiographs, with the x-ray beam centered on the radiocapitellar joint, usually provide sufficient information for the diagnosis and treatment of radial head fractures.
- Bilateral posteroanterior radiographs of both wrists in neutral rotation should be performed to evaluate ulnar variance in patients with wrist discomfort or a comminuted radial head fracture, since there is a higher incidence of an associated interosseous ligament injury in these patients.[6]
- Computed tomography with sagittal, coronal, and 3D reconstructions may assist with preoperative planning and can help the surgeon predict whether a displaced radial head fracture can be repaired with open reduction and internal fixation or if an arthroplasty will likely be needed.

DIFFERENTIAL DIAGNOSIS

- Acute radial head fractures
- Other fractures or dislocations about the elbow (eg, supracondylar, capitellar, coronoid, osteochondral fractures)
- Radial head nonunion or malunion, posttraumatic arthritis
- Congenital dislocation of the radial head
- Forearm or elbow instability

- Lateral epicondylitis
- Rheumatoid arthritis or osteoarthritis
- Synovitis, inflammatory or infectious
- Tumors

NONOPERATIVE MANAGEMENT

- The indications for surgical management of radial head fractures are not well defined in the literature. Fragment size, number of fracture fragments, degree of displacement, and bone quality influence decision making regarding the optimal management.
- Nondisplaced fractures or small (less than 33% of radial head) minimally displaced fractures (less than 2 mm) can be treated with early motion with an excellent outcome in the majority of patients.
- Associated injuries and a block to motion are also important factors to consider when deciding between nonoperative and surgical management.

SURGICAL MANAGEMENT

- Small displaced fractures that cause painful crepitus or limited motion are managed with fragment excision if they are too small (typically less than 25% of the diameter of the radial head) or osteopenic to be internally fixated.
- Larger displaced fractures are typically managed with ORIF with good outcomes in most patients.
- Radial head fractures that are displaced but too comminuted to be anatomically reduced and stably fixed and that are too large to consider fragment excision (involve more than a quarter to a third of the radial head) should be managed by radial head excision with or without arthroplasty.
- Patients who are known to have, or are likely to have, an associated ligamentous injury of the elbow or forearm should have a radial head arthroplasty because radial head excision is contraindicated (**FIG 2**).
- The decision as to what fracture is reconstructable depends on surgeon factors (eg, experience), patient factors (eg, osteoporosis), and fracture factors (eg, fragment number and size, comminution, associated soft tissue injuries). The final decision is often made only at the time of surgery.
- Other indications for radial head arthroplasty include radial head nonunion or malunion, primary or secondary management of forearm or elbow instability (eg, Essex-Lopresti injury), rheumatoid arthritis or osteoarthritis, and tumors.

Preoperative Planning

- Currently available devices include spacer implants, press-fit and ingrowth stems, and bipolar and ceramic articulations.
- Silicone radial head implants offer little in the way of axial or valgus stability to the elbow and have been complicated by a high incidence of implant wear, fragmentation, and silicone synovitis leading to generalized joint damage. As a result, they have fallen out of favor and have been replaced by metallic implants.
- Most metallic radial head implants that have been developed and used to date employ a monoblock design, making size matching suboptimal and implant insertion often difficult because of the need to subluxate the elbow to allow for insertion of these devices.[10]
- Recently, modular metallic radial head prostheses have become available with separate heads and stems, allowing improved size matching of the native radial head and neck[18] and easier placement in the setting of competent lateral ligaments.[17]

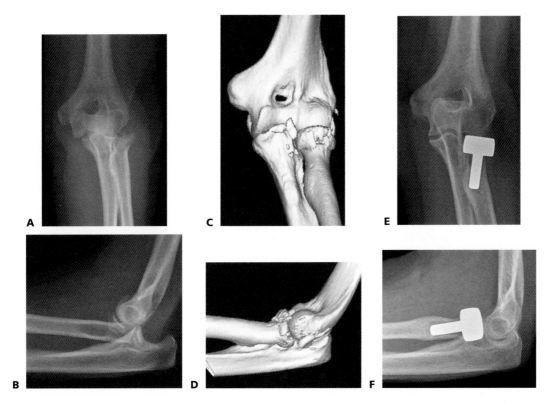

FIG 2 • **A,B.** AP and lateral radiographs of a 54-year-old woman who sustained a posterolateral elbow dislocation associated with a comminuted fracture of the radial head and coronoid—the "terrible triad." **C,D.** Preoperative 3D reconstruction images demonstrating a comminuted radial head fracture with a small undisplaced coronoid fracture. **E,F.** Postoperative radiographs after modular radial head arthroplasty (Evolve, Wright Medical Technology, Arlington, TN) and repair of the lateral collateral ligament. Medial collateral ligament and coronoid repairs were not required since the elbow was sufficiently stable at the end of the procedure. A good functional outcome was achieved at the final follow-up.

■ Precise implant sizing and placement are critical with these devices to ensure correct capitellar tracking and to avoid a cam effect with forearm rotation, which may cause premature capitellar wear due to shearing of the cartilage and stem loosening due to increased loading of the stem–bone interface.

■ Preoperative radiographic templating of the contralateral normal radial head should be employed in the setting of a secondary radial head replacement but is not needed for acute fractures because the excised radial head is available for accurate implant sizing.

Positioning

■ The patient is placed supine on the operating table and a sandbag is placed beneath the ipsilateral scapula to assist in positioning the arm across the chest.

■ Alternatively, the patient can be positioned in a lateral position with the affected arm held over a bolster.[2]

■ Prophylactic intravenous antibiotics are administered.

■ General or regional anesthesia is employed.

■ A sterile tourniquet is applied.

SURGICAL APPROACH

- A midline posterior elbow incision is made just lateral to the tip of the olecranon (**TECH FIG 1A**).

- A full-thickness lateral fasciocutaneous flap is elevated on the deep fascia. This extensile incision decreases the risk of cutaneous nerve injury and provides access to the radial head, coronoid, and medial and lateral collateral

ligaments for the management of more complex injuries (**TECH FIG 1B**).[8,22]

- Alternatively, a lateral skin incision centered over the lateral epicondyle and passing obliquely over the radial head can be used (see Tech Fig 1A).

TECHNIQUES

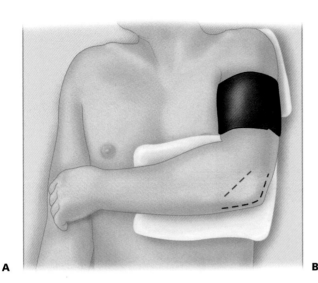

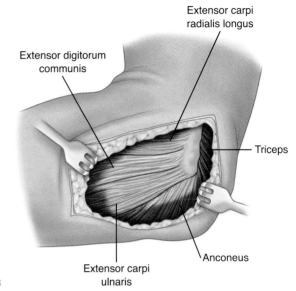

TECH FIG 1 • A. The patient is placed supine on the operating table and a sandbag is placed beneath the ipsilateral scapula to assist in positioning the arm across the chest. The posterior incision is indicated in red. Alternatively, a lateral skin incision centered over the lateral epicondyle and passing obliquely over the radial head can be used (blue). **B.** A midline posterior elbow incision made just lateral to the tip of the olecranon. A full-thickness lateral fasciocutaneous flap is elevated on the deep fascia. This extensile incision allows access to both the lateral and medial aspects of the elbow, in case of more complex injuries, and reduces the incidence of cutaneous nerve injury.

COMMON EXTENSOR SPLIT

- The extensor digitorum communis tendon is identified.
  - The landmarks for this plane are a line joining the lateral epicondyle and the tubercle of Lister.
- The extensor digitorum communis tendon is split longitudinally at the middle aspect of the radial head, and the underlying radial collateral and annular ligaments are incised (**TECH FIG 2A**).
  - Dissection should stay anterior to the lateral ulnar collateral ligament to prevent the development of posterolateral rotatory instability (see Fig 1).
  - The forearm is maintained in pronation to move the posterior interosseous nerve more distal and medial during the surgical approach.[7]
- If further exposure is required:
  - The humeral origin of the radial collateral ligament and the overlying extensor muscles are elevated anteriorly off the lateral epicondyle to improve the exposure if needed (**TECH FIG 2B**).
  - Release of the posterior component of the lateral collateral ligament can be considered, but careful ligament repair is required at the end of the procedure in order to restore the varus and posterolateral rotatory stability of the elbow.[9]

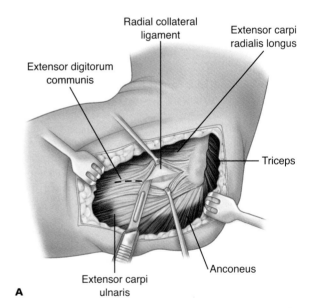

TECH FIG 2 • A. The extensor digitorum communis tendon is split longitudinally at the middle aspect of the radial head and the underlying radial collateral and annular ligaments are incised. The forearm is pronated to protect the posterior interosseous nerve. *(continued)*

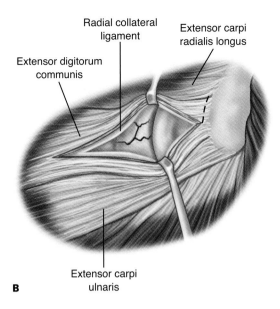

Extensor digitorum communis

Radial collateral ligament

Extensor carpi radialis longus

Extensor carpi ulnaris

B

TECH FIG 2 • *(continued)* **B.** The humeral origin of the radial collateral ligament and the overlying extensor muscles are elevated anteriorly off the lateral epicondyle to improve the exposure if needed.

PREPARATION OF THE RADIAL HEAD AND NECK

- All fragments of the radial head are removed, as well as a minimal amount of radial neck at a right angle to the medullary canal, to make a smooth surface for seating of the prosthetic radial head.
    - Complete fragment excision can be confirmed with the use of an image intensifier.
- The capitellum is evaluated for chondral injuries or osteochondral fractures.
- The radial head prosthesis is sized in one of several ways:
    - The resected radial head is reassembled in the provided sizing template to assist in the accurate sizing of the prosthesis (**TECH FIG 3A–C**).
    - The diameter of radial head prosthesis should be based on the size of the articular dish. This is typically 2 mm smaller than the outer diameter of the excised radial head.

- Alternatively, if the radial head has been previously excised, radiographic templating of the contralateral normal radial head may be used to determine the appropriate diameter and height of the radial head implant.
- If the native radial head is in between available implant sizes, the implant diameter or thickness should be downsized.
- The radial neck is delivered laterally using a Hohmann retractor carefully placed around the posterior aspect of the proximal radial neck (**TECH FIG 3D**).
    - An anteriorly based retractor should be avoided because of the risk of injury from pressure on the posterior interosseous nerve.
- The medullary canal of the radial neck is reamed using hand reamers until cortical contact is encountered.
    - A trial stem one size smaller than the rasp is inserted to achieve a nontight press-fit.

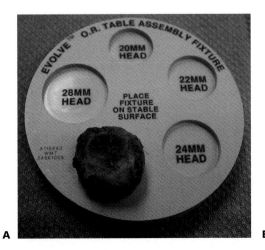

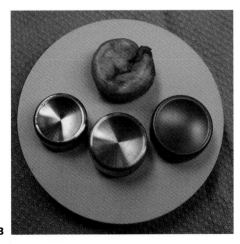

A   **B**

TECH FIG 3 • The resected radial head is reassembled in the provided sizing template (**A**) to assist in the accurate sizing of the prosthesis in terms of diameter (**B**) *(continued)*

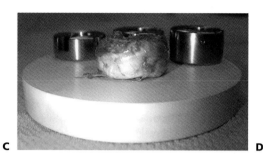

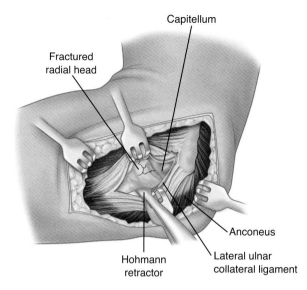

Capitellum

Fractured radial head

Anconeus

Hohmann retractor

Lateral ulnar collateral ligament

TECH FIG 3 • *(continued)* and height (**C**), and to ensure that all the fragments have been removed from the elbow. **D.** The radial neck is delivered laterally using a Hohmann retractor carefully placed around the posterior aspect of the proximal radial neck. An anteriorly based retractor should be avoided because of the risk of injury to the posterior interosseous nerve.

RADIAL HEAD REPLACEMENT

- A trial head is inserted onto the stem, and the diameter, height, tracking, and congruency of the prosthesis are evaluated both visually and with the aid of an image intensifier.
  - The radial head prosthesis should articulate at the same height as the radial notch of the ulna and about 1 mm distal to the tip of the coronoid (**TECH FIG 4A**).
  - The alignment of the distal radioulnar joint, ulnar variance, as well as the width of the lateral and medial portions of the ulnohumeral joint, are checked and compared to the contralateral wrist and elbow, respectively, under fluoroscopy.
  - Overlengthening the radiocapitellar joint with a radial head implant that is too thick should be avoided

  to reduce the risk of cartilage wear on the capitellum from excessive pressure; a nonparallel medial ulnohumeral joint space that is wider laterally is suggestive of overstuffing.
  - Some modular and bipolar implants allow insertion of the stem first, then placement of the head onto the stem with coupling in situ, which significantly reduces the surgical exposure needed (**TECH FIG 4B**).
- If the prosthesis is maltracking on the capitellum with forearm rotation, a smaller stem size should be trialed to ensure that the articulation of the radial head with the capitellum is controlled by the annular ligament and articular congruency and not dictated by the proximal radial shaft.

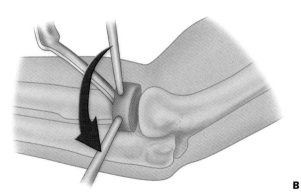

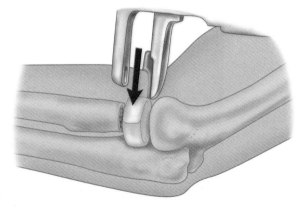

TECH FIG 4 • A. A trial stem is inserted. A trial head is inserted onto the stem and the diameter, height, tracking, and congruency of the prosthesis are evaluated both visually and with the aid of an image intensifier. **B.** Some modular and bipolar implants ellow insertion of the stem first, then placement of the head onto the stem with coupling in situ, which significantly reduces the surgical exposure needed.

LATERAL SOFT TISSUE CLOSURE

- After radial head replacement, the lateral collateral ligament and extensor muscle origins are repaired back to the lateral condyle.
- If the posterior half of the lateral collateral ligament is still attached to the lateral epicondyle, then the anterior half of the lateral collateral ligament (the annular ligament and radial collateral ligament) and extensor muscles are repaired to the posterior half using interrupted absorbable sutures (**TECH FIG 5A**).
- If the lateral collateral ligament and extensor origin have been completely detached either by the injury or surgical exposure, they should be securely repaired less equalize to the lateral epicondyle using drill holes through bone and nonabsorbable sutures or suture anchors.

- A single drill hole is placed at the axis of motion (the center of the arc of curvature of the capitellum) and connected to two drill holes placed anterior and posterior to the lateral supracondylar ridge.
- A locking (Krackow) suture technique is employed to gain a secure hold of the lateral collateral ligament and common extensor muscle fascia (**TECH FIG 5B–D**).
- The ligament sutures are pulled into the holes drilled in the distal humerus using suture retrievers and the forearm is pronated, and varus forces are avoided, while tensioning the sutures before tying (**TECH FIG 5E**).
- The knots should be left anterior or posterior to the lateral supracondylar ridge to avoid prominence.

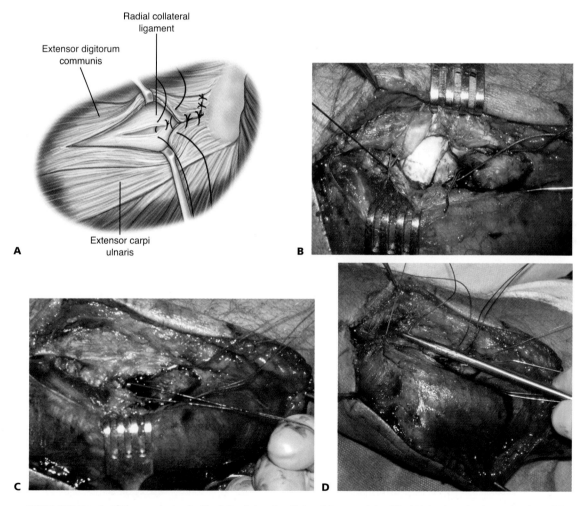

TECH FIG 5 • A. If the posterior half of the lateral collateral ligament is still attached to the lateral epicondyle, then the anterior half of it (the annular ligament and radial collateral ligament) and extensor muscles are repaired to the posterior half using interrupted absorbable sutures. *ECU,* extensor carpi ulnaris; *EDC,* extensor digitorum communis. **B–D.** If the lateral collateral ligament and extensor origin have been completely disrupted by the injury or detached by the surgical exposure, they should be securely repaired to the lateral epicondyle. A single drill hole is placed at the center of the arc of curvature of the capitellum and connected to two drill holes placed anterior and posterior to the lateral supracondylar ridge. A locking (Krackow) suture technique is employed to gain a secure hold of the lateral collateral ligament (**B**) as well as of the annular ligament (**C**). **D.** A second stitch is used in a similar manner to repair the common extensor muscle fascia. *(continued)*

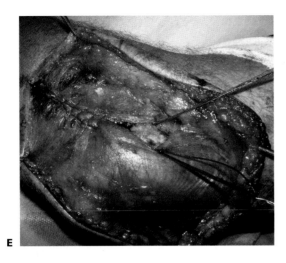

E

TECH FIG 5 • *(continued)* **E.** The sutures are pulled into the holes drilled in the distal humerus using suture retrievers, tensioned while keeping the forearm pronated and while avoiding varus forces, and eventually tied over the lateral supracondylar ridge.

COMPLETION

- After replacement arthroplasty and lateral soft tissue closure, the elbow should be placed through an arc of flexion–extension while carefully evaluating for elbow stability in pronation, neutral, and supination.[2]
- Pronation is generally beneficial if the lateral ligaments are deficient,[9] supination if the medial ligaments are deficient,[1] and neutral position if both sides have been injured.

- In patients who have an associated elbow dislocation, additional repair of the medial collateral ligament and flexor pronator origin should be performed if the elbow subluxates at 40 degrees or more of flexion.
- Tourniquet deflation and hemostasis should be secured before wound closure.

KÖCHER APPROACH

- Alternatively, the radial head may be approached by using the Köcher interval[20] between the extensor carpi ulnaris and anconeus.
- The fascial interval between these muscles is identified by noting the diverging direction of the muscle groups and small vascular perforators that exit at this interval (**TECH FIG 6**).
- Care should be taken to preserve the lateral ulnar collateral ligament, which is vulnerable as the dissection is carried deeper through the capsule.

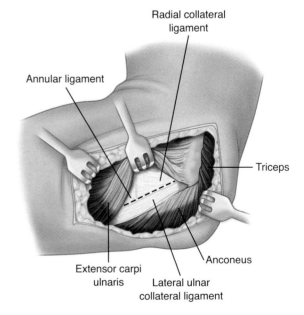

TECH FIG 6 • The extensor carpi ulnaris is elevated anteriorly and an arthrotomy is performed at the midportion of the radial head. Care should be taken to preserve the lateral ulnar collateral ligament, which is vulnerable as the dissection is carried deeper through the capsule.

PEARLS AND PITFALLS

Indications	▪ Displaced unreconstructable fracture of the radial head with known or probable associated medial or lateral collateral or interosseous ligament injury
Pearls	▪ A preoperative radiographic template of the contralateral native radial head should be used in the setting of a secondary radial head replacement.
	▪ Dissection should stay anterior to the lateral ulnar collateral ligament to prevent the development of posterolateral rotatory instability.
	▪ The radial head should be sized based on the diameter of the articular dish and thickness of the excised radial head.
	▪ The radial head implant is typically 2 mm smaller than the outer diameter of the radial head.
	▪ Radial head articular surface height should be at the level of the proximal radioulnar joint.
	▪ If the radial head does not track well on the capitellum, the stem should be downsized.
	▪ If the native radial head is in between implant sizes, the implant should, in general, be downsized.
	▪ Intraoperative fluoroscopy is used to assess the alignment of the radiocapitellar and distal radioulnar joints and to avoid overlengthening of the radius.
Pitfalls	▪ Hohmann retractors should not be used around the anterior aspect of the radial neck and the forearm should be kept pronated to avoid damage to the posterior interosseous nerve.
	▪ The surgeon should avoid overstuffing the thickness or diameter of the radial head because of the risk of capitellar wear and pain. Filling the gap between the capitellum and radial neck is not a useful landmark for prosthesis thickness because lateral soft tissues are often deficient owing to the surgical exposure or initial injury.

POSTOPERATIVE CARE

▪ The elbow with stable ligaments should be splinted using anterior plaster slabs in extension and elevated for 24 to 48 hours to diminish swelling, decrease tension on the posterior wound, and minimize the tendency to develop a flexion contracture.

▪ In the setting of a more tenuous ligamentous repair or the presence of some residual instability at the end of the operative procedure, the elbow should initially be splinted in 60 to 90 degrees of flexion in the optimal position of forearm rotation to maintain stability.

▪ Perioperative antibiotics are continued for 24 hours postoperatively.

▪ Indomethacin 25 mg three times daily for 3 weeks may be considered in patients undergoing radial head arthroplasty to decrease postoperative pain, reduce swelling, and potentially lower the incidence of heterotopic ossification.

▪ Indomethacin should be avoided in elderly patients and those with a history of peptic ulcer disease, asthma, known allergy, or other contraindications to anti-inflammatory medications.

▪ For an isolated radial head replacement treated with a lateral ulnar collateral ligament-sparing approach, active range of motion should be initiated on the day after surgery.

  ▪ A collar and cuff with the elbow maintained at 90 degrees is employed for comfort between exercises.

  ▪ A static progressive extension splint is fabricated for nighttime use for patients without associated ligamentous disruptions and is employed for a period of 12 weeks. The splint is adjusted weekly as extension improves.

  ▪ In patients with associated elbow dislocations or residual instability, extension splinting is not implemented until 6 weeks after surgery.

▪ Patients with associated fractures, dislocations, or ligamentous injuries should commence active flexion and extension motion within a safe arc 1 day postoperatively.

  ▪ Active forearm rotation is performed with the elbow in flexion to minimize stress on the medial or lateral ligamentous injuries or repairs.

  ▪ Extension is performed with the forearm in the appropriate rotational position—that is, pronation if the lateral ligaments are deficient,[9] supination if the medial ligaments are deficient,[1] and neutral position if both sides have been injured.

▪ A resting splint with the elbow maintained at 90 degrees and the forearm in the appropriate position of forearm rotation is employed for 3 to 6 weeks.

▪ Passive stretching is not permitted for 6 weeks to reduce the incidence of heterotopic ossification.

▪ Strengthening exercises are initiated once the ligament injuries and any associated fractures have adequately healed, usually at 8 weeks postoperatively.

OUTCOMES

▪ Silicone radial head arthroplasty, while initially successful in many patients,[5,24] has fallen out of favor because of problems with residual instability and arthritis, implant fracture, and silicone synovitis due to particulate debris.[25]

▪ While the short- and medium-term results of metallic radial head implants are encouraging, there is a paucity of literature demonstrating the long-term outcome with respect to loosening, capitellar wear, and arthritis.

▪ Metallic radial head replacement in elbows with intact ligaments restores the kinematics and stability similar to that measured with a native radial head. Moreover, when the fractured radial head occurs in combination with ligamentous and soft tissue disruption, a metallic prosthesis restores elbow stability, with only mild residual deficits in strength and motion.

▪ Moro et al[21] reported the functional outcome of 25 cases managed with a metallic radial head arthroplasty for unreconstructable fractures of the radial head at an average follow-up of 39 months. The results were rated as 17 good or excellent, 5 fair, and 3 poor.

  ▪ The radial head prosthesis restored elbow stability when the fractured radial head occurred in combination with a dislocation of the elbow, rupture of the medial collateral ligament, fracture of the coronoid, or fracture of the proximal ulna.

  ▪ There were mild residual deficits in strength and motion, and no patient required removal of the implant.

■ Harrington et al[12] reported their experience with metallic radial head arthroplasty in 20 patients at an average follow-up of 12 years. The results were excellent or good in 16 and fair or poor in 4.

■ Improvements in radial head arthroplasty designs, sizing, and implantation techniques may lead to improved outcomes for unreconstructable radial head fractures.

COMPLICATIONS

■ Posterior interosseous nerve injury can occur as a consequence of dissection distal to the radial tuberosity and placement of anterior retractors around the distal radial neck.

■ Infection

■ Loss of motion, mainly terminal extension due to capsular contracture, heterotopic ossification, or retained cartilaginous or osseous fragments

■ Prosthetic loosening or polyethylene wear

■ Capitellar wear and pain due to implant overstuffing

■ Complex regional pain syndrome

■ Instability or recurrent dislocations of the elbow due to an inadequate or failed ligament repair

■ Osteoarthritis of the capitellum as a consequence of articular cartilage damage from the initial injury, from component insertion, from persistent instability, or due to loading from a radial head implant that is too thick.

REFERENCES

1. Armstrong AD, Dunning CE, Faber KJ, et al. Rehabilitation of the medial collateral ligament-deficient elbow: an in vitro biomechanical study. J Hand Surg Am 2000;25A:1051–1057.
2. Bain GI, Ashwood N, Baird R, et al. Management of Mason type III radial head fractures with a titanium prosthesis, ligament repair, and early mobilization. J Bone Joint Surg Am 2005;87A:136–147.
3. Beingessner DM, Dunning CE, Gordon KD, et al. The effect of radial head excision and arthroplasty on elbow kinematics and stability. J Bone Joint Surg Am 2004;86A:1730–1739.
4. Boulas HJ, Morrey BF. Biomechanical evaluation of the elbow following radial head fracture: comparison of open reduction and internal fixation versus excision, Silastic replacement and non-operative management. Ann Chir Main 1998;17:314–320.
5. Carn RM, Medige J, Curtain D, et al. Silicone rubber replacement of the severely fractured radial head. Clin Orthop Relat Res 1986;209:259–269.
6. Davidson PA, Moseley JB Jr, Tullos HS. Radial head fracture: a potentially complex injury. Clin Orthop Relat Res 1993;297:224–230.
7. Diliberti T, Botte MJ, Abrams RA. Anatomical considerations regarding the posterior interosseous nerve during posterolateral approaches to the proximal part of the radius. J Bone Joint Surg Am 2000;82A:809–813.
8. Dowdy PA, Bain GI, King GJ, et al. The midline posterior elbow incision: an anatomical appraisal. J Bone Joint Surg Br 1995;77B:696–699.
9. Dunning CE, Zarzour ZD, Patterson SD, et al. Muscle forces and pronation stabilize the lateral ligament deficient elbow. Clin Orthop Relat Res 2001;388:118–124.
10. Gupta GG, Lucas G, Hahn DL. Biomechanical and computer analysis of radial head prostheses. J Shoulder Elbow Surg 1997;6:37–48.
11. Halls AA, Travill A. Transmission of pressures across the elbow joint. Anat Rec 1964;150:243–248.
12. Harrington IJ, Sekyi-Otu A, Barrington TW, et al. The functional outcome with metallic radial head implants in the treatment of unstable elbow fractures: a long-term review. J Trauma 2001;50:46–52.
13. Ikeda M, Oka Y. Function after early radial head resection for fracture: a retrospective evaluation of 15 patients followed for 3–18 years. Acta Orthop Scand 2000;71:191–194.
14. Janssen RP, Vetger J. Resection of the radial head after Mason type III fracture of the elbow. J Bone Joint Surg Br 1998;80B:231–233.
15. Jensen SL, Olsen BS, Sojbjerg JO. Elbow joint kinematics after excision of the radial head. J Shoulder Elbow Surg 1999;8:238–241.
16. Johnston GW. A follow-up of one hundred cases of fracture of the head of the radius with a review of the literature. Ulster Med J 1962;31:51–56.
17. King GJ. Management of radial head fractures with implant arthroplasty. J Am Soc Surg Hand 2004;4:11–26.
18. King GJ, Zarzour ZD, Patterson SD, et al. An anthropometric study of the radial head: implications in the design of a prosthesis. J Arthroplasty 2001;16:112–116.
19. King GJ, Zarzour ZD, Rath DA, et al. Metallic radial head arthroplasty improves valgus stability of the elbow. Clin Orthop Relat Res 1999;368:114–125.
20. Köcher T. Textbook of Operative Surgery. London: Adam and Charles Black, 1911.
21. Moro JK, Werier J, MacDermid JC, et al. Arthroplasty with a metal radial head for unreconstructible fractures of the radial head. J Bone Joint Surg Am 2001;83A:1201–1211.
22. Patterson SD, Bain GI, Mehta JA. Surgical approaches to the elbow. Clin Orthop Relat Res 2000;370:19–33.
23. Pomianowski S, Morrey BF, Neale PG, et al. Contribution of monoblock and bipolar radial head prostheses to valgus stability of the elbow. J Bone Joint Surg Am 2001;83A:1829–1834.
24. Swanson AB, Jaeger SH, La Rochelle D. Comminuted fractures of the radial head: the role of silicone-implant replacement arthroplasty. J Bone Joint Surg Am 1981;63A:1039–1049.
25. Vanderwilde RS, Morrey BF, Melberg MW, et al. Inflammatory arthritis after failure of silicone rubber replacement of the radial head. J Bone Joint Surg Br 1994;76B:78–81.

Chapter 37

Open Reduction and Internal Fixation of Olecranon Fractures

David Ring

DEFINITION

- Fracture of the olecranon process is common, usually displaced, and nearly always treated operatively.
- Important injury characteristics include displacement, comminution, and subluxation or dislocation of the elbow, and all are accounted for in the Mayo classification (**FIG 1**).[6]
- Fracture-dislocations of the olecranon can be anterior (trans-olecranon) or posterior (the most proximal type of posterior Monteggia according to Jupiter and colleagues[3]) in direction.[2,3,9,10]
- Open injuries are unusual.

ANATOMY

- The greater sigmoid notch of the ulna is formed by the coronoid and olecranon processes and forms a nearly 180-degree arc capturing the trochlea.
- The region between the coronoid and olecranon articular facets is the nonarticular transverse groove of the olecranon, a common location of fracture and a place where precise articular reduction is not critical.
- The triceps has a broad and thick insertion from just superior to the point of the olecranon and the tip of the olecranon process that can be used to enhance fixation of small, osteoporotic, or fragmented fractures and can be split longitudinally, if needed, when applying a plate.

PATHOGENESIS

- Fractures of the olecranon are most often the result of a direct blow to the point of the elbow, but occasionally they result from indirect forces during a fall on the outstretched hand.

NATURAL HISTORY

- Stable nondisplaced or minimally displaced fractures are uncommon.
- The majority of olecranon fractures are displaced and benefit from operative treatment.
- The occasional untreated displaced simple olecranon fracture demonstrates a slight flexion contracture, some weakness of extension, no arthrosis, and little if any pain.
- In contrast, undertreated or poorly treated fracture-dislocations lead to severe arthrosis with or without instability.
- Even well-treated complex injuries are at risk for stiffness, heterotopic ossification, arthrosis, and occasionally nonunion.

PATIENT HISTORY AND PHYSICAL FINDINGS

- Knowledge of the characteristics of the patient (age, gender, medical health) and the injury (mechanism, energy) will help the surgeon understand the injury and determine optimal treatment.
- First the patient is assessed for life-threatening injuries (ATLS protocol) and any medical problems that may have contributed to the injury.
- A secondary survey is performed to identify any other fractures, ipsilateral arm injuries in particular.
- The skin is carefully inspected for any wounds associated with the fracture.
- The pulses are palpated, capillary refill inspected, and an Allen test performed if necessary.
- Peripheral nerve function is assessed.
- Patients with high-energy injuries, particularly those with ipsilateral wrist or forearm injuries, are at risk for compartment syndrome. If the clinical examination is suggestive or unreliable (owing to problems with mental status), compartment pressure monitoring should be performed.

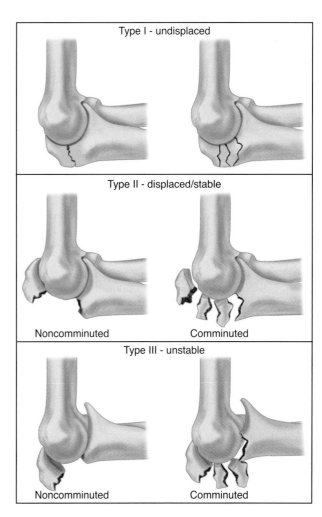

FIG 1 • The Mayo classification of olecranon fractures accounts for the factors that will influence treatment decisions: displacement, comminution, and dislocation or subluxation of the articulations.

IMAGING AND OTHER DIAGNOSTIC STUDIES

▪ Anteroposterior (AP) and lateral radiographs are used for initial characterization of the injury.
▪ Radiographs after reduction or splinting, or oblique views can be useful.
▪ Computed tomography (CT) is useful for characterization of fracture-dislocations. In particular, 3D CT reconstructions can be useful for assessment of the coronoid and radial head.

DIFFERENTIAL DIAGNOSIS

▪ Elbow dislocation
▪ Monteggia and Essex-Lopresti fracture-dislocations of the forearm
▪ Distal humerus fracture

NONOPERATIVE MANAGEMENT

▪ Nonoperative management is appropriate for the rare fracture of the olecranon that is less than 2 millimeters displaced with the elbow flexed 90 degrees.
▪ Four weeks of splint immobilization followed by active assisted mobilization of the elbow will usually result in a healed fracture and good elbow function.

SURGICAL MANAGEMENT

▪ The vast majority of olecranon fractures are displaced and merit operative treatment.

▪ Transverse, noncomminuted fractures not associated with fracture-dislocation are treated with tension band wiring.[4,8]
▪ Comminuted fractures and fracture-dislocations are treated with dorsal contoured plate and screw fixation.[1–3]
▪ The treatment of fracture-dislocations requires attention to the coronoid, radial head, and lateral collateral ligament.[2,9–11]

Preoperative Planning

▪ The fracture characteristics that determine treatment are defined on radiographs and CT.
▪ Templating the surgery with tracings of the radiographs is a useful way of running through the surgery in detail before performing it, familiarizing oneself with the anatomy, anticipating problems, and ensuring that all of the implants and equipment that might be necessary are available.

Positioning

▪ In most patients a lateral decubitus position with the arm over a bolster or support is best.
▪ Some patients with fracture-dislocations that require both medial and lateral access may be positioned supine with the arm supported on a hand table.
▪ A sterile pneumatic tourniquet is used.

Approach

▪ A dorsal longitudinal skin incision is used.

TENSION BAND WIRING

Reduction and Kirschner Wire Fixation

▪ Blood clot and periosteum are cleared from the fracture site to facilitate reduction.
▪ Limited periosteal elevation is performed at the fracture site to monitor reduction.
▪ A large tenaculum clamp is used to secure the fracture in a reduced position (**TECH FIG 1A,B**). A drill hole can be made in the dorsal cortex of the distal fragment to facilitate clamp application.

▪ Two 1.0-mm smooth Kirschner wires are drilled across the fracture site (**TECH FIG 1C**).
  ▪ If these are drilled obliquely from dorsal proximal to volar distal, they will exit the anterior ulnar cortex distal to the coronoid process, providing an anchoring point of cortical bone to limit the potential for pin migration.
  ▪ In anticipation of later impaction of the proximal ends of the wires, the Kirschner wires should be retracted 5 to 10 mm after drilling through the anterior ulnar cortex.

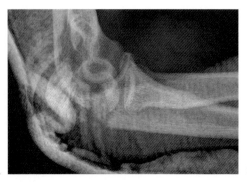
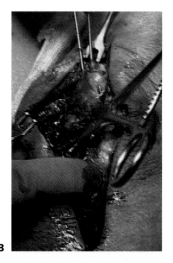

TECH FIG 1 • A. A lateral radiograph with the arm in plaster shows a transverse, noncomminuted fracture of the olecranon. **B.** An open reduction is held with a fracture reduction forceps. *(continued)*

A   **B**

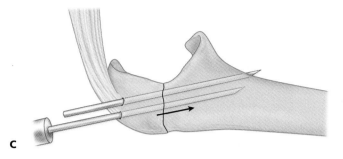

C

TECH FIG 1 • *(continued)* **C.** Two 1-mm Kirschner wires are drilled obliquely across the fracture site so that they exit the anterior ulnar cortex distal to the coronoid process. (**A,B:** Copyright David Ring, MD.)

Wiring

- The apex of the ulnar diaphysis just distal to the flat portion of the proximal ulna is drilled with a 2.0-mm drill, with or without prior subperiosteal dissection.
  - When two wires are used, a second drill hole is made a centimeter more distal.
- If one wire is used, it should be 18 gauge. My preference is to use two 22-gauge stainless steel wires to limit the size of the knots, which may diminish implant prominence. The wires are passed through the drill holes. A large-bore needle can be used to facilitate passage of the wire through the drill hole (**TECH FIG 2A**).
- The two tension wires are each passed over the dorsal ulna in a figure 8 fashion, then around the Kirschner wires, and underneath the insertion of the triceps tendon using a large-bore needle (**TECH FIG 2B**).

- Each wire is tensioned both medially and laterally by twisting the wire with a needle holder (**TECH FIG 2C,D**).
  - This should be done to take up slack only. These small wires will break if they are firmly tightened, which is not necessary.
  - The tightening should be done in a place that will make the wire knots less prominent.
  - After tightening the knots are trimmed and bent into the soft tissues to either side.
- The Kirschner wires are then bent 180 degrees and trimmed.
- These bent ends are then impacted into the proximal olecranon, beneath the triceps insertion, using an osteotome (**TECH FIG 2E–H**).

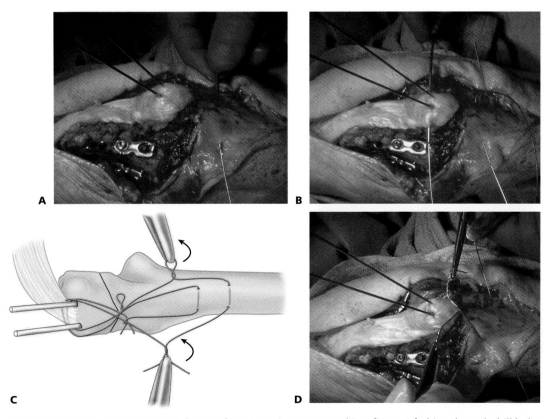

A   B

C   D

TECH FIG 2 • A. Two 22-gauge stainless steel tension wires are passed in a figure 8 fashion through drill holes in the ulnar shaft. **B.** They engage the triceps insertion proximally. **C,D.** The wires are tensioned on both sides. These do not need to be tight, but simply snug, with all slack taken up. Attempts to tighten these smaller 22-gauge wires will break them. *(continued)*

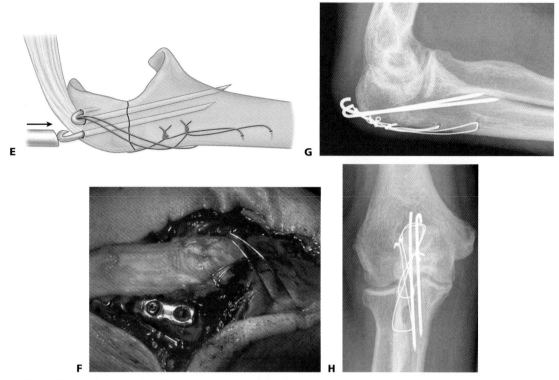

TECH FIG 2 • *(continued)* **E.** The proximal ends of the Kirschner wires are bent 180 degrees and impacted into the olecranon process, beneath the triceps insertion. **F.** The resulting fixation has a relatively low profile and is unlikely to migrate. **G,H.** Even these small wires are strong enough for active exercises to regain elbow motion. (**A,B,D,F–H:** Copyright David Ring, MD.)

PLATE AND SCREW FIXATION OF OLECRANON FRACTURES

- Contour the plate to wrap around the proximal aspect of the olecranon or use a precontoured plate (**TECH FIG 3A–C**).
- A straight plate will have only two or three screws in metaphyseal bone proximal to the fracture.
- Bending the plate around the proximal aspect of the olecranon provides additional screws in the proximal fragment. The most proximal screws can be very long, crossing the fracture line into the distal fragment. In some cases,

these screws can be directed to engage one of the cortices of the distal fragment, such as the anterior ulnar cortex.

- A plate contoured to wrap around the proximal ulna can be placed on top of the triceps insertion. Alternatively, the triceps insertion can be incised longitudinally and partially elevated medially and laterally sufficiently to allow direct plate contact with bone.
- If the proximal (olecranon) fragment is small, fragmented, or osteoporotic, it can be useful to add a figure

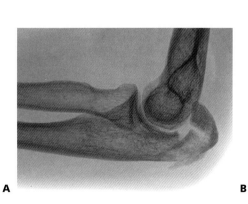
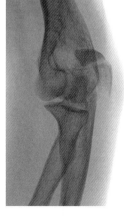
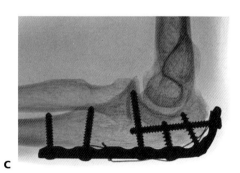

TECH FIG 3 • **A.** A lateral radiograph illustrates a comminuted olecranon fracture with a small proximal olecranon fragment. **B.** An oblique view shows the fragmentation. **C.** A 3.5-mm limited-contact dynamic compression plate and screws contoured to wrap around the dorsal surface of the olecranon is used for fixation. *(continued)*

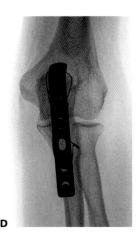

D

TECH FIG 3 • *(continued)* **D.** A 22-gauge stainless steel wire engages the triceps insertion—this is useful when the olecranon fragment is small, fragmented, or osteopenic. (Copyright David Ring, MD.)

8 tension wire that engages the triceps insertion and passes over the top of the plate and around one of the screws at the metaphyseal level.

- Distally, a dorsal plate will lie directly on the apex of the ulnar diaphysis. The muscle need only be split sufficiently to gain access to this apex—there is no need to elevate the muscle or periosteum off either the medial or lateral flat aspect of the ulna.
- No attempt is made to precisely realign intervening fragmentation—once the relationship of the coronoid and olecranon facets is restored and the overall alignment is restored, the remaining fragments are bridged, leaving their soft tissue attachments intact.
  - Bone grafts are rarely necessary if the soft tissue attachments are preserved.
- If the olecranon fragment is small, osteoporotic, or fragmented, a wire engaging the triceps insertion should be used to reinforce the fixation (**TECH FIG 3D**).
  - The plate and screws will serve to hold the coronoid and olecranon facets in proper alignment and bridge fragmentation, and the wire will help ensure fixation even if screw purchase is lost.

PLATE AND SCREW FIXATION OF FRACTURE-DISLOCATIONS OF THE OLECRANON

Exposure

- In the setting of a fracture-dislocation of the olecranon (**TECH FIG 4A**), fractures of the radial head and coronoid process can be evaluated and often definitively treated through the exposure provided by the fracture of the olecranon process.
  - With little additional dissection, the olecranon fragment can be mobilized proximally as one would do with an olecranon osteotomy, providing exposure of the coronoid through the ulnohumeral joint.
- If the exposure of the radial head through the posterior injury is inadequate, a separate muscle interval (eg, Köcher or Kaplan intervals) accessed by the elevation of a broad lateral skin flap can be used.
- If the exposure of the coronoid is inadequate through posterior injury and olecranon fracture, a separate medial or lateral exposure can be developed.

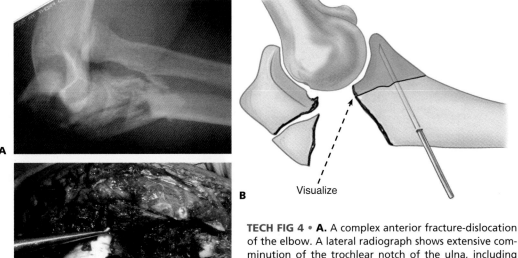

A

B

Visualize

C

TECH FIG 4 • **A.** A complex anterior fracture-dislocation of the elbow. A lateral radiograph shows extensive comminution of the trochlear notch of the ulna, including the coronoid, and anterior displacement of the forearm. **B,C.** The coronoid fragments are connected to the dorsal metaphyseal fragments in this patient, which facilitates reduction and fixation. (**A,C:** Copyright David Ring, MD.)

- A medial exposure, between the two heads of the flexor carpi ulnaris, or by splitting the flexor-pronator mass more anteriorly, or by elevating the entire flexor–pronator mass from dorsal to volar, may be needed to address a complex fracture of the coronoid, particularly one that involves the anteromedial facet of the coronoid process.
- When the lateral collateral ligament is injured, it is usually avulsed from the lateral epicondyle. This facilitates repair that can be performed using suture anchors or suture placed through drill holes in the bone.
- The fracture of the coronoid can often be reduced directly through the elbow joint using the limited access provided by the olecranon fracture (**TECH FIG 4B,C**).

Fixation

- Provisional fixation can be obtained using Kirschner wires to attach the fragments either to the metaphyseal or diaphyseal fragments of the ulna, or to the trochlea of the distal humerus when there is extensive fragmentation of the proximal ulna.
- An alternative to keep in mind when there is extensive fragmentation of the proximal ulna is the use of a skeletal distractor (a temporary external fixator; **TECH FIG 5A**).
  - External fixation applied between a wire driven through the olecranon fragment and up into the trochlea and a second wire in the distal ulnar diaphysis can often obtain reduction indirectly when distraction is applied between the pins.
  - Definitive fixation can usually be obtained with screws applied under image intensifier guidance.
- The screws are placed through the plate when there is extensive fragmentation of the proximal ulna.
- A second, medial plate may be useful when the coronoid is fragmented.
- If the coronoid fracture is very comminuted and cannot be securely repaired, the ulnohumeral joint should be protected with temporary hinged or static external fixation, or temporary pin fixation of the ulnohumeral joint, depending on the equipment and expertise available.
- A long plate is contoured to wrap around the proximal olecranon (**TECH FIG 5B**).
  - A very long plate should be considered (between 12 and 16 holes), particularly when there is extensive fragmentation or the bone quality is poor.
- When the olecranon is fragmented or osteoporotic, a plate and screws alone may not provide reliable fixation.
  - In this situation, it can be useful to use ancillary tension wire fixation to control the olecranon fragments through the triceps insertion (**TECH FIG 5C**).

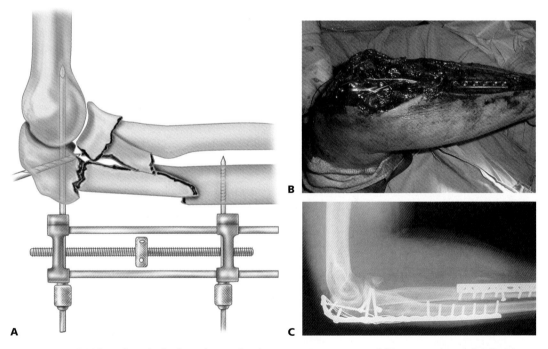

TECH FIG 5 • A. When there is diaphyseal comminution, a temporary external fixator may be useful. **B.** A long, 3.5-mm limited-contact dynamic compression plate is used for fixation. A 22-gauge stainless steel wire is used to enhance fixation of the comminuted olecranon fragments. **C.** The comminution extending into the diaphysis heals with the bridging plate. The trochlear notch is restored with good elbow function. (**B,C:** Copyright David Ring, MD.)

PEARLS AND PITFALLS

Prominence of olecranon hardware	■ The use of two small (22-gauge) wires rather than one large one will results in smaller knots. Care taken to place the Kirschner wires below the triceps insertion and impacting them into bone will limit prominence and the potential for migration.[5,8]
Narrowing of trochlear notch	■ The surgeon should not use a tension wire alone on a comminuted fracture. An intact articular surface to absorb compressive forces with active motion is mandatory for tension band wiring to be effective.
Plate loosening	■ The surgeon should use a dorsal plate contoured to wrap around the olecranon, providing a greater number of screws and screws at different, nearly orthogonal angles. Use of a medial or lateral plate should be avoided.[10,11]
Loss of fixation of the proximal (olecranon) fragment	■ Screw fixation alone should not be trusted if the fragment is small, fragmented, or osteoporotic. A tension wire engaging the triceps insertion should be added.
Failure to recognize a complex injury	■ The surgeon should be vigilant for subluxation or dislocation of the elbow, fracture of the coronoid or radial head, and injury to the lateral collateral ligament. When identified, each injury is treated accordingly. The olecranon and proximal ulna is always secured with a plate and screws.

POSTOPERATIVE CARE

■ When good fixation is obtained (which occurs in most patients), active assisted and gravity-assisted elbow and forearm exercises can be initiated immediately after surgery. A delay of several days for comfort is reasonable.

■ If the lateral collateral ligament was repaired, the patient must be instructed not to abduct the shoulder for the first month.

■ If the fixation is tenuous, it is reasonable to immobilize the arm in a splint for a month or so before beginning exercises.

OUTCOMES

■ Nonunion is nearly unheard of after simple olecranon fractures, and early implant failure is usually due to noncompliance.[6]

■ The appeal of tension band wiring has been limited by prominence of the implants; however, if the techniques described herein are followed, few patients will request a second surgery specifically for implant removal.[8]

■ Macko and Szabo pointed out that it was initial implant prominence and not migration that led to implant-related problems after tension band wiring of olecranon fractures.[5]

■ In any case, a second surgery for implant removal is not unreasonable, and it may not be appropriate to consider this a complication.

■ Some surgeons have considered plate-and-screw fixation of simple, noncomminuted olecranon fractures.[1] However, plates can also cause symptoms, and if only a few screws can be placed in the olecranon fragment, particularly in the setting of fragmentation or osteoporosis, it may be preferable to use the soft tissue attachments to enhance fixation rather than relying on implant–bone purchase alone.

■ Medial and lateral plates have been associated with early failure, malunion, and nonunion in the treatment of complex proximal ulna fractures.[10,11]

■ Dorsal plates perform better, but the elbow is often compromised in the setting of such complex injuries.

COMPLICATIONS

■ Implant loosening
■ Implant breakage
■ Nonunion
■ Malunion
■ Instability
■ Arthrosis

REFERENCES

1. Bailey CS, MacDermid J, Patterson SD, et al. Outcome of plate fixation of olecranon fractures. J Orthop Trauma 2001;15:542–548.
2. Doornberg J, Ring D, Jupiter JB. Effective treatment of fracture-dislocations of the olecranon requires a stable trochlear notch. Clin Orthop Relat Res 2004;429:292–300.
3. Jupiter JB, Leibovic SJ, Ribbans W, et al. The posterior Monteggia lesion. J Orthop Trauma 1991;5:395–402.
4. Karlsson M, Hasserius R, Besjakov J, et al. Comparison of tension-band and figure-of-eight wiring techniques for treatment of olecranon fractures. J Shoulder Elbow Surg 2002;11:377–382.
5. Macko D, Szabo RM. Complications of tension-band wiring of olecranon fractures. J Bone Joint Surg Am 1985;67A:1396–1401.
6. Morrey BF. Current concepts in the treatment of fractures of the radial head, the olecranon, and the coronoid. J Bone Joint Surg Am 1995;77A:316–327.
7. O'Driscoll SW, Jupiter JB, Cohen M, et al. Difficult elbow fractures: pearls and pitfalls. AAOS Instruct Course Lect 2003;52:113–134.
8. Ring D, Gulotta L, Chin K, et al. Olecranon osteotomy for exposure of fractures and nonunions of the distal humerus. J Orthop Trauma 2004;18:446–449.
9. Ring D, Jupiter JB, Sanders RW, et al. Trans-olecranon fracture-dislocation of the elbow. J Orthop Trauma 1997;11:545–550.
10. Ring D, Jupiter JB, Simpson NS. Monteggia fractures in adults. J Bone Joint Surg Am 1998;80A:1733–1744.
11. Ring D, Tavakolian J, Kloen P, et al. Loss of alignment after surgical treatment of posterior Monteggia fractures: salvage with dorsal contoured plating. J Hand Surg Am 2004;29A:694–702.

Chapter 38

Management of Simple Elbow Dislocation

Bradford O. Parsons

DEFINITION

- Simple elbow dislocation is a dislocation of the ulnohumeral joint without concomitant fracture.
- Complex instability denotes the presence of a fracture associated with dislocation.
- The elbow is the second most commonly dislocated large joint (excluding phalanx dislocations and so forth).

PATHOANATOMY

- Elbow stability is conferred by both the osseous anatomy as well as the ligamentous anatomy.
- Primary stabilizers of the ulnohumeral joint include the osseous architecture of the joint, including the coronoid process and greater sigmoid notch of the ulna, and the trochlea of the humerus.
  - The anterior band of the medial collateral ligament (aMCL) and the lateral ulnar collateral ligament (LUCL) are the primary ligamentous stabilizers of the elbow.[9,12]
  - The aMCL originates on the anterior inferior face of the medial epicondyle and inserts on the sublime tubercle of the ulna.
  - The LUCL originates from an isometric point on the lateral supracondylar column and traverses across the inferior aspect of the radial head, inserting on the supinator crest of the ulna.[8]
- Secondary stabilizers include the radial head and dynamic constraints such as the flexor and extensor muscles of the forearm.
  - The anterior joint capsule is also felt to play a role in ulnohumeral stability.
- O'Driscoll[12] has proposed the term "posterolateral rotatory instability" (PLRI) to describe the series of pathologic events that result in ulnohumeral dislocation.
  - PLRI is felt to start with disruption of the LUCL and progresses medially with tearing of the anterior and posterior capsules. This allows the ulna to "perch" on the distal humerus. Further soft tissue or osseous injury results in dislocation[13] (**FIG 1A**).
    - Most traumatic injuries to the LUCL result in avulsion of the ligament from the lateral humerus (**FIG 1B**).
  - As forces continue from lateral to medial across the joint, the anterior and posterior capsular tissues and eventually the MCL may be disrupted.
    - It is possible to dislocate the ulnohumeral joint with disruption of the LUCL and preservation of the aMCL.[12]
- Common fractures that occur with elbow dislocation include radial head or neck and coronoid fractures, although any fracture about the elbow may be observed.
  - Radial head fractures are usually readily apparent on plain radiographs.
  - Coronoid fractures may be subtle, and even a "fleck" of coronoid is often a hallmark of a more significant injury (eg, "terrible triad" injury), and its importance should not be underestimated.
- Recently, a variant of elbow instability termed postero-*medial* rotatory instability (PMRI) has been described, which is a consequence of LUCL injury and medial coronoid facet fracture. This injury pattern is most commonly observed *without* radial head fracture, making it potentially very subtle on plain radiographs. A computed tomography (CT) scan can delineate this injury in detail and should be obtained if any suspicion exists (**FIG 1C–E**).[2,11]

ETIOLOGY AND CLASSIFICATION

- Most elbow dislocations occur with a fall on an outstretched arm.
- Forces of valgus, extension, supination, and axial load across the joint can result in the ulna rotating away from the humerus, disrupting lateral–anterior soft tissues initially, and dislocating the elbow.
- Simple elbow dislocations are classified by the direction of displacement of the ulna in reference to the humerus, with posterolateral dislocation the most common.
  - Less common variants include anterior, medial, or lateral dislocations.

PATIENT HISTORY AND PHYSICAL FINDINGS

- History is aimed at determining the timeline and mechanism of injury, frequency of dislocations, and previous treatment.
- Unlike the shoulder, recurrent instability of the elbow is rare after an initial simple dislocation that was treated expediently.
  - Recurrent instability is more common in association with fractures (eg, the "terrible triad" injury).
  - Chronic instability, although rare in the United States, does occasionally occur, and management often requires reconstructive surgery or elbow replacement. Closed treatment is rarely successful in these patients.
- Iatrogenic injury of the LUCL (during procedures such as open tennis elbow release or radial head fracture management) is a known cause of recurrent PLRI. However, these patients often complain of subtle lateral elbow pain due to subluxation of the joint with activities, such as rising from a chair, but rarely have recurrent dislocation.
- Examination at the time of injury requires attention to the neurovascular anatomy.
  - Nerve injury can occur after elbow dislocation, and a thorough neurologic examination of the extremity is mandatory before any treatment of the dislocation.
    - Most nerve injuries are neuropraxia that often resolve.
    - The ulnar nerve is most frequently involved, although median or radial nerve injury may also occur.[14]
- The dislocated elbow has obvious deformity, with the elbow often held in a varus position and the forearm supinated.

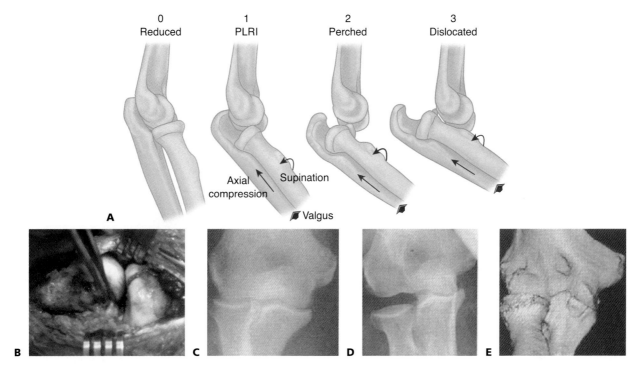

FIG 1 • A. Posterolateral rotatory instability follows a typical progression of disruption, allowing the joint to become perched and then dislocate as soft tissue injury progresses. **B.** Intraoperative photograph demonstrating avulsion of the origin of the lateral ulnar collateral ligament (LUCL) after traumatic dislocation of the elbow. The origin of the LUCL and the extensor muscles are avulsed as one layer, held by the forceps. **C–E.** Posteromedial rotatory instability is a variant of elbow instability in which the elbow dislocates, rupturing the LUCL, and the medial coronoid sustains an impaction fracture **C,D**. In this injury pattern, the radial head remains intact, making appropriate diagnosis of the severity of the injury difficult on standard radiographs. CT scans help better delineate the injury pattern. **E.** Impaction fracture can be seen on the 3D CT reconstruction. (**A:** Adapted from O'Driscoll SW, Morrey BF, Korinek S, et al. Elbow subluxation and dislocation: a spectrum of instability. Clin Orthop Relat Res 1982;280:194. **C–E:** Copyright the Mayo Foundation, Rochester, MN.)

■ After initial reduction, the neurovascular status of the limb is re-evaluated. Loss of neurologic function after closed reduction is rare but can be an indication for surgical exploration to rule out an entrapped nerve.

■ Stability of the joint is assessed based on the amount of extension obtainable and association of pronation or supination with instability (see the treatment algorithm section).

  ■ It is helpful to evaluate the stability throughout the elbow range of motion while the patient is still anesthetized, as this may guide treatment (examination under anesthesia).

  ■ Stressing of the lateral soft tissues is performed with the lateral pivot-shift maneuver, which can be performed under anesthesia and with fluoroscopic imaging[12] (**FIG 2**).

    ■ This test can be used to assess the degree of posterolateral rotatory instability, and may aid in determining treatment.

■ Medial ecchymosis may be a sign of an aMCL injury, and often is apparent 3 to 5 days after dislocation when the MCL has been injured.

IMAGING AND OTHER DIAGNOSTIC STUDIES

■ Standard orthogonal radiographs of the elbow are obtained before and after reduction to assess for fracture and confirm relocation of the joint.

  ■ Congruency of the trochlea–ulna and radial head–capitellum is assessed.

■ Valgus stress views, once the joint is reduced, may help demonstrate an aMCL injury.

  ■ With the elbow flexed 30 degrees and the forearm in pronation, a valgus stress is placed under fluoroscopic evaluation to see if the medial ulnohumeral joint opens compared to the resting state.

■ Varus stress views are often not helpful.

■ CT scans with 3D reconstructions are obtained in any situation where a fracture may be suspected, as it is critical to identify PMRI variants or subtle coronoid fractures, which may be an indication for surgical management.

■ Magnetic resonance imaging (MRI) is usually not necessary in the management of simple dislocation, although if questions regarding the integrity of the MCL exist, an MRI can delineate this structure well.

NONOPERATIVE MANAGEMENT

■ Most simple dislocations may be managed nonoperatively with splinting or bracing, guided by the degree of instability determined during the examination under anesthesia after reduction.[12]

■ Once reduced, elbow stability is assessed during flexion–extension in neutral forearm rotation.

  ■ If the elbow is stable throughout an arc of motion, it is immobilized in a sling or splint for 3 to 5 days for comfort and then range-of-motion exercises are begun.

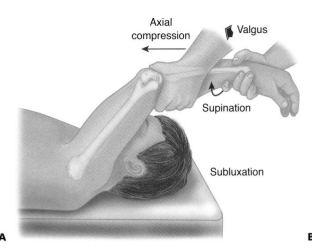

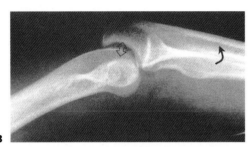

A   **B**

FIG 2 • A. The lateral pivot-shift maneuver is performed with the patient's arm positioned overhead, and a supination–valgus stress is applied. As the elbow is brought into flexion the joint reduces, often with a clunk. **B.** When performed under fluoroscopy, subluxation of the radial head posterior to the capitellum can be observed, consistent with posterolateral rotatory instability. (**B:** From O'Driscoll SW, Bell DF, Morrey BF. Posterolateral rotatory instability of the elbow. J Bone Joint Surg Am 1991;73A:440–446.)

■ If instability is present in less than 30 degrees of flexion, the forearm is pronated and stability is reassessed.

  ■ If pronation confers stability, then a hinged orthosis that maintains forearm pronation is used, after 3 to 5 days of splinting, to allow protected range of motion.

■ Elbows that sublux (confirmed by fluoroscopic imaging) in less than 30 degrees of flexion and pronation of the forearm are managed with a brief period of splinting, followed by a hinged orthosis that controls rotation of the forearm and has an extension block.

■ Elbows that are unstable in more than 30 degrees of flexion and pronation often are managed surgically.

■ Hinged bracing is maintained for 6 weeks, with progressive advancement of extension and rotation, as allowed by stability of the joint.

  ■ Weekly radiographs are needed to ensure maintenance of a congruent joint during the first 4 to 6 weeks.

■ After 6 weeks bracing is discontinued and terminal stretching to regain motion is used if flexion contractures exist.

SURGICAL MANAGEMENT

Indications

■ Surgical management is indicated in elbows that are unstable, even when placed in flexion (more than 30 degrees) and pronation, elbows that recurrently sublux or dislocate during the treatment protocol, or those with associated fractures ("complex" instability).

■ Management of simple dislocation requires repair or reconstruction of those ligamentous injuries resulting in instability. By definition, simple dislocation occurs without fracture.

■ An algorithmic approach to ligament repair is used to stabilize the elbow. The LUCL is felt to be the primary lesion of dislocation, and therefore this ligament is addressed first, followed by assessment of stability.

■ The LUCL usually avulses from its origin during dislocation, and therefore most often can be repaired after acute injury.

  ■ Repair may be performed via bone tunnels in the humerus or with suture anchors, depending on the surgeon's preference.

■ Reconstruction of the LUCL is rarely needed in acute management but is more commonly needed in chronic instability.

  ■ Reconstruction, when necessary, uses autograft (either palmaris or gracilis) or allograft.

■ Often, repair or reconstruction of the LUCL confers stability, even in the face of MCL injury, as the intact radial head is a secondary stabilizer to valgus instability.

■ Persistent instability after LUCL repair is rare and is more commonly observed with fracture-dislocations or chronic instability.

  ■ If persistent instability exists, the MCL is repaired or reconstructed, a hinged external fixator is placed, or both are performed.

■ This section will discuss the surgical technique of LUCL repair and reconstruction.

Preoperative Planning

■ Planning should include the possibility of reconstruction of the LUCL using autograft, which will be harvested at surgery, or by having allograft available.

  ■ If autograft is to be harvested, a tendon stripper is needed.

  ■ For allograft we routinely use semitendinosus tendon.

■ A hinged external fixator should be available in the rare case that the elbow remains unstable after ligamentous repair or reconstruction.

■ 2.0- and 3.2-mm drill bits or burrs are used to make bone tunnels for LUCL repair or reconstruction.

  ■ Alternatively, some surgeons prefer suture anchor repair of ligament avulsions; if desired, these should be available.

■ Fluoroscopy is useful for confirming reduction and is required for placement of a hinged external fixator.

■ A sterile tourniquet is used if exposure of the proximal humerus is necessary for placement of proximal external fixator pins.

Patient Positioning

■ Patients are positioned supine with the arm on a radiolucent hand table.

▪ A small bump is placed under the scapula to aid in arm positioning.

▪ The forequarter is draped free to ensure the entire brachium is kept in the surgical field.

▪ If hamstring autograft is to be used for LUCL, the leg should be draped free and a bump is placed under the hemipelvis to aid in exposure.

LATERAL ULNAR COLLATERAL LIGAMENT REPAIR

Surgical Approach and Arthrotomy

▪ Tourniquet control is used during this procedure.

▪ Two different surgical approaches are used to manage elbow instability.

▪ Often, a posterior midline skin incision can be used to gain access to both the medial and lateral aspects of the joint; therefore, it is a very extensile approach to the elbow.

▪ Alternatively, a "column" incision, centered over the lateral epicondyle, may be used (**TECH FIG 1A**). If medial-sided exposure is needed, a similar "column" incision may be made over the medial epicondyle to gain access.

▪ There are benefits to both approaches, and currently no data exist delineating which approach is better.
  ▪ For simple dislocation we routinely use a lateral column approach.

▪ After skin incision, skin flaps are raised anteroposterior at the level of the deep fascia.

▪ Often the lateral soft tissues are avulsed off the epicondyle, exposing the joint. Occasionally, however, the extensor origin is intact with an underlying ligament injury.
  ▪ If the extensor muscles are intact, the interval between the extensor carpi ulnaris (ECU) and anconeus (the Köcher approach), which directly overlies the LUCL, is used. This interval is often readily identified by the presence of a "fat stripe" in the deep fascia (**TECH FIG 1B**).

▪ The elbow joint is then exposed by incising the proximal capsule along the lateral column of the humerus, continuing distally along the radial neck (through the supinator muscle and underling capsule) in line with the ECU–anconeus interval.
  ▪ The posterior interosseous nerve (PIN) is at risk with this exposure, and therefore the forearm is kept in pronation to protect the PIN.

▪ The radiocapitellar joint and coronoid are inspected to confirm no fractures are present and that no soft tissue is interposed in the joint, preventing reduction.

▪ Once the joint is clear of debris, the ability to obtain a concentric reduction is confirmed with fluoroscopy.

Ligament Repair

▪ The origin of the LUCL is identified.
  ▪ Often, the LUCL is avulsed from the isometric point on the lateral capitellum, and the origin can be identified by a "fold" of tissue on the deep surface of the capsule (**TECH FIG 2A**).

▪ Starting at the origin, a running no. 2 nonabsorbable Krackow locking suture is placed along the anterior and posterior aspect of the ligament. Once placed, the suture–ligament construct is tensioned to confirm the integrity of the insertion onto the ulna.
  ▪ A common mistake is to start the repair at the level of the proximal origin of the superficial tissue, which is not the origin of the LUCL but part of the extensor origin.

▪ The isometric origin on the humerus is then identified in the center of the capitellum, not the lateral epicondyle (**TECH FIG 2B,C**).
  ▪ Confirmation of the isometric point is made by clamping the limbs of the running suture at the point of isometry and then flexing and extending the elbow to confirm proper placement.

▪ A 2.0-mm burr is used to make a humeral bone tunnel.
  ▪ It is critical to make the most anterior aspect of the bone tunnel at the isometric point, not the center of the tunnel, as this small translation can result in a lax LUCL repair (**TECH FIG 2D**).

▪ Two "exit" tunnels (in a Y configuration), one anterior and one posterior to the lateral column, are then made

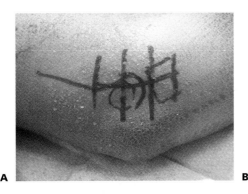
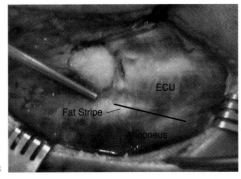

TECH FIG 1 ▪ A. Lateral column skin incision. The lateral incision is centered over the epicondyle and radiocapitellar joint and is often the primary incision, as the lateral ulnar collateral ligament (LUCL) rupture is thought to be the primary injury in simple dislocations. **B.** The deep interval between the extensor carpi ulnaris and anconeus is used to gain exposure to the joint. This is often identified by a "fat stripe" in the fascia. Care should be taken not to violate the LUCL, which traverses in line with this interval deep to the fascia and supinator muscle.

TECHNIQUES

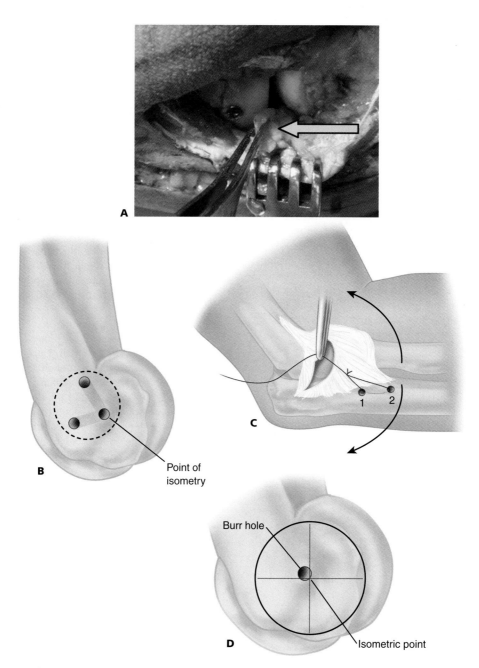

TECH FIG 2 • A. The origin of the lateral ulnar collateral ligament (LUCL), which often avulses during elbow dislocation, is identified by a "fold" of tissue on the deep surface of the capsule. The isometric point of the joint is in the center of rotation of the capitellum (**B**), and confirmation is made using the previously placed sutures in the ligament remnant to ensure that an isometric repair will be obtained (**C**). **D.** It is important to make the humeral tunnel so that the most anterior aspect of the tunnel is placed at the isometric point. Exit holes for the humeral tunnel are made anterior and posterior to the lateral supracondylar ridge (**B**).

with a 2.0-mm drill bit or burr, connected to the distal humeral tunnel at the isometric point.

■ Once the humeral tunnels are completed, the limbs of the running suture are passed through the humeral tunnels.

■ The joint is concentrically reduced with fluoroscopic confirmation and the LUCL repair sutures are then tied with the joint reduced and the elbow in 30 degrees of flexion and neutral rotation.

■ The elbow is ranged through an arc of motion to assess stability, with careful attention placed on the radial head's articulation with the capitellum, looking for posterior sag in extension, indicating either a lax LUCL or a nonisometric repair.

■ If the elbow is stable through an arc of motion, the extensor origin is repaired with interrupted, heavy (no. 0) nonabsorbable suture and the skin is closed in layers.

LATERAL ULNAR COLLATERAL LIGAMENT RECONSTRUCTION

- Occasionally, the native LUCL is damaged beyond repair (more often with iatrogenic PLRI than with primary instability) or attenuated after recurrent or chronic elbow instability, and reconstruction is necessary.
- Autograft palmaris or gracilis or allograft may be used.
- Autograft and allograft options should be discussed with the patient and decisions made preoperatively. We routinely use semitendinosus allograft unless the patient desires autograft.
- This section will cover the technique of ligament graft reconstruction once tendon graft has been harvested.

Bone Tunnel Preparation

- We use a "docking" technique, similar to those described for MCL reconstruction,[1] for LUCL reconstruction.
- The insertion of the LUCL is at the supinator crest of the ulna, and reconstruction begins with creation of the ulnar tunnels at the supinator crest.
- Reflecting the supinator origin from the ulna posterior to the radial head exposes the supinator crest.
  - The forearm is held in pronation to protect the PIN.
- Once the crest is exposed, the ulnar tunnel is made at the level of the radial head using two 3.4-mm burr holes placed 1 cm apart. Care is taken to connect the holes using small curettes or awls without fracturing the roof of the tunnel (**TECH FIG 3**).
- Once the ulnar tunnel is made, a suture is placed in the tunnel to aid in graft passage and to help identify the isometric point on the humerus, similar to the technique described with ligament repair.
- Once the isometric origin on the humerus is confirmed, humeral bone tunnels are made as mentioned in the LUCL repair section.
  - With LUCL reconstruction the isometric tunnel is deepened to about 1 cm to allow graft docking.
  - Further, the docking tunnel is widened using a 3.4-mm burr to be able to accept both limbs of the graft.
  - It is important to widen the docking hole anterior and proximal to the isometric point, as the most posterior aspect of the tunnel needs to be at the isometric point.

Graft Preparation

- One end of the graft is freshened and tubularized using a no. 2 nonabsorbable suture in a running Krackow fashion.
- The graft is then passed through the ulnar bone tunnels using the passage suture previously placed.
- The limb of the graft with locking suture is then fully docked into the humeral origin, and the joint is reduced.
- The final length of the graft is determined by tensioning the graft and identifying the point at which the free limb of the graft meets the isometric origin. This point is marked on the graft.
  - Care should be taken to ensure appropriate graft tension and length by fully docking the first limb and then marking the free limb at the point of initial contact with the humerus, thereby allowing some overlap of graft limbs in the humeral tunnel but minimizing the likelihood of slack in the final construct.
- The marked graft end is then freshened and tubularized in an identical fashion as the other limb.

Final Reconstruction

- Once the graft is placed and ready for final tensioning and fixation, the capsule and remnant of the LUCL is repaired back to the humerus in an effort to make the ligament reconstruction extra-articular, if possible.
- Each limb of the graft is then placed into the isometric docking tunnel on the humerus with corresponding limbs from each locking suture exiting the proximal humeral tunnels.
  - Both limbs of locking suture from one end of the graft are passed through one proximal tunnel in the humerus, followed by the limbs from the other end of the graft through the second proximal tunnel.
- The joint is then reduced and the graft is finally tensioned to ensure there is no slack and neither graft end has "bottomed out" in the humeral docking tunnel.
- The locking sutures are then tied together over the lateral column of the distal humerus with the joint concentrically reduced in 30 degrees of flexion and neutral rotation.
- The joint is then ranged and stability assessed. If the joint is stable, no further reconstruction is necessary and the extensor muscles are repaired using a nonabsorbable interrupted stitch, followed by skin closure.

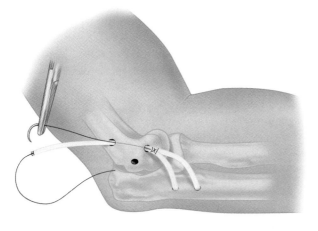

TECH FIG 3 • The insertion of the lateral ulnar collateral ligament is the supinator crest of the ulna. Reconstruction uses an ulnar tunnel in the supinator crest made at the level of the radial head. Holes are made about 1 cm apart and connected to form a tunnel.

HINGED EXTERNAL FIXATION

- A hinged fixator may be necessary in chronic dislocations, some fracture-dislocations, or rarely in patients with persistent instability after LUCL repair or reconstruction for simple dislocation.[4,16]
- Once any soft tissue blocking reduction is removed and a concentric reduction can be obtained, the fixator is placed.
- All hinged elbow fixators are constructed around the axis or rotation of the elbow to allow range of motion to occur while maintaining a concentric reduction.
  - Most implants are built around an axis pin, placed in this center of rotation.
  - The center of rotation is identified as the center of the capitellum on a lateral aspect of the elbow, and on the medial side it is just anteroinferior to the medial epicondyle, in the center of curvature of the trochlea (**TECH FIG 4**).
  - The axis pin is placed through both of these points, parallel to the joint surface, and the position is confirmed by fluoroscopy.

- After placement of the axis pin, the humeral and ulnar pins are placed after confirmation of concentric reduction of the elbow is made.
- Once the external fixator is fully constructed, the elbow is taken through an arc of motion and maintenance of reduction is confirmed.
- Fixators are kept on for 6 to 8 weeks.
- Meticulous pin care is necessary to minimize pin tract infections or loosening.

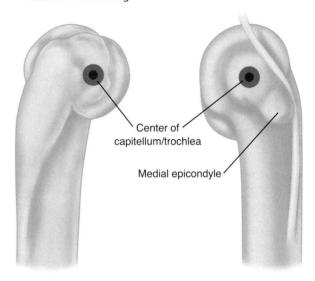

Center of capitellum/trochlea

Medial epicondyle

TECH FIG 4 • The center of rotation of the elbow, along which an axis pin for hinged fixators is placed, is identified by the center of the capitellum and just anteroinferior to the medial epicondyle.

PEARLS AND PITFALLS

- LUCL avulsion is the primary ligamentous injury in most simple dislocations of the elbow.
- If the radial head and coronoid are intact (as is the case in a simple dislocation), the MCL rarely needs to be repaired or reconstructed, as the radial head acts as a secondary stabilizer in the elbow with a repaired lateral ligament complex.
- The LUCL origin can be identified by a capsular fold of tissue. This is the point at which repair sutures should be placed, not at the origin of the more superficial extensor tendons.
- The isometric origin of the LUCL is in the center of the capitellum, as projected onto the lateral column, and repair or reconstruction needs to be brought to this point to have an isometric ligament.
- Bone tunnels in the humerus for repair or reconstruction are made so the anteroinferior aspect of the tunnel is at the isometric origin.
- A hinged external fixator may be necessary in management of elbow dislocation, especially chronic or recurrent situations, and should be available.
- All hinged fixators are constructed around the axis of rotation of the elbow, identified by a line between the isometric point on the lateral capitellum and the center of rotation of the trochlea on the medial aspect of the joint.
- Stiffness is the most common adverse sequela of elbow dislocation, and therefore range of motion should be started as soon as soft tissue and skin healing allows, with care taken to avoid varus or valgus stress.

POSTOPERATIVE CARE

- After operative stabilization without external fixation, the elbow is splinted in flexion for 3 to 5 days to allow wound healing.
- Range-of-motion exercises are then begun in flexion, extension, and rotation, with care taken to avoid varus or valgus stress.
  - A hinged orthosis can be helpful in protecting the ligament repair or reconstruction.
- Active and passive motion is continued for 6 weeks, when strengthening is added.

- Residual contractures, often loss of extension, can be managed with static splinting and terminal stretching.

OUTCOMES

- Most series have reported the results of closed management of simple dislocation.
  - Mehlhoff and colleagues[7] reported the results of 52 simple dislocations managed, with most patients having normal elbows. Length of immobilization, especially greater then 3 weeks, was found to be more likely to result in persistent loss of extension.

Similarly, Eygendaal and colleagues[3] reported the long-term results of 50 patients after closed management of simple dislocations. Sixty-two percent of patients described their elbow function as good or excellent, and 24 of 50 (48%) patients had loss of extension of 5 to 10 degrees.

Some series have examined the surgical management of PLRI, often as a result of recurrent instability after traumatic dislocation.

Nestor and colleagues[10] reported the results of 11 patients with recurrent PLRI managed with either repair or reconstruction of the LUCL. Ten of 11 (91%) remained stable and 7 of 11 (64%) had an excellent result.

More recently, Sanchez-Sotelo and colleagues[15] reported the results of 44 patients treated for recurrent PLRI (9 occurred after simple dislocation). Thirty-two (75%) of the patients had an excellent result by Mayo score.

Lee and Teo[5] found that in patients with chronic PLRI, reconstruction offered more predictable outcomes over repair.

COMPLICATIONS

- Stiffness[3,7]
- Heterotopic ossification[6]
- Neurovascular injury[14]
- Recurrent instability[3,7]
- Compartment syndrome
- Hematoma or infection

REFERENCES

1. Dodson CC, Thomas A, Dines JS, et al. Medial ulnar collateral ligament reconstruction of the elbow in throwing athletes. Am J Sports Med 2006;34:1926–1932.
2. Doornberg JN, Ring DC. Fracture of the anteromedial facet of the coronoid process. J Bone Joint Surg Am 2006;88A:2216–2224.
3. Eygendaal D, Verdegaal SH, Obermann WR, et al. Posterolateral dislocation of the elbow joint: relationship to medial instability. J Bone Joint Surg Am 2000;82A:555–560.
4. Jupiter JB, Ring D. Treatment of unreduced elbow dislocations with hinged external fixation. J Bone Joint Surg Am 2002;84A:1630–1635.
5. Lee BP, Teo LH. Surgical reconstruction for posterolateral rotatory instability of the elbow. J Shoulder Elbow Surg 2003;12:476–479.
6. Linscheid RL, Wheeler DK. Elbow dislocations. JAMA 1965;194:1171–1176.
7. Mehlhoff TL, Noble PC, Bennett JB, et al. Simple dislocation of the elbow in the adult. Results after closed treatment. J Bone Joint Surg Am 1988;70A:244–249.
8. Morrey BF, An KN. Functional anatomy of the ligaments of the elbow. Clin Orthop Relat Res 1985;201:84–90.
9. Morrey BF, Tanaka S, An KN. Valgus stability of the elbow: a definition of primary and secondary constraints. Clin Orthop Relat Res 1991;265:187–195.
10. Nestor BJ, O'Driscoll SW, Morrey BF. Ligamentous reconstruction for posterolateral rotatory instability of the elbow. J Bone Joint Surg Am 1992;74A:1235–1241.
11. O'Driscoll SW. Acute, recurrent, and chronic elbow instabilities. In: Norris TR, ed. Orthopaedic Knowledge Update: Shoulder and Elbow 2. Rosemont, IL: American Academy of Orthopaedic Surgeons, 2002:313–323.
12. O'Driscoll SW, Bell DF, Morrey BF. Posterolateral rotatory instability of the elbow. J Bone Joint Surg Am 1991;73A:440–446.
13. O'Driscoll SW, Morrey BF, Korinek S, et al. Elbow subluxation and dislocation: a spectrum of instability. Clin Orthop Relat Res 1992;280:186–197.
14. Rana NA, Kenwright J, Taylor RG, et al. Complete lesion of the median nerve associated with dislocation of the elbow joint. Acta Orthop Scand 1974;45:365–369.
15. Sanchez-Sotelo J, Morrey BF, O'Driscoll SW. Ligamentous repair and reconstruction for posterolateral rotatory instability of the elbow. J Bone Joint Surg Br 2005;87B:54–61.
16. Tan V, Daluiski A, Capo J, et al. Hinged elbow external fixators: indications and uses. J Am Acad Orthop Surg 2005;13:503–514.

Chapter 39

Open Reduction and Internal Fixation of Fracture-Dislocations of the Elbow With Complex Instability

Jubin B. Payandeh and Michael D. McKee

DEFINITION

▪ Simple dislocations of the elbow can most often be treated successfully with closed means: reduction and short-term immobilization followed by early motion.

▪ Fracture-dislocations of the elbow are more troublesome in that they often require operative intervention.

▪ Fractures associated with elbow dislocations often involve the radial head and coronoid. When both are combined with dislocation, this is termed the "terrible triad."

▪ The principle of treating fracture-dislocations of the elbow is to provide sufficient stability through reconstruction of bony and ligamentous restraints such that early motion can be instituted without recurrent instability.

▪ Failure to achieve this will result in either recurrent instability or severe stiffness after prolonged immobilization.

ANATOMY

▪ Posterolateral dislocations of the elbow are associated with disruption of the medial and lateral collateral ligaments.

▪ The medial collateral ligament (MCL) is the primary stabilizer to valgus stress (**FIG 1**).

▪ The lateral collateral ligament (LCL) is the primary stabilizer to posterolateral rotatory instability. Most often the disruption is from the lateral epicondyle, leaving a characteristic bare spot. Less commonly, the ligament may rupture mid-substance.[5] Secondary restraints on the lateral side that may also be disrupted are the common extensor origin and the posterolateral capsule.

▪ Radial head fractures have been classified by Mason:
  ▪ Type I: small or marginal fracture with minimal displacement
  ▪ Type II: marginal fracture with displacement
  ▪ Type III: comminuted fractures of the head and neck[2]

▪ Coronoid fractures have been classified by Regan and Morrey[9] (**FIG 2**):
  ▪ Type I: tip fractures (not avulsions)
  ▪ Type II: less than 50% of the coronoid
  ▪ Type III: more than 50% of the coronoid
    ▪ The insertion of the MCL is at the base of the coronoid and it may be involved in type III fractures[1]

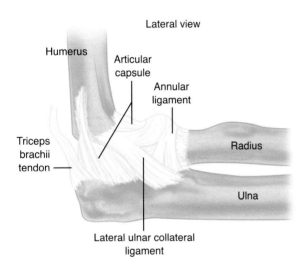

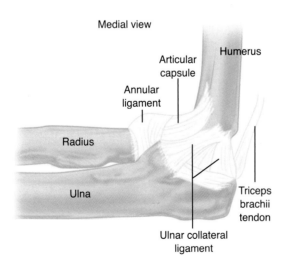

FIG 1 • The medial and collateral ligament complexes of the elbow. Note their points of attachment on the distal humerus and proximal ulna.

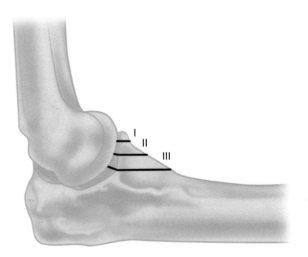

FIG 2 • Lateral view of the elbow depicting the different types of coronoid fractures.

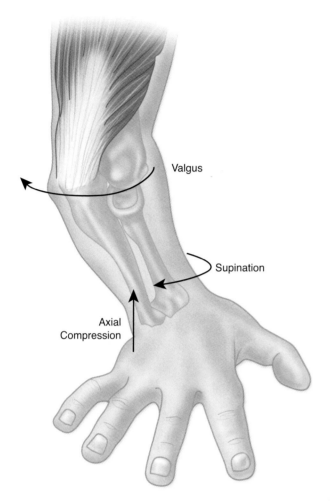

FIG 3 • Typical mechanism of elbow fracture dislocation. Note the forces at play on the elbow.

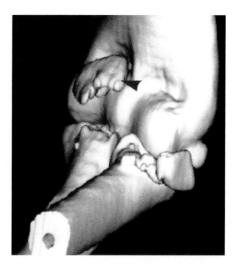

FIG 4 • Three-dimensional CT reconstruction of "terrible triad" injury. The *arrow* represents the large coronoid fragment anterior to the elbow. (From Pugh DMW, Wild LM, Schemitsch EH, et al. Standard surgical protocol to treat elbow dislocations with radial head and coronoid fractures. J Bone Joint Surg Am 2004;86A:1122–1130.)

PATHOGENESIS

- Fracture-dislocations of the elbow occur during falls onto an outstretched hand, falls from a height, motor vehicle accidents, or other high-energy trauma (**FIG 3**).
- Typically there is a hyperextension and valgus stress applied to the pronated arm.

NATURAL HISTORY

- Elbow dislocations with associated coronoid or radial head fractures have a poor natural history. Redislocation or subluxation is likely with closed treatment.
- Treatment of the radial head fracture by excision alone in the context of an elbow dislocation has a high rate of failure due to recurrent instability.
- Problems of recurrent instability, arthrosis, and severe stiffness lead to poor functional results.[10]

PATIENT HISTORY AND PHYSICAL FINDINGS

- Fracture-dislocations of the elbow are acute and traumatic, so the history should be straightforward.
- It is not unusual for these injuries to occur with high-energy trauma, so a diligent search for other musculoskeletal and

systemic injuries must accompany evaluation of the elbow. The ipsilateral shoulder and wrist should be evaluated.
- The evaluation and documentation of peripheral nerve and vascular function in the injured extremity is critical.

IMAGING AND OTHER DIAGNOSTIC STUDIES

- High-quality plain radiographs in the anteroposterior (AP) and lateral plane should be obtained before and after closed reduction.
  - Cast material can obscure bony detail after closed reduction.
- If there is any evidence of forearm or wrist pain associated with the elbow injury, these should be imaged as well.
- Computed tomography (CT) scans with reformatted images and 3D reconstructions are helpful in understanding the configuration of bony injuries and are helpful in treatment planning (**FIG 4**).

DIFFERENTIAL DIAGNOSIS

- Radial head or neck fractures without associated dislocation
- Coronoid fracture associated with posteromedial instability. This results from a varus force and is associated with rupture of the LCL. The radial head is not fractured, making diagnosis more difficult.

NONOPERATIVE MANAGEMENT

- Initial treatment involves closed reduction and splinting with radiographs to confirm reduction (**FIG 5**).
- If reduction cannot be maintained because of bone or soft tissue injury, repeated attempts at closed reduction should not be attempted. This is thought to contribute to the formation of heterotopic ossification.
- The ability of nonoperative management to meet treatment goals in these situations is rare and surgery is indicated in almost all cases.

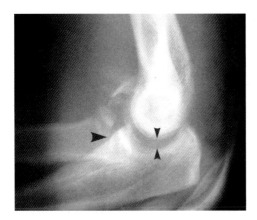

FIG 5 • Radiograph revealing nonconcentric reduction after closed reduction. The *small arrows* highlight the nonconcentric reduction of the ulnohumeral joint. (From Pugh DMW, Wild LM, Schemitsch EH, et al. Standard surgical protocol to treat elbow dislocations with radial head and coronoid fractures. J Bone Joint Surg Am 2004;86A:1122–1130.)

SURGICAL MANAGEMENT

- The goals of surgery are to obtain and maintain a concentric and stable reduction of the ulnohumeral and radiocapitellar joint such that early motion within a flexion–extension arc of 30 to 130 degrees can be initiated. Early motion is key to avoid elbow stiffness and resultant poor function.
- Management of elbow dislocations with associated radial head and coronoid fractures should follow an established protocol (Table 1) that has produced reliable results.[8]
- The radial head is an important secondary stabilizer of the elbow to valgus stress and posterior instability.[7]
  - It is also a longitudinal stabilizer of the forearm to proximal translation.
  - If fractured in this setting, it must be fixed or replaced, as excision leads to recurrent instability and unacceptable results.[10]

Preoperative Planning

- Before surgery, the surgeon must ensure that the proper equipment and implants are available.

Table 1	Treatment Protocol for Elbow Dislocation With Associated Radial Head and Coronoid Fractures		
Step	**Action**		
1	Fix the coronoid fracture		
2	Fix or replace the radial head		
3	Repair the lateral collateral ligament		
4	Assess elbow stability within 30 to 130 degrees of flexion–extension with the forearm in full pronation		
5	If the elbow remains unstable, consider fixing the medial collateral ligament		
6	Failing this, apply a hinged external fixator to maintain concentric reduction and allow for early motion		

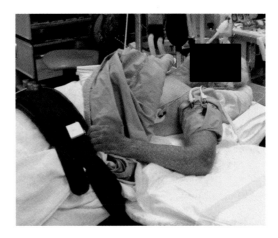

FIG 6 • Patient positioned supine with hand table.

- Coronoid fractures are fixed with small fragment or cannulated screws of appropriate size.
- Radial head and neck fracture fixation is accomplished with small fragment plates and screws.
  - We often use countersunk Herbert screws to fix articular head fragments.
  - A metallic, modular radial head implant system should be available if primary osteosynthesis cannot be achieved.
- An image intensifier is helpful during surgery. Films confirming concentric reduction and the proper positioning of implanted hardware should always be obtained before leaving the operating room.
- In rare instances in which bony and ligamentous repair fails to restore sufficient elbow stability, dynamic hinged external fixation is used.
  - This is a highly specialized technique that may not be appropriate for all surgeons.
  - In that case, static external fixation and patient referral is an appropriate alternative.

Positioning

- Most commonly, the patient is positioned supine on the operating table under general anesthesia.
- The operative limb is supported on a hand table and a tourniquet is applied to the upper arm before preparation and draping (**FIG 6**).
- Alternatively, the lateral decubitus position can be used with the operative limb supported by a padded bolster. This position is used if hinged fixation is deemed likely.

Approach

- The lateral approach is the workhorse for treatment of these injuries where the coronoid, radial head, and LCL can be addressed. A direct lateral incision with the patient supine and the arm on a hand table is used.
- Landmarks and skin incision are shown in FIGURE 7A.
- The surgeon should use the traumatic dissection that occurred at the time of injury to gain exposure of the elbow.
- Typically the LCL has been avulsed from the lateral distal humerus, leaving a bare spot (**FIG 7B**).[8]
- Some cases require a medial approach as well for either medial ligament reconstruction or plating of a coronoid

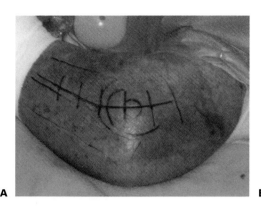
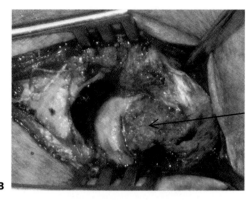

FIG 7 • **A.** Landmarks and skin incision. The underlying bones have been represented and the position of the lateral skin incision is marked with the *hashed line*. **B.** Avulsion of lateral collateral ligament. The *arrow* is pointing to the bare spot on the distal lateral humerus where the lateral collateral ligament complex has been avulsed.

fracture. This can be accomplished through a second medial incision.

■ The ulnar nerve is at risk in this approach and should be identified and protected. The common flexor origin is split distal to the medial epicondyle to expose the coronoid medially.

■ Alternatively, a posterior skin incision can be used with elevation of full-thickness flaps at the fascial level to approach both laterally and medially.

■ The patient can be placed in the lateral decubitus position or supine with the arm across the chest for this approach.

LATERAL EXPOSURE

■ Make an incision along the lateral supracondylar ridge of the humerus curving at the lateral epicondyle toward the radial head and neck.

■ At the fascial level, elevate full-thickness flaps and insert a self-retaining retractor (**TECH FIG 1**).

■ Split the common extensor origin in line with its fibers.

■ Make use of the traumatic dissection that occurred at the time of injury.

■ Most commonly, the LCL will have avulsed from the distal humerus, leaving a bare spot. The common extensor origin is avulsed as well two thirds of the time.[7]

■ Reconstruction occurs in an orderly fashion from deep to superficial.

■ If the radial head is to be replaced, its excision provides excellent exposure of the coronoid through the lateral approach.

■ If, on the other hand, it is to be fixed, set free fragments aside to allow access to the coronoid.

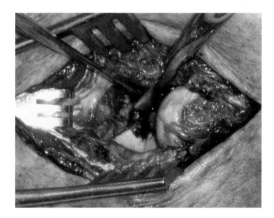

TECH FIG 1 • Lateral approach. In this case, the radial neck was fractured and the head has been removed. An excellent view of the coronoid is achieved. Here a type I coronoid fracture is present.

ORIF OF CORONOID FRACTURE

Type I Coronoid Fractures

■ For type I fractures, we recommend fixation with a nonabsorbable (no. 2 braided) suture passed through the anterior elbow capsule just above the bony fragment (**TECH FIG 2**).

■ Two parallel drill holes are made from the dorsal surface of the ulna through a separate small incision and directed toward the coronoid tip. These are made with a small drill or Kirschner wire.

■ Once the suture is passed through the capsule, its ends are brought out each of the drill holes and tied over the ulna to plicate the anterior elbow capsule.

■ The suture ends can be retrieved through the drill holes using an eyeleted Kirschner wire, a Keith needle, or a suture retriever.

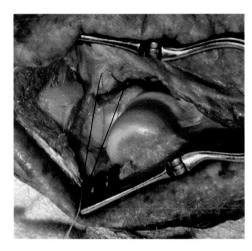

TECH FIG 2 • Suture fixation of a type I coronoid fracture. The suture is passed through the anterior capsule above the coronoid. Its ends will be passed through the proximal ulna and tied over the dorsal surface. This type of fixation is used if the coronoid fragment is too small to accept a screw. (From McKee MD, Pugh DM, Wild LM, et al. Standard surgical protocol to treat elbow dislocation with radial head and coronoid fractures. J Bone Joint Surg Am 2005;87A:22–32.)

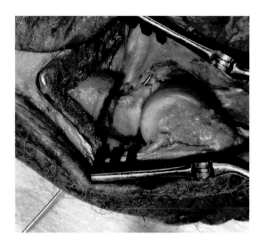

TECH FIG 3 • Coronoid fracture held reduced with Kirschner wire. (From McKee MD, Pugh DM, Wild LM, et al. Standard surgical protocol to treat elbow dislocation with radial head and coronoid fractures. J Bone Joint Surg Am 2005; 87A:22–32.)

Type II and III Coronoid Fractures

- Type II and III coronoid fractures can be fixed with one or two cannulated screws. Regular, partially threaded, cancellous screws can also be used.
- Once the fracture has been débrided such that it can be anatomically reduced, pass a guidewire from the dorsal surface of the proximal ulna such that it exits at the fracture site.
  - Back the guidewire up until it is just buried, and reduce the fracture.
- Hold the fragment reduced with a pointed instrument such as a dental pick and advance the wire across the fracture site into the fragment (**TECH FIG 3**). If there is enough space, insert a second wire across the fracture.

- Once one or two guidewires are in place, they are replaced with appropriate-length screws, cannulated or regular. It is critical to tap the fragment before screw placement to avoid splitting the fragment on screw insertion.
- Coronoid fractures that are comminuted may be difficult to treat. Typically, the largest fragment with articular cartilage is fixed.
- If screw fixation is not possible or access is difficult due to an intact radial head, the coronoid can also be addressed through a medial approach.
  - A medial incision along the supracondylar ridge is used.
  - The ulnar nerve is identified and protected.
  - The common flexor origin is split to gain access to the coronoid on the proximal ulna.
  - From the medial side, a buttress or spring plate can be used to secure a comminuted fracture.

RADIAL HEAD OR NECK FRACTURE

- Radial head fracture is addressed after treatment of the coronoid injury because once the head is fixed or replaced, access to the coronoid from the lateral approach is limited.
- The decision to fix a radial head is largely based on the fracture configuration. If fracture comminution is limited such that the head is in two or three fragments, reduction and fixation is usually possible.
  - Fractures that are comminuted or with articular surface damage require replacement.
- Expose the head and neck as necessary for fracture reduction and fixation by extending the Köcher interval.
- The posterior interosseous nerve is at risk during more distal radial neck exposures. Its distance from the operative site can be maximized by keeping the forearm in full pronation.

ORIF of Radial Head Fractures

- For radial head fragments, reduce and hold the fragment to the intact head with a pointed reduction clamp.
- We secure the fragments with Herbert screws. The fragments can be held temporarily with a 2-mm Kirschner wire and then replaced with a Herbert screw.
  - If the screw is inserted through articular cartilage, its head must be countersunk.
- Radial neck fractures, once reduced, can be held provisionally with a Kirschner wire.
- Definitive fixation is with a small fragment T plate over the "safe zone" (**TECH FIG 4**).
  - Care is taken to not injure the posterior interosseous nerve while exposing the shaft or by trapping it under the plate distally.
- If the radial head cannot be reconstructed, it is replaced.

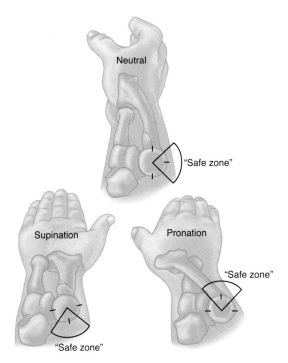

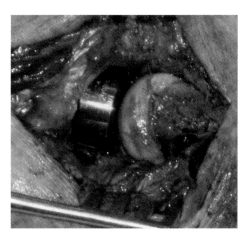

TECH FIG 5 • Radial head implant. An appropriately sized radial head implant has been inserted. It is held reduced with the forearm in full pronation. Note the anatomic alignment with the capitellum.

TECH FIG 4 • The "safe zone" for plating radial neck fractures. The 90-degree arc outlined does not articulate with the proximal ulna throughout the full range of forearm rotation. Plating a radial neck fracture in this zone will not interfere with rotation.

Radial Head Replacement

- The replacement used must be metallic as silicone implants are inadequate both biomechanically and biologically.[6]
  - We use a modular implant such that the stem diameter can be varied independent of the head diameter and thickness.

- If required, cut the proximal radius at the level of the neck with a micro-sagittal saw.
- Ream the canal of the proximal radius to cortical bone with sequentially larger reamers.
- Radial head size can be judged by assembling the fractured fragments that have been removed. In general, downsizing the head slightly is recommended such that the elbow joint is not overstuffed.
- A trial implant should be inserted to test stability and motion. Elbow range of motion, both flexion–extension and forearm rotation, should be checked. View the articulation between the proximal radius and ulna to see if the diameter of the implant seems appropriate.
- Once satisfied with sizing, the definitive implant is inserted (**TECH FIG 5**).

REPAIR OF THE LATERAL COLLATERAL LIGAMENT COMPLEX

- Repair of the LCL complex is critical to re-establish elbow stability (**TECH FIG 6A**).
- It is most often avulsed from the distal humerus. Its anatomic attachment point is slightly posterior to the lateral epicondyle at the center of the arc of the capitellum.

- The LCL is a discrete structure deep to the common extensor origin, which runs from the lateral epicondyle to the supinator crest of the ulna (**TECH FIG 6B**).
- Use a no. 2, braided, nonabsorbable suture for the repair.

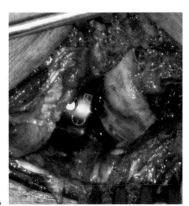

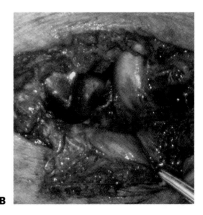

TECH FIG 6 • **A.** Elbow instability associated with deficient lateral collateral ligament. Without repair of the lateral collateral ligament, the radial head subluxes into a posterolateral position with forearm supination. Note that the radial head and capitellum are no longer in normal alignment. **B.** The lateral collateral ligament is held by the forceps. It is a distinct structure easily identified in this acutely injured elbow. (*continued*)

A **B**

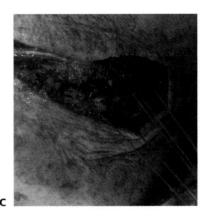

TECH FIG 6 • (*continued*) **C.** Sutures passed for lateral collateral ligament repair.

- The ligament can be reattached to the distal humerus through bone tunnels or using suture anchors. We prefer bony tunnels.
- Using a drill, Kirschner wire, or pointed towel clip, make holes in the distal lateral humerus above the epicondyle.
- Pass the suture through the holes and into the lateral ligament such that it will tighten on tying the sutures.
- At least two, preferably three, sutures through bone are required. Pass, cut, and snap all of the sutures (**TECH FIG 6C**).
  - Ensure that the elbow is now held in 90 degrees of flexion and full forearm pronation.
  - Incorporate the more superficial common extensor origin in the repair.
- Tie the sutures once they have all been passed and then close the lateral wound in layers.

PERSISTENT INSTABILITY

- On occasion, repair of the coronoid, radial head, and LCL from the lateral approach is insufficient to restore elbow stability such that early motion may be initiated.
- In these cases, further efforts must be made to obtain such stability.
- Repair of the MCL through a separate medial incision is one option if a lateral approach has been used for coronoid and radial head fracture fixation.
  - Alternatively, a posterior skin incision can be used with full-thickness flaps created to access both sides. Positioning the patient in the lateral decubitus position facilitates this approach.
- A deep approach to the medial aspect of the elbow puts the ulnar nerve at risk, and it must be identified and protected during the procedure.
- Usually the MCL is torn in its mid-substance. Suture repair of this is often unsatisfying. Using a graft to replace the MCL is not recommended in the acute injury setting.
- If elbow stability remains insufficient, applying a hinged fixator is the final option.[3]
  - If the hinge is not available or the surgeon is not familiar with its use, a static fixator can be applied to maintain elbow reduction.

Hinged External Fixation

- Application of the hinged fixator starts with the insertion of a guide pin through the center of elbow rotation.

- Insert the pin from medial to lateral starting at the medial epicondyle through a small incision and protect the ulnar nerve. The pin should be directed through the center of the capitellum.
- After pin insertion, the elbow is held reduced while the frame is assembled around it.
- The hinge slides over the guide pin on either side of the elbow. Three-quarter rings are attached proximal and distal to the elbow.
- Insert two half-pins in the humerus above the elbow through small open incisions over the posterior surface by bluntly spreading the triceps fibers.
- Insert two half-pins in the ulna over its subcutaneous border dorsally.
- Attach the pins to the rings and tighten all parts of the hinged fixator.
- Verify that the elbow remains reduced in the frame through 30 to 130 degrees of motion. The forearm is maintained in pronation to protect the lateral ligament repair.
- Lock the elbow at 90 degrees in the hinge for the initial postoperative course.
- Obtain plain radiographs in the operating room before the conclusion of the procedure.

PEARLS AND PITFALLS

Indications	■ Elbow dislocations with associated fractures of the coronoid or radial head must be recognized as complex dislocations. They usually require surgical treatment.
Goals of treatment	■ The goals are to obtain a concentric reduction with sufficient elbow stability such that early range of motion is possible, and to avoid persistent instability, elbow stiffness, and arthritis.
Coronoid fractures	■ Repair of coronoid fractures is technically demanding but necessary for successful treatment.
Radial head	■ The surgeon should be prepared to replace the radial head if necessary with a metal, modular prosthesis. ■ Excision alone is not an option.

Lateral ligaments	■ Repair of the lateral ligaments is important to impart the necessary stability for early motion and to avoid late posterolateral rotatory instability.
Physiotherapy	■ It is important to emphasize to the patient the need to be diligent with rehabilitation and exercises, as this will have a great effect on the end result.

POSTOPERATIVE CARE

■ The injured elbow is placed in a well-padded plaster splint at 90 degrees of flexion and full pronation. The patient is given a sling for comfort.

■ AP and lateral radiographs are obtained in the operating room to ensure congruent reduction and verify hardware placement.

■ The patient typically stays in hospital one night to receive adequate analgesia and prophylactic antibiotics.

■ We do not routinely give prophylaxis for heterotopic ossification unless the patient has a concomitant head injury: in this case, indomethacin 25 mg three times a day is prescribed with a cytoprotective agent for 3 weeks.

■ The patient returns to our clinic at 7 to 10 days postoperatively for staple removal. The splint is typically removed at this point.

■ Range-of-motion exercises are initiated at this time under the supervision of a physiotherapist.

■ Active and active-assisted flexion–extension between 30 and 130 degrees and forearm rotation with the elbow at 90 degrees of flexion is initiated.

■ A lightweight resting splint is made for the injured elbow that is removed for hygiene and physiotherapy.

■ The patient returns at 4, 8, and 12 weeks after surgery for clinical review with plain radiographs. Thereafter the interval of clinic visits is widened, but we follow our patients out to 2 years.

■ At 4 weeks we allow unrestricted range of motion and at 8 weeks unrestricted strengthening.

■ Evidence of fracture union is usually present between 6 and 8 weeks.

■ Progress with range of motion can be slow and frustrating for the patient but does not plateau until 1 year of follow-up.

OUTCOMES

■ Following the protocol outlined for fracture-dislocations of the elbow should yield satisfactory functional results.

■ Pugh et al[8] reported the results of this treatment protocol for 36 elbows at 34 months.

■ The flexion–extension arc averaged 112 degrees and rotation 136 degrees.

■ Fifteen patients had excellent results, 13 good, 7 fair, and 1 poor by the Mayo Elbow Performance Score.

■ Eight patients had a complication requiring reoperation.

COMPLICATIONS

■ The most likely complication after treatment is unacceptable elbow stiffness with a resultant nonfunctional range of motion.

■ An acceptable range is 30 to 130 degrees of flexion.

■ At about 1 year after surgery, once motion has plateaued, patients are candidates for release with hardware removal if they are not happy with their range of motion and the flexion–extension arc is less than 100 degrees.

■ This is done through the lateral approach with an anterior and posterior capsulectomy plus manipulation under anesthesia.

■ A radial head implant in place can be downsized to improve motion, but it should not be simply removed. The lateral ligament complex is preserved.

■ In our series, this was necessary in 11% of cases.[8]

■ Synostosis around the elbow is another possible cause of rotational forearm stiffness.

■ A resection can be planned to improve motion.

■ CT scanning preoperatively helps to define the extent of the lesion. Resection is technically demanding.

■ Superficial and deep wound infection is possible after repair. Immediate and aggressive treatment is recommended with antibiotics initially and irrigation with débridement if rapid improvement is not seen.

■ Persistent instability is rare but may occur despite best efforts at repair.

■ Posttraumatic arthritis may be a long-term problem.

REFERENCES

1. Cage DJ, Abrams RA, Callahan JJ, et al. Soft tissue attachments of the ulnar coronoid process: an anatomic study with radiographic correlation. Clin Orthop Relat Res 1995;320:154–158.

2. Mason ML. Some observations on fractures of the head of the radius with a review of one hundred cases. Br J Surg 1954;42:123–132.

3. McKee MD, Bowden SH, King GJ, et al. Management of recurrent, complex instability of the elbow with a hinged external fixator. J Bone Joint Surg Br 1998;80B:1031–1036.

4. McKee MD, Pugh DM, Wild LM, et al. Standard surgical protocol to treat elbow dislocation with radial head and coronoid fractures. J Bone Joint Surg Am 2005;87A:22–32.

5. McKee MD, Schemitsch EH, Sala MJ, et al. The pathoanatomy of lateral ligamentous disruption in complex elbow instability. J Shoulder Elbow Surg 2003;12:391–396.

6. Moro JK, Werier J, MacDermid JC, et al. Arthroplasty with a metal radial head for unreconstructable fractures of the radial head. J Bone Joint Surg Am 2001;83A:1201–1211.

7. Morrey BF, Tanaka S, An KN. Valgus stability of the elbow: a definition of primary and secondary constraints. Clin Orthop Relat Res 1991;265:187–195.

8. Pugh DMW, Wild LM, Schemitsch EH, et al. Standard surgical protocol to treat elbow dislocations with radial head and coronoid fractures. J Bone Joint Surg Am 2004;86A:1122–1130.

9. Regan W, Morrey B. Fractures of the coronoid process of the ulna. J Bone Joint Surg Am 1989;71:1248–1254.

10. Ring D, Jupiter JB, Zilberfarb J. Posterior dislocation of the elbow with fractures of the radial head and coronoid. J Bone Joint Surg Am 2002;84A:547–551.

Chapter 40 | Monteggia Fractures in Adults

Matthew L. Ramsey

DEFINITION

- This injury was initially reported by Giovanni Monteggia in 1814 as a fracture of the ulna associated with an anterior dislocation of the radial head.[6]
- The term "Monteggia lesions" was coined by Bado to describe any fracture of the ulna associated with a dislocation of the radiocapitellar joint.[1]
- The Bado classification of Monteggia lesions,[1] with the Jupiter subclassification of type II fractures,[4] is shown in Table 1.
- Equivalent injuries in adults
  - Variable pathology that is thought to be equivalent to injuries classified by the Bado system
  - Equivalent injuries do not always fall within the traditional definition of a Monteggia fracture in that they do not always have a concomitant radiocapitellar dislocation. Therefore, it can be argued that these injuries are not necessarily equivalent to Monteggia fractures.
  - Type I and II injuries are the only ones that have equivalent injury patterns.

PATHOGENESIS

- The exact mechanism of injury for Monteggia fractures is controversial.
- Proposed mechanisms of injury for type I injuries include the following:
  - Direct blow to the posterior aspect of the elbow
  - Fall on outstretched arm with hyperpronated hand (forearm pronation levers radial head anteriorly)
  - Fall on outstretched arm
  - Violent contraction of biceps pulling radial head anteriorly
- Proposed mechanism for type II injuries: hypothesized to occur when a supination force tensions the ligaments that are stronger than bone
- Proposed mechanism for type III injuries: direct blow to the inside of the elbow with or without rotation

PATIENT HISTORY AND PHYSICAL FINDINGS

- The initial examination should systematically evaluate:
  - Skin integrity
  - Neurovascular status of the extremity
  - Bony injury
- Ulna fracture
  - Injury pattern
    - Noncomminuted
    - Comminution
    - Associated injury to key structural elements of the ulna (coronoid, olecranon)
- Radial head injury
  - Isolated dislocation without fracture
  - Radial head or neck fracture

IMAGING AND OTHER DIAGNOSTIC STUDIES

- Plain radiographs (**FIG 1**): Orthogonal radiographs of the elbow, forearm, and wrist are required.
  - Ulna fracture is easily identified.
  - Radial head fracture or dislocation can be subtle, especially if radial head dislocation reduces.
- Computed tomography (CT) scans can be helpful to determine the extent of the bony injury and the location of fracture fragments. They are particularly helpful in fractures involving the coronoid, olecranon, and radial head.
- 3D CT reconstructions provide information on the spatial relationship of fracture fragments in comminuted fractures.

DIFFERENTIAL DIAGNOSIS

- Isolated ulna fracture
  - Nightstick fracture
  - Olecranon fracture
- Fracture-dislocation of the elbow ("terrible triad" injury)
- Transolecranon fracture-dislocation

NONOPERATIVE MANAGEMENT

- Monteggia fracture-dislocations in the adult population are generally treated surgically.
- Improved fixation methods and surgical technique have remarkably improved the results of surgery, making it a more reliable treatment option.

SURGICAL MANAGEMENT

Preoperative Planning

- The timing of surgery depends on the condition of the soft tissues and the availability of necessary equipment and personnel.
- The surgeon should define all injuries that need to be addressed.
- Equipment requirements:
  - Small fragment plates and screws or anatomic plating system
  - Minifragment system
  - Threaded Kirchner wires
  - Radial head replacement
- Bone graft (allograft or autograft)

Patient Positioning

- Lateral decubitus position with the arm over a padded arm support (**FIG 2**)
- Supine positioning is an alternative approach (although it is not preferred because of difficulty in maintaining the arm across the chest). If this approach is used, a saline bag under the ipsilateral shoulder will help keep the arm across the chest.

Table 1	Bado Classification of Monteggia Lesions, With Jupiter Subclassification of Type II Fractures

Type	Description	Illustration
I	Anterior dislocation of the radial head with fracture of the diaphysis of the ulna with anterior angulation of the ulna fracture (most common type of lesion)	
II	Posterior or posterolateral dislocation of the radial head with fracture of the ulnar diaphysis with posterior angulation of the ulna fracture	
IIA	Fracture at the level of the trochlear notch (ulna fracture involves the distal part of the olecranon and coronoid)	
IIB	Ulna fracture is at the metaphyseal–diaphyseal junction, distal to the coronoid	
IIC	Ulna fracture is diaphyseal	
IID	Comminuted fractures involving more than one region	

Table 1 *(continued)*

Type	Description	Illustration
III	Lateral or anterolateral dislocation of the radial head with fracture of the ulnar metaphysis	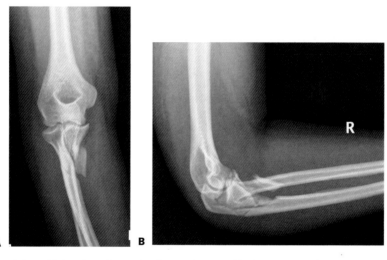
IV	Anterior dislocation of the radial head with a fracture of the proximal third of the radius and ulna at the same level	

Adapted from Bado J. The Monteggia lesion. Clin Orthop Relat Res 1967;50:717; and Jupiter JB, Leibovic SJ, Ribbans W, et al. The posterior Monteggia lesion. J Orthop Trauma 1991;5:395–402.

FIG 1 • Plain AP and lateral radiographs typically demonstrate fracture pattern.

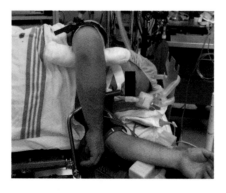

FIG 2 • Lateral decubitus positioning is preferred.

SURGICAL APPROACH

- A midline posterior skin incision is placed lateral to the tip of the olecranon (**TECH FIG 1A**).

- Subcutaneous flaps are elevated on the fascia of the forearm. The medial antebrachial cutaneous nerve does not need to be identified if dissection is performed on the fascia of the flexor–pronator muscles since it is mobilized with the medial skin flap.

- The interval between the flexor carpi ulnaris (FCU) and anconeus is developed along the subcutaneous border of the ulna to expose the fracture site. The amount of dissection required for exposure is dictated by the fracture pattern and the type of fixation to be used (**TECH FIG 1B**).

- If the radial head needs to be addressed surgically, the anconeus can be mobilized more extensively through a Boyd approach (**TECH FIG 1C**). If the ulna fracture permits, the radial head can be fixed through the fracture bed of the ulna before definitive fixation of the ulna. Once the ulna is fixed, access to the radial head is not possible.

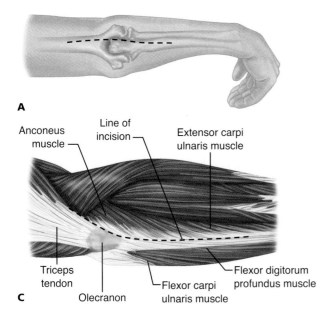

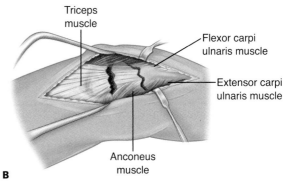

TECH FIG 1 • A. Posterior midline incision positioned just off the lateral aspect of the olecranon. **B.** Deep surgical interval uses the internervous plane between the anconeus and flexor carpi ulnaris. **C.** Exposure of the radial head can be accomplished by releasing the anconeus from the humerus and reflecting it proximally to expose the radial head.

RADIAL HEAD MANAGEMENT

- Radial head fractures are typically fixed before the ulna fracture is addressed. If the lesser sigmoid notch of the ulna is involved, determining radial length if radial head replacement is required can be difficult. Therefore, fractures are generally fixed before the ulna while replacement may need to be performed after ulnar fixation is completed in order to establish appropriate radial head sizing.

- Reconstructable fractures of the radial head are fixed (**TECH FIG 2A,B**).

- Unreconstructable fractures of the radial head are replaced (**TECH FIG 2C**).

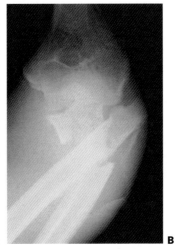

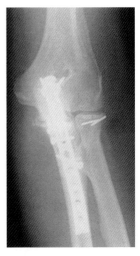

TECH FIG 2 • A,B. Preoperative and postoperative radiographs demonstrating open reduction and internal fixation of the radial head component of the Monteggia fracture. (*continued*)

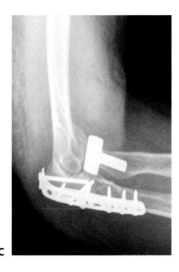

TECH FIG 2 • (*continued*) **C.** Postoperative radiograph of a Monteggia fracture in which the radial head fracture needed to be replaced.

ULNA FRACTURE FIXATION

No Articular Involvement of the Ulnohumeral Joint

- Ulna fractures distal to the coronoid can be plated laterally or on the subcutaneous border of the ulna.
- Lateral plate placement is preferred by some to prevent hardware prominence.

Articular Involvement of the Ulnohumeral Joint

- Fractures extending proximal to the coronoid require the plate be placed on the subcutaneous border of the ulna to accommodate the complex geometry of this region.
- In general, the ulna fracture is reconstructed from distal to proximal. Ensure that any associated injury to the coronoid is identified and addressed.
- The fracture is reconstructed by fixing the distal fragments; this may require interfragmentary fixation or subarticular Kirchner wires **(TECH FIG 3A)**. As fixation progresses proximally, reconstruction of the coronoid and greater sigmoid notch is performed. Particular attention is directed at anatomic reconstruction of the articular surface.
- Coronoid involvement with a Monteggia fracture-dislocation often extends distally into the volar cortex of the ulna, as opposed to the axial-plane fracture patterns characterized by Regan and Morrey[9] **(TECH FIG 3B)**.
- Larger fragments can be definitively fixed with antegrade lag screws from the dorsal aspect of the ulnar or can be provisionally fixed with threaded wires and ultimately definitively fixed once the plate is applied to the dorsal aspect of the ulna.
- Coronoid fracture exposure can typically be obtained through the olecranon fracture. If this does not provide sufficient exposure, the FCU can be elevated from the dorsal aspect of the ulna.
- The final fragment to be fixed is the olecranon fragment. The attached triceps will obscure fracture reduction if reduced before distal reconstruction **(TECH FIG 3C)**.

- Definitive fixation is performed with a dorsal plate. The triceps is partially split to allow the proximal aspect of the plate to oppose the olecranon **(TECH FIG 3D)**.

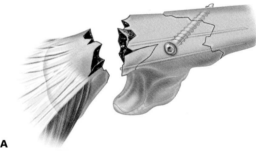

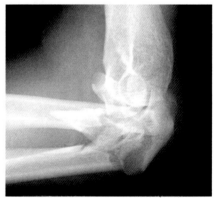

TECH FIG 3 • **A.** Monteggia fractures with articular involvement should be fixed distal to proximal. Fixation may require intramedullary Kirschner wires or interfragmentary fixation. **B.** Coronoid fracture often extends into the volar cortex of the ulnar. (*continued*)

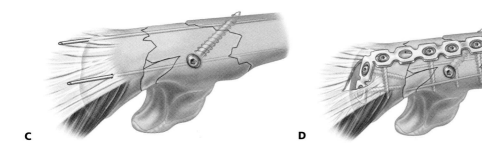

C **D**

TECH FIG 3 • (continued) **C.** The olecranon fragment with attached triceps is reduced and provisionally held with medial and lateral Kirschner wires pending definitive fixation. **D.** Final fixation for most Monteggia fractures is with a rigid plate applied to the dorsal cortex.

WOUND CLOSURE

- The tourniquet is deflated and hemostasis is obtained.
- The fascia between the FCU and anconeus is closed with interrupted absorbable 0 or 1 suture.
- Subcutaneous tissues are closed with 3-0 absorbable suture and skin is closed with staples.

- I prefer to close the wound over a drain placed in the subcutaneous tissues to avoid hematoma.
- A well-padded dressing is applied and an anterior splint is placed with the elbow in full extension.

PEARLS AND PITFALLS

Indications	▪ Monteggia fracture-dislocations in adults require surgical intervention.
Goals of treatment	▪ The first goal is to restore ulnar length and location of the radial head. When the articulation is involved, the goal is to obtain a concentric reduction with sufficient elbow stability that early range of motion is possible. ▪ The second goal is to avoid complications that compromise function.
Ulna fractures	▪ Fractures distal to the coronoid need only to be fixed such that ulnar length is re-established. ▪ When plating these fractures, avoiding malreduction of the ulna is critical to reduction of the radial head. Failure to re-establish ulnar geometry can result in persistent subluxation or dislocation of the radial head (**FIG 3**). ▪ Fractures involving the articulation require stable fixation to re-establish a competent joint.
Radial head	▪ Radial head fractures are fixed or replaced.
Physical therapy	▪ Early range of motion is the goal of treatment but may be delayed if fixation is questionable.

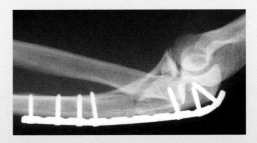

FIG 3 • Malunion of the ulna with resulting apex dorsal angulation results in dislocation of the radial head.

POSTOPERATIVE CARE

▪ The arm is splinted in full extension to take pressure off the posterior soft tissues.

▪ If a drain is used, the splint and dressing are removed when the drain output is less than 30 mL in 8 hours. If no drain is used, the dressing is removed on postoperative day 1.

▪ Active or active-assisted flexion and gravity-assisted extension is begun once the surgical dressings are removed.

▪ If fixation is tenuous because of poor-quality bone or comminution, mobilization is delayed.

OUTCOMES

▪ Historically, the results of operative treatment of Monteggia fracture-dislocations have been unpredictable.[3,7,8,11]

▪ The advent of rigid internal fixation has improved the results of operative treatment.[2,4,7]

▪ Certain factors have been associated with a poor clinical result[5]:

▪ Bado type II injury
▪ Jupiter type IIa injury
▪ Fracture of the radial head
▪ Coronoid fracture
▪ Complications requiring further surgery

COMPLICATIONS

▪ Complications associated with Monteggia fracture-dislocations occur with frequency. A multicenter study evaluating Monteggia fracture-dislocations in adults demonstrated complications in 43% of the patients treated, with an unsatisfactory outcome in 46% of the patients treated.[10]

▪ Radial nerve palsy
  ▪ Most commonly posterior interosseous nerve
  ▪ Causes of injury include:
    ▪ Compression at the arcade of Frosche
    ▪ Direct trauma
    ▪ Traction with lateral displacement of the radial head

▪ Most common with type III fractures
  ▪ Complete resolution typically occurs.

▪ Malunion
  ▪ Most common in type II fractures with volar comminution that is not appreciated or addressed

▪ If radial head subluxation persists, malunion must be considered.

▪ Nonunion
  ▪ Causes of nonunion include:
    ▪ Infection
    ▪ Inadequate internal fixation
  ▪ Compression plate fixation required, particularly if fracture is comminuted
  ▪ Semitubular and reconstruction plates are not structurally strong enough.

▪ Radioulnar synostosis
  ▪ Seen with high-energy injuries with associated comminution
  ▪ Higher incidence if radial head fracture associated with ulna fracture at the same level
  ▪ Boyd approach implicated since the radius and ulna are exposed through the same incision

REFERENCES

1. Bado J. The Monteggia lesion. Clin Orthop Relat Res 1967;50:71.
2. Boyd H, Boals J. The Monteggia lesion: a review of 159 cases. Clin Orthop Relat Res 1969;66:94–100.
3. Bruce H, Harvey JJ, Wilson JJ. Monteggia fractures. J Bone Joint Surg Am 1974;56A:1563–1576.
4. Jupiter JB, Leibovic SJ, Ribbans W, et al. The posterior Monteggia lesion. J Orthop Trauma 1991;5:395–402.
5. Konrad GG, Kundel K, Kreuz PC, et al. Monteggia fractures in adults: long-term results and prognostic factors. J Bone Joint Surg Br 2007;89B:354–360.
6. Monteggia GB. *Instituzioni Chirurgiche.* 2nd ed. Milan: G. Masperp, 1813–1815.
7. Reckling F. Unstable fracture-dislocations of the forearm (Monteggia and Galeazzi lesions). J Bone Joint Surg Am 1982;64A:857–863.
8. Reckling FW, Cordell LD. Unstable fracture-dislocations of the forearm: the Monteggia and Galeazzi lesions. Arch Surg 1968;96:999–1007.
9. Regan W, Morrey B. Fractures of the coronoid process of the ulna. J Bone Joint Surg Am 1989;71A:1348–1354.
10. Reynders P, De Groote W, Rondia J, et al. Monteggia lesions in adults: a multicenter Bota study. Acta Orthop Belg 1996;62(Suppl 1):78–83.
11. Speed J, Boyd H. Treatment of fractures of ulna with dislocation of the head of radius (Monteggia fracture). JAMA 1940;115:1699–1705.

Chapter 41

Lateral Collateral Ligament Reconstruction of the Elbow

Jason A. Stein and Anand M. Murthi

DEFINITION

- Lateral collateral ligament (LCL) injuries most often occur after significant elbow trauma, most commonly dislocation.
- Attenuation of the LCL can also occur after multiple surgeries to the lateral side of the elbow and after multiple corticosteroid injections[4] and has recently been reported to occur in patients who have residual cubitus varus after malunion of supracondylar humerus fractures.[7]
- Significant injury to the LCL complex can result in posterolateral rotatory instability (PLRI).

ANATOMY

- The LCL is made up of four major components: the lateral ulnar collateral ligament (LUCL), also called the radial ulnohumeral ligament (RUHL); the radial collateral ligament proper (RCL); the annular ligament; and the accessory collateral ligament (**FIG 1**).
- The ligaments originate from a broad band over the lateral epicondyle, deep to the extensor muscle mass, and separate distally into more discrete structures.
- The RUHL is the most important stabilizer against PLRI, and it attaches distally on the supinator crest of the ulna.[6]
- The RCL is more anterior and primarily resists varus stress.
- The annular ligament sweeps around the radial head and stabilizes the proximal radioulnar joint.
- The capsule acts as a static stabilizer, especially at the anterior portion, while the arm is extended.
- The anconeus and extensor muscle groups act as dynamic stabilizers.

PATHOGENESIS

- Multiple studies have shown that injury to the LCL can lead to PLRI, which is the first stage in elbow instability that can lead to frank elbow dislocation.

- It is controversial whether injury to the RUHL alone can lead to PLRI or whether further injury to the LCL complex is necessary.[5]
- When the forearm is supinated and slightly flexed, a valgus stress with an attenuated LCL causes the ulnohumeral joint to rotate, compresses the radiocapitellar joint, and ultimately causes the radial head to subluxate or dislocate posteriorly.

NATURAL HISTORY

- PLRI is not a new condition, but it has only recently been described and studied.
- The prevalence and natural history of this condition are currently not known.

PATIENT HISTORY AND PHYSICAL FINDINGS

- Patients typically report trauma but may have had recurrent lateral epicondylitis or previous surgery.
- Elderly patients may not have frank dislocation of the elbow, but 75% of patients younger than 20 years report elbow dislocation.[5]
- Patients report mechanical-type symptoms (clicking, popping, and slipping) during elbow supination and extension and rarely report recurrent dislocations.
- Physical examination can be difficult; provocative tests are described below. It is often necessary to conduct these tests with the patient under anesthesia or with the aid of fluoroscopy.
  - Inspection for effusion: With acute injuries, effusion is likely to be present, but in more chronic situations, it may be absent.
  - Range of motion (ROM): Locking of the elbow could represent loose bodies; stiffness may indicate intrinsic capsular contracture.

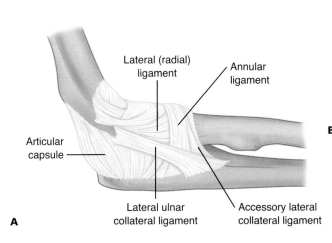

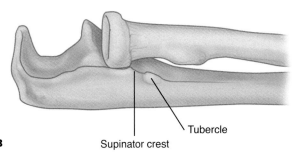

FIG 1 • A. The lateral collateral ligament complex is made up of four major components: the lateral ulnar collateral ligament, also called the radial ulnohumeral ligament; the radial collateral ligament proper; the annular ligament; and the accessory collateral ligament. **B.** Osseous anatomy of the lateral collateral ligament insertion.

351

■ Supine lateral pivot-shift test: When the elbow is slightly flexed, the radial head can be palpated to subluxate or frankly dislocate, and as the elbow flexes past 40 degrees, it relocates, often with a palpable clunk.[6] This test is difficult to perform on an awake patient because often apprehension is felt and the patient does not allow the test to continue.

■ Prone pivot-shift test: Radial head or ulnohumeral subluxation constitutes a positive test, same as the supine lateral pivot-shift test. Examination under anesthesia may be required.

■ Push-up test: Reproduction of the patient's symptoms of apprehension during supination and not pronation constitutes a positive test. Inability to complete the push-up also constitutes a positive test.

■ Chair push-up: Elicited pain constitutes a positive test.

■ Table-top relocation test: Elicited pain or apprehension as the elbow reaches 40 degrees constitutes a positive test.

■ Elbow drawer test: Ulnohumeral subluxation constitutes a positive test.

■ A thorough examination of the elbow should also be completed to rule out other injuries.

■ Valgus instability with the forearm in pronation and 30 degrees of flexion suggests medial collateral ligament (MCL) injury.

■ Lateral epicondylitis or radial tunnel syndrome can present with tenderness over the proximal extensor mass and with resisted extension of the wrist (Thompson test) and long finger.

■ Loose bodies may present with crepitus or locking of the elbow during ROM.

IMAGING AND OTHER DIAGNOSTIC STUDIES

■ Standard anteroposterior (AP) and lateral view radiographs often indicate normal findings but may reveal small lateral epicondyle avulsion fractures and radiocapitellar wear.

■ Stress AP and lateral view radiographs may reveal widening of the ulnohumeral joint and posterior subluxation of the radial head (**FIG 2A**).

■ Magnetic resonance imaging (MRI), especially with intra-articular contrast enhancement, may reveal injuries to the LCL complex. The proximal extensor mass requires attention (**FIG 2B**).

■ Diagnostic arthroscopy of the elbow can be performed, although we do not recommend routine diagnostic arthroscopy for this injury.

■ The drive-through sign occurs when the scope can easily be "driven through" the lateral gutter into the ulnohumeral joint from the posterolateral portal.

■ The pivot-shift test also can be performed during arthroscopy, and the radial head will subluxate posteriorly.

DIFFERENTIAL DIAGNOSIS

■ Lateral epicondylitis
■ Loose bodies
■ Elbow fracture-dislocation
■ MCL injury
■ Radial head dislocation

NONOPERATIVE MANAGEMENT

■ If the injury is diagnosed early, immobilization in a hinged elbow brace in pronation for 4 to 6 weeks may prevent chronic instability.[3]

■ Removable neoprene sleeves may offer support.

■ A trial of elbow extensor strengthening can be performed.

SURGICAL MANAGEMENT

Indications

■ Recurrent symptomatic PLRI despite nonoperative treatment

Preoperative Planning

■ All imaging studies should be reviewed and informed consent obtained.

■ An examination of the elbow should be performed with the patient under anesthesia, especially the pivot-shift test.

■ If there is any doubt regarding the diagnosis, a pivot-shift test should be performed under fluoroscopy.

Positioning

■ The patient is placed supine on the operating room table.

■ The arm can be placed on an arm board or across the patient's chest with a sterile tourniquet applied to the upper arm and the entire arm draped free (**FIG 3**).

■ During the approach, the forearm should be pronated to protect the posterior interosseous nerve.

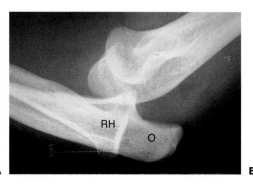

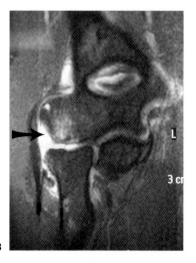

FIG 2 • **A.** Lateral view stress radiograph reveals complete ulnohumeral and radial head (*RH*) rotatory instability. *O*, olecranon. **B.** Coronal oblique view magnetic resonance image of elbow (with contrast enhancement). Lateral collateral ligament disruption can be seen (*arrow*).

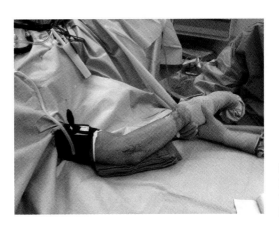

Approach

- The main approach is the Köcher interval between the anconeus and extensor carpi ulnaris muscles.
- This can be accomplished through a lateral skin incision or through a utilitarian posterior incision.
  - A posterior incision should be considered if a medial approach will also be needed to repair concomitant ligamentous or bony injury.

FIG 3 • The patient is placed supine on the operating room table. The arm is placed on an arm board with a sterile tourniquet applied to the upper arm and the entire arm draped free. During the approach, the forearm should be pronated to protect the posterior interosseous nerve.

FIGURE 8 YOKE TECHNIQUE

Surgical Approach

- A 10-cm incision is made over the Köcher interval.
  - The interval between the anconeus and the extensor carpi ulnaris is developed, and the remainder of the LCL complex is identified along with the supinator crest and the lateral epicondyle.
- The lateral epicondyle and 2 cm of the supracondylar ridge are exposed.

Tunnel Placement

- Two drill holes for the graft insertion site are made in the ulna.
  - One is drilled near the tubercle of the supinator crest (palpate in supination and varus stress), the other 1.25 cm proximal to that, near the insertion of the annular ligament (**TECH FIG 1A**).
- A suture is passed through the two holes and tied to itself. The suture is then held up against the lateral epicondyle as the elbow is ranged in flexion and extension to determine its isometric point.

- The isometric ligament insertion occurs at the point where the suture does NOT move.
- The isometric point is usually more anteroinferior than expected (**TECH FIG 1B,C**).
- A Y-shaped tunnel is made with the base exiting at the isometric point.
  - The hole is widened to accept a three-ply graft. (Palmaris longus is usually harvested; if not present, gracilis or allograft is used.) A 16-cm graft is usually sufficient.

Graft Passage and Tensioning and Wound Closure

- The graft is passed through the ulnar tunnel with enough length to just reach the isometric point.
  - The end is then sutured to the long end of the graft (the Yoke stitch).
  - The long end is then passed through the isometric point and exits the superior humeral tunnel (**TECH FIG 2A**).

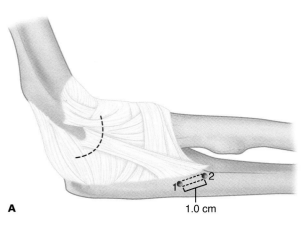

A   1.0 cm

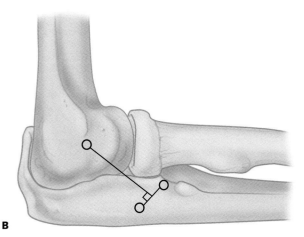

B

TECH FIG 1 • **A.** Two drill holes for the graft insertion site are made in the ulna. One is drilled near the tubercle of the supinator crest (palpate while varus and supination applied); the other is drilled 1.25 cm proximal, near the insertion of the annular ligament. *1*, proximal hole near insertion of annular ligament; *2*, tubercle of supinator crest. **B.** The ulnar holes should lie perpendicular to the intended direction of the lateral ulnar collateral ligament. *(continued)*

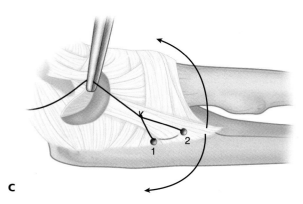

C

TECH FIG 1 • *(continued)* **C.** A suture is passed through the two holes and tied to itself. The suture is then held up with a hemostat against the lateral epicondyle as the elbow is ranged in flexion and extension to determine its isometric point. No movement occurs if the suture is at the isometric point.

- The long end is wrapped around the supracondylar ridge and passed through the distal tunnel, exiting back through the isometric point and into the ulnar tunnel.
  - The graft is then tensioned in 40 degrees of flexion, full pronation, and axial tension.
  - If the graft is not long enough to reach the ulnar tunnel, it can be sutured back to itself (**TECH FIG 2B**).
- The reconstruction can be reinforced by weaving a no. 2 Fiberwire suture (Arthrex, Inc., Naples, FL) from distal to proximal through the course of the figure 8, thus sewing the graft to itself.
- Plicate the anterior and posterior capsule as needed.
- The extensor origin is repaired to the lateral epicondyle, and the extensor carpi ulnaris fascia is reapproximated to the anconeus muscle with absorbable sutures.

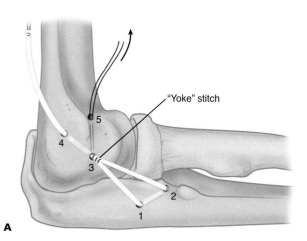

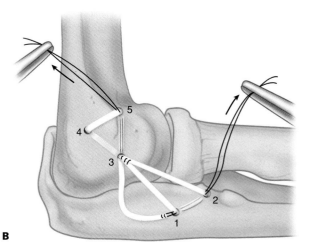

TECH FIG 2 • **A.** A Y-shaped tunnel is made with the base exiting at the isometric point (*3*). The hole is widened to accept a three-ply graft. The tendon graft is passed through the ulnar tunnel (*1→2*) with enough length to just reach the isometric point. The end is then sutured to the long end of the graft (the Yoke stitch). The long end is then passed through the isometric point and exits the superior humeral tunnel (*3→4*). **B.** The long end is then passed through the distal tunnel, exiting back through the isometric point (*5→3*) and into the ulnar tunnel (*3→1→2*). The graft is then tensioned in 40 degrees of flexion, full pronation, and axial tension. If the graft is not long enough to reach the ulnar tunnel, it can be sutured back to itself.

SPLIT ANCONEUS FASCIA TRANSFER

- We have developed a reproducible technique for LCL reconstruction that has proved biomechanical strength and reproducibility.
- Advantages include using only local autograft tissue and the minimal creation of bone tunnels.[1,2]

Surgical Approach

- A 6- to 8-cm skin incision is made over the Köcher interval, exposing the underlying Köcher interval between the extensor carpi ulnaris and anconeus (**TECH FIG 3A,B**).

- The interval between the anconeus and extensor carpi ulnaris muscles is developed, taking care to preserve the remainder of the underlying LCL complex.
  - The annular ligament, lateral epicondyle, and 2 cm of supracondylar ridge are isolated (**TECH FIG 3C**).

Graft Preparation

- The anconeus and distal triceps fascia are isolated in continuity. A 1.0-cm-wide by 8.0-cm-long band of fascia is mobilized off the underlying muscle, leaving the ulnar insertion intact (**TECH FIG 4A,B**).

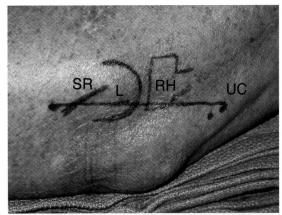

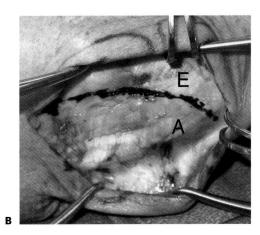

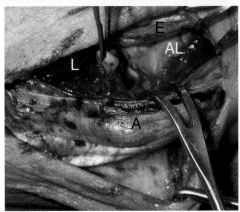

TECH FIG 3 • A. A 6- to 8-cm skin incision is made over the Kocher interval. *SR*, supracondylar ridge; *L*, lateral epicondyle; *RH*, radial head; *UC*, ulnar crest. **B.** The underlying Kocher interval between the extensor carpi ulnaris (*E*) and anconeus (*A*) is exposed. **C.** The interval between the anconeus (*A*) and the extensor carpi ulnaris (*E*) is developed, taking care to preserve the remainder of the underlying lateral collateral ligament complex (held in forceps). The annular ligament (*AL*), lateral epicondyle (*L*), and 2 cm of the supracondylar ridge are isolated.

■ The band is then divided longitudinally into two bands of equal width (**TECH FIG 4C**).

■ The anterior band is passed through an incision just distal to the annular ligament while the posterior band is passed under the anconeus muscle (**TECH FIG 4D**).

■ The isometric point of the lateral epicondyle is then located by holding the two bands against the epicondyle while ranging the elbow (**TECH FIG 4E**).

■ The final lengths of the fascial bands are estimated by holding the bands along their respective paths. The bands are then trimmed appropriately to prevent them from "bottoming out" prematurely in the humeral docking tunnel.

■ Separate Krackow sutures are placed in each band with no. 0 FiberWire suture.

Tunnel Preparation

■ A 5-mm round burr is used to create a 1.5-cm-long (depth) docking tunnel into the humerus at the isometric point. A 1-mm side-cutting burr is then used to make anterior and posterior bone bridge holes. The holes are separated by 1.5 cm. Individual suture lassos are placed from proximal to distal into the docking tunnel from the separate humeral tunnels (**TECH FIG 5**).

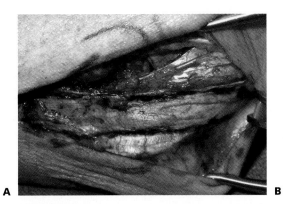

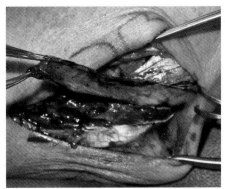

TECH FIG 4 • A. The anconeus and distal triceps fascia are isolated in continuity. **B.** A 1.0-cm-wide by 8.0-cm-long band of fascia is mobilized off the underlying muscle, leaving the ulnar insertion. *(continued)*

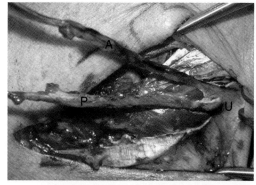

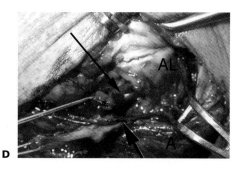

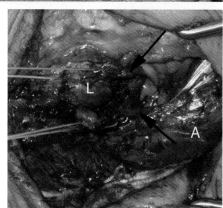

TECH FIG 4 • *(continued)* **C.** The split anconeus fascia band is then divided longitudinally into two bands of equal width. *A*, anterior band; *P*, posterior band; *U*, ulnar insertion point. **D.** The anterior band (*thin arrow*) is passed through an incision just distal to the annular ligament (*AL*) while the posterior band (*thick arrow*) is passed under the anconeus muscle (*A*). **E.** The isometric point of the lateral epicondyle (*L*) is then located by holding the two bands against the epicondyle while ranging the elbow. The point of minimal tension loss in either band while ranging the elbow is the optimal isometric point. *Arrows*, anterior and posterior split anconeus fascia bands.

Graft Passage and Tensioning and Wound Closure

- The anterior band sutures are brought out the anterior humeral exit hole by using suture passers. The posterior band passes superficial to the annular ligament, and its sutures are brought out the posterior humeral exit tunnel.
- The ends of the fascial bands are docked into the humeral tunnel, and the grafts are tensioned with the elbow in 40 degrees of flexion, in full pronation, and with a valgus stress.
- The sutures are then tied over the bony bridge on the supracondylar ridge (**TECH FIG 6A**).
- The extensor origin is then repaired to the lateral epicondyle and the extensor carpi ulnaris fascia is reapproximated to the anconeus muscle with absorbable sutures.
- The skin is closed with a running subcuticular suture (**TECH FIG 6B**).

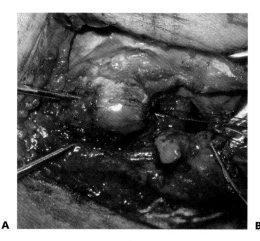

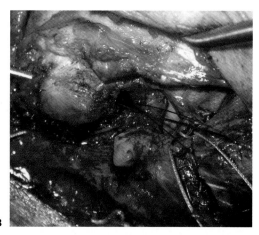

TECH FIG 5 • A. Suture lassos passed through exit holes out distal docking tunnel. *SCR*, supracondylar ridge. **B.** Suture lasso wires exiting docking tunnel.

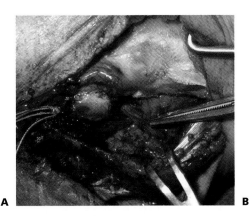 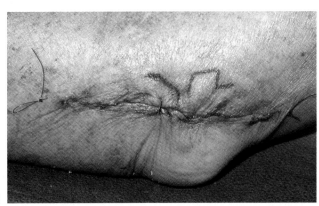

TECH FIG 6 • **A.** The ends of the fascial bands are docked into the humeral tunnel, and the grafts are tensioned with the elbow in 40 degrees of flexion, full pronation, and valgus stress. Sutures are then tied over the bony bridge on the supracondylar ridge (clamp on posterior band). **B.** The incision is closed with subcuticular suture.

DOCKING TECHNIQUE

- As previously discussed, the Köcher approach is used for the docking technique.
- Preparation of the ulnar drill holes is described in the section on the figure 8 yoke technique elsewhere in this chapter.
- A 5-mm round burr is used to create a 1.5-cm-long (depth) docking tunnel into the humerus at the isometric point. A 1-mm side-cutting burr is then used to make anterior and posterior bone bridge holes. The holes are separated by 1.5 cm. Individual suture lassos are placed from proximal to distal into the docking tunnel from the separate humeral tunnels (see Tech Fig 5).
- After passage of the graft through the ulnar tunnels, the final lengths of the two graft strands are estimated by holding the strands against the docking tunnel with the arm in the "reduced" position of 40 degrees of flexion, full pronation, and axial tension.

- The strands are then trimmed appropriately to prevent the strands from "bottoming out" prematurely in the humeral docking tunnel.
  - Separate Krackow sutures are placed in each graft strand with no. 0 FiberWire suture for 1 cm.
- The anterior graft strand sutures are brought out the anterior humeral exit hole by using suture passers. The posterior graft strand sutures are brought out the posterior humeral exit tunnel.
- The ends of the humeral graft portion are docked into the humeral tunnel, and the grafts are tensioned with the elbow in 40 degrees of flexion, in full pronation, and with a valgus stress.
- The sutures are then tied over the bony bridge on the supracondylar ridge.
- Standard incision closure is performed.

DIRECT REPAIR

- As previously discussed, the Köcher approach is used for direct repair.
- If the LCL complex is intact but avulsed from its ulnar or humeral attachments (or both), it can be directly repaired to its correct anatomic location with suture anchors or bone tunnels.
- A running locked no. 2 FiberWire suture is placed into the detached LCL complex and repaired back to its origin on the lateral epicondyle through the anterior and posterior drill holes (**TECH FIG 7**).
- A careful repair of the extensor origin and the interval between the anconeus and the extensor carpi ulnaris is performed.

TECH FIG 7 • Primary lateral ulnar collateral ligament repair. Running locked suture placed through detached lateral ulnar collateral ligament. A relaxing incision can be made at its attachment to the base of the annular ligament. Repair through drill holes in the lateral epicondyle.

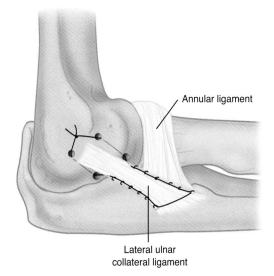

Annular ligament

Lateral ulnar
collateral ligament

PEARLS AND PITFALLS

Indications	▪ Iatrogenic causes (eg, "tennis elbow" surgery) very common ▪ Careful history and physical examination to exclude other pathologic conditions ▪ History of numerous lateral elbow corticosteroid injections
Split anconeus fascia technique: exposure	▪ Isolate Köcher interval; fatty stripe within interval. ▪ Anconeus fibers oblique to extensor carpi ulnaris ▪ Identify LCL disruption. ▪ Isolate annular ligament; protect posterior interosseous nerve.
Splint anconeus fascia preparation	▪ Be careful to harvest long enough fascial band (proximal to humeral bone tunnels). ▪ Be careful not to detach from ulnar insertion. ▪ Isolate LCL complex isometric point of origin. ▪ Harvest fascial band in line with old LUCL.
Figure 8 yoke technique	▪ Carefully isolate isometric point on lateral epicondyle, usually more anterior and inferior; err on inferior placement. ▪ Make ulnar tunnel perpendicular to direction of LUCL. ▪ Chamfer bone tunnels to prevent graft impingement and breakage.
Bone tunnel preparation	▪ Maintain sufficient bony bridge between tunnels. ▪ Smooth edges to prevent graft irritation.
Arm position for final graft tensioning	▪ 40 degrees of elbow flexion ▪ Full pronation ▪ Axial load, valgus stress

POSTOPERATIVE CARE

▪ Stage I (0 to 3 weeks)
  ▪ Elbow immobilization in posterior splint or brace at 40 degrees of flexion
  ▪ Wrist and hand isometrics as tolerated
  ▪ Shoulder active and passive ROM
▪ Stage II (3 to 6 weeks)
  ▪ Hinged elbow brace or orthoplast splint, with limits set by surgeon
  ▪ Begin flexor–pronator isometrics
  ▪ Continue with wrist and hand strengthening
  ▪ Continue shoulder as above
  ▪ Active-assisted ROM: 20 to 120 degrees of flexion; keep forearm pronated at all times
▪ Stage III (6 to 12 weeks)
  ▪ Discontinue immobilization
  ▪ Passive ROM and active-assisted ROM to full motion, including supination
  ▪ Begin unrestricted strengthening of flexor–pronators and extensors
▪ Stage IV (3 to 6 months)
  ▪ Avoid varus stress to elbow and ballistic movement in terminal elbow ranges
  ▪ Begin shoulder strengthening with light resistance (emphasis on cuff)
  ▪ Start total body conditioning
  ▪ Terminal elbow stretching in flexion and extension
  ▪ Resistive elbow exercises as tolerated

OUTCOMES

▪ Nestor et al[5] have shown successful functional outcomes in patients using the figure 8 reconstruction technique with reproducible results.

▪ Our early experience with the split anconeus fascia reconstruction technique has shown excellent results, with no failures to date in 22 patients at an average follow-up of 2 years. All elbows have achieved stability without loss of motion.

COMPLICATIONS

▪ Recurrent elbow instability
▪ Elbow stiffness
▪ Infection
▪ Graft harvest site morbidity (if remote autograft is used for reconstruction)
▪ Humerus stress fracture through bone tunnels
▪ Ulnar stress fracture through bone tunnels
▪ Bone bridge compromise

REFERENCES

1. Chebli CA, Murthi AM. Lateral collateral ligament complex: anatomic and biomechanical testing. 73rd Annual Meeting and Scientific Program of the American Academy of Orthopaedic Surgeons, Chicago, March 2006.
2. Chebli CM, Murthi AM. Split anconeus fascia transfer for reconstruction of the elbow lateral collateral ligament complex: anatomic and biomechanical testing. 22nd Open Meeting of the American Shoulder and Elbow Surgeons. Chicago, IL, March 2006.
3. Cohen MS, Hastings H II. Acute elbow dislocation: evaluation and management. J Am Acad Orthop Surg 1998;6:15–23.
4. Kalainov DM, Cohen MS. Posterolateral rotatory instability of the elbow in association with lateral epicondylitis: a report of three cases. J Bone Joint Surg Am 2005;87A:1120–1125.
5. Nestor BJ, O'Driscoll SW, Morrey BF. Ligamentous reconstruction for posterolateral rotatory instability of the elbow. J Bone Joint Surg Am 1992;74A:1235–1241.
6. O'Driscoll SW, Bell DF, Morrey BF. Posterolateral rotatory instability of the elbow. J Bone Joint Surg Am 1991;73A:440–446.
7. O'Driscoll SW, Spinner RJ, McKee MD, et al. Tardy posterolateral rotatory instability of the elbow due to cubitus varus. J Bone Joint Surg Am 2001;83A:1358–1369.

Chapter 42

Ulnohumeral (Outerbridge-Kashiwagi) Arthroplasty

Filippos S. Giannoulis, Alexander H. Payatakes, and Dean G. Sotereanos

DEFINITION

- Primary osteoarthritis of the elbow is a relatively uncommon but limiting disorder that affects mostly middle-aged men who use the upper extremity in a repetitive fashion. Typically, patients are heavy manual workers or athletes. Osteoarthritis affects the elbow less frequently than other major joints.
- Early stages of arthritis of the elbow may be characterized primarily by pain at the extremes of motion, with some loss of terminal extension and flexion. Some patients present with pain carrying an object with the arm in extension. More advanced stages may present with pain and crepitus throughout the range of motion, stiffness, or locking. Rotation of the forearm may be spared, depending on radiohumeral involvement.
- Radiographs show osteophyte formation on the coronoid and olecranon but relatively preserved joint space at the early stages. More advanced stages may be associated with significant joint space narrowing.
- Multiple operative techniques have been described for treatment of primary osteoarthritis of the elbow: débridement arthroplasty, interposition arthroplasty, the Outerbridge-Kashiwagi procedure, arthroscopic débridement, and total elbow replacement.
  - Ulnohumeral (Outerbridge-Kashiwagi) arthroplasty was first described in 1978 and became popular a few years later. It is based on a posterior approach to the elbow, removal of olecranon spur and bony overgrowth of the olecranon fossa, and drilling of a hole in this fossa with a trephine to expose the anterior capsule and excise the coronoid osteophyte.

ANATOMY

- The elbow joint consists of three separate articulations: the ulnohumeral, the radiocapitellar, and the proximal radioulnar joints.
- The elbow has two main functions: position the hand in space and stabilize the upper extremity for motor activities and power.
- The normal range of elbow flexion–extension is 0 to 150 degrees and normal forearm pronation–supination is 80 and 80 degrees.
- A 100-degree flexion–extension arc of motion, from 30 to 130 degrees, is quoted for normal activities of daily living. Functional forearm rotation is quoted as 100 degrees, with 50 degrees pronation and 50 degrees supination.
- The condyles articulate at the elbow joint, as the trochlea medially and the capitellum laterally. The articular surface is angled about 30 degrees anterior to the axis of the humeral shaft and has a slight valgus position, about 6 degrees, compared to the epicondylar axis.

- The coronoid fossa and the olecranon fossa, just proximal to the articular surface, accommodate the coronoid process and olecranon process of the ulna in the extremes of flexion and extension, respectively.
- The olecranon and coronoid process coalesce to form the greater sigmoid notch, the articulating portion of the proximal ulna. It is often not completely covered with articular cartilage centrally.

PATHOGENESIS

- Symptomatic osteoarthritis of the elbow has been found to affect about 2% of the general population and represents only 1% to 2% of all patients diagnosed with degenerative arthritis.
- It has a predilection for males, with a ratio of 4 or 5 to 1. It is most commonly seen in middle-aged and older patients.
- The majority of patients experience symptoms in their dominant extremity.
- The exact etiology of primary degenerative elbow arthritis is still unknown. It is generally attributed to overuse. About 60% of patients report employment or hobbies or sports requiring repetitive use of the limb. The few younger patients who present likely have a predisposing condition such as osteochondritis dissecans.
- There are characteristic pathologic changes that occur within the elbow joint: osteophyte formation on the olecranon, olecranon fossa, coronoid, and coronoid fossa.
  - In early stages the joint space is relatively preserved. The periarticular bone is typically hard.
  - Very often, loose bodies may be present into the joint and cause clicking or locking of the elbow, or both.
  - Capsular contracture and fibrosis of the anterior capsule contribute to loss of extension.

NATURAL HISTORY

- Early stages of primary osteoarthritis of the elbow are characterized by pain at the extremes of motion and some loss of terminal extension and flexion. As the severity of the arthritis progresses, pain, stiffness, and loss of range of motion increase.
- When symptoms do not improve with nonoperative treatment, surgical intervention is indicated.
- Because osteoarthritis is a progressive disease, symptoms and pathologic condition may recur. The most common problem is recurrence of impingement pain and flexion contractures.
- Prognostic factors include the etiology of arthritis, the degree of motion loss, mid-arc versus end-range discomfort, the presence of loose bodies, mechanical symptoms, and the presence or absence of cubital tunnel syndrome.

PATIENT HISTORY AND PHYSICAL FINDINGS

- The typical patient with primary degenerative elbow arthritis is a man older than 45 years of age, exposed to repetitive manual labor, who presents with pain at the end ranges of motion, especially in extension.
- Younger patients also may provide a history of sports such as weightlifting, boxing, and other throwing-intensive activities. Arthritic elbows in athletes frequently will include a spectrum of pathologic changes, such as loose bodies and bone spurs.
- Some patients report a history of chronic use of crutches or wheelchairs.
- The chief complaint is pain, especially terminal extension pain, as a result of mechanical impingement.
  - Patients usually feel pain while carrying objects with the elbow in full extension.
  - The intensity of pain is mild to moderate and only occasionally is described as severe.
  - Pain is not usually noted in the mid-range of motion until later stages of arthritis.
- Loss of motion is the most common presenting symptom.
  - Loss of extension is often partially the result of posterior olecranon and humeral osteophytes or anterior capsule contracture.
  - Loss of flexion is secondary to osteophytes on the coronoid or its fossa and to loose bodies.
  - Supination–pronation is not restricted or is only minimally restricted, owing to limited involvement of the radiohumeral joint.
- Catching or locking may be present with articular incongruity, or when loose bodies are present.
- Crepitus may be present throughout the range of motion.
- Swelling may occur but is not typical.

- Ulnar nerve symptoms may also be present owing to excessive osteophyte formation. They should actively be sought out because they may influence treatment decisions and even direct the surgical approach.
- Physical examination may reveal a positive Tinel sign and a positive elbow flexion test, with decreased sensation and weakness in the ulnar nerve distribution. Cubital tunnel syndrome may be present in up to 20% of patients.

IMAGING AND OTHER DIAGNOSTIC STUDIES

- Anteroposterior (AP), lateral, and oblique radiographs (**FIG 1**) are diagnostic and illustrate characteristic features of the condition.
  - The AP view should be taken with the beam perpendicular to the distal humerus for distal humerus pathology and perpendicular to the radial head for proximal forearm pathology. These views will show ossification and osteophyte formation of the olecranon and coronoid fossa.
  - The lateral view should be taken in 90 degrees of flexion with the forearm in neutral rotation. This view will show an anterior osteophyte on the coronoid fossa and process and a posterior osteophyte on the olecranon fossa and process.
  - The lateral oblique view provides better visualization of the radiocapitellar joint, medial epicondyle, and radioulnar joint.
  - The medial oblique view provides better visualization of the trochlea, olecranon fossa, and coronoid tip.
  - A cubital tunnel view may be useful if there is ulnar nerve symptomatology.
- A lateral tomogram and computed tomography are helpful for preoperative planning to assess the presence and location of loose bodies and subtle osteophyte formation (especially in earlier stages).

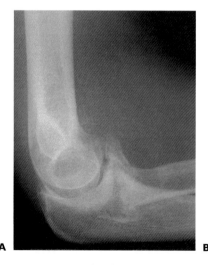 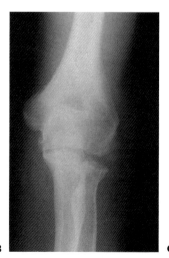 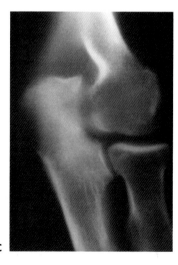

A   B   C

FIG 1 • A. Lateral radiograph of a 50-year-old heavy laborer's elbow. The patient had severe pain at the extremes of motion. The radiograph reveals characteristic osteophytes of the olecranon and of the coronoid process. **B.** AP radiograph of the elbow (same patient). This view shows ossification and osteophytes of the olecranon and coronoid fossa. **C.** Lateral oblique radiograph. This view provides better visualization of the radiocapitellar and radioulnar joint. There is an osteophyte at the tip of the olecranon, which causes pain during full extension.

DIFFERENTIAL DIAGNOSIS

▪ Posttraumatic arthritis
▪ Rheumatoid (inflammatory) arthritis

NONOPERATIVE MANAGEMENT

▪ Nonoperative treatment may be helpful in the early stages.
▪ Patients should limit activities that require heavy elbow use.
▪ Physical therapy is used to maintain range of motion and strength. Modalities such as heat and cold may be effective.
▪ Nonsteroidal anti-inflammatory drugs can decrease pain and are of some value. Intra-articular corticosteroid injections may also improve symptoms, but their benefits are usually temporary.
▪ Avoidance of pressure on the cubital tunnel and avoidance of prolonged elbow flexion are recommended if ulnar nerve symptoms are present.

SURGICAL MANAGEMENT

▪ Surgical treatment is indicated when symptoms do not improve with appropriate nonoperative management.
▪ The procedure is indicated in patients with pain in terminal extension or flexion (or both), radiographic evidence of coronoid or olecranon osteophytes (or both), ulnar neuropathy, and functional limitations due to pain or loss of motion.
▪ The procedure is contraindicated in patients with pain throughout the entire arc of motion, marked limitation of motion with an arc of less than 40 degrees, or severe involvement of the radiohumeral or proximal radioulnar joints.

Preoperative Planning

▪ It is very important to carefully review all radiographs (AP, lateral, oblique) before surgery to assess the severity of arthritic changes and evaluate for the presence of loose bodies. A lateral tomogram or CT scan may assist in this evaluation. Care should be taken not to overlook any loose bodies, as these may lead to persistent mechanical symptoms postoperatively.
▪ Specific attention should be paid to the presence of ulnar nerve pathology. If present, this must be addressed at the time of the procedure.

Positioning

▪ There are two options for positioning:
  ▪ The patient may be positioned in the lateral decubitus position with the elbow flexed at 90 degrees and resting on an armrest.

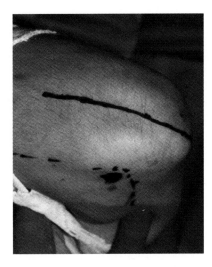

FIG 2 ▪ With the patient in the lateral decubitus position, the elbow is flexed at 90 degrees and is resting on pillows (authors' preferred method). A posterior approach is used via a straight skin incision, which extends distally about 4 cm and proximally 6 to 8 cm from the tip of the olecranon. Note the marked medial epicondyle.

  ▪ Alternatively, the patient may be placed supine with a sandbag underneath the scapula. The elbow is flexed at 90 degrees and brought across the chest. The patient is rotated about 35 degrees for better access to the posterior aspect of the affected elbow.

Approach

▪ A posterior approach is used. The incision is straight, starting 6 to 8 cm proximal to the tip of the olecranon and extending 4 cm distal to the olecranon (**FIG 2**).
▪ Dissection is carried down to the triceps fascia.
▪ The triceps tendon can be split or reflected. In the original description, the triceps muscle is split along the midline, exposing the posterior aspect of the elbow to the lateral and medial supracondylar ridges. Alternatively, the medial margin of the triceps tendon may be reflected from the olecranon.
▪ The decision to reflect or to split the tendon can be determined based on the size of the distal part of the triceps and the need to explore and decompress the ulnar nerve. If the muscle is very bulky, reflection will not provide adequate exposure.

EXPOSURE

▪ After the skin incision is made, the subcutaneous tissue is reflected from the medial aspect of the triceps.
▪ The ulnar nerve is identified and decompressed at the cubital tunnel if there is evidence of ulnar nerve pathology.
▪ The triceps muscle–tendon unit is split longitudinally or reflected.

▪ The triceps is elevated from the posterior aspect of the distal humerus by blunt dissection using a periosteal elevator.
▪ A capsulotomy is then performed (**TECH FIG 1**).

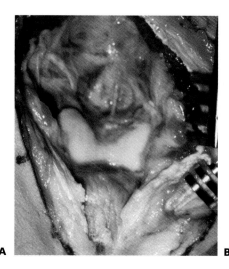
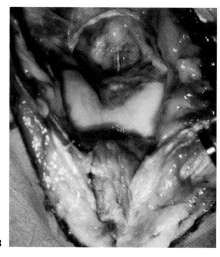

TECH FIG 1 • The triceps muscle has been split to expose the posterior joint. The prominent olecranon osteophyte and the tip of the olecranon process are then removed. The initial cut should be made with an oscillating saw to provide optimal orientation. The osteotomy of the olecranon is completed with an osteotome parallel to each face of the trochlea.

OSTEOPHYTE REMOVAL AND OLECRANON RESECTION

- To minimize impingement in extension, the posterior osteophyte and the tip of the olecranon are removed using an oscillating saw. An osteotome is then used to complete the resection. The orientation of the osteotomy should be parallel to each face of the trochlea.

- A rongeur is used to smooth the edges.
- A hole is drilled in the olecranon fossa to gain access to the anterior elbow compartment and the coronoid process. This requires removal of osteophytes around the olecranon fossa (**TECH FIG 2**).

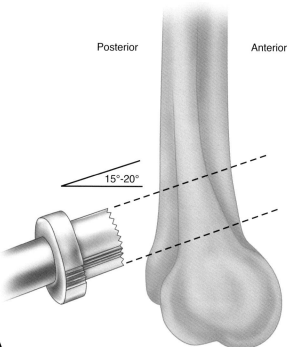
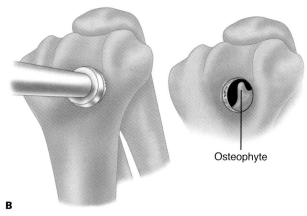

TECH FIG 2 • A neurosurgical dowel is used to make a hole and remove the ossified olecranon fossa. Care should be taken for proper placement of the foraminectomy. The dowel should follow the curvature of the trochlea.

FORAMINECTOMY

- A 1.5-cm neurosurgical dowel is applied to a reaming drill bit, and a drill hole is developed. Proper placement of this foraminectomy is of great importance. The dowel should follow the curvature of the trochlea.

- Once the foraminectomy is complete, a core of bone is removed from the distal humerus. This may include osteophytes from the anterior aspect of the joint (**TECH FIG 3A,B**).

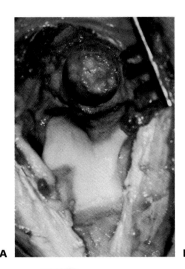

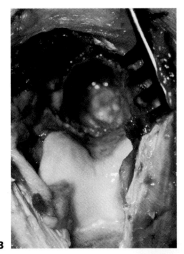

A **B**

TECH FIG 3 • A,B. Once the foraminectomy is completed, the core of bone is removed from the distal humerus. This allows access to the anterior elbow compartment and to the coronoid. At this time, loose bodies of the anterior compartment may be identified and removed. **C.** With maximum elbow flexion, the anterior osteophyte from the coronoid process is removed, using a curved osteotome. **D.** An instrument is then introduced through the foramen and the osteophyte and a portion of the coronoid are removed.

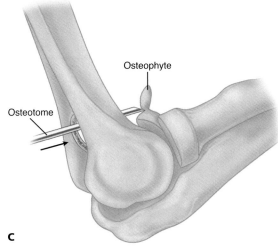

Osteophyte

Osteotome

C

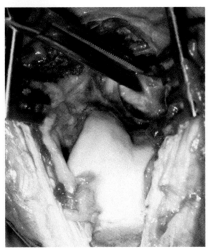

D

- This hole is used to clean debris and remove loose bodies from the anterior aspect of the elbow (**TECH FIG 3C,D**).
- With maximum elbow flexion, the anterior osteophyte from the coronoid process is removed using a curved osteotome.
- Occasionally it is necessary to strip the anterior capsule from the anterior humerus using a blunt periosteal elevator, to regain better extension.

- Care must be taken to ensure that no osteophytes or loose bodies are overlooked.
- Bone wax is used to cover the margins of the foramen, and Gelfoam is inserted into the defect to fill the dead space.
- The wound is meticulously irrigated and closed in standard fashion.
- The elbow is carefully manipulated to maximize the total arc of motion.

PEARLS AND PITFALLS

Indications	▪ Primary osteoarthritis of the elbow presenting with pain at the extremes of motion due to osteophyte formation on the olecranon or coronoid process (or both) and in the olecranon or coronoid fossa (or both)
Contraindications	▪ Severe involvement of the radiohumeral joint ▪ Pain throughout the entire arc of motion
Assessment	▪ Careful selection of patients is important. ▪ Appropriate imaging studies should be obtained to identify all loose bodies or osteophytes. A preoperative lateral tomogram may be indicated. ▪ The surgeon should always evaluate for coexisting ulnar nerve pathology, which should be addressed during surgery.
Operation	▪ Proper placement of foraminectomy ▪ Meticulous inspection of posterior and anterior aspects of the joint ▪ Removal of all loose bodies and osteophytes

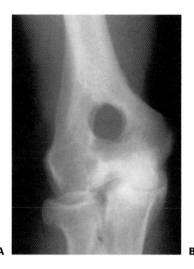
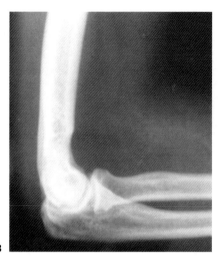

FIG 3 • AP and lateral radiographs after ulno-humeral arthroplasty has been performed. The hole of the foraminectomized distal humerus can be easily seen. There are no osteophytes of the olecranon and coronoid process and the patient has gained a much better arc of motion without pain.

POSTOPERATIVE CARE

■ A splint is applied with the elbow in 15 degrees of extension for 1 week.
■ Active range of motion is allowed 7 to 10 days after surgery.
■ The patient is re-evaluated at 3 weeks, 6 weeks, and 3 months after surgery.
■ Continuous passive motion can be initiated on the day of surgery and is discontinued after 3 weeks.

OUTCOMES

■ A review of the literature shows satisfactory results in over 80% of patients.
■ Satisfactory pain relief is achieved in about 90% of patients.
■ Extension improves by about 10 to 15 degrees and flexion improves by about 10 degrees. Overall improvement in the motion arc is about 20 to 25 degrees (**FIG 3**).
■ There have been no reports of postoperative instability.

COMPLICATIONS

■ The complication rate for this procedure is very low, in contrast to most reconstructive procedures of the elbow.
■ The recurrence rate is less than 10%.
■ Iatrogenic ulnar nerve palsy is unusual, but can occur as a result of overzealous use of retractors intraoperatively.
■ Improper placement of the foraminectomy may result in a column fracture.

REFERENCES

1. Antuna SA, Morrey BF, Adams RA, et al. Ulnohumeral arthroplasty for primary degenerative arthritis of the elbow. J Bone Joint Surg Am 2002;84A:2168–2173.
2. Forster MC, Clark DI, Lunn PG. Elbow osteoarthritis: prognostic indicators in ulnohumeral debridement—the Outerbridge-Kashiwagi procedure. J Shoulder Elbow Surg 2001;10:557–560.
3. Kashiwagi D. Intra-articular changes of the osteoarthritic elbow, especially about the fossa olecrani. J Jpn Orthop Assoc 1978;52:1367–1382.
4. Kashiwagi D. Outerbridge-Kashiwagi arthroplasty for osteoarthritis of the elbow. In Kashiwagi D, ed. Elbow joint. Proceedings of the International Congress, Kobi, Japan. Amsterdam: Elsevier Science Publishers, 1986:177–188.
5. Minami M, Kato S, Kashiwagi D. Outerbridge-Kashiwagi's method for arthroplasty of osteoarthritis of the elbow: 44 elbows followed for 8–16 years. J Orthop Sci 1996;1:11–15.
6. Morrey BF. Primary degenerative arthritis of the elbow: treatment by ulnohumeral arthroplasty. J Bone Joint Surg Br 1992;74B:409–413.
7. Morrey BF. Primary degenerative arthritis of the elbow: ulnohumeral arthroplasty. In: Morrey BF, ed. The Elbow and Its Disorders. Philadelphia: WB Saunders, 2000:799–808.
8. Morrey BF. Ulnohumeral arthroplasty. In: Morrey BF, ed. Master Techniques in Orthopaedic Surgery: The Elbow. New York: Raven Press Ltd, 1994:277–289.
9. O'Driscoll SW. Elbow arthritis: treatment options. J Am Acad Orthop Surg 1993;1:106.
10. Tsuge K, Mizuseki T. Debridement arthroplasty for advanced primary osteoarthritis of the elbow. J Bone Joint Surg Br 1994;76B:641–646.
11. Tsuge K, Murakami T, Yasunaga Y, et al. Arthroplasty of the elbow: twenty years experience of a new approach. J Bone Joint Surg Br 1987;69B:116–120.
12. Vingerhoeds B, Degreef I, De Smet L. Debridement arthroplasty for osteoarthritis of the elbow (Outerbridge-Kashiwagi procedure). Acta Orthop Belg 2004;70:306–310.

Chapter 43

Lateral Columnar Release for Extracapsular Elbow Contracture

Leonid I. Katolik and Mark S. Cohen

DEFINITION

- Extrinsic elbow contracture refers to elbow stiffness secondary to fibrosis, thickening, and, occasionally, ossification of the elbow capsule and periarticular soft tissues.
- In contrast to intrinsic contracture, the articular surface is either uninvolved or minimally involved, without the presence of intra-articular adhesions or articular cartilage destruction.
- While a distinction is made between extrinsic and intrinsic causes of contracture, these entities often overlap.

ANATOMY

- The elbow is a compound uniaxial synovial joint comprising three highly congruous articulations.
- The ulnohumeral joint is a ginglymus, or hinge, joint. The radiocapitellar and proximal radioulnar joints are gliding joints.
- All three articulations exist within a single capsule and are further stabilized by the proximity of the articular surface and capsule to the intracapsular ligaments and overlying extracapsular musculature.

PATHOGENESIS

- The propensity for elbow stiffness after even trivial elbow trauma is well recognized. After even seemingly trivial injuries, the capsule can undergo structural and biochemical alterations leading to thickening, decreased compliance, and loss of motion.
- Causes of extrinsic elbow contracture include capsular contracture, damage to and fibrosis of the flexor–extensor muscular origins, collateral ligament scarring, heterotopic bone, and skin contracture.
- Prolonged immobilization after trauma may be a separate risk factor for the development of stiffness.

NATURAL HISTORY

- Little consensus exists regarding the natural history of capsular contracture. It is felt that appropriate recognition and treatment of acute elbow injuries, avoidance of prolonged immobilization, and early active range of motion may limit the severity of posttraumatic extrinsic contracture.
- Patients typically do not tolerate elbow stiffness well since adjacent joints do not provide adequate compensatory motion.
  - Morrey[10] showed that the performance of most activities of daily living requires a functional arc of motion from 30 to 130 degrees.
  - Vasen and colleagues[11] have demonstrated that volunteers with uninjured elbows may adapt to a functional arc of motion from 70 to 120 degrees to perform 12 tasks of daily living.
  - Patients typically request treatment for elbow contracture when loss of extension approaches 40 degrees and flexion does not exceed 120 degrees.
  - Patients who do not improve with a concerted effort at nonoperative treatment often require surgical release.

- Stiffness of the elbow typically is incited by soft tissue trauma, hemarthrosis, and the patient's response to pain. Elbow trauma may cause tearing and contusion of the periarticular soft tissues. The patient typically holds the injured elbow in a flexed position to reduce pain. A fibrous tissue response then ensues within the hematoma and damaged muscular tissues. This fibrous tissue may ossify. In addition, overly aggressive therapy may further exacerbate these injuries, potentiating the cycle of pain, swelling, and limitation in motion that leads ultimately to frank contracture.
- Collateral ligament injury may contribute to contracture. Primary fibrosis may develop within the collateral ligaments because of the initial injury. Alternatively, secondary fibrosis may result from immobilization and scar formation.
- Significant injury to the anterior joint capsule and the overlying brachialis muscle may also result in capsular hypertrophy and fibrotic reaction contributing to ankylosis. This is particularly common in association with fracture-dislocations of the elbow.

PATIENT HISTORY AND PHYSICAL FINDINGS

- The cause of contracture should generally be easily elucidated from the history. Particular notation should be made of concomitant injuries, including closed head injury or associated burn injury.
- The duration and possible progression of symptoms should be noted.
- The impact of the contracture on the patient's upper extremity function and any limitations in activities of daily living should be noted.
- Any previous treatment for contracture should be elucidated. This should include the appropriateness, duration, and results of prior physical therapy, splinting, intra-articular injections, and surgeries.
- For patients with prior elbow surgery, the presence and type of any residual internal fixation devices should be noted. In addition, attention should be paid to any remote history of elbow infection.
- Physical examination should include a general physical examination as well as a detailed examination of the involved extremity.
  - Attention must be paid to the examination of the skin and soft tissue envelope about the elbow, with notation made of prior incisions, skin grafts, flaps, or areas of wound breakdown.
- Elbow motion should be measured with a goniometer and active and passive motion should be compared.
- Notation should be made whether motion improves with the forearm in full pronation, which may suggest posterolateral rotatory instability. This effectively "spins" the forearm away from the humerus, causing gapping of the ulnohumeral joint and posterior subluxation of the radial head from the

capitellum. While frank dislocation is not possible in the unanesthetized patient, guarding is effectively a positive sign.
- While rare, symptomatic incompetence of the ulnar collateral ligament may elucidated by examination.
- Strength of the involved limb should be assessed, as a joint without adequate strength is unlikely to maintain motion after release.
- Since many posttraumatic and inflammatory contractures about the elbow are associated with ulnar nerve symptoms, a careful neurologic examination should be performed. A positive Tinel test over the cubital tunnel as well as a positive elbow flexion test should increase the suspicion for concomitant ulnar nerve pathology.

IMAGING AND OTHER DIAGNOSTIC STUDIES

- Anteroposterior (AP) and lateral radiographs are often all that is needed for preoperative planning (**FIG 1**).
- Cross-sectional imaging with computed tomography is helpful in visualizing the articular surfaces, particularly after fracture.
  - We advocate the use of computed tomography for preoperative planning in cases of moderate to severe heterotopic ossification.
- Extracapsular contracture is typically not painful through the remaining arc of motion and is not painful at rest. If pain is a significant component of the patient's symptoms, serologic workup for infection, including a complete blood count, erythrocyte sedimentation rate, and C-reactive protein, is indicated.

DIFFERENTIAL DIAGNOSIS

- Conversion disorder
- Infection
- Inflammatory arthropathy
- Intracapsular contracture

NONOPERATIVE MANAGEMENT

- Alternative measures to improve elbow stiffness include conservative modalities to decrease joint swelling and inflammation and relax or stretch contracted soft tissues. For protracted swelling, edema control sleeves, ice, elevation, active motion (including the forearm, wrist, and hand), and oral agents such as anti-inflammatory medication can be useful.
- A short-term oral prednisone taper can be very effective in difficult cases. In addition, one can consider an intra-articular cortisone injection to decrease inflammation and joint synovitis.

- Rarely, when patients exhibit guarding and involuntary co-contraction, biofeedback may be a helpful adjunct.
- Dynamic splints, which apply a constant tension to the soft tissues, may be helpful.
- Patient-adjusted static braces appear to be more effective. These braces use the principle of passive progressive stretch, allowing for stress relaxation of the soft tissues. They are applied for much shorter periods of time and are better tolerated by patients.

SURGICAL MANAGEMENT

- To improve elbow flexion, one must release any soft tissue structures posteriorly that might be tethering the joint. These include the posterior joint capsule and the triceps muscle and tendon, which can become adherent to the humerus.
  - Any bony or soft tissue impingement also must be removed anteriorly, including osteophytes off the coronoid process and any bony or soft tissue overgrowth in both the coronoid and radial fossae.
  - There must be a concavity above the humeral trochlea to accept both the coronoid centrally and the radial head laterally for full flexion to occur.
- Similarly, to improve elbow extension, posterior impingement must be removed between the olecranon tip and the olecranon fossa.
  - Anteriorly, any tethering soft tissues must be released, namely the anterior joint capsule and any adhesions between the brachialis and the humerus.

Preoperative Planning

- All radiographic studies should be reviewed.
- The presence and type of any retained implants is noted.
- Range-of-motion and pivot-shift testing is performed under anesthesia as well as under live fluoroscopy.

Positioning

- Patients are positioned supine with the arm on a hand table.
- The patient's torso is brought to the edge of the operating table to ensure adequate elbow exposure for fluoroscopic imaging.
- A towel bump may be placed under the medial elbow.

Approach

- A direct posterior skin incision or a lateral incision is used.
  - A direct posterior incision has been criticized for an increased propensity toward postoperative seroma formation.

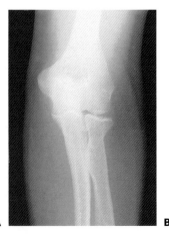 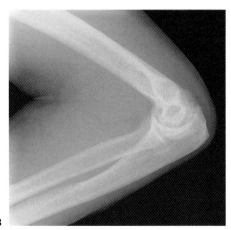

A   B

FIG 1 • Routine preoperative AP (**A**) and lateral (**B**) radiographs are obtained in all cases. Contracture may occur after subtle injury. This patient developed stiffness after nonoperative treatment of a nondisplaced radial neck fracture.

■ It has the advantage of being a utilitarian incision that allows access to the medial and lateral sides simultaneously.

■ Advantages to the lateral exposure include its simplicity, less extensor and flexor–pronator disruption, and access to all three joint articulations.

■ The main disadvantage of the lateral exposure is the inability to address the ulnar nerve when indicated.

■ The deep interval for exposure of the anterior capsule lies between the extensor carpi radialis longus (ECRL) proximally and the extensor carpi radialis brevis (ECRB) distally. Posterior access is achieved between the triceps and the humerus.

SURGICAL APPROACH

■ The procedure can be performed under general anesthesia or under regional anesthesia with a long-acting regional block.

■ For the posterior incision, care is taken to avoid placing the line of incision directly over the prominence of the olecranon. Full-thickness fasciocutaneous flaps are elevated laterally to expose the extensor muscle mass.

■ For a lateral incision, an extended Köcher approach is used, beginning along the lateral supracondylar ridge of the humerus and passing distally in the interval between the anconeus and the extensor carpi ulnaris (ECU).

POSTERIOR RELEASE

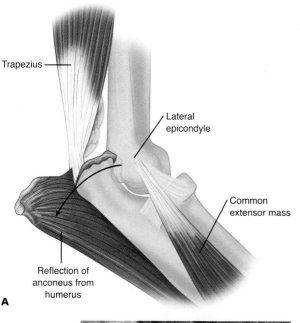

Trapezius

Lateral epicondyle

Common extensor mass

Reflection of anconeus from humerus

A

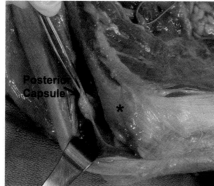

Posterior Capsule

*

B

■ The Köcher interval between the anconeus and ECU is developed.

■ The anconeus is reflected posteriorly in continuity with the triceps. This exposes the posterior and posterolateral joint capsule (**TECH FIG 1A,B**).

■ A triceps tenolysis is carried out with an elevator, releasing any adhesions between the muscle and the posterior humerus. The humeroulnar joint is identified posteriorly and the olecranon fossa is cleared of any fibrous tissue or scar that would restrict terminal extension. The tip of the olecranon is removed if there was evidence of overgrowth or impingement (**TECH FIG 1C**).

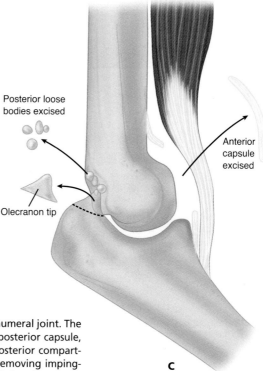

Posterior loose bodies excised

Anterior capsule excised

Olecranon tip

C

TECH FIG 1 • **A,B.** Exposure of the lateral and posterior ulnohumeral joint. The anconeus and triceps are reflected posteriorly, exposing the posterior capsule, olecranon tip, and olecranon fossa. **C.** Visualization of the posterior compartment permits débridement of the posterior joint, including removing impinging tissue of osteophytes in the olecranon fossa and the tip of the olecranon.

- The posterior aspect of the radiocapitellar joint is inspected after excision of the elbow capsule just proximal to the conjoined lateral collateral and annular ligament complex through the "soft spot" on the lateral side of the elbow. The proximal edge of this complex lies along the proximal border of the radial head.

ANTERIOR RELEASE

- Once the posterior release is completed, dissection is carried anteriorly. The anterior interval proximally is between the lateral supracondylar column and the brachioradialis and ECRL. Distally the interval is between the ECRL and extensor digitorum communis (EDC) (**TECH FIG 2A**).
- The brachialis is then mobilized off the humerus and anterior capsule with an elevator, releasing any adhesions between the muscle and the anterior humerus (**TECH FIG 2B**).
- The brachioradialis and ECRL released from the lateral supracondylar ridge of the humerus (**TECH FIG 2C**).
- This dissection is continued distally between the ECRL and ECRB, allowing exposure of the anterior capsule with preservation of the lateral collateral ligament and the origins of the ECRB, the EDC and minimi, and the ECU from the lateral epicondyle.

- Dissection is then carried out beneath the elbow capsule between the joint and the brachialis. The capsule is excised as far as the medial side of the joint.
- The radial and coronoid fossae are cleared of fibrous tissue and the tip of the coronoid is removed if overgrowth or impingement was noted in flexion. Loose bodies are removed (**TECH FIG 2D,E**).
- After release of the anterior capsule, gentle extension of the elbow with applied pressure usually brings the joint out to nearly full extension.
- In longstanding cases of contracture, the brachialis muscle can be tight, inhibiting full terminal elbow extension. This myostatic contracture can be stretched for several minutes during the procedure and requires attention at subsequent physiotherapy (**TECH FIG 2F**).

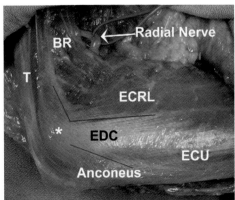

A

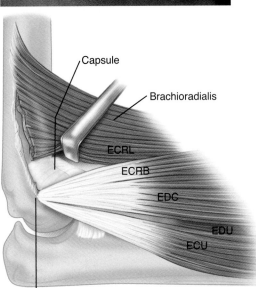

B
Lateral epicondyle

TECH FIG 2 • A. The lateral view of a dissected elbow. Blue lines mark the fascial intervals for access to the anterior and posterior aspect of the joint, which leaves the extensor carpi ulnaris (ECU), extensor digitorum communis (EDC), and extensor carpi radialis longus (ECRL) origins intact as well as the underlying lateral collateral ligament complex. The anterior elbow capsule is exposed by releasing the extensor carpi radialis longus from the lateral supracondylar ridge. Distally the exposure continues between the ECRL and ECRB. *T*, triceps; *BR*, brachioradialis. **B,C.** The anterior exposure for release. The anterior capsule is exposed by detaching the humeral origin of the ECRL proximally and the interval between the ECRL and ECRB distally. The brachialis is released from the anterior capsule. The capsule should be visualized all the way over to the medial joint with all muscle reflected anteriorly. *(continued)*

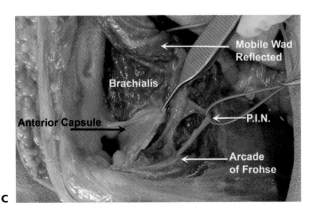

C

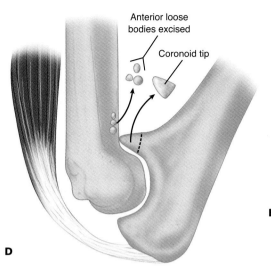

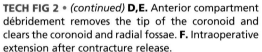

Anterior loose
bodies excised

Coronoid tip

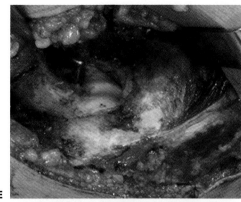

E

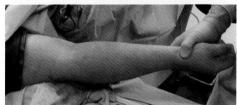

F

TECH FIG 2 • *(continued)* **D,E.** Anterior compartment débridement removes the tip of the coronoid and clears the coronoid and radial fossae. **F.** Intraoperative extension after contracture release.

PEARLS AND PITFALLS

Indications	■ The importance of prolonged postoperative rehabilitation cannot be stressed enough. A program of active and passive range of motion, weighted elbow stretches with wrist weights, formal therapy, and patient-adjusted elbow bracing is common for 3 to 6 months after surgery. ■ Postoperative gains may easily be lost in the patient who is not fully committed to rehabilitation or who does not have access to regular supervised therapy.
Ulnar nerve	■ Patients with preoperative signs and symptoms of ulnar nerve irritability should undergo neurolysis and transposition of the ulnar nerve. Although no strict guidelines exist, patients with preoperative flexion less than 100 degrees generally undergo concurrent ulnar nerve release even in the absence of preoperative symptoms.
Median nerve and brachial artery	■ These structures are generally well protected by the brachialis muscle. Their safety is increased if dissection proceeds in the interval between the elbow capsule and the brachialis.
Radial nerve injury	■ The posterior interosseous nerve may be encountered as extracapsular dissection proceeds distal to the radiocapitellar joint. Care must be taken with more distal dissection, and a firm understanding of neural anatomy is mandatory before attempting capsular release. Except in cases of significant anterolateral heterotopic ossification, we do not routinely dissect and isolate the radial nerve from proximal to distal.
Iatrogenic posterolateral rotatory instability	■ Instability may be induced with overly aggressive dissection about the lateral condyle. Care should be taken to stay anterior to the origin of the extensor carpi radialis brevis.

POSTOPERATIVE CARE

■ Although several rehabilitation programs may be effective, we have found continuous passive motion, begun immediately in the recovery room and used continuously until the following morning, to be helpful in maintaining the motion gained at surgery (**FIG 2A**).

■ Formal therapy is begun on postoperative day 1.

   ■ The dressing is removed and edema control modalities (eg, an edema sleeve or Ace wrap, ice) are used to limit swelling.

   ■ Active and gentle passive elbow motion is combined with intermittent continuous passive motion.

   ■ To help maintain extension, weighted passive stretches using a two-pound wrist weight with the arm extended over a bolster are performed several times daily for 10 to 15 minutes as tolerated.

   ■ Because the collateral ligaments are not released at surgery, no restrictions are typically placed on therapy.

■ Static progressive elbow bracing is begun early in the postoperative period. The brace is worn for about 30 minutes, two

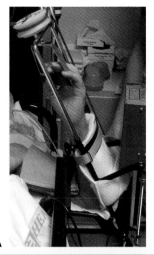

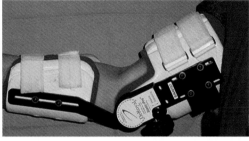

FIG 2 • **A.** Elbow continuous passive motion device. **B.** Patient-adjusted static elbow brace.

or three times a day. Flexion and extension are alternated based on the preoperative deficit and the early progress of the elbow (**FIG 2B**).

■ A nonsteroidal anti-inflammatory agent (Indocin) is commonly prescribed as a prophylaxis against heterotopic ossification for several weeks postoperatively. This also helps to limit inflammation of the joint and soft tissues during rehabilitation.

■ Patients are typically discharged home on postoperative day 1. Home therapy is performed daily thereafter, including active and passive exercises, continuous passive motion, weighted stretches, and patient-adjusted bracing.

  ■ Progress should be closely monitored by a therapist who is familiar with the protocol. The physician must also follow these patients closely.

■ Although the bulk of ultimate elbow motion is gained during the first 6 to 8 weeks, patients can continue to make gains in terminal flexion and extension for several months postoperatively. This is especially true for elbow flexion.

■ Continuous passive motion is typically discontinued at 3 to 4 weeks, but bracing is continued for several months as required. As long as the patient is able to obtain full elbow flexion and extension once per day (eg, in the brace), a favorable prognosis exists with respect to the ultimate outcome if vigilance is maintained.

OUTCOMES

■ In appropriate patients, release of the contracted elbow can be a reliable and satisfying procedure with predictable results.

■ We reviewed our results for 22 patents treated for posttraumatic elbow stiffness using a soft tissue release of the elbow through a lateral approach. The average length of follow-up was 29 months.

  ■ Total elbow motion improved in all subjects. Extension increased from an average of 39 ± 10 degrees preoperatively to 8 ± 6 degrees at follow-up. Elbow flexion increased from 113 ± 18 degrees preoperatively to 137 ± 9 degrees at follow-up. Thus, total ulnohumeral joint motion increased an average of 55 degrees (P <0.001).

  ■ Elbow pain, as determined by visual analogue scales, decreased in all patients. Elbow function, as determined by standardized scales, also significantly improved.

  ■ Radiographic analysis revealed no patients with regrowth of excised osteophytes or loose bodies at follow-up.

COMPLICATIONS

■ Ulnar nerve

  ■ The most common complication after elbow release surgery involves the ulnar nerve. This may be related in part to improved elbow flexion after surgery, as ulnar nerve tension increases with flexion. This may precipitate symptoms in a nerve that is already subclinically compromised.

  ■ Patients with preoperative signs and symptoms of ulnar nerve irritability should undergo neurolysis and transposition of the ulnar nerve.

  ■ Although no strict guidelines exist, patients with preoperative flexion less than 100 degrees generally undergo concurrent ulnar nerve release even in the absence of preoperative symptoms.

■ Median nerve and brachial artery

  ■ Although generally well protected by the brachialis muscle, these structures are at risk with anterior dissection. Their safety is increased if dissection proceeds in the interval between the elbow capsule and the brachialis.

  ■ In addition, transient median neuritis is known to occur in our practices after release. This is likely due to stretch of the median nerve with extension of the severely contracted elbow.

■ Radial nerve injury

  ■ The posterior interosseous nerve may be encountered as extracapsular dissection proceeds distal to the radiocapitellar joint.

  ■ Except in cases of significant anterolateral heterotopic ossification, the radial nerve does not typically require identification.

■ Persistent stiffness

  ■ The importance of prolonged postoperative rehabilitation cannot be stressed enough. A program of active and passive range of motion, weighted elbow stretches with wrist weights, formal therapy, and patient-adjusted elbow bracing is common for 3 to 6 months after surgery. All of our patients meet preoperatively both with the therapists at our home institutions as well as with their local therapists.

REFERENCES

1. Cohen MS, Hastings H. Post-traumatic contracture of the elbow: operative release using a lateral collateral sparing approach. J Bone Joint Surg Br 1998;80B:805–812.
2. Cohen MS, Hastings H. Capsular release for contracture of the elbow: operative technique and functional results. Orthop Clin North Am 1999;30:133–139.
3. Cohen MS, Hastings, H. Rotatory instability of the elbow: the anatomy and role of the lateral stabilizers. J Bone Joint Surg Am 1997;79A:225–233.

4. Gates HS, Sullivan FL, Urbaniak JR. Anterior capsulotomy and continuous passive motion in the treatment post-traumatic flexion contracture of the elbow. J Bone Joint Surg Am 1992;74A:1229–1234.

5. Green DP, McCoy H. Turnbuckle orthotic correction of elbow flexion contractures after acute injuries. J Bone Joint Surg Am 1979;61A:1092–1095.

6. Jupiter JB, O'Driscoll SW, Cohen MS. The assessment and management of the stiff elbow. AAOS Instr Course Lect 2003;52:93–112.

7. Kasparyan NG, Hotchkiss RN. Dynamic skeletal fixation in the upper extremity. Hand Clin 1997;13:643–663.

8. Mansat P, Morrey BF. The column procedure: a limited lateral approach for extrinsic contracture of the elbow. J Bone Joint Surg Am 1998;80A:1603–1615.

9. Modabber MR, Jupiter JB. Current concepts review: reconstruction for posttraumatic conditions of the elbow joint. J Bone Joint Surg Am 1995;77A:1431–1446.

10. Morrey BF. Post-traumatic contracture of the elbow: operative treatment, including distraction arthroplasty. J Bone Joint Surg Am 1990;72A:601–618.

11. Vasen AP, Lacey SH, Keith MW, Shaffer JW. Functional range of motion of the elbow. J Hand Surg Am 1995;20(2):288–292.

Chapter 44

Extrinsic Contracture Release: Medial Over-the-Top Approach

Pierre Mansat, Aymeric André, and Nicolas Bonnevialle

DEFINITION

▪ Multiple techniques have been described for the release of elbow contractures. The medial approach has the advantages of direct access to both the anterior and posterior aspects of the ulnohumeral joint, and direct visualization of the ulnar nerve.

▪ Medial-based releases were initially proposed by Wilner,[24] whose technique involved medial epicondylectomy and wide dissection.

   ▪ Weiss[23] subsequently has described splitting the flexor pronator mass rather than complete release of the flexor pronator mass.

   ▪ Hotchkiss[12] popularized this approach to deal with extrinsic contracture of the elbow and ulnar nerve involvement.

   ▪ Itoh et al[10] and Wada et al[22] underlined the importance of the posterior oblique band of the medial collateral ligament as a critical structure to identify and release if an extension contracture exists.

ANATOMY

▪ The medial compartment of the elbow includes the medial side of the ulnohumeral joint, the medial collateral ligament, the flexor–pronator mass, the ulnar nerve, and the medial antebrachial cutaneous nerve (**FIG 1A**).

▪ The medial ulnohumeral joint is composed of the medial column, the medial epicondyle, the medial side of the proximal aspect of the ulna, and the coronoid process.

▪ The medial collateral ligament consists of three parts: anterior, posterior, and transverse segments (**FIG 1B**).

   ▪ The anterior bundle is the most discrete component, the posterior portion being a thickening of the posterior capsule, and is well defined only in about 90 degrees of flexion.

   ▪ The transverse component appears to contribute little or nothing to elbow stability.

   ▪ The medial collateral ligament originates from a broad anteroinferior surface of the epicondyle but not from the condylar elements of the trochlea just inferior to the axis of rotation.[18] The ulnar nerve rests on the posterior aspect of the medial epicondyle, but it is not intimately related to the fibers of the anterior bundle of the medial collateral ligament itself.

▪ The flexor–pronator mass includes the pronator teres, the most proximal of the flexor pronator group; the flexor carpi radialis, which originates just inferior to the origin of the pronator teres at the anteroinferior aspect of the medial epicondyle; the palmaris longus muscle, which arises from the medial epicondyle and from the septa it shares with the flexor carpi radialis and flexor carpi ulnaris; the flexor carpi ulnaris, which is the most posterior of the common flexor tendons originating from the medial epicondyle and from the medial border of the coronoid and the proximal medial aspect of the

ulna; and the flexor digitorum superficialis, which is the deepest from the common flexor tendon but superficial to the flexor digitorum profundus.

IMAGING AND OTHER DIAGNOSTIC STUDIES

▪ Diagnosis of the contracture is usually made by identifying a characteristic history and performing a physical examination.

▪ Joint involvement is confirmed by plain radiographs. The anteroposterior (AP) view gives good visualization of the joint line, but the lateral view demonstrates osteophytes on the coronoid and at the tip of the olecranon, even when the joint space is preserved.

▪ The details of the extent of the involvement are best observed on computed tomography.

▪ Transverse imaging by magnetic resonance imaging (MRI) has little utility in our practice.

NONOPERATIVE MANAGEMENT

▪ Several options have been proposed for the treatment of elbow contracture.

▪ Nonoperative treatment with mobilization of the elbow through the use of alternating flexion and extension splints[17] or dynamic splints[8] sometimes provides a good result if it is begun soon after the contracture develops.

▪ Manipulation with the patient under anesthesia has also been recommended, but loss of motion and ulnar nerve injury have been reported.[6]

▪ Recently, botulinum toxin has been used to release muscle contracture in order to improve elbow rehabilitation.[20]

▪ Nonoperative treatment usually is successful only for extrinsic stiffness that has been present for 6 months or less, however, and the results are unpredictable. With failure of nonoperative treatment, surgical release may be indicated. Some reports of this being done through an arthroscopic procedure recently appeared. Most surgeons employ an open procedure, and several have been described.

SURGICAL MANAGEMENT

Indications

▪ Contracture release
▪ Stiff elbow
▪ Degenerative arthritis with anterior and posteromedial osteophytes
▪ Ulnar nerve symptoms

Advantages

▪ Allows exposure, protection, and transposition of the ulnar nerve
▪ Preserves the anterior band of the medial collateral ligament
▪ Affords access to the coronoid with intact radial head

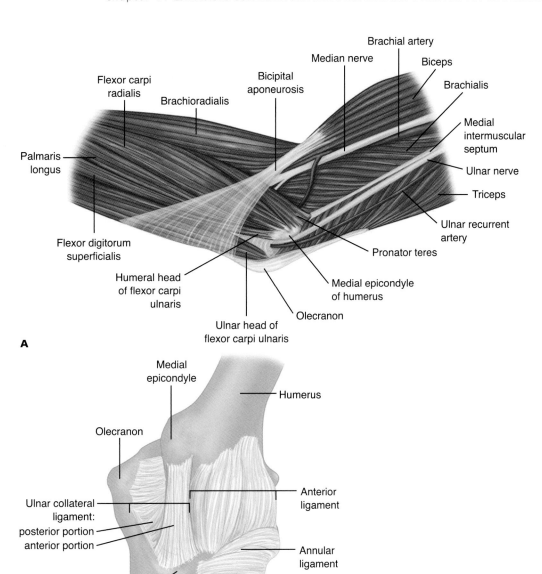

FIG 1 • Superficial (**A**) and deep (**B**) anatomy of the medial side of the elbow.

Disadvantages

■ Difficulty in removing heterotopic bone on the lateral side of the joint
■ Affords poor access to radial head

Preoperative Planning

■ Before surgery, the decision must be made to approach the capsule from the lateral or medial aspect.
    ■ If the ulnar nerve is to be addressed or there is extensive medial or coronoid arthrosis, the medial approach is of value.

■ If the radiohumeral joint is involved or if a simple release is all that is required, the lateral "column" procedure is carried out.

Positioning

■ The patient is usually positioned supine, supported by an elbow or a hand table.
■ Two folded towels should be placed under the scapula.
■ A sterile tourniquet is positioned.

■ To expose the posterior joint, the patient's shoulder should have fairly free external rotation; otherwise, the arm should be positioned over the chest.

Approach

■ The skin incision may be a posterior skin incision or a midline medial one (**FIG 2**).

■ The key to this exposure is identification of the medial supracondylar ridge of the humerus.

■ At this level, the surgeon can locate the medial intermuscular septum, the origin of the flexor–pronator muscle mass, and the ulnar nerve.

■ This site also serves as the starting point of the anterior and posterior subperiosteal extracapsular dissection of the joint.

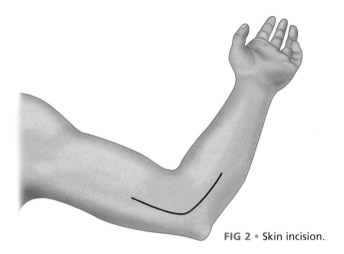

FIG 2 • Skin incision.

EXPOSING THE ULNAR NERVE AND THE MEDIAL FASCIA

■ Once the medial intermuscular septum is identified, the medial antebrachial cutaneous nerve is identified, traced distally, and protected.

■ The branching pattern varies, however, so it is occasionally necessary to divide the nerve to gain full exposure and to adequately mobilize the ulnar nerve, especially in revision surgery.

■ If this is necessary, the nerve is divided as proximally as the skin incision will allow, ensuring that the cut end lies in the subcutaneous fat (**TECH FIG 1**).

■ If previously anterior transposition was performed, the ulnar nerve should be fully identified and mobilized before proceeding.

■ The surgeon must be prepared to extend the previous incision proximally, as necessary.

■ In this setting, the nerve is often flattened over the medial flexor–pronator muscle mass, or it can "subluxate" to a posterior position.

■ This dissection requires patience and may take considerable time. Dissection of the nerve needs to be carried distally far enough to allow the nerve to sit in the anterior position without being kinked distal to the epicondyle.

■ The septum is excised from the insertion on the supracondylar ridge to the proximal extent of the wound, usually about 5 to 8 cm.

■ Many of the veins and perforating arteries at the most distal portion of the septum require cauterization.

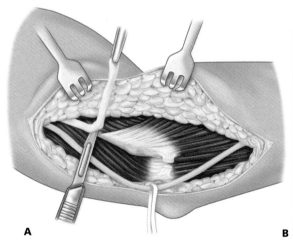
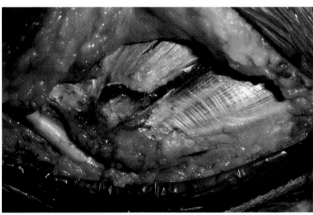

TECH FIG 1 • Exposure of the ulnar nerve and medial fascia.

EXPOSING THE ANTERIOR CAPSULE FOR EXCISION AND INCISION

■ Once the septum has been excised, the flexor–pronator muscle mass should be divided parallel to the fibers, leaving roughly a 1.5-cm span of flexor carpi ulnaris tendon attached to the epicondyle (**TECH FIG 2A,B**).

■ The surgeon then returns the supracondylar ridge and begins elevating the anterior muscle with a Cobb elevator.

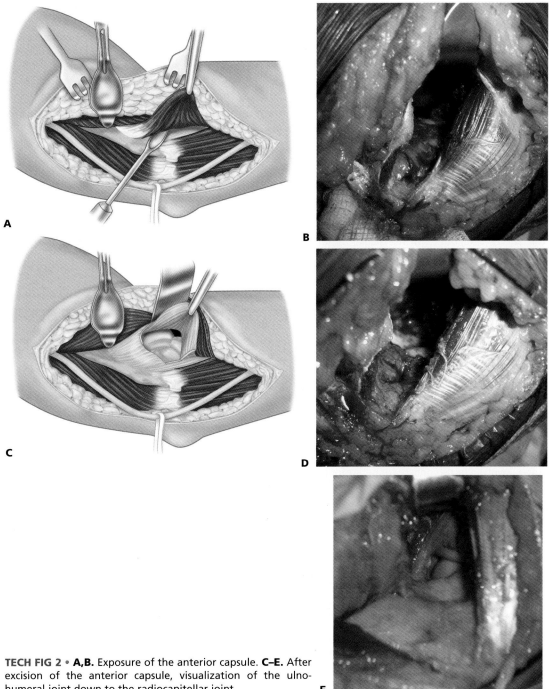

TECH FIG 2 • A,B. Exposure of the anterior capsule. **C–E.** After excision of the anterior capsule, visualization of the ulno-humeral joint down to the radiocapitellar joint.

- Subperiosteally, the anterior structures of the distal humeral region proximal to the capsule are elevated to allow placement of a wide Bennett retractor. As the elevator moves from medial to lateral, the handle of the elevator is lifted carefully, keeping the blade of the elevator along the surface of the bone.
  - When heterotopic ossification along the lateral distal humerus is profuse, the radial nerve is at risk if it is entrapped in the scar on the surface of the bone.
  - A separate approach to the lateral side is sometimes needed.
- The median nerve, brachial vein, and artery are superficial to the brachialis muscle.

- A small cuff of tissue of the flexor–pronator origin can be left on the supracondylar ridge as the muscle is elevated. This facilitates reattachment during closing.
- A proximal, transverse incision in the lacertus fibrosus may also be needed to adequately mobilize this layer of muscle.
- Once the Bennett retractor is in place and the medial portion of the flexor–pronator has been incised, the plane between muscle and capsule should be carefully elevated.
  - As this plane is developed, the brachialis muscle is encountered from the underside. This muscle should be kept anterior and elevated from the capsule and anterior surface of the distal humerus.

- Finding this plane requires careful attention.
- The dissection of the capsule from the brachialis muscle proceeds both laterally and distally.
- At this point, it is helpful to feel for the coronoid process by gently flexing and extending the elbow. The first few times that this approach is used, the coronoid seems quite deep and far distal.
  - A deep, narrow retractor is often helpful to allow the operator to see down to the level of the coronoid.
- The extreme anteromedial corner of the exposure deserves special comment.
  - In a contracture release, the anteromedial portion often requires release.
  - To see this area, a small, narrow retractor can be inserted to retract the medial collateral ligament, pulling it medially and posteriorly.
  - This affords visualization of the medial capsule and protection of the anterior medial collateral ligament.

- The anterior capsule should be excised (**TECH FIG 2C–E**) to the extent that that is practical and safe.
  - When first performing this procedure, it is helpful first to incise the capsule from the medial to the lateral aspect along the anterior surface of the joint.
  - Once this edge of the capsule is incised, it can be lifted and excised as far distally as is safe. From this vantage, and after capsule excision, the radial head and capitellum can be visualized and freed of scar, as needed.
- In cases of primary osteoarthritis of the elbow, removing the large spur from the coronoid is crucial.
  - Using the Cobb elevator, the brachialis muscle can be elevated anteriorly for 2 cm from the coronoid process.
  - With the elevator held in position, protecting the brachialis but anterior to the coronoid, the large osteophyte can be removed with an osteotome.
  - The brachialis insertion is well distal to the tip of the coronoid.

EXPOSING AND EXCISING THE POSTERIOR CAPSULE AND BONE SPURS

- The posterior capsule of the joint is exposed. The supracondylar ridge is again identified (**TECH FIG 3**).
  - Using the Cobb elevator, the triceps is elevated from the posterior distal surface of the humerus.
  - The exposure should extend far enough proximal to permit use of a Bennett retractor.
- The posterior capsule can be separated from the triceps as the elevator sweeps from proximal to distal. The posterior medial joint line should also be identified, as it is often involved by osteophytes or heterotopic bone.

- In contracture release, the posterior capsule and posterior band of the medial collateral ligament should be excised.
- The medial joint line up to the anterior band of the medial collateral ligament should also be exposed and the capsule excised. This area is the floor of the cubital tunnel.
- In contracture release and in primary osteoarthritis, the tip of the olecranon usually must be excised to achieve full extension.
  - The posteromedial joint line is easily visualized, but the posterolateral side must also be carefully palpated to ensure clearance.

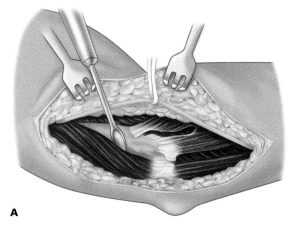

A

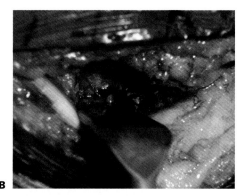

B

TECH FIG 3 • Exposure of the posterior compartment.

ULNAR NERVE TRANSPOSITION

- After being reattached to the medial supracondylar region, the ulnar nerve should be transposed and secured with a fascial sling to prevent posterior subluxation.
  - The sling can be fashioned by elevating two overlapping rectangular flaps of fascia or by using a medially based flap attached to the underlying subcutaneous tissue.

- Once this maneuver is completed, the nerve must not be compressed or kinked.
- The joint should be flexed and extended to ensure that the nerve is free to move.

CLOSURE

- The flexor–pronator mass should be reattached to the supracondylar ridge with nonabsorbable braided 1-0 or 0 suture.
    - If a large enough cuff of tissue was left on the medial epicondyle, no holes need be drilled in bone.
    - Otherwise, drill holes in the edge of the supracondylar ridge can be made to secure the flexor–pronator mass (**TECH FIG 4**).

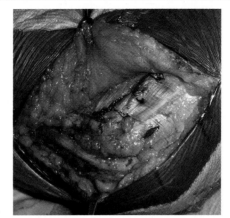

TECH FIG 4 • Closure.

PEARLS AND PITFALLS

Wrong incision	▪ Identification of the medial supracondylar ridge
Injury to the medial antebrachial cutaneous nerve	▪ Identification of the medial antebrachial cutaneous nerve
Injury to the ulnar nerve	▪ Identification, mobilization, and protection of the ulnar nerve
Disinsertion of the flexor–pronator mass from the medial epicondyle	▪ The flexor–pronator muscle mass should be divided parallel to the fibers.
Injury to the anterior vessels and nerves	▪ A Bennett retractor is placed between the anterior muscle and the capsule.
Section of the anterior band of the medial collateral ligament	▪ A small, narrow retractor is inserted to retract the medial collateral ligament, pulling it medially and posteriorly.

POSTOPERATIVE CARE

▪ If the neurologic examination findings in the recovery room are normal, a brachial plexus block is established and maintained with a continuous pump through a percutaneous catheter.

 ▪ The arm is elevated as much as possible, and mechanical continuous passive motion exercise is begun the day of surgery and adjusted to provide as much motion as pain or the machine itself allows.

 ▪ After 2 days the plexus block is discontinued, and, at day 3, the continuous passive motion machine is stopped.

▪ Physical therapy is not used, but a detailed program of splint therapy is prescribed.

 ▪ Adjustable splints are prescribed, depending on the motion before and after the procedure. The splints include a hyperextension or a hyperflexion brace, or both.

 ▪ A detailed discussion regarding heat, ice, and anti-inflammatory medication, along with a visual schedule for bracing, is provided.

 ▪ During the first 3 months, the patient sleeps with the splint adjusted to maximize flexion or extension, whichever is more needed; it should not be so uncomfortable as to prevent sleeping for at least 6 hours.

 ▪ Because the principal objective is to gain motion but to avoid pain, swelling, and inflammation, routine use of an anti-inflammatory medication is prescribed.

 ▪ Therapy with splints is continued for about 3 months, during which time the patient is seen at 2- to 4-week intervals, if possible.

 ▪ After 4 weeks, an arc of about 80 degrees of motion is obtained, and the amount of time that each splint is worn is gradually decreased.

 ▪ Splinting at night is continued for as long as 6 months if flexion contracture tends to recur when the splint is not used.

 ▪ Patients are advised that it may take a year to realize full correction.

OUTCOMES

▪ Recent reports on the results of surgical arthrolysis reveal an absolute gain in the flexion–extension arc between 30 and 60 degrees.[1,3–5,7,9–11,14–16,19,21]

 ▪ A functional arc of motion between 30 and 130 degrees is obtained in more than 50% of cases, and some improvement in motion in more than 90% of the cases has been reported in the literature.[1,3–5,7,9–11,14–16,19,21]

 ▪ In Europe, a combined lateral and medial approach has been used for many years, and gains in flexion arc have averaged between 40 and 72 degrees (in about 400 procedures).[1,3,7,14] Some preferred a posterior extensile approach if medial and lateral exposures are anticipated.

 ▪ The importance of sequential release of tissues has been emphasized, based on an experience with 44 of 46 patients

(95%) who were satisfied with such an approach.[13] The preoperative arc improved from 45 to 99 degrees.

■ The authors emphasize the need to release the exostosis and the collateral ligament when contracted, especially noting the need to release the posterior portion of the medial collateral ligament and decompress the ulnar nerve when ulnar nerve symptoms exist preoperatively.[13]

■ Using a medial approach, Wada et al[22] obtained improvement of the mean arc of movement of 64 degrees. A functional arc of flexion–extension (30 to 130 degrees) was obtained in 7 of the 14 elbows. None of the patients developed symptoms related to the ulnar nerve. According to those authors, the medial approach has several advantages over both the anterior and lateral approaches:

■ Pathologic changes in the posterior oblique bundle of the medial collateral ligament can be observed and excised under direct vision.

■ Anterior and posterior exposure is possible through one medial incision, through which a complete soft tissue release and excision of part of the olecranon and coronoid process can be undertaken if necessary. Additional lateral exposure is indicated only if the medial approach has proved to be inadequate.

■ In the medial approach, the ulnar nerve is routinely released and protected under direct vision, which decreases the risk of damage.

COMPLICATIONS

■ A most important emerging consideration of the proper treatment of elbow stiffness is the vulnerability of the ulnar nerve.

■ The most common cause of failure of treatment has been in patients whose preoperative ulnar nerve symptoms were not appreciated or addressed, or patients in whom ulnar nerve symptoms developed postoperatively without adequate treatment. This is attributable to traction neuritis caused by the abrupt increase in elbow flexion or extension during the operation.

■ Even in the absence of preoperative neurologic symptoms, the nerve may be compromised subclinically and become symptomatic as elbow motion increases after surgery. Therefore, all patients who have stiff elbows must be evaluated for the presence or absence of ulnar nerve symptoms.

■ Antuna et al[2] recommended that elbows with preoperative flexion limited to 90 to 100 degrees in which we expect to improve the motion by 30 or 40 degrees must be treated with inspection and often prophylactic decompression or translocation of the nerve, depending on the appearance of the nerve once the surgical procedure is finished.

■ Furthermore, all patients with preoperative ulnar nerve symptoms, even if they are mild, are treated with mobilization of the nerve.

■ These authors stated that manipulation of the elbow in the early postoperative period must be avoided if the nerve has not been decompressed or translocated.

REFERENCES

1. Allieu Y. Raideurs et arthrolyses du coude. Rev Chir Orthop 1989; 75(Suppl I):156–166.
2. Antuna SA, Morrey BF, Adams RA, et al. Ulnohumeral arthroplasty for primary degenerative arthritis of the elbow: long-term outcome and complications. J Bone Joint Surg Am 2002;84A:2168–2173.
3. Chantelot C, Fontaine C, Migaud H, et al. Etude retrospective de 23 arthrolyses du coude pour raideur post-traumatique: facteurs prédictifs du résultat. Rev Chir Orthop 1999;85:823–827.
4. Cikes A, Jolles BM, Farron A. Open elbow arthrolysis for posttraumatic elbow stiffness. J Orthop Trauma 2006;20:405–409.
5. Cohen MS, Hastings H II. Posttraumatic contracture of the elbow: operative release using a lateral collateral ligament sparing approach. J Bone Joint Surg Br 1998;80B:805–812.
6. Duke JB, Tessler RH, Dell PC. Manipulation of the stiff elbow with patient under anesthesia. J Hand Surg Am 1991;16:19–24.
7. Esteve P, Valentin P, Deburge A, et al. Raideurs et ankyloses post-traumatiques du coude. Rev Chir Orthop 1971;57(Suppl I):25–86.
8. Gelinas JJ, Faber KJ, Patterson SD, et al. The effectiveness of turnbuckle splinting for elbow constractures. J Bone Joint Surg Br 2000; 82B:74–78.
9. Husband JB, Hastings H. The lateral approach for operative release of post-traumatic contracture of the elbow. J Bone Joint Surg Am 1990;72A:1353–1358.
10. Itoh Y, Saegusa K, Ishiguro T, et al. Operation for the stiff elbow. Int Orthop 1989;13:263–268.
11. Mansat P, Morrey BF. The "column procedure": a limited surgical approach for the treatment of stiff elbows. J Bone Joint Surg Am 1998;80A:1603–1615.
12. Mansat P, Morrey BF, Hotchkiss RN. Extrinsic contracture: the column procedure, lateral and medial capsular releases. In Morrey BF, ed. The Elbow and Its Disorders, 3rd ed. Philaelphia: WB Saunders, 2000:447–456.
13. Marti RH, Kerkhoffs GM, Maas M, et al. Progressive surgical release of a posttraumatic stiff elbow: technique and outcome after 2–18 years in 46 patients. Acta Orthop Scand 2002;73:144–150.
14. Merle D'Aubigne R, Kerboul M. Les opérations mobilisatrices des raideurs et ankylose du coude. Rev Chir Orthop 1966;52:427–448.
15. Morrey BF. Post-traumatic contracture of the elbow: operative treatment, including distraction arthroplasty. J Bone Joint Surg Am 1990; 72A:601–618.
16. Morrey BF. The posttraumatic stiff elbow. Clin Orthop Relat Res 2005;431:26–35.
17. Morrey BF. The use of splints for the stiff elbows. Perspect Orthop Surg 1990;1:141–144.
18. O'Driscoll SW, Horii E, Morrey BF. Anatomy of the attachment of the medial ulnar collateral ligament. J Hand Surg Am 1992;17:164.
19. Park MJ, Kim HG, Lee JY. Surgical treatment of post-traumatic stiffness of the elbow. J Bone Joint Surg Br 2004;86B:1158–1162.
20. Rosenwasser M. Sequellae of fractures of the elbow. 11th Trauma Course, AIOD, Strasbourg, 2005.
21. Urbaniak JR, Hansen PE, Beissinger SF, et al. Correction of posttraumatic flexion contracture of the elbow by anterior capsulotomy. J Bone Joint Surg Am 1985;67A:1160–1164.
22. Wada T, Ishii S, Usui M, et al. The medial approach for operative release of post-traumatic contracture of the elbow. J Bone Joint Surg Br 2000;82B:68–73.
23. Weiss AP, Sachar K. Soft tissue contractures about the elbow. Hand Clin 1994;10:439–451.
24. Wilner P. Anterior capsulectomy for contractures of the elbow. J Int Coll Surg 1948;11:359–361.

Chapter 45

Total Elbow Arthroplasty for Rheumatoid Arthritis

Bryan J. Loeffler and Patrick M. Connor

DEFINITION

- Rheumatoid arthritis (RA) is a chronic, systemic, inflammatory condition of unknown etiology affecting 1% to 2% of the population.
  - It affects females two to three times as frequently as males, and the incidence increases with age, typically peaking between 35 and 50 years of age.
- Peripheral joints are often affected in a symmetric pattern.
- The elbow is affected in about 20% to 70% of patients with RA, with a wide spectrum of severity.
  - Ninety percent of these patients also have hand and wrist involvement, and 80% also have shoulder involvement.
- Juvenile rheumatoid arthritis (JRA) is diagnosed based on the presence of arthritis, synovitis, or both in at least one joint lasting for more than 6 weeks in an individual less than 16 years old.
- Compared with adult-onset RA, JRA is complicated by severe osseous destruction, deformity, and soft tissue contractures.

PATHOGENESIS

- The cause of RA is unknown.
  - Infectious etiologies have been proposed, but no microorganism has been proven to be causative.
  - Genetic and twin studies have demonstrated that a genetic predisposition clearly exists, and the disease is also associated with autoimmune phenomena.
- In patients with RA, numerous cell types, including B lymphocytes, CD4 T cells, mononuclear phagocytes, neutrophils, fibroblasts, and osteoclasts, have been shown to produce abnormally high levels of various cytokines, chemokines, and other inflammatory mediators.
- The result is inflammatory-mediated proliferation of synovial tissue, leading to soft tissue and finally bony destruction.

NATURAL HISTORY

- Overall, the disease progresses from predominantly soft tissue (synovial) inflammation to articular cartilage damage and ultimately subchondral and periarticular bone destruction.
- Manifestations of RA are initiated by synovitis and synovial hyperplasia resulting in pannus formation. This correlates with a boggy, inflamed elbow that is painful and with limited range of motion.
- Synovial proliferation coupled with joint capsule distention may produce a compressive neuropathy with pain, paresthesias, or weakness in the ulnar or radial nerve distributions, or both.
- Degeneration may progress to ligamentous erosion or disruption, or both. Clinically, the patient experiences progressive instability as ligamentous integrity is compromised.
  - It may affect the annular ligament and produce radial head instability with anterior displacement.
- Eventually the medial and lateral collateral ligament complexes may be disrupted, thus causing further instability.
- Prolonged synovitis leads to erosion of the cartilage followed by subchondral cyst and marginal osteophyte formation; the result is end-stage arthritis.
- End-stage disease is marked by severe damage to subchondral bone and gross joint instability. At this stage, patients typically have a painful, weak, and functionally unstable elbow.

PATIENT HISTORY AND PHYSICAL FINDINGS

- Patients typically describe a history of a swollen, tender, and warm elbow with diminished and painful range of motion.
  - This may be accompanied by a report of progressively declining function, constitutional complaints, and often polyarticular involvement.
- In early stages of the disease, the elbow may appear more boggy, with impressive soft tissue swelling and erythema about the elbow.
- As the disease progresses to later stages, soft tissue swelling may become less prominent, and the elbow becomes more stiff and painful.

Differences in Examination Findings Between Rheumatoid Arthritis and Juvenile Rheumatoid Arthritis

- Elbows affected by JRA obviously occur in younger patients as compared with elbows affected by RA.
- Patients with JRA also have stiffer elbows and therefore typically do not have instability.
- Often JRA patients have more joints affected by the rheumatoid process, but they also demonstrate a greater tolerance for pain.

IMAGING AND OTHER DIAGNOSTIC STUDIES

- Anteroposterior (AP) and lateral radiographs of the elbow are obtained to assess the degree of rheumatoid involvement and for preoperative planning (**FIG 1**). No further studies are typically required.

Classification

- Although several classification systems have been proposed, the most commonly used is the Mayo Radiographic Classification System (Table 1).[6]
  - It allows monitoring of disease progression and often correlates well with clinical examination findings and patients' functional limitations.
  - The grading system is based on bone quality, joint space, and bony architecture and delineates four grades of progression in order of increasing severity.

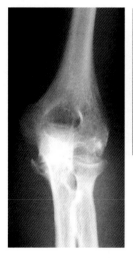

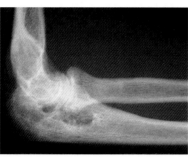

FIG 1 • Preoperative AP and lateral radiographs of a 38-year-old woman with juvenile rheumatoid arthritis demonstrating advanced changes of osteopenia, joint space narrowing, and changes in subchondral architecture.

DIFFERENTIAL DIAGNOSIS

- Calcium pyrophosphate deposition disease
- Osteoarthritis
- Polymyalgia rheumatica
- Psoriatic arthritis
- Systemic lupus erythematosus
- Fibromyalgia

NONOPERATIVE MANAGEMENT

- Optimal care of the patient with RA requires a team-based approach between the orthopaedic surgeon, rheumatologist, and physical therapists to coordinate the full gamut of nonsurgical and surgical treatment options.

Medical Therapy

- The medical management of RA continues to evolve at an impressive rate.
- The mainstays of medical therapy are the classes of drugs known as disease modifying antirheumatic drugs (DMARDs).
  - These include older agents such as gold salts as well as newer agents such as methotrexate, sulfasalazine, anti-tumor necrosis factor (anti-TNF) medications, and other immunomodulators. Such medications may be given alone or as part of combination therapy.
- Other medications prescribed to abate symptoms include nonsteroidal anti-inflammatories (NSAIDs) and steroids.
- Judicious use of intra-articular steroid injections also plays a role in symptom management.
- The importance of early referral to a rheumatologist for medical management cannot be overemphasized. Aggressive management of the synovitis can limit or delay the onset and severity of joint involvement. The most reliable and effective responses to the DMARDs are observed with therapy initiated in the early stages of the disease.

Physical Therapy

- The goal of physical therapy is to encourage range of motion, functional strength, and maintenance of activities of daily living. This is accomplished by activity modification, rest, ice, and gentle exercise.

- The primary objective of nonoperative management of the rheumatoid elbow is to minimize soft tissue swelling and to optimize range of motion, as preoperative range of motion is often predictive of postoperative total arc of motion after arthroscopic synovectomy as well as total elbow arthroplasty.

SURGICAL MANAGEMENT

- Surgical management of the rheumatoid elbow primarily consists of synovectomy and total elbow arthroplasty.

Surgical Management of the Elbow Before Total Elbow Arthroplasty

- For early disease states, excellent clinical results may be achieved with synovectomy performed using open or arthroscopic techniques.
- The goal of synovectomy is to relieve pain and swelling. Although this procedure has not necessarily been shown to alter the natural history of the disease, it reliably produces symptomatic relief for 5 or more years in the majority of cases performed on elbows in the early stages of the disease process.[3]
- The arthroscopic approach is advantageous over the more traditional open approach in that it is less invasive, is associated with less perioperative morbidity, and also allows predictable access to the sacciform recess. When open synovectomy is performed, the radial head must be excised to access and completely débride the diseased synovial tissue that exists in this region.
- Open synovectomy has traditionally been accompanied by radial head excision due to (1) ubiquitous radiocapitellar and proximal radioulnar joint articular destruction and (2) the need to surgically expose the sacciform recess for the requisite complete synovectomy.
  - It has been shown that routine radial head excision may predispose some patients with RA to increasing valgus elbow instability due to the loss of the stabilizing effect of the radial head (particularly if the medial collateral ligament is adversely affected by the rheumatoid process).[7]
  - Now that the entire synovial proliferation around the radial neck can be accessed arthroscopically, a combined arthroscopic radial head excision is performed only in patients with stable elbows and preoperative elbow symptoms with forearm rotation. Otherwise, a complete arthroscopic synovectomy is performed without excising the radial head.
- In addition, the minimally invasive nature of an arthroscopic approach yields the potential advantages of less pain, faster recovery with earlier range of motion, and a lower rate of infection compared with an open procedure.
- An arthroscopic anterior capsular release may be performed at the time of the arthroscopic synovectomy to improve elbow extension. A posterior olecranon-plasty may also be performed to re-establish normal concavity of the olecranon fossa.
- Posteromedial capsule release should be avoided to prevent the risk of iatrogenic ulnar nerve injury. If an elbow requires a release of the posterior capsule to regain elbow flexion (typically those with 100 degrees or less of preoperative flexion), then the surgeon should consider performing an open

Table 1	Mayo Radiographic Classification System		
Grade	**Radiographic Appearance**	**Description**	**Implications**
I		Synovitis in a normal-appearing joint with mild to moderate osteopenia	Often correlates with impressive soft tissue swelling on clinical examination
II		Loss of joint space, but maintenance of the subchondral architecture	Varying degrees of soft tissue swelling are present
III		Marked by complete loss of joint space	The synovitis has "burned out" and the elbow is typically more stiff
IIIA IIIB IV		Bony architecture is maintained Associated bone loss Severe bony destruction	Patients often have severe pain and functional limitations; functional instability may also be present if the joint's bony architecture is destroyed.
V		Presence of bony ankylosis of the ulnohumeral joint	Most commonly seen with juvenile rheumatoid arthritis

(Adapted from Morrey BF, Adams RA. Semiconstrained arthroplasty for the treatment of rheumatoid arthritis of the elbow. J Bone Joint Surg Am 1992;74A:479–490; and from Connor PM, Morrey BF. Total elbow arthroplasty in patients who have juvenile rheumatoid arthritis. J Bone Joint Surg Am 1998;80A:678–688.)

ulnar nerve decompression and subcutaneous transposition followed by complete posterior capsule release (including the posteromedial band of the medial collateral ligament).

Total Elbow Arthroplasty

■ This procedures is indicated primarily for advanced (grade III or IV) RA of the elbow in patients with significant pain and limitations in activities of daily living.

■ Absolute contraindications include active infection, upper extremity paralysis, and a patient's refusal or inability to abide by postoperative activity restrictions.

■ Relative contraindications include presence of infection at a remote site and a history of infected elbow or elbow prosthesis.

Preoperative Planning

■ AP and lateral radiographs of the elbow are reviewed to assess humeral bow and medullary canal diameter as well as angulation and diameter of the ulnar medullary canal.

  ■ Preoperative radiographic templates may be helpful to assess preoperative radiographic magnification.

■ In particular for JRA patients, the canal width may be very small, and therefore the surgeon must ensure that appropriately sized implants as well as intramedullary guidewires and reamers are available.

■ If an ipsilateral total shoulder arthroplasty has been performed or is anticipated, use of a 4-inch humeral implant and a humeral cement restrictor should be considered.

■ Preoperative limitations in forearm rotation may be due in part to ipsilateral distal radioulnar joint pathology. Thus, radiographs should also be obtained on the ipsilateral shoulder and wrist.

Implant Selection for Total Elbow Arthroplasty

■ Implant options have traditionally been classified as linked (semiconstrained) or unlinked.

  ■ These terms are being used with decreasing frequency, however, as unlinked implant designs have been developed that have precisely contoured components that create a degree of constraint.

  ■ Linked, semiconstrained implants have about 7 degrees of varus–valgus "play" and 7 degrees of axial rotation, while unconstrained implants consist of unlinked, resurfacing components.

  ■ The stability of unconstrained implants depends on soft tissue and ligamentous integrity, while such tissues may be destroyed by the rheumatoid inflammatory process or surgically released with semiconstrained implants without compromising stability.

■ Although no prospective comparisons between linked (semiconstrained) and unlinked implants have yet been performed, both appear to have similar survivorship records.

  ■ The semiconstrained design is preferred because it is equally effective in pain relief and in improving range of motion and function, while preserving stability without an observed increase in aseptic loosening.[5]

  ■ The Techniques section below focuses on implantation of a linked (semiconstrained) implant.

Sequence and Timing of Total Elbow Arthroplasty in the Patient with Polyarticular Involvement

■ Because RA typically affects multiple joint articulations, the timing of elbow arthroplasty should be considered with regard to the need for arthroplasties of other joints.

■ In general, the most disabling articulation should be addressed first. In the case of equivocal involvement in the elbow and a lower extremity joint in which arthroplasty is planned, the surgeon must consider the postoperative effects of surgery and plan accordingly.

■ If total elbow arthroplasty is performed first, at least 3 to 6 months should pass before lower extremity reconstruction is performed to allow adequate healing in the elbow. If the lower extremity will be addressed first, total elbow arthroplasty should be delayed until assistive ambulatory devices, which may put strain on the elbow, are no longer required.

  ■ Patients with total elbow arthroplasty should not weight bear with crutches. A walker may be used, provided it does not increase strain on the elbow. This may be achieved by raising the walker's arm rests to an appropriate height such that when the forearms are placed on the arm rests, the elbow may not be extended beyond 90 degrees of flexion.

Assessment of the Cervical Spine

■ Because nearly 90% of patients with RA have cervical spine involvement, about 30% of whom have significant subluxation, the cervical spine must be evaluated before any surgery in which intubation is likely.

  ■ Cervical spine radiographs should be routinely obtained.

  ■ If patients have neck pain, decreased range of motion, myelopathic symptoms, or radiographic evidence of instability, a magnetic resonance imaging (MRI) study should be ordered with concomitant referral to a spine surgeon to consider addressing the cervical spine pathology before elbow surgery.

Temporary Cessation of Medications Before Total Elbow Arthroplasty

■ Tumor necrosis factor (TNF) inhibitors affect the immune system and have been found to increase the risk of developing a prosthetic joint infection.

  ■ In general, anti-TNF agents are typically stopped for a short period before surgery and for about 2 weeks after surgery to reduce the risk of perioperative morbidity.

■ Patients on chronic NSAIDs should stop taking those medications about 2 weeks before surgery to reduce the risk of increased bleeding.

■ For patients on chronic steroids, stress-dose steroids may be required perioperatively.

■ Communications with the patient's rheumatologist and the anesthesiologist are imperative to coordinate these efforts.

Positioning

■ Intravenous antibiotics are administered 30 to 60 minutes before the incision.

■ The patient is placed in a supine position on the operating table with a rolled towel under the ipsilateral scapula.

■ The entire operative extremity and shoulder girdle is prepared and draped; a sterile tourniquet is placed.

■ The arm is exsanguinated and the tourniquet inflated.

Approach

■ Although multiple approaches may be used, the Bryan-Morrey approach (triceps–anconeus "slide") is preferred.

INCISION AND EXPOSURE

- A straight incision, measuring about 15 cm, is made centered between the lateral epicondyle and the tip of the olecranon.
- The ulnar nerve is carefully identified and isolated along the medial aspect of the triceps.
- Proximal neurolysis of the nerve is achieved by incising the fascia from the medial head of the triceps to the medial intermuscular septum and then mobilized to beyond its first motor branch distally by splitting the cubital tunnel retinaculum, which includes the band of Osborne (the fascia between the two heads of the flexor carpi ulnaris [FCU]) and the FCU fascia (**TECH FIG 1A,B**).
- The intermuscular septum is excised and a deep pocket of subcutaneous tissue over the flexor pronator group distally and anterior to the triceps proximally is created.
  - The nerve is then anteriorly transposed into this subcutaneous tissue pocket; it must be protected throughout the operation.
- An incision is then made over the medial aspect of the ulna between the anconeus and FCU. The anconeus is subperiosteally elevated off the ulna.
- The medial aspect of the triceps is then retracted along with the fibers of the posterior capsule to tension the Sharpey fibers at their ulnar insertion (**TECH FIG 1C,D**).

- These fibers are then sharply dissected, and the triceps in continuity with the anconeus is reflected from medial to lateral (**TECH FIG 1E**).
- The lateral ulnar collateral ligament complex is released from its humeral attachment, thus allowing the extensor mechanism to be completely reflected to the lateral aspect of the humerus (**TECH FIG 1F**).
- If ulnohumeral ankylosis is present, as is sometimes the case in JRA patients, a saw or osteotome may be necessary to re-establish the joint line and to create the osteotomy at the appropriate center of rotation of the ulnohumeral joint.
- The elbow is then progressively flexed, exposing the medial collateral ligament, which is then released subperiosteally from its humeral attachment (**TECH FIG 1G**).
- The tip of the olecranon is removed with a rongeur or oscillating saw, depending on the quality of the bone, and the humerus is then externally rotated and the elbow fully flexed to adequately expose the articulating surfaces of the humerus, ulna, and radial head.

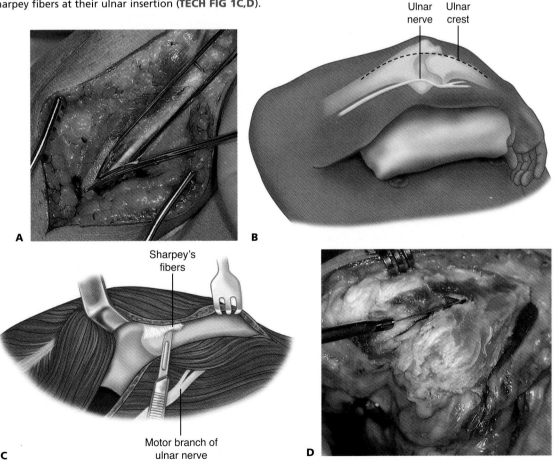

TECH FIG 1 • **A,B.** The ulnar nerve is identified along the medial border of the triceps, and a vessel loop is placed. **C,D.** Under tension, the medial and ulnar border of the triceps (**C**) and the anconeus (**D**) are incised from their insertions into the olecranon. *(continued)*

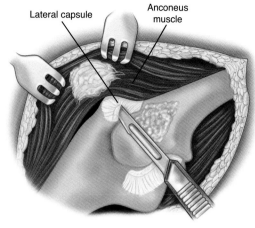

Lateral capsule

Anconeus muscle

E

TECH FIG 1 • (continued) E. The fibers of the extensor mechanism are further reflected laterally. **F.** The extensor mechanism is slid lateral to the lateral condyle. **G.** The medial collateral ligament is released to give the elbow maximal motion and to facilitate complete exposure of the ulnohumeral joint.

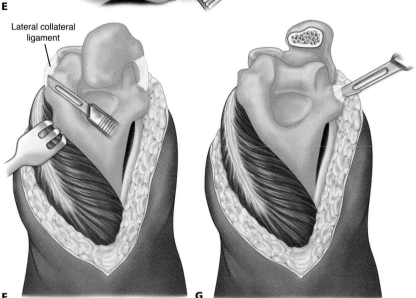

Lateral collateral ligament

F

G

HUMERAL PREPARATION

- The midportion of the trochlea is then removed, with an oscillating saw if the bone is dense or with a rongeur if the bone is soft, up to the roof of the olecranon fossa.
- The removed bone should be preserved for the anterior, distal humeral bone graft needed later in the procedure (**TECH FIG 2A**).
- The roof of the olecranon is entered with a rongeur or burr, and a small twist reamer is then used to identify the humeral medullary canal (**TECH FIG 2B,C**).
- For patients with severe stiffness, the effect of humeral shortening should be considered.
  - Hughes et al[4] developed a biomechanical model that demonstrated that resecting 1 cm or less of humeral bone has little effect on triceps strength.
    - With the elbow in 30 degrees of flexion, resecting 1 to 2 cm reduced triceps strength by 17% to 40%, while shortening of 3 cm reduced extension strength by 63%.
    - Therefore, the humerus should not be shortened by greater than 2 cm.

- An alignment stem is then placed down the canal. The handle of the alignment stem is then replaced by the humeral cutting jig (**TECH FIG 2D,E**).
- An oscillating saw is used to make oblique cuts along the edges of the jig, with the tip of the saw pointing away from the midline of the humerus to avoid cross-hatching at the junction of the column and the olecranon fossa (**TECH FIG 2F**).
  - Care must be taken as this area may be very thin in patients with RA, and thus susceptible to fracture.
- With the midportion of the trochlea removed, a thin rasp or intramedullary guide is used to again identify the humeral canal.
  - Progressive 6-inch rasps are typically used unless an ipsilateral shoulder arthroplasty has been performed or is planned (**TECH FIG 2G**).
    - In these cases, consider using a 4-inch humeral component.
- The anterior capsule is completely subperiosteally released from the anterior aspect of the humerus to accommodate the flange of the humeral component and to allow unencumbered postoperative elbow extension.

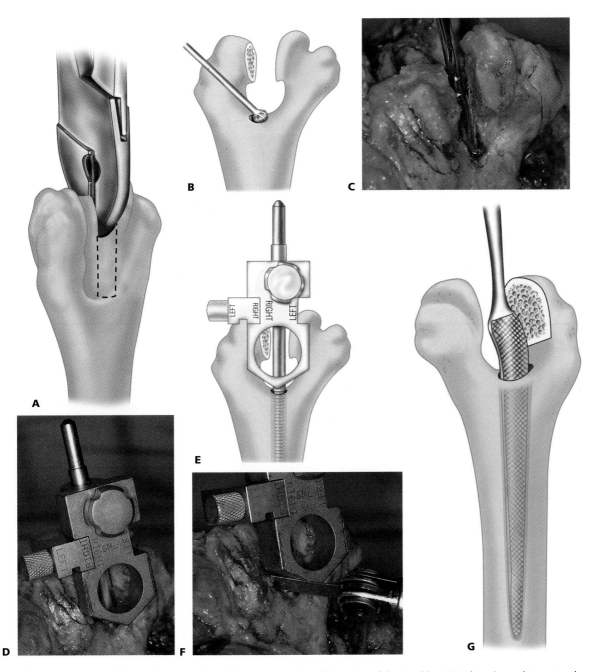

TECH FIG 2 • **A.** For soft bone, a rongeur is used to remove the midportion of the trochlea. **B.** A burr is used to enter the roof of the olecranon. **C.** Then a twist reamer is used to identify the medullary canal. **D,E.** The humeral cutting jig is aligned as a template for removal of the distal humeral articulation. **F.** An oscillating saw is placed at an oblique angle to the jig to accurately remove the articulating surface of the distal humerus while avoiding cross-hatching of the supracondylar columns. **G.** An appropriately sized rasp is used for the humeral canal.

ULNAR PREPARATION

- It is important to fully expose the greater sigmoid notch.
- A high-speed burr is angled 45 degrees relative to the axis of the ulnar shaft at the junction of the sigmoid fossa and coronoid to identify the ulnar medullary canal (**TECH FIG 3A,B**).
- Again, a twist reamer is used to further identify the canal, and an appropriately sized ulnar rasp is then inserted.
- The ulnar bow should be acknowledged and palpated while inserting the ulnar rasps to avoid ulnar perforation.
  - During advancement of the rasp, it is important to maintain proper rotation of the rasp so that the handle is perpendicular to the flat, dorsal aspect of the proximal ulna (**TECH FIG 3C,D**).
- Alternatively, reaming should be considered if the canal is very small, as may be the case in JRA patients.

- The ulnar canal is thus prepared, and the ulnar component is inserted to the depth such that the center of the ulnar component is midway between the tips of the olecranon and coronoid to reproduce the elbow's axis of rotation (**TECH FIG 3E**).
- A rongeur is then used to remove the tip of the coronoid.
- Because proximal radioulnar arthritis is ubiquitous in patients with RA and JRA, and the Conrad-Morrey total elbow arthroplasty does not require proximal radioulnar and radiocapitellar reconstruction, a radial head excision is performed.
- This may be performed by rotating the forearm and using a rongeur to progressively excise the radial head from an axial orientation, while holding the elbow in full flexion.

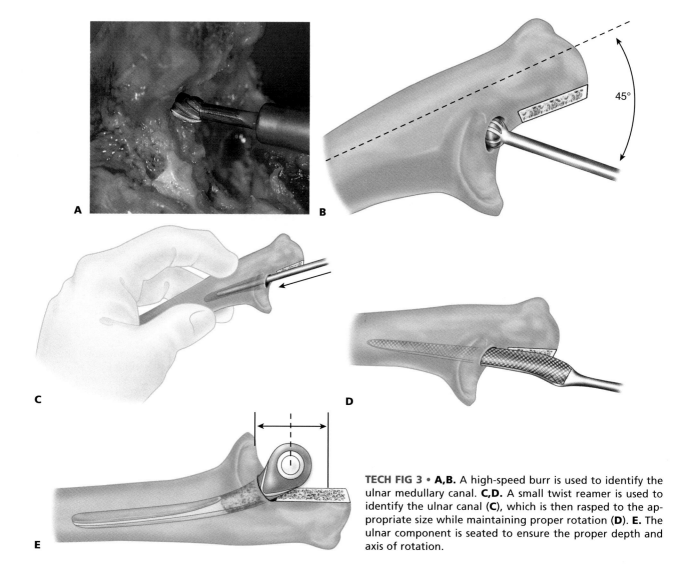

TECH FIG 3 • A,B. A high-speed burr is used to identify the ulnar medullary canal. **C,D.** A small twist reamer is used to identify the ulnar canal (**C**), which is then rasped to the appropriate size while maintaining proper rotation (**D**). **E.** The ulnar component is seated to ensure the proper depth and axis of rotation.

TRIAL REDUCTION

- The humeral component is then inserted and a trial reduction is performed.
- Range of motion is tested and should be full without limitation in the flexion–extension plane.
    - If range of motion is limited owing to inadequate soft tissue release, this should be addressed at this time.
- The components should also be evaluated for bony impingement, which may commonly occur posteriorly (olecranon impingement on the humerus) or anteriorly (coronoid tip on the anterior flange of the humeral component; **TECH FIG 4**).
    - Any impinging bone should be removed with a rongeur.
- After satisfactory trial reduction, the provisional components are removed.

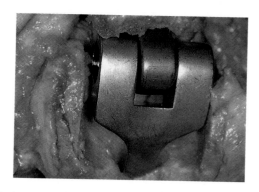

TECH FIG 4 • A trial reduction of the components is performed and range of motion is assessed to evaluate for bony impingement.

CEMENTING

- Both medullary canals are then pulse lavaged and dried.
- Based on the trial components used, the length of the cement applicator is measured to equal that of the humeral component.
    - The tip of the applicator is cut at this level to ensure appropriate depth of the cement down the humeral canal (**TECH FIG 5**).

- It is recommended that cementing of the components be performed simultaneously.
    - Two packs of cement with antibiotics are mixed and injected with a runny consistency.
    - The humeral cement is placed first, followed by the ulnar cement and then the ulnar component.
    - Remove excess cement.

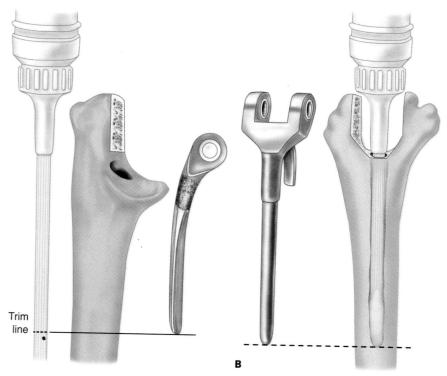

Trim
line

A

B

TECH FIG 5 • Simultaneous cementing of the humeral and ulnar medullary canals is recommended.

HUMERAL COMPONENT AND BONE GRAFT

- A small (about 2 cm × 2 cm and 2- to 4-mm thick) piece of the removed trochlea is used for the anterior bone graft.
- This bone graft is wedged between the anterior aspect of the humerus and the flange as the humeral component is placed (**TECH FIG 6**).
- This provides the humeral component with rotational stability as well as additional stability in the AP plane.
- Once again, excess cement is removed at this time.

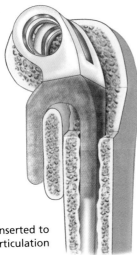

TECH FIG 6 • The humeral component is inserted to the optimal depth that allows proper articulation with the ulnar component.

ASSEMBLY AND IMPACTION

- The components are then linked with the use of two interlocking cross-pins, which are placed from opposite directions (**TECH FIG 7A**).
- If humeral bowing or a small canal exists, a slight bow can be placed in the proximal aspect of the humeral component to ensure proper fit (**TECH FIG 7B,C**).
- After coupling the prosthesis, the components must be seated; the elbow is flexed to 90 degrees and the humeral component is then impacted such that the distal aspect of the humeral component is roughly at or slightly proximal to the contour of the distal capitellum (**TECH FIG 7D,E**).
- Range of motion is checked and a full arc of motion is confirmed.
- The elbow is taken through several arcs of flexion—extension to "normalize" the rotational version of components to one another.
- Hold the elbow in full extension until the cement cures.

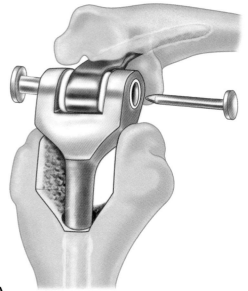

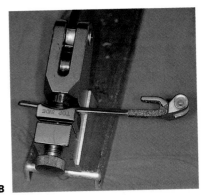

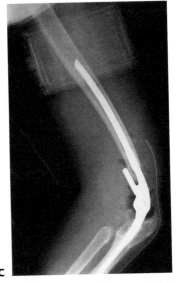

A **B** **C**

TECH FIG 7 • **A.** The ulnar and humeral components are linked by two interlocking cross-pins, which are placed from opposite sides. **B,C.** A slight bow may be created in the proximal aspect of the humeral component if humeral bowing or a small canal is present. *(continued)*

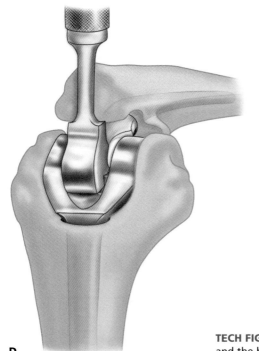

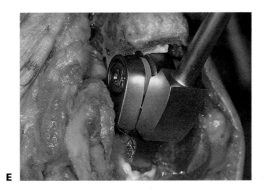

D

E

TECH FIG 7 • *(continued)* **D,E.** The elbow is flexed to 90 degrees and the humeral component is then impacted.

TRICEPS REATTACHMENT

- Small cruciate and transverse drill holes are placed through the olecranon at the site of triceps reattachment, and a heavy, nonabsorbable suture is placed on a Keith needle and then brought through the distal medial cruciate drill hole and out the proximal lateral hole (**TECH FIG 8A–C**).

- The elbow is flexed to about 60 degrees and the extensor mechanism is reduced over the tip of the olecranon; consider slightly overreducing the extensor mechanism medially to minimize the potential for postoperative lateral subluxation.

- The suture is woven through the triceps tendon in a locking, crisscross pattern such that the suture emerges at the proximal medial hole (**TECH FIG 8D**).

- The suture is then passed through this hole and out the distal medial hole such that it is located directly across from the initial suture end.

- These suture ends are then passed again through the forearm extensor fascia and tied together.

- Two reinforcing sutures are then passed through the transverse holes and extensor fascia before being tied together.

- Avoid knots directly over the subcutaneous border of the proximal ulna.

- The tourniquet is then deflated and hemostasis is achieved.

- The medial soft tissue extensor mechanism is then reapproximated.

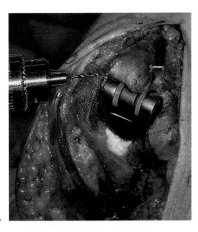

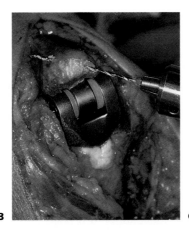

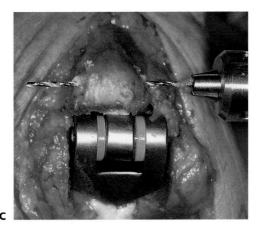

A

B

C

TECH FIG 8 • Cruciate (**A,B**) and transverse (**C**) drill holes are placed in the ulna for triceps reattachment. *(continued)*

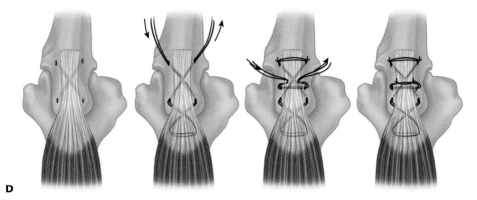

D

TECH FIG 8 • *(continued)* **D.** Suture is passed through the proximal ulna and then woven through the triceps tendon before being tied together.

ULNAR NERVE TRANSPOSITION AND WOUND CLOSURE

- The protected nerve is in the subcutaneous tissue pocket previously created, and dermal sutures are placed to protect and secure the nerve (**TECH FIG 9**).
- Wounds are closed in layers, and a drain is placed. Staples are used to close the skin.
- A volar splint is placed with the elbow in full extension, making sure to adequately pad the anterior aspect of the splint both proximally and distally to prevent skin breakdown.

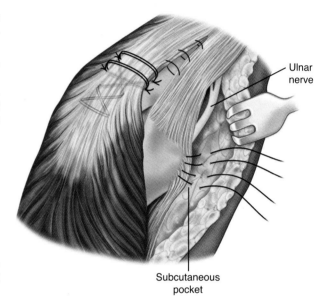

Ulnar nerve

Subcutaneous pocket

TECH FIG 9 • The ulnar nerve is transposed into the subcutaneous tissue of the medial epicondylar region and secured with sutures in the dermal layer.

PEARLS AND PITFALLS

Approach and exposure	■ Take your time with the Bryan-Morrey approach; maintaining subperiosteal elevation of the extensor mechanism will make for a better postoperative extensor mechanism repair. ■ Obtain complete ulnohumeral dissociation before bony preparation. This includes complete releases of the lateral ulnar collateral ligament and medial collateral ligament complexes, and a complete anterior capsule release. ■ Consider reflection of common flexors or extensors if severe deformities or arthrofibrosis is present.
Humeral preparation	■ Shorten the humerus by 1 cm or less to augment postoperative range of motion without compromising strength. ■ Use a burr distally to open up the humeral canal if needed, rather than forcing with rasps.
Radial and ulnar preparation	■ Excise the radial head and the tip of the coronoid. ■ Always palpate the ulna and consider the ulnar bow before ulnar preparation to avoid perforation. ■ Have guidewires and reamers (5.0, 5.5, 6.0, 6.5) available if needed.
Cementing	■ Review the cement technique and order mentally before proceeding; use cement that does not rapidly set.
Triceps reattachment	■ Overreduce the triceps–anconeus repair medially.
Postoperative care	■ Use a postoperative extension splint for 24 to 36 hours. ■ Make all efforts to reduce postoperative swelling.

POSTOPERATIVE CARE

▪ Postoperatively, the anteriorly placed splint maintains the elbow in full extension for about 24 to 36 hours.

▪ The elbow is elevated overnight and on postoperative day 1.

▪ The drain is removed on postoperative day 1 or when output is less than 30 mL in an 8-hour period.

▪ After splint removal, open-chain active-assisted range of motion is allowed. A formal physical therapy consultation is not usually required.

▪ The patient is restricted to no pushing and no overhead activities for 3 months to protect the triceps. In addition, no repetitive lifting of objects heavier than 5 pounds and no lifting greater than 10 pounds in a single event is allowed for life.

▪ A collar and cuff are provided for comfort.

OUTCOMES

▪ Successful outcomes for total elbow arthroplasty are judged based on relief of pain and improved range of motion, stability, and function.

▪ The Mayo Elbow Performance Score assigns numeric values to each of these categories to produce scores for each of these criteria as well as an overall score.[6] Outcomes are often compared using this system.

▪ Total elbow arthroplasty for RA

▪ In the largest study with the longest follow-up in the literature, Gill and Morrey[2] reported 86% good or excellent results with a 13% reoperation rate on 69 patients with RA treated with a semiconstrained total elbow arthroplasty. Forty-four of these patients were followed for more than 10 years.

▪ The prosthetic survival rate was 92.4% at 10 years of follow-up, thus approaching the success of lower extremity arthroplasty.

▪ Total elbow arthroplasty for JRA

▪ Connor and Morrey[1] reported 87% good or excellent results on 19 patients (24 elbows) followed for a mean of 7.4 years.

▪ The mean improvement in the Mayo Elbow Performance Score was 59 points, 96% had little or no pain, and there was no evidence of loosening in any prostheses at the latest follow-up.

▪ The mean flexion–extension arc of motion improved by only 27 degrees (from 67 to 90 degrees) in this study, but these outcomes were reported before shortening of the humerus for severely contracted elbows was routinely performed.

COMPLICATIONS

▪ Infection
▪ Aseptic loosening
▪ Mechanical failure
▪ Short term
▪ Long term
▪ Ulnar nerve injury
▪ Triceps weakness or avulsion
▪ Ulnar component fracture
▪ Ulnar fracture
▪ Wound healing problems

REFERENCES

1. Connor PM, Morrey BF. Total elbow arthroplasty in patients who have juvenile rheumatoid arthritis. J Bone Joint Surg Am 1998;80A:678–688.

2. Gill DR, Morrey BF. The Coonrad-Morrey total elbow arthroplasty in patients who have rheumatoid arthritis: a ten- to fifteen-year follow-up study. J Bone Joint Surg Am 1998;80A:1327–1335.

3. Horiuchi K, Momohara S, Tomatsu T, et al. Arthroscopic synovectomy of the elbow in rheumatoid arthritis. J Bone Joint Surg Am 2002;84A:342–347.

4. Hughes RE, Schneeberger AG, An KN, et al. Reduction of triceps muscle force after shortening of the distal humerus: a computational model. J Shoulder Elbow Surg 1997;6:444–448.

5. Little CP, Graham AJ, Karatzas G, et al. Outcomes of total elbow arthroplasty for rheumatoid arthritis: comparative study of three implants. J Bone Joint Surg Am 2005;87A:2439–2448.

6. Morrey BF, Adams RA. Semiconstrained arthroplasty for the treatment of rheumatoid arthritis of the elbow. J Bone Joint Surg Am 1992;74A:479–490.

7. Rymaszewski LA, Mackay I, Amis AA, et al. Long-term effects of excision of the radial head in rheumatoid arthritis. J Bone Joint Surg Br 1979;66B:109–113.

Chapter 46

Elbow Replacement for Acute Trauma

Srinath Kamineni

DEFINITION

▪ Most comminuted elbow fractures have significant associated soft tissue injuries, which are often of equal or greater importance to the bony element.

▪ The key point in determining how to treat acute elbow fractures is to assume that all fractures will be anatomically reduced and fixed.

▪ An acute elbow replacement should be considered only if it is felt that open reduction and internal fixation is unlikely to achieve a predictably good functional outcome.

▪ In the vast majority of cases, elbow replacements for the treatment of acute fractures should be limited to the physiologically elderly patient with low demands and osteoporotic bone stock.

ANATOMY

▪ The bony anatomy of the elbow consists of the distal humerus, proximal ulna, and proximal radius.

▪ Important soft tissue stabilizers include the medial and lateral ligamentous complexes and surrounding musculature, especially the brachialis, common flexor and common extensor masses, and triceps.

▪ The ulnar nerve is tethered to the medial condylar–epicondylar fragment by the cubital tunnel retinaculum distally and the arcade of Struthers proximally.

PATHOGENESIS

▪ Elbow injuries are often the result of direct impact—for example, a direct blow on the elbow during a fall.

▪ Knowing the energy of the fracture is important to gauge the likelihood of associated injuries.

▪ Less energy is required to create a comminuted fracture in elderly and osteoporotic individuals, but muscular injuries of the triceps and brachialis are common, with a subsequent influence on the functional outcome.

▪ The ulnar nerve displaces with the medial fragment. As a consequence, the nerve may kink, leading to a local nerve injury. Nerve lacerations are an uncommon consequence of comminuted distal humeral fractures.

NATURAL HISTORY

▪ Most distal humeral fractures are treatable with either open reduction and internal fixation (ORIF) or nonoperative management. The challenging fracture subgroups are those that involve the articular surfaces and are comminuted.

▪ Many direct and indirect soft tissue complications may ensue, including neurovascular entrapment,[2,6] muscle tears leading to myositis ossificans,[6,11,15] and soft tissue contracture with joint stiffness.

▪ There is some evidence to suggest that congruently reducing and fixing a comminuted intra-articular distal humeral fracture

does not eliminate the risk of posttraumatic arthritis,[7] although, where possible, ORIF should remain the primary goal.

PATIENT HISTORY AND PHYSICAL FINDINGS

▪ The physical examination (**FIG 1**) should be performed gently in the presence of fractures, especially when comminution suggests the possibility of neurovascular injury if the examination is too vigorous.

▪ A complete examination of the elbow should also include evaluation of associated injuries. It should begin away from the elbow, progressing toward it.

▪ The following associated injuries should be ruled out:

▪ Distal radial and scaphoid fractures: Since the most common mechanism of injury is a fall onto an outstretched hand, the energy transfer of the fall begins in the extended wrist, through the distal radius and scaphoid. Direct palpation of the distal radius should be done and anatomic snuffbox tenderness should be elicited. Palpation of the scaphoid tubercle and ulnar and radial deviation of the wrist may also identify a scaphoid injury.

▪ Distal radioulnar joint disruption: Ballottement of the ulnar head should be done in the volar and dorsal directions, in pronation and supination. A disrupted joint is often painful with such ballottement, and the ulnar head may be prominent with the forearm in pronation.

▪ Fracture extension beyond the elbow: The examiner should palpate the ulna shaft, along its subcutaneous border, from the wrist to the olecranon.

▪ Interosseous membrane injury: Palpating the interval between the bones of the forearm is not a sensitive examination but can raise suspicion for an Essex-Lopresti injury,

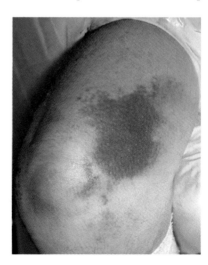

FIG 1 • Typical appearance of an elbow with an underlying fracture with extensive swelling and bruising.

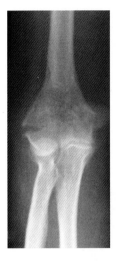
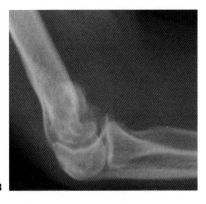

FIG 2 • Standard AP and lateral plain radiographs.

leading to further imaging. If an interosseous membrane disruption is present, this will influence the type of implant used for elbow replacement (one with a radial head replacement), but the pathology is not commonly described.

IMAGING AND DIAGNOSTIC STUDIES

■ Plain radiographs, including anteroposterior (AP) and lateral views (**FIG 2**) of the elbow and both wrists, should be obtained. The elbow view may have to be taken in a protective splint or plaster back-slab for patient comfort.
■ Elbow radiographs will allow initial assessment of the degree of comminution and may indicate the presence of decreased bone mineral density.
■ Bilateral wrist views will indicate the presence of an axial (interosseous membrane) injury if the ulnar head is in positive variance compared to the contralateral uninjured wrist.
■ Plain tomograms are of use in improving the understanding of the fracture configuration, but an alternative would be a computed tomography (CT) scan. With the latter the surgeon can view a three-dimensional reconstruction, which is a useful surgical planning tool.
■ If there is evidence on physical examination of a neurologic injury, it is prudent to document its extent with a carefully performed neurologic examination.

DIFFERENTIAL DIAGNOSIS

■ Nonunion
■ Ligamentous disruption
■ Fracture-dislocation

NONOPERATIVE MANAGEMENT

■ The "bag-of-bones" technique is a nonoperative method of treatment described by Eastwood that encourages the compressive molding of the comminuted distal humeral fracture fragments.
■ Subsequent rehabilitation with collar and cuff support achieves substandard but acceptable results only in the elderly and debilitated group of patients who have almost no demand on elbow function.
■ This type of treatment does not achieve acceptable results with respect to stability and strength in younger patients.

SURGICAL MANAGEMENT

Open Reduction and Internal Fixation

■ ORIF has been widely documented for comminuted fractures of the distal humerus.
■ Some reported series demonstrate good results with fixation of such challenging fractures, with better results predominantly in the younger age groups.[12,16] Rarely are good results achieved in the elderly, osteoporotic group.[7]
■ Many series report less-than-satisfactory outcomes in the elderly treated by operative fixation.[12]
■ A direct comparison of internal fixation to primary total elbow replacement in the elderly osteoporotic group revealed that replacement produced no poor results and no need for revision surgery at 2 years of follow-up. The internal fixation group produced three poor results requiring revision to a total elbow replacement.[4]

Elbow Arthroplasty

■ When a distal humerus fracture is not reconstructable, arthroplasty becomes a valid treatment option.
■ Elbow replacement following a failed attempt at fixation has proven to have a significantly worse outcome than if the arthroplasty was performed initially.[3]
■ There are a number of studies that support the concept of an acute total elbow arthroplasty in select patients with comminuted fractures of the distal humerus.[1,3,9]
■ The more traditional form of replacement for the elderly and low-demand population with an unreconstructable distal humerus fracture is the total elbow arthroplasty.
■ A more recent innovation has been the replacement of the distal humerus (hemiarthroplasty) to preserve an intact ulna and radial head.[13] This procedure is not FDA approved and so should be considered experimental and not for general consideration, especially since the elbow joint is variable and highly congruent in its topography, which differs from many of the standard implants used for acute fractures.

Indications and Contraindications

■ Indications for acute total elbow arthroplasty
  ■ Comminuted, unreconstructable distal humerus fracture
  ■ Physiologically elderly patient
  ■ Low-demand patient
■ Indications for acute elbow hemiarthroplasty
  ■ Unreconstructable distal humeral fracture (C3)
  ■ Unreconstructable combined fractures of capitellum and trochlea
  ■ Very low bicondylar T fracture of distal humerus
    ■ Young patient
    ■ Active patient
  ■ Repairable or intact collateral ligaments (may require reconstruction of the medial and lateral supracondylar columns)
  ■ Repairable or intact radial head
■ Absolute contraindications for acute joint replacement
  ■ Infection (overt)
  ■ Lack of soft tissue coverage (skin, muscle)
■ Relative contraindications for acute joint replacement
  ■ Infection in distant body part
  ■ Contaminated wound
  ■ Neurologic injury involving the elbow flexors

Preoperative Planning

■ Standard radiographs should be obtained (AP and lateral).

■ If doubt exists regarding the ability to anatomically repair the fracture, then a CT scan should be requested to assess the degree of comminution and the fracture line orientation.

■ An assessment of humeral shaft bone loss is important in planning the implant design that might be considered. If the degree of loss is greater than the articular condylar fragments, an implant that has the ability to restore humeral length will be more appropriate. If an unreconstructable fracture of the humeral articular surfaces without humeral shaft bone loss is encountered, an implant with the ability to resurface the articular surfaces as a hemiarthroplasty or a resurfacing ulnotrochlear replacement can be considered, but the former implantation technique should be regarded as an off-label and experimental procedure.

■ Humeral shaft length loss of 2 cm can be tolerated and standard implants used.

■ Humeral shaft length loss of greater than 2 cm can be restored with implant designs with anterior flanges, especially those with extended flanges that allow restoration of humeral length.

■ The surgeon should assess the intramedullary canal dimensions of the humerus and ulna. This will help to plan the requirement of extra-small diameter.

■ Neurovascular status of the limb should be fully assessed and documented in the clinical notes.

Patient Positioning

■ Two methods of patient positioning can be used, depending on surgeon comfort and the access required:

  ■ Supine: The arm is draped for maximum maneuverability. During the procedure the arm is supported on a large rolled towel placed on the patient's upper thorax, carefully avoiding the endotracheal tube, stabilized by an assistant. In this position the surgeon stands on the side of the patient's injured limb (**FIG 3A**).

  ■ Lateral decubitus: The arm is positioned on an arm support, thereby minimizing the need for an assistant, but this set-up is less maneuverable. In this position the surgeon stands on the opposite side of the patient's injured limb (**FIG 3B**).

Surgical Approach

■ Two main surgical approaches are useful for acute total elbow arthroplasty:

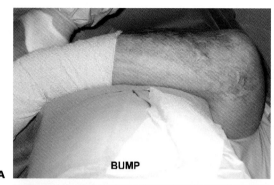

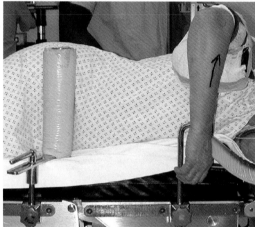

FIG 3 ● **A.** Patient positioned in a supine position. The elbow is isolated and placed on a roll of towel placed on the patient's chest, and stabilized by an assistant. The surgeon must take care to avoid the neck and anesthetic equipment. **B.** Patient positioned in a lateral decubitus position with the elbow draped over an arm support.

  ■ Triceps-splitting approach
  ■ Bryan-Morrey approach

■ The triceps should be carefully managed in either approach, and it often has a thin tendon, especially in older patients and those with rheumatoid arthritis. The triceps tendon should be dissected from the olecranon with a small curved scalpel blade, maintained perpendicular to the interface between the tendon and bone.

INCISION AND DISSECTION

■ Make a midline longitudinal skin incision (**TECH FIG 1A**), with a gentle curve to avoid the olecranon weight-bearing prominence. Extend the incision 5 cm distal to and proximal to the prominence of the olecranon tip.

■ Develop the full-thickness medial and lateral skin flaps (**TECH FIG 1B**) and define the medial and lateral borders of the triceps (**TECH FIG 1C,D**).

■ At the medial border, define and partially neurolyse the ulnar nerve, and mark and handle it with a tied ves-

sel loop (without an attached hemostat, since its constant weight may cause inadvert nerve injury) (**TECH FIG 1E**).

■ With the nerve visualized and handled to safety, remain in the medial gutter to extend the dissection distally to define the medial fracture fragment. Transect the medial collateral ligament in its entirety, and remove all soft tissue from this bony fragment and remove the latter (**TECH FIG 1F**).

TECHNIQUES

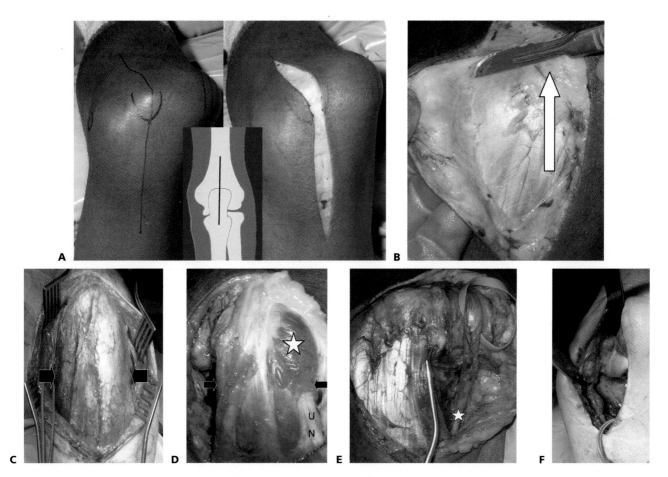

TECH FIG 1 • A. Skin incision is posterior longitudinal, with or without a small diversion to avoid the "point" of the olecranon. **B.** Raising the skin should aim to maintain the full thickness of the flaps by using the "flat knife" technique. **C.** The medial and lateral borders of the triceps are defined (*arrows*). **D.** This patient had an anconeus epitrochlearis (*star*) in relation to the ulna nerve (UN). **E.** A vessel loop is used to maneuver the nerve without an attached clip. **F.** The medial fragment of the fracture is removed once all the soft tissues are released from it, and the nerve is gently retracted to ensure tension-free removal.

TRICEPS MANAGEMENT

Triceps Preserving

- With the ulnar nerve gently medially retracted, use a periosteal elevator to define the plane between the triceps and the posterior humerus, from the medial to the lateral border, exiting posterior to the lateral intermuscular septum. Use this elevator to lift the triceps, with blunt dissection, by sliding the shaft of the elevator proximal and distal in the interface (**TECH FIG 2A**).
- Develop the lateral triceps–lateral intermuscular septum margin and resect the lateral fracture fragments, having firstly cleared them of soft tissue attachments (**TECH FIG 2B**).
  - While in the lateral corridor, visualize the radial head and resect sufficient head to prevent abutment on the prosthesis.
- From the lateral margin of the humeral shaft, raise the brachialis from 2 to 3 cm of the anterior surface.

Modified Bryan-Morrey Approach

- Preserving the integrity of the triceps insertion makes component insertion more difficult. An alternative approach for managing the triceps is to reflect it from the tip of the olecranon from medial to lateral, thereby improving exposure (**TECH FIG 3**).
- Define the medial triceps border and dissect the ulna nerve free from its connections, while protecting it in a vessel loop. The nerve is transposed into a subcutaneous pocket.
- The medial triceps is dissected to its ulna attachment. Release the triceps from the medial condylar fragments and transect the medial collateral ligament. Free the medial fragments from soft tissue attachments and remove the medial fragments between the triceps and a gently anteriorly retracted ulnar nerve.

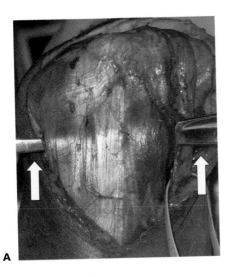
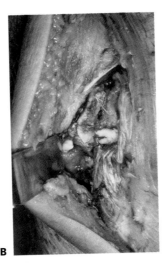

TECH FIG 2 • A. A periosteal elevator is introduced between the triceps and the humeral shaft and the two structures are separated by sliding the elevator proximally and then distally to the level of the triceps insertion. **B.** The lateral corridor is defined and lateral fragments are removed.

- Develop the interval between the anconeus and flexor carpi ulnaris along the subcutaneous border of the ulna.
- The triceps tendon is sharply elevated from the olecranon, in continuity with the anconeus, and subluxed laterally. Take care to release the Sharpey fibers adjacent to the bone in order to retain the flap thickness. Further access is

afforded by raising the anconeus from its ulnar attachment while maintaining its attachment distally.

- As the triceps is reflected laterally, the lateral condylar fragments are identified and removed by releasing the lateral collateral ligament and common extensor tendon.

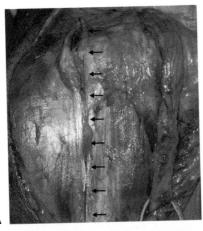
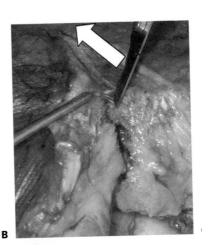
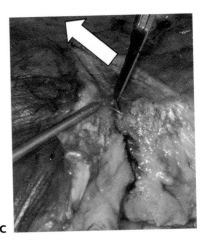
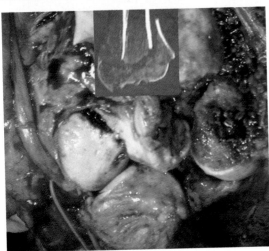

TECH FIG 3 • A. The triceps is split through its central tendon, in line with the fibers. The tendinous portion is dissected from the olecranon to gain access to the ulna. **B,C.** To dissect the Sharpey fibers off the ulna, the surgeon uses the scalpel parallel to the ulna surface and maintains the release directly adjacent to the bone. **D.** Comminuted distal humeral fracture in an osteoporotic elderly woman, with CT imaging confirming significant articular comminution. This is the view through the triceps split.

BONE PREPARATION

- Identify the olecranon fossa (if any part of it still exists). This landmark is the seating point for the base of the anterior flange of the Coonrad-Morrey humeral component (**TECH FIG 4A**). If the olecranon fossa is not present owing to a greater degree of comminution, an extended-flange humeral component can be used.
- Release the anterior capsule and any soft tissue from the anterior surface of the distal humerus. This provides a site for the anterior humeral bone graft.
- The posterior flat surface of the humerus is identified since this plane approximates the axis of rotation of the distal humerus (**TECH FIG 4B**). Humeral canal preparation is completed with the canal broaches provided with the implant system being used.
- The ulnar canal preparation commences with removal of the tip of the olecranon. The intramedullary canal is entered at the base of the coronoid (**TECH FIG 4C,D**).
- The entry point is enlarged up toward the coronoid with a burr to allow easier component insertion without cortical abutment, which leads to malalignment (**TECH FIG 4E**).

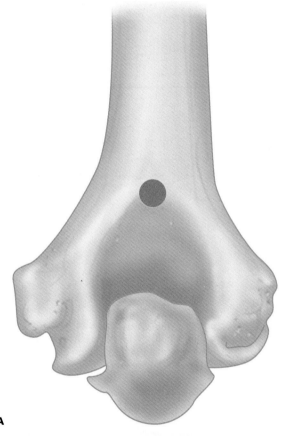

A

TECH FIG 4 • A. The humeral component entry point, the apex of the olecranon fossa, is identified and humeral canal preparation is commenced by opening the canal with a bone nibbler or burr. **B.** The posterior flat surface of the humeral shaft is identified and the component is aligned. **C,D.** Ulnar canal preparation is commenced by opening the canal at the base of the coronoid process with a drill or burr. *(continued)*

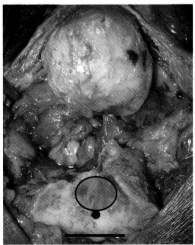

B

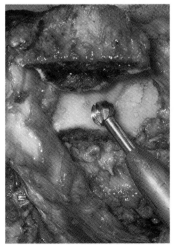

C

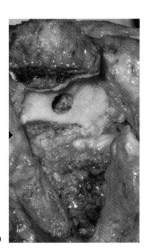

D

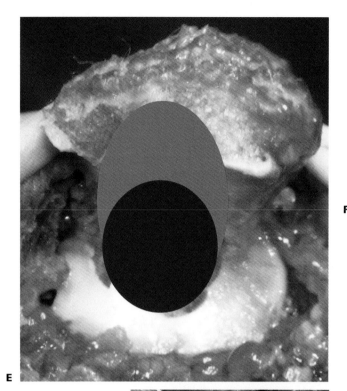

E

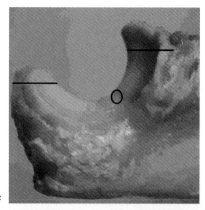

F

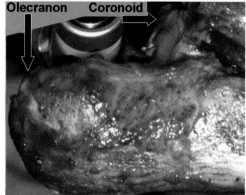

Olecranon   Coronoid

G

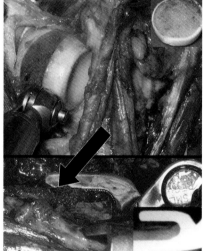

H

TECH FIG 4 • *(continued)* **E.** The trajectory of the ulnar component (*black ring*) is prepared by rasping the entry track posteriorly into the ulna with a rasp or bone nibbler (*gray crescent*). **F,G.** The tip of the coronoid should be resected sufficiently to prevent abutment on the humeral flange during full flexion. Also shown are the resections of the olecranon and the entry point for the ulnar stem insertion. **H.** The partially resected radial head is used as a bone graft for incorporation behind the humeral flange.

- During intramedullary preparation, the broaches must parallel the subcutaneous border of the ulna. This ensures that the track of insertion of the ulna parallels the intramedullary canal.

- The tip of the coronoid is removed to avoid impingement during terminal flexion (**TECH FIG 4F,G**).
- The radial head does not need to be resected if there is no disease of the proximal radioulnar joint (**TECH FIG 4H**).

IMPLANT INSERTION AND TENSIONING

- With the canal preparation completed (**TECH FIG 5A**), including pulse lavage of the medullary canals and cement restrictor placement, implant insertion can commence (**TECH FIG 5B,C**).
- Humeral insertion
  - When bone loss is at or below the level of the olecranon fossa, standard humeral insertion can occur. If bone loss occurs above the olecranon fossa

(greater than 2 cm), then humeral length must be restored.
- Prepare a wedge-shaped bone "cookie" for placement behind the humeral flange.
- Inject antibiotic cement into the humerus.
- When inserting the humeral component, place the bone graft behind the anterior flange. Because the humeral condyles have been resected, the implant can

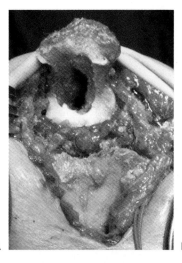
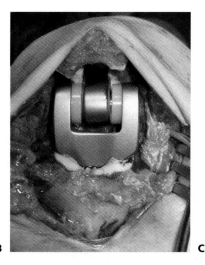
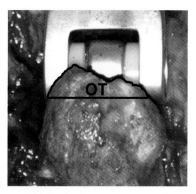

TECH FIG 5 • A. The prepared bony surfaces, with the fracture fragments removed, and just before implantation. **B.** The linked Coonrad-Morrey replacement is cemented and linked in situ. **C.** If in terminal extension there is abutment of the tip of the olecranon on the implant, the surgeon resects the olecranon tip (OT) but should not approach the triceps insertion footprint.

be completely seated and coupled once the cement has hardened.
- Maintain the component orientation relative to the posterior flat surface of the distal humerus.
- Seat the component and flange until the flange is completely engaged with the anterior cortex.

- Ulnar component insertion
  - Inject antibiotic cement into the ulnar canal.
  - The ulnar component is inserted such that the axis of rotation is recreated and the implant is perpendicular to the dorsal flat surface of the olecranon.

TRICEPS REATTACHMENT

- The triceps is reattached using a nonabsorbable suture in a running locking mode (eg, running Krakow stitch) to achieve predictable purchase (**TECH FIG 6A,B**).
- Avoid capturing large amounts of triceps muscle fibers within the locking loops.
- The triceps tendon should be reattached to the flat of the olecranon process, not to the tip (**TECH FIG 6C,D**). Pass the sutures through bone tunnels (oblique crossing) that begin on the periphery of the flat reattachment area of the olecranon (**TECH FIG 6E**).
- Avoid tying the sutures directly over the midline of the proximal ulna, which is a source of painful symptoms and may require knot removal. Place the knot under the anconeus.
- When tensioning the triceps at reattachment, place the elbow at 30 to 45 degrees of flexion while tying the knot.
- Use a separate absorbable suture to "cinch" the triceps footprint onto the reattachment area (**TECH FIG 6F**).

TECH FIG 6 • A,B. A running locking stitch is used to improve triceps purchase when reattaching the muscle to the ulna. **A.** An example of a running locking stitch on either side of the split tendon. **B.** A locking stitch that locks both sides of the split together with one continuous locking suture. It is then reinforced with a reversed across-split locking suture. *(continued)*

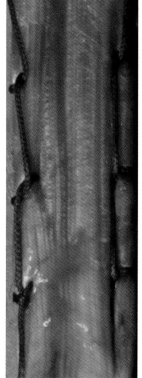
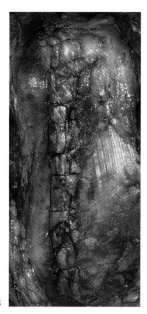

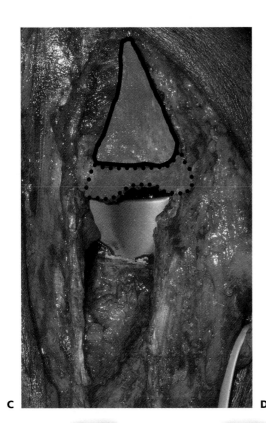

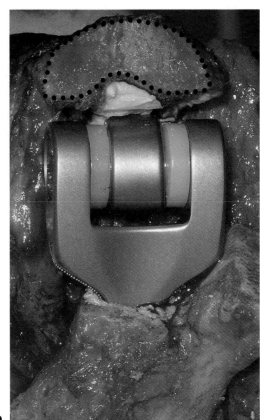

C

D

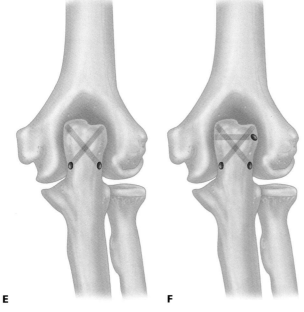

E

F

TECH FIG 6 • *(continued)* **C,D.** The triceps footprint to which reattachment should be attempted is predominantly on the flat part of the ulna or olecranon process, and not the tip, which is resected to prevent posterior abutment. **E.** Drill holes (1.5 to 2 mm) are oriented in a crossing fashion to secure the triceps to the footprint area. **F.** A separate "cinch" suture is used to increase the security and the area of contact between the triceps and the ulna, thereby improving healing potential.

WOUND CLOSURE

- The ulnar nerve is transposed into an anterior subcutaneous location.
- Reapproximate the triceps to the flexor and extensor masses with absorbable suture. Do not overtighten this repair, as it will restrict motion.

- The use of a subcutaneous drain is a matter of surgeon preference. However, there is no literature demonstrating the efficacy of a postoperative drain in preventing hematoma.

PEARLS AND PITFALLS

Indications	▪ A complete history and physical examination should be performed, with specific questions about any bone mineral density problems and healing tendency. ▪ Care must be taken to address associated pathology at the elbow, wrist, and shoulder.
Planning	▪ The surgeon should attempt fracture osteosynthesis when physiologically the patient has adequate bone stock and demand on the elbow. ▪ Arthroplasty should be available in the physiologically older and lower-demand patient, with a view to converting the decision to an acute arthroplasty if the osteosynthesis potential is tenuous.
Exposure	▪ Initial definition and protection of the ulnar nerve are important. Careful dissection of the nerve from the cubital tunnel restraints will allow freedom to move the nerve without risking traction injury during the remainder of the procedure. ▪ If the exposure involves removing the triceps from its ulnar attachment (Bryan-Morrey or TRAP approach), the site of Sharpey fiber attachment should be marked and reattached anatomically. ▪ During a tendon-splitting approach, the distal triceps tendon should be split within the structure of the tendon and should not involve the muscular belly.
Inspection	▪ A thorough inspection of the ulna and radial articular surface should be performed to investigate the possibility of a hemiarthroplasty replacement in the appropriately selected younger patient. ▪ The surgeon should observe the state of the ulnar nerve and muscles around the elbow (especially triceps and brachialis); this will help to explain altered nerve function in the former, and weakness and possible myositis ossificans and stiffness in the latter.
Bone preparation	▪ If the humeral columns are intact, then an attempt at preservation should be made, with their extensor and flexor mass attachments, during a total elbow replacement.
Implantation	▪ When planning length and implantation, the surgeon should pay careful attention to the tension and lever arms of the main motor drivers; the brachialis and triceps need some tension to function well, but if over-tensioned the elbow will be stiff and if under-tensioned the elbow will be weak.
Wound closure	▪ Drains should not be used because of the superficial nature of the elbow and the risk of deep infection. However, the surgeon should pay close attention to hemostasis, and for the first 12 hours a moderately tight bandage should be used to avoid hematoma formation. The dressing is reduced the next day.
Rehabilitation	▪ With triceps reattachment, the surgeon should be cautious to avoid overzealous rehabilitation for fear of compromising triceps healing, with subsequent avulsions or extension weakness.

POSTOPERATIVE CARE

▪ A volar plaster or thermoplastic splint is used to maintain the elbow in full extension for the first several days. This avoids tension on the incision and on the triceps reattachment.
▪ The arm is elevated on pillows or with a Bradford sling overnight to prevent edema.
▪ Nonsteroidal anti-inflammatories are avoided because of their detrimental effects on tissue healing (bone to tendon and bone to bone).
▪ On the second day after surgery the dressing is removed and the compliant patient should commence gentle active antigravity flexion, with passive gravity-assisted extension.
▪ Graduated and targeted motion is prescribed, with greater than 90 degrees of elbow flexion attempted after 5 weeks. This allows sufficient time for the triceps to adhere and heal (incompletely) to the ulna. Aggressive flexion too early may result in triceps avulsion or pull-out. Triceps antigravity exercises can commence after 5 weeks.
▪ Always, at each patient interaction, the surgeon should reiterate the restrictions of use with an elbow arthroplasty: limited internal (varus) and external (valgus) rotatory torques, 2-pound repetitive and 10-pound single-event lifting.

COMPLICATIONS

▪ Triceps avulsion
▪ Stiffness
  ▪ Overlengthened implantation
  ▪ Overtensioned triceps reattachment

  ▪ Overzealous closure of triceps to flexor–extensor compartments
  ▪ Inadequate soft tissue release
▪ Impingement
  ▪ Radial head on humeral component (distal yolk)
  ▪ Coronoid on humeral component (anterior yolk)
  ▪ Olecranon process on posterior humerus
▪ Deep venous thrombosis
▪ Infection
▪ Periprosthetic fracture
  ▪ Osteoporotic bone
  ▪ Stem–canal mismatched sizes
  ▪ Stem–canal mismatched curvature
  ▪ Inadequate opening for ulna component at coronoid base
▪ Ulna nerve neuropathy or injury

OUTCOMES

▪ Cobb and Morrey[1] reported 15 excellent and 5 good results, with one patient with inadequate data, in a cohort of patients with acute distal humeral fractures (average age 72 years) at 3.3 years of follow-up.
▪ Ray et al[14] reported 5 excellent and 2 good functional results in a group of patients with an average age of 81 years at 2 to 4 years of follow-up.
▪ Gambirasio et al[5] reported excellent functional results in a cohort of 10 elderly patients with osteoporotic intra-articular fractures.

■ Frankle et al[4] compared the outcomes of patients over age 65 with comminuted intra-articular distal humeral fractures treated with ORIF versus acute total elbow replacements. The ORIF group had 8 excellent results, 12 good results, 1 fair result, and 3 poor results, with 3 patients requiring conversion to elbow replacement. All 12 acute primary elbow replacements achieved excellent (n = 11) or good (n = 1) results.

■ Kamineni and Morrey[8] reported an average Mayo Elbow Performance Score (MEPS) of 93/100 in a series of 49 acute distal humeral fractures (average patient age 67 years) at 7 years of follow-up. The average arc of motion was 107 degrees.

■ Lee et al[10] reported seven acute elbow replacements for distal humeral fractures in patients with an average age of 73 years. The average arc of motion was 89 degrees and the average MEPS was 94/100 at an average follow-up of 25 months.

REFERENCES

1. Cobb TK, Morrey BF. Total elbow arthroplasty as primary treatment for distal humeral fractures in elderly patients. J Bone Joint Surg Am 1997;79A:826–832.
2. Faierman E, Wang J, Jupiter JB. Secondary ulnar nerve palsy in adults after elbow trauma: a report of two cases. J Hand Surg Am 2001;26A:675–678.
3. Frankle MA, Herscovici D Jr, DiPasquale TG, et al. A comparison of open reduction and internal fixation and primary total elbow arthroplasty in the treatment of intraarticular fractures of the distal humerus in women older than 65 years. J Shoulder Elbow Surg 1999;9:455.
4. Frankle MA, Herscovici D Jr, DiPasquale TG, et al. A comparison of open reduction and internal fixation and primary total elbow arthroplasty in the treatment of intraarticular distal humerus fractures in women older than age 65. J Orthop Trauma 2003;17:473–480.
5. Gambirasio R, Riand N, Stern R, Hall JE. Total elbow replacement for complex fractures of the distal humerus: an option for the elderly patient. J Bone Joint Surg Br 2001;83B:974–978.
6. Holmes JC, Skolnick MD, et al. Untreated median-nerve entrapment in bone after fracture of the distal end of the humerus: postmortem findings after forty-seven years. J Bone Joint Surg Am 1979;61A:309–310.
7. Huang TL, Chiu FY, Chuang TY, et al. The results of open reduction and internal fixation in elderly patients with severe fractures of the distal humerus: a critical analysis of the results. J Trauma 2005;58:62–69.
8. Kamineni S, Morrey BF. Distal humeral fractures treated with non-custom total elbow replacement. J Bone Joint Surg Am 2004;86A:940–947.
9. Kamineni S, Morrey BF. Distal humeral fractures treated with non-custom total elbow replacement: surgical technique. J Bone Joint Surg Am 2005;87A:41–50.
10. Lee KT, Lai CH, Singh S. Results of total elbow arthroplasty in the treatment of distal humerus fractures in elderly Asian patients. J Trauma 2006;61:889–892.
11. Mohan K. Myositis ossificans traumatica of the elbow. Int Surg 1972;57:475–478.
12. Pajarinen J, Bjorkenheim JM. Operative treatment of type C intercondylar fractures of the distal humerus: results after a mean follow-up of 2 years in a series of 18 patients. J Shoulder Elbow Surg 2002;11:48–52.
13. Parsons M, O'Brien R, Hughes JS. Elbow hemiarthroplasty for acute and salvage reconstruction of intra-articular distal humerus fractures. Tech Shoulder Elbow Surg 2005;2:87–97.
14. Ray PS, Kakarlapudi K, Rajsekhar C, et al. Total elbow arthroplasty as primary treatment for distal humeral fractures in elderly patients. Injury 2000;31:687–692.
15. Thompson HC 3rd, Garcia A. Myositis ossificans: aftermath of elbow injuries. Clin Orthop Relat Res 1967;50:129–134.
16. Zhao J, Wang X, Zhang Q. Surgical treatment of comminuted intra-articular fractures of the distal humerus with double tension band osteosynthesis. Orthopedics 2000;23:449–452.

Chapter 47

Management of Primary Degenerative Arthritis of the Elbow: Linkable Total Elbow Replacement

Bassem Elhassan, Matthew L. Ramsey, and Scott P. Steinmann

DEFINITION

- Primary degenerative arthritis of the elbow is an uncommon problem.[1]
  - It occurs in less than 2% of the population[29] and principally affects the dominant extremity in middle-aged manual laborers.[1,3,17,23,29]
  - The disorder predominates in men and is rarely seen in women, with an incidence of 4 to 5:1.[8]
  - The dominant extremity is involved in 80% to 90% of symptomatic patients. Bilateral involvement of the elbow is noted in 25% to 60% of patients.[6]
  - It has also been reported in people who require continuous use of a wheelchair or crutches, in athletes, and in patients with a history of osteochondritis dissecans of the elbow.[21,25]
- The pattern of pathologic changes in primary degenerative arthritis is different than the age-related changes of the distal humerus and the radiohumeral joint.[6,26]
- The current understanding of the disease process in primary degenerative arthritis has led to treatment algorithms designed to address the pathologic process short of joint replacement.
- The role of total elbow arthroplasty (TEA) for patients with primary degenerative arthritis of the elbow is limited, in large part because of the younger age and increased activity levels of patients with this condition.

PATHOGENESIS

- The exact pathogenesis of primary osteoarthritis of the elbow is still unknown. It is generally believed that overuse plays a key role in the onset of the disease process. However, younger patients with this disease often have predisposing conditions such as osteochondritis dissecans.[11]
- The degenerative changes of the elbow joint are usually more advanced in the radiohumeral joint, where bare bone is often in wide contact, and the capitellum appears to have been shaved obliquely (**FIG 1**).[6]
  - This is due to the high axial, shearing, and rotational stresses at this articulation, which result in marked erosion of the capitellum and hypertrophic callus formation in a skirt-like pattern on the radial neck.[32]
- The ulnohumeral joint is usually less involved in the beginning of the disease process, but involvement becomes more pronounced with more advanced disease.[21]
  - The central aspect of the ulnohumeral joint is characteristically spared. The anterior and posterior involvement of this joint is usually manifested by fibrosis of the anterior capsule in the form of a cord-like band and hypertrophy of the olecranon.
  - Osteophytes are seen over the olecranon, especially medially, the coronoid process, and the coronoid fossa.

- These changes in the radiohumeral and ulnohumeral joints lead to the loss and fragmentation of the cartilaginous joint surfaces with distortion, cyst formation, and bone sclerosis.[2]
  - Kashiwagi[9] noted that the early stage of the disease is characterized by small, round bony protuberances; the early stage progresses into various shapes of osteophytes and bony sclerosis with more advanced cases.
  - Suvarna and Stanley[30] reported on the progressive fibrosis of the local marrow, increased thickness of all the bony components of the olecranon fossa, and increases in anterior and posterior fibrous tissues.

PATIENT HISTORY AND PHYSICAL FINDINGS

- Despite considerable radiographic severity, many patients with osteoarthritis of the elbow report minimal symptoms.[11]
- Trauma rarely underlies the onset of degenerative arthritis. However, trivial injury often brings the problem to the patient's attention.
- Characteristic manifestations of primary degenerative arthritis of the elbow are well described.[22,24] These include:
  - Progressive loss of motion

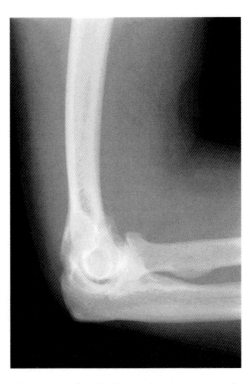

FIG 1 • Lateral view of right elbow, showing advanced osteoarthritis specifically involving the radiocapitellar joint. Notice osteophyte formation anteriorly and posteriorly.

403

- Mechanical symptoms of locking and catching caused by intra-articular loose bodies (occurs in about 10% of patients)[9]
- Pain at the extremes of motion due to mechanical impingement of osteophytes (pain occurs most frequently at terminal extension, although about 50% of patients also have pain during terminal flexion)
- Pain throughout the arc of motion indicates significant involvement of the ulnohumeral joint; this typically occurs late in the disease process.
- Ulnar neuropathy
  - Medial joint pain in patients with advanced osteoarthritis of the elbow might be the first manifestation of ulnar neuropathy.
  - Up to 20% of patients with primary osteoarthritis of the elbow have some degree of ulnar neuropathy.[1]
  - The proximity of the ulnar nerve to the arthritic posteromedial aspect of the ulnohumeral joint makes it susceptible to impingement.
  - The expansion of the capsule as a result of synovitis and the presence of osteophytes in that area of the joint result in direct compression and ischemia of the ulnar nerve.
  - Acute onset of cubital tunnel syndrome in patients with osteoarthritis of the elbow might be also the first manifestation of a medial elbow ganglion.[10]
- Radiocapitellar symptoms: With more progressive disease, the patients may have pain with forearm rotation and throughout the range of elbow motion. This could lead to disability in this patient population as well in the older laborers who extensively use their upper extremity.[6,16,33]

PHYSICAL FINDINGS

- Physical examination findings depend on the extent of the patient's disease.
- Range of motion
  - The flexion-extension arc will demonstrate loss of extension greater than flexion and will average about 30 to 120 degrees.
    - The midrange of the flexion–extension arc is typically pain-free in the early stages of the disease.
  - A painful midrange of motion and crepitus indicate more extensive involvement of the ulnohumeral joint.
  - The arc of pronation–supination is rarely affected early in the disease process. Involvement of the proximal radioulnar and radiohumeral joint later in the disease process may limit forearm rotation.
- Forced motion at the extremes of flexion and extension will often cause pain, particularly in extension.
- Ulnar nerve symptoms need to be thoroughly evaluated. Symptoms of ulnar neuropathy associated with primary degenerative arthritis of the elbow include:
  - Decreased sensation and weakness
  - Positive Tinel sign at the cubital tunnel
  - Positive elbow hyperflexion test

IMAGING AND OTHER DIAGNOSTIC STUDIES

- Some characteristic radiographic features are seen on the anteroposterior and lateral radiographs of the elbow:
  - Radiocapitellar narrowing (noted in 25% to 50% of patients)
  - Ossification and osteophyte formation in the olecranon fossa in almost all patients with osteoarthritis of the elbow[15,21]
  - Osteophyte formation of the coronoid and olecranon processes
  - Loose bodies and fluffy densities might be observed filling the coronoid and olecranon fossae (**FIG 2A,B**).
  - Radiographs do not allow for accurate visualization of all osteophytes.
- A cubital tunnel view is obtained if there is ulnar nerve irritation to look for impinging osteophytes or loose bodies.[4,6,7]
- Computed tomography (CT) helps in delineating the detailed structural anatomy of the articular surface of the elbow with an accurate determination of the locations of the osteophytes and loose bodies (**FIG 2C**).
  - When contemplating surgical treatment of the osteoarthritic elbow, a CT is quite helpful for determining which osteophytes need to be removed.

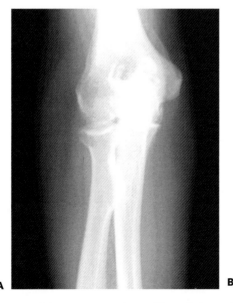

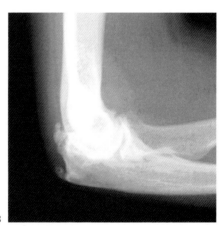

A **B**

FIG 2 • A,B. Anteroposterior and lateral views of a right osteoarthritic elbow show narrowing of the joint line and subchondral sclerosis, with formation of osteophytes in the coronoid, capitellar, and olecranon fossae. *(continued)*

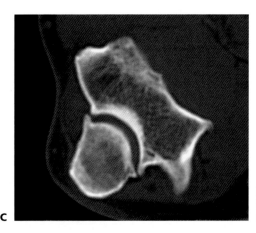

FIG 2 • *(continued)* **C.** Computed tomography of the elbow demonstrating marginal osteophytes on the ulna and olecranon fossa.

- Three-dimensional reconstructions provide additional detail on osteophytic deformity and facilitate preoperative planning of removal.
- MRI does not provide any useful information in primary osteoarthritis of the elbow and is rarely indicated.

NONOPERATIVE MANAGEMENT

- Because of their young age, most patients with primary osteoarthritis of the elbow tend to be active and involved in manual labor, which will place a great demand on any kind of prosthetic replacement.
- Early in the course of the disease, treatment by nonsurgical measures should be followed.[21]
  - This consists of activity modification, physical therapy, anti-inflammatory medications, and possibly steroid injection or visco-supplementation.[13]

SURGICAL MANAGEMENT

Indications

- If nonoperative treatment fails to improve symptoms, surgery may be indicated.
- Several surgical options exist for the management of primary degenerative arthritis of the elbow. Surgery is directed toward addressing the pathology contributing to the predominant complaints of the patient.
- The surgical techniques depend on:
  - Degree of osteophyte formation
  - Degree and direction of motion loss
  - Associated loose bodies
  - Associated ulnar nerve symptoms
  - Degree of ulnohumeral involvement resulting in pain through the midrange of motion

Arthroscopic Débridement

- Arthroscopic management of degenerative arthritis of the elbow is discussed in detail in Chapter SM-22.
- In general, arthroscopic débridement for degenerative arthritis of the elbow can be performed for moderate to severe disease when there are no midrange symptoms, indicating limited involvement of the ulnohumeral joint.
- Advantages of arthroscopy include the ability to visualize the entire joint and limited morbidity from surgery.
  - Savoie et al reported good results with extensive arthroscopic débridement involving capsular release, fenestration of the distal part of the humerus, and removal of osteophytes.[28]

- Disadvantages of arthroscopy include potential neurovascular injury and difficulty assessing the normal anatomic relationships, resulting in inadequate débridement, compared with open débridement and release.
- Contraindications to arthroscopic treatment include altered neurovascular anatomy, limited surgical expertise, and advanced involvement of the ulnohumeral joint.

Open Débridement

- Open débridement can be performed for all patients with primary degenerative arthritis of the elbow.
- Open joint débridement should be considered in patients with advanced disease or when the treating surgeon has limited experience with arthroscopic techniques.
- Options for open débridement of the elbow include:
  - Outerbridge-Kashiwagi arthroplasty (see Chap. SE-42)
  - Lateral column approach for débridement (see Chap. SE-43)
  - Medial over-the-top approach for débridement (see Chap. SE-44)

Total Elbow Arthroplasty

- TEA for the treatment of primary osteoarthritis of the elbow is performed sparingly in carefully selected patients. In general, the patient population with primary degenerative arthritis of the elbow includes relatively young men who are physically active in their occupation and want to remain so. TEA is contraindicated in high-demand patients.
- The indications for TEA for primary degenerative arthritis of the elbow include patients older than 65 years with low physical demands and a painful arc of motion. These patients should have attempted and failed all other appropriate treatment options.

Implant Choices

- Unlinked (resurfacing) and linked (semiconstrained) designs may be appropriate in patients with primary degenerative arthritis of the elbow.
- The current literature supports the use of linked implant designs for primary degenerative arthritis. However, osteoarthritis may be the best indication for the use of an unlinked implant.
- Linked implants
  - Current linked designs with a semiconstrained, loose-hinged articulation allow varying degrees of varus–valgus motion and rotational laxity (**FIG 3A**).
  - Muscle activation about the elbow protects against excessive loading, thereby reducing aseptic loosening.

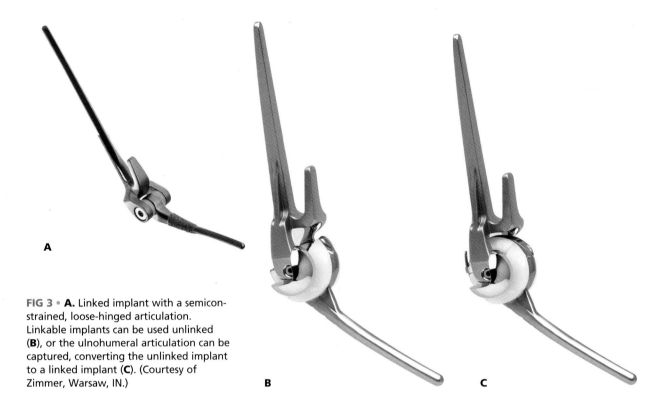

A

B

C

FIG 3 • **A.** Linked implant with a semiconstrained, loose-hinged articulation. Linkable implants can be used unlinked (**B**), or the ulnohumeral articulation can be captured, converting the unlinked implant to a linked implant (**C**). (Courtesy of Zimmer, Warsaw, IN.)

- Unlinked implants
    - Anatomic requirements for the use of unlinked implants include:
        - Competence of the medial and lateral collateral ligaments
        - Minimal deformity of the subchondral architecture
        - Integrity of the medial and lateral supracondylar columns
    - Maintenance of the collateral ligaments and surrounding muscles helps absorb forces across the elbow, thereby reducing stress on the bone–cement interface. This has the theoretical, but unproven, advantage of offloading stresses on the implant.
    - Some authors believe that this potential advantage may allow this implant type to be used in a higher-demand patient population. However, this potential advantage is yet unproven. Therefore, the indications for total elbow replacement are still limited in this patient population to patients willing to adopt low physical demands.
    - The major complication of unlinked implants is instability.
    - If an unlinked implant is considered in this patient population, the ability to convert to a linked replacement (linkable) has obvious advantages.
- Linkable implants
    - These devices permit implantation in an unlinked fashion, taking advantage of the benefits of an unlinked design (**FIG 3B**).
    - The ulnohumeral articulation can be captured, thereby converting the unlinked implant to a linked implant by placing an ulnar cap on the ulnar component (**FIG 3C**). This can be performed at the time of implantation of the unlinked implant if stability cannot be established or at a point distant to the initial implantation if instability becomes an issue.

Patient Positioning

- The patient is positioned supine on the operating room table with a bump under the ipsilateral scapula. The arm is positioned across the chest and supported on a bolster (**FIG 4**).
- A tourniquet is applied to the arm. The use of a sterile tourniquet increases the "zone of sterility" and allows removal for more proximal exposure if needed.

Approach

- The surgical technique for linked arthroplasty is discussed in other chapters. Please refer to these chapters for the specific technical details of implantation of a linked, semiconstrained implant. This chapter will discuss an unlinked total elbow system, which can be converted to a linked implant if required for stability.

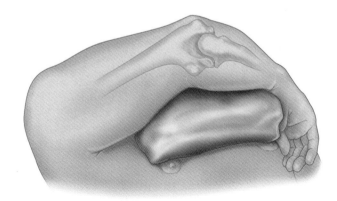

FIG 4 • Patient positioning with the arm across the chest supported on a bolster.

SURGICAL EXPOSURE

- A straight posterior, midline incision placed just off the medial tip of the olecranon is used (**TECH FIG 1**).
- Full-thickness flaps are elevated. The extent of flap elevation is based on how the triceps is to be managed surgically.
- The ulnar nerve is identified, protected with help of a Penrose drain, and transposed anteriorly.

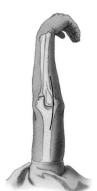

TECH FIG 1 • Straight posterior midline skin incision is placed off the medial aspect of the olecranon. (Courtesy of Tornier, Inc., Edina, MN.)

TRICEPS MANAGEMENT

- Surgical management of the triceps is a matter of surgeon preference. The general methods of triceps management are triceps-sparing, triceps-reflecting, and triceps-splitting approaches.
  - Triceps-sparing approaches leave the triceps attached to the tip of the olecranon. The advantage of this type of approach is that it prevents triceps weakness postoperatively, but it sacrifices surgical exposure.
  - Triceps-reflecting approaches subperiosteally elevate the triceps from its attachment on the ulna; it must be carefully reattached and protected postoperatively. However, surgical exposure is facilitated with these approaches.
  - Triceps-splitting approaches violate the attachment of the triceps to the ulna yet provide the advantages of improved visualization of the joint.
- Triceps-splitting approach
  - A triceps-splitting approach is performed by completing a midline split in the triceps muscle and tendon, which is carried distally onto the ulna along the subcutaneous border of the ulna between the anconeus and the flexor carpi ulnaris (**TECH FIG 2A**).
- The medial triceps is elevated in continuity with the flexor carpi ulnaris while the lateral triceps is elevated in continuity with the anconeus. Care must be taken when elevating the medial triceps flap. The medial triceps attachment to the triceps is tenuous in comparison to the lateral triceps flap, which is much more robust.
- The medial collateral ligament (anterior bundle) and lateral collateral ligament complex are tagged and released from their humeral attachment (**TECH FIG 2B**).
- The shoulder is externally rotated and the elbow is flexed, allowing the ulna to separate from the humerus (**TECH FIG 2C**).

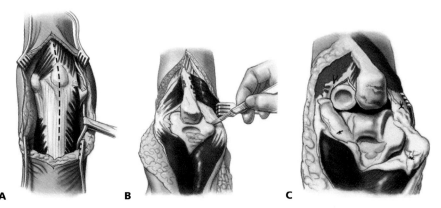

A   **B**   **C**

TECH FIG 2 • **A.** Triceps-splitting approach carried from the subcutaneous border of the ulna proximally into the triceps tendon. The medial and lateral triceps are subperiosteally elevated from the olecranon. **B.** The medial and lateral collateral ligaments are released from their humeral attachment and tagged for later repair. **C.** The elbow is dislocated with flexion of the joint, allowing the ulna to separate from the humerus. This separation provides exposure for component insertion. (Courtesy of Tornier, Inc., Edina, MN.)

IMPLANTATION

Humeral Preparation

■ Sizing of the implant to the patient's native anatomy is critical. Trial spools should be compared to the distal humerus and the proximal radioulnar joint for appropriate sizing (**TECH FIG 3A,B**). If the native joint size is between spool sizes, the smaller spool is selected.

■ The medial and lateral points of the axis of rotation through the distal humerus are determined and an axis pin is placed through these two points, thereby replicating the axis. A drill guide aids in reproducing these points (**TECH FIG 3C**).

■ The central portion of the distal humerus articulation is removed, the intramedullary canal is opened, and a rod is placed in the intramedullary canal. The axis pin is replaced to determine the offset of the intramedullary canal relative to the flexion–extension axis (**TECH FIG 3D,E**).

■ A distal humeral cutting block is used to precisely prepare the distal humerus relative to the intramedullary canal and the flexion–extension axis (**TECH FIG 3F,G**).

■ The humeral canal is sequentially broached to the size selected for the articular spool.

Ulnar Preparation

■ Preparation of the ulna is based on the flexion–extension axis of the proximal radius and ulna. The selected size spool is attached to the cutting guide, and the guide is tightened with set screws (**TECH FIG 4A**). Care must be taken to maintain the relationship of the trochlea and capitellar portions of the spool with the native greater sigmoid notch and radial head.

■ A bell saw is used to resect a small portion of the articular surface and subchondral bone of the ulna (**TECH FIG 4B**).

■ If the radial head is going to be replaced, a sagittal saw is used to resect the radial head through the cutting guide. The canal is broached and a trial radial head component is inserted.

■ The ulnar canal is opened and sequentially broached to the same size as the selected humeral component.

Component Placement

■ If the replacement is going to be unlinked, a short ulnar component can be used. If the implant is going to be linked, a standard (longer) stem is selected. If a standard ulnar component is going to be used, flexible reamers may be required to prepare the ulna.

■ Trial reduction is performed to assess the alignment, stability, and tracking of the components.

■ If the components are going to be inserted unlinked, the collateral ligaments are reattached to the anatomic origin through the humeral implant. An accessory box stitch could be placed through the ulna and humeral component to support the collateral ligament repair.

■ The canals are lavaged and cement restrictors are placed in the humerus and ulna.

■ Antibiotic-impregnated cement is injected into the canals. Methylene blue is added to the cement to facilitate cement removal if required in the future.

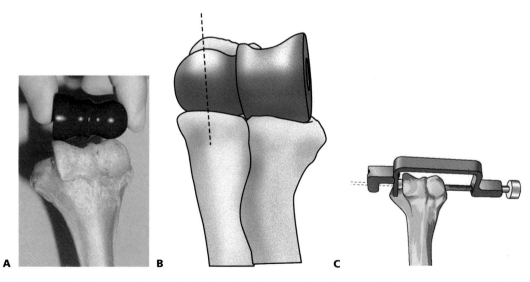

TECH FIG 3 • The anatomic spool is sized against the native distal humerus (**A**) and the proximal radioulnar articulation (**B**). **C.** The native flexion–extension axis is determined. A drill guide assists in accurately establishing the flexion–extension axis. Next, the offset of the distal humeral articulation with respect to the intramedullary canal is determined. *(continued)*

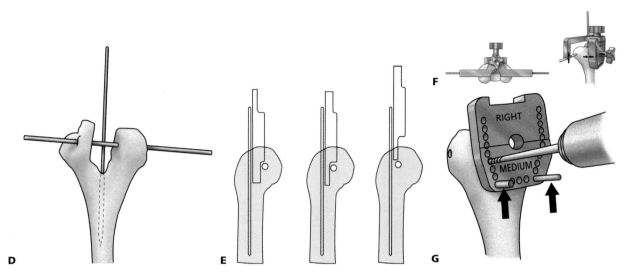

D   E   G   F

TECH FIG 3 • *(continued)* D. The relationship between the axis of flexion–extension and the intramedullary canal is determined. **E.** Measurement guides are used to determine whether the offset is anterior, posterior, or neutral. **F.** A cutting block is placed relative to the flexion–extension axis. **G.** The cutting block is fixed to the humerus with pins and the guide is removed. Once all of the holes are drilled, the cutting block is removed and the holes are connected with an oscillating saw. (Courtesy of Tornier, Inc., Edina, MN.)

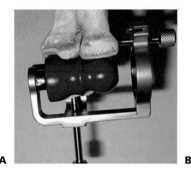

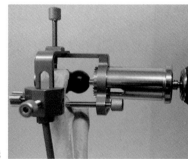

A   B

TECH FIG 4 • A. The selected anatomic spool is attached to the ulnar cutting jig. The set screws are tightened, taking care to ensure the anatomic spool stays firmly opposed to the native radius and ulna. **B.** With the ulnar cutting guide properly aligned, a bell saw is used to prepare the proximal ulna. The radial head can also be removed using the same cutting jig. (Courtesy of Tornier, Inc., Edina, MN.)

LIGAMENT REPAIR

- A locking stitch is used to repair the collateral ligaments through the cannulated humeral bolt (**TECH FIG 5A**).

- Further support is achieved using a cerclage stitch passed through the humeral bolt and a transverse drill hole in the ulna (**TECH FIG 5B**).

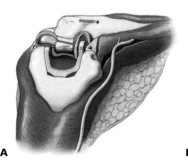

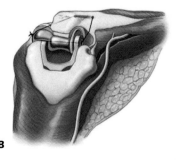

A   B

TECH FIG 5 • A. The medial and lateral collateral ligaments are reattached to the epicondyles using a locking stitch that is passed through the cannulated humeral screw. **B.** The collateral ligament repair is reinforced with a box stitch passed through the cannulated humeral screw and a transverse hole placed through the proximal ulna. (Courtesy of Tornier, Inc., Edina, MN.)

TRICEPS REPAIR

- Triceps repair is crucial for the stability of unlinked devices.
- The triceps is reattached through two crossing drill holes and one transverse drill hole in the olecranon.
- A grasping suture (Krackow stitch) is used and passed through the crossing drill holes.
- A cerclage stitch is passed through the transverse drill hole around the triceps attachment (**TECH FIG 6**).

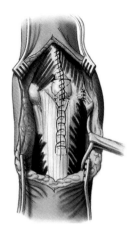

TECH FIG 6 • The triceps is repaired to the ulna through drill holes. The split in the triceps and between the anconeus and flexor carpi ulnaris is closed side to side with interrupted or running suture. (Courtesy of Tornier, Inc., Edina, MN.)

WOUND CLOSURE

- The ulnar nerve is transposed into an anterior subcutaneous pouch.
- The wound is closed over a drain placed in the subcutaneous position.

POSTOPERATIVE CARE

- The arm is placed in a well-padded postoperative dressing and the arm is immobilized in about 90 degrees of flexion for the first several days.
- A resting elbow splint at 90 degrees with the wrist included is fabricated before discharge to protect the soft tissue repair while it heals.

OUTCOMES

- Most studies in the literature reporting on TEA involve large numbers of patients, mostly with rheumatoid arthritis or other inflammatory pathologies but very few patients with primary osteoarthritis.
  - This makes it difficult to make accurate conclusions on the value of this treatment option for this population of patients.[5,14,20,27]
  - There are few studies in the English literature reporting specifically on the outcome and complications of TEA as a treatment option for patients with primary osteoarthritis of the elbow.[4,13]
- Kozak[13] reported on the Mayo clinic experience.
  - Over a 13-year period, only 5 of 493 patients (<1%) who underwent TEA had the procedure performed for primary osteoarthritis of the elbow.
  - A linked Coonrad-Morrey implant (Zimmer, Warsaw, IN) was used in three patients and an unlinked Pritchard elbow resurfacing system (ERS) (DePuy, Warsaw, IN) was used in the other two patients.
    - The average age of the patients was 67 and follow-up ranged from 37 to 121 months.
    - Two minor and four major complications were reported in four elbows, two of which required revision.

- This rate of complications, according to the authors, is much higher than the rate of complications reported in TEA performed for other reasons in the same institution during the same period of time, including revision TEA, posttraumatic arthritis, nonunion of distal humerus, and rheumatoid arthritis.[12,18,19]
- Espag et al[4] reported on 11 Souter-Strathclyde cemented unlinked primary TEAs in 10 patients with osteoarthritis of the elbow.
  - The diagnosis was primary osteoarthritis of the elbow in nine patients and posttraumatic osteoarthritis in two patients.
  - The average age of the patients was 66 years; mean follow-up was 68 months.
  - Only one patient required revision after 97 months for ulnar component loosening.
  - All patients reported good symptomatic relief of pain and a significant increase in range of motion, and all patients considered the procedure to be successful.
  - The authors compared these results with the result of Souter-Strathclyde TEA used in patients with rheumatoid arthritis.[27,31]
- The revision rate in their series (9%) performed for ulnar component loosening compares favorably with the revision rate with the rheumatoid patients (5% to 21%), in which the main indications for revision included dislocation, and perioperative fracture.
  - The authors attributed the decrease in the incidence of peri- and postoperative fracture to the good amount of bone stock in patients with primary osteoarthritis of the elbow, which makes the risk of fracture very minimal.
  - As evident from this review, the outcome studies of TEA in patients with primary osteoarthritis of the elbow are very limited. The above-mentioned studies included a

small number of patients, and no final recommendation could be drawn at this time.

■ It is hoped that a greater understanding of elbow anatomy and kinematics will lead to advances in prosthetic design and surgical technique.

  ■ The newer anatomic unlinked implants may improve the outcome of elbow replacement in younger patients.[7]

  ■ More outcome studies are needed on these implants or any other modern implants before openly recommending elbow replacement in younger active patients with primary osteoarthritis of the elbow.

REFERENCES

1. Antuna SA, Morrey BF, Adams RA, et al. Ulnohumeral arthroplasty for primary degenerative arthritis of the elbow: long-term outcome and complications. J Bone Joint Surg Am 2002;84A:2168–2173.
2. Bullough PG. Atlas of Orthopedic Pathology, 2nd ed. New York: Gower Medical Publishing, 1992;10:4–10.
3. Doherty M, Preston B. Primary osteoarthritis of the elbow. Ann Rheum Dis 1989;48:743–747.
4. Espag MP, Black DL, Clark DI, et al. Early results of the Souter-Strathclyde unlinked total elbow arthroplasty in patients with osteoarthritis. J Bone Joint Surg Br 2003;85B:351–353.
5. Ewald FC. Total elbow replacement. Orthop Clin North Am 1975;3:685–696.
6. Goodfellow JW, Bullough PG. The pattern of aging of the articular cartilage of the elbow joint. J Bone Joint Surg Br 1967;49B:175–181.
7. Gramstad GD, King GJ, O'Driscoll SW, et al. Elbow arthroplasty using a convertible implant. Tech Hand Up Extrem Surg 2005;9:153–163.
8. Kahiwagi D. Intra-articular changes of the osteoarthritis of the elbow. Orthop Clin North Am 1995;26:691–706.
9. Kashiwagi D. Osteoarthritis of the elbow joint: intra-articular changes and the special operative procedure, Outbridge-Kashiwagi method (O-K method). In: Kashiwagi D, ed. Elbow Joint. Amsterdam: Elsevier Science Publishers Biomedical Division, 1985:177–188.
10. Kato H, Hirayama T, Minami A, et al. Cubital tunnel syndrome associated with medial elbow ganglia and osteoarthritis of the elbow. J Bone Joint Surg Am 2002;84A:1413–1419.
11. Kellgren JH, Larence JS. Radiological assessment of osteoarthrosis. Ann Rheum Dis 1957;16:494–501.
12. King GJW, Adams RA, Morrey BF. Total elbow arthroplasty: revision with use of a non-custom semiconstrained prosthesis. J Bone Joint Surg Am 1997;79A:394–398.
13. Kozak TK, Adams RA, Morrey BF. Total elbow arthroplasty in primary osteoarthritis of the elbow. J Arthroplasty 1998;13:837–842.
14. Kraay MJ, Figgie MP, Inglis AE, et al. Primary semiconstrained total elbow arthroplasty. J Bone Joint Surg Br 1994;76B:636–640.
15. London JT. Kinematics of the elbow. J Bone Joint Surg Am 1981;63A:529–535.
16. Meachim G. Age changes in articular cartilage. Clin Orthop Relat Res 1969;64:33–44.
17. Mintz G, Fraga A. Severe osteoarthritis of the elbow in foundry workers. Arch Environ Health 1973;27:78–80.
18. Morrey BF, Adams RA, Bryan RS. Total replacement for post-traumatic arthritis of the elbow. J Bone Joint Surg Br 1991;73B:607–612.
19. Morrey BF, Adams RA. Semiconstrained elbow replacement arthroplasty for distal humeral non-union. J Bone Joint Surg Br 1995;77B:67–72.
20. Morrey BF, Bryan RS, Dobyns JH, et al. Total elbow arthroplasty. J Bone Joint Surg Am 1981;81A:80–84.
21. Morrey BF. Primary degenerative arthritis of the elbow. J Bone Joint Surg Br 1992;74B:409–413.
22. O'Driscoll SW. Arthroscopic treatment for osteoarthritis of the elbow. Orthop Clin North Am 1995;26:691–706.
23. O'Driscoll SW. Elbow arthritis: treatment options. J Am Acad Orthop Surg 1993;1:106–116.
24. Ogilvie-Harris DJ, Schemitsch E. Arthroscopy of the elbow for removal of loose bodies. Arthroscopy 1993;9:5–8.
25. Oka Y. Debridement for osteoarthritis of the elbow in athletes. Int Orthop 1999;23:91–94.
26. Ortner DJ. Description and classification of degenerative bone changes in the distal joint surfaces of the humerus. Am J Phys Anthrop 1968;28:139–155.
27. Rozing P. Souter-Strathclyde total elbow arthroplasty. J Bone Joint Surg Br 2000;82B:1129–1134.
28. Savoie FH III, Nunley PD, Field LD. Arthroscopic management of the arthritic elbow: indications, technique, and results. J Shoulder Elbow Surg 1999;8:214–219.
29. Stanley D. Prevalence and etiology of symptomatic elbow osteoarthritis. J Shoulder Elbow Surg 1994;3:386–389.
30. Suvarna SK, Stanley D. The histologic changes of the olecranon fossa membrane in primary osteoarthritis of the elbow. J Shoulder Elbow Surg 2004;13:555–557.
31. Trail IA, Nuttal D, Stanley JK. Survivorship and radiological analysis of the standard Souter-Strathyclyde total elbow arthroplasty. J Bone Joint Surg Br 1999;81B:80–84.
32. Tsuge K, Mizuseki T. Debridement arthroplasty for advanced primary osteoarthritis of the elbow: results of a new technique used for 29 elbows. J Bone Joint Surg Br 1994;76B:641–646.
33. Wadworth TG. Osteoarthritis. In: Wadworth TG, ed. The Elbow. Edinburgh: Churchill Livingstone, 1982:292–293.

Chapter 48

Surgical Management of Traumatic Conditions of the Elbow

Matthew L. Ramsey

DEFINITION AND PATHOGENESIS

- Posttraumatic conditions of the elbow represent a variety of disorders involving the elbow as a result of previous injury. Included among the posttraumatic conditions are:
  - Posttraumatic arthritis
    - Primary pathology involves posttraumatic degeneration of the articular surface.
    - Secondary pathologies can include contracture, loose bodies, and heterotopic bone.
  - Nonunion of the distal humerus
    - Total elbow arthroplasty (TEA) is considered when reconstruction of the nonunion is deemed impossible or undesirable.
  - Dysfunctional instability of the elbow
    - This is a special clinical situation where the fulcrum for stable elbow function is lost. The forearm may be dissociated from the brachium (**FIG 1**).
  - Chronic instability (dislocation)
    - Chronic ligamentous instability of the elbow can lead to articular degeneration, particularly in the elderly, osteopenic patient.
- Treatment for posttraumatic conditions is individualized depending on the underlying pathology as well as the functional demands and age of the patient.

PATIENT HISTORY AND PHYSICAL FINDINGS

- The patient history is directed at gaining information about the initial injury, treatments undertaken, complications of treatment, presenting complaints, and patient expectations.
  - Detailed investigation of the patient's symptoms should include questions regarding the degree of pain, presence of instability or stiffness, and mechanical symptoms of catching, or locking.
- The physical examination of the elbow should follow a systematic approach:
  - Inspection of the elbow
    - Presence and location of previous skin incisions or persistent wounds
    - Alignment of the extremity at rest
    - Prominent hardware
  - Range of motion (ROM)
    - Active ROM is assessed and compared to the opposite side. The degree of motion, smoothness of motion, and feel of the endpoint are established.
    - Normal active ROM varies, but it should be symmetrical with the opposite unaffected side. Range of motion should be from near full extension (may have hyperextension) to 130 to 140 degrees of flexion. Normal forearm rotation is an arc of 170 degrees, with slightly more supination than pronation.
    - Functional ROM has been defined as a flexion–extension arc from 30 degrees to 130 degrees and a

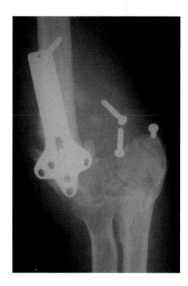

FIG 1 • Radiograph demonstrating dissociation of the forearm from the brachium in a patient with an inadequately treated fracture of the distal humerus with resultant nonunion.

pronation–supination arc from 50 degrees of pronation and 50 degrees of supination.[10]
  - Passive range of motion (PROM) is then assessed and compared to the active motion arc.
- Palpation of the elbow should systematically review all of the bony and soft tissue structures of the elbow.
  - The ulnar nerve needs to be carefully assessed. If previously surgically manipulated, its location should be identified if possible.
  - Motor function of the elbow should be assessed, in particular the flexor (biceps and brachialis) and extensor (triceps) function.

IMAGING AND OTHER DIAGNOSTIC STUDIES

- Orthogonal radiographic views of the elbow are mandatory (**FIG 2**).
  - A good lateral radiograph can typically be obtained.
  - A useful anteroposterior (AP) radiograph can be difficult, particularly if the patient has significant flexion contracture. A poor AP radiograph can make assessment of the joint space difficult, typically resulting in overestimating the amount of joint destruction.
- Oblique radiographs can be helpful in obtaining more detail.
- CT scans are particularly helpful in assessing the integrity of the bone and establishing whether the joint space is reasonably preserved.
  - Three-dimensional reconstructions provide a better understanding of any deformity.
- Magnetic resonance imaging is rarely needed in the assessment of a posttraumatic joint and is therefore used sparingly.

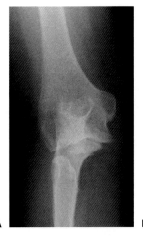
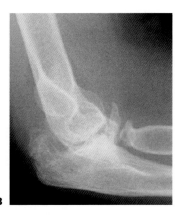

FIG 2 • AP and lateral radiographs of the elbow in a patient with posttraumatic arthritis of the elbow.

DIFFERENTIAL DIAGNOSIS

- Nonunion or malunion of the distal humerus
- Posttraumatic stiffness of the elbow
- Chronic dislocation of the elbow

NONOPERATIVE MANAGEMENT

- The success of nonoperative management depends on specific features of the pathology and the motivation and goals of the patient.
- Activity modification is used to reduce the forces across the elbow.
- Range of motion of the elbow should be maintained. Aggressive efforts to regain lost motion can aggravate the joint.
- External bracing is occasionally used to support an unstable extremity. However, in general, bracing is poorly tolerated and functionally limiting.

SURGICAL MANAGEMENT

- Surgical management of traumatic conditions of the elbow is directed at addressing the underlying cause of disability and should take into consideration the patient's age, physical requirements, and expectations.

Surgical Options

Interposition Arthroplasty[2,7]

- Indications
  - Patients with pain or loss of range of motion who have failed to respond to nonoperative management
  - Posttraumatic arthritis in patients who are either too young for TEA or who are unwilling to accept the functional restrictions with TEA
  - The patients who do best following interposition are those with painful loss of motion when there is no requirement for aggressive, heavy use of the extremity.
- Contraindications
  - Active infection (septic arthritis with persistent infection)
  - Grossly unstable elbow
  - Marked angular deformity
  - Pain without associated functional loss

- Inadequate bone stock
- Patients unable or unwilling to follow postoperative instructions

Total Elbow Replacement[3–5,8,11,14,15]

- Patients with posttraumatic conditions of the elbow tend to be younger than other patients undergoing TEA.
- In this group of patients, TEA should be considered in patients who:
  - Have failed to respond to appropriate nonoperative management
  - Are not appropriate candidates for other surgical options
  - Are willing to adopt a more sedentary lifestyle
  - Have no absolute contraindications to the procedure

Preoperative Planning

Interposition Arthroplasty

- Graft options
  - Achilles tendon allograft has the advantage of no donor site morbidity. It can also be used to reconstruct the collateral ligaments if necessary.
  - Dermis or fascia lata autogenous graft
  - Dermal tissue allograft
- Revision
  - The salvage for a failed interposition arthroplasty is a TEA.[1]
  - Interposition arthroplasty should not be undertaken unless the surgeon is comfortable performing a total elbow replacement in the face of failure.

Total Elbow Replacement

- Implants are described in terms of their physical linkage (linked, unlinked, or linkable) and based on their constraint (constrained, semiconstrained, minimally constrained).
  - Linkage is determined by whether the components are physically linked.
  - Constraint is a more poorly defined quality of the implant. It depends on the geometry of the implant and its interaction with stabilizing soft tissues about the elbow.[6]
- Implant selection in posttraumatic arthritis
  - Linked (semiconstrained) designs: Linked implants have the advantage of being universally applicable to all posttraumatic conditions of the elbow.
  - Unlinked designs: The requirement for the use of unlinked designs in posttraumatic conditions of the elbow is integrity of the collateral ligaments and limited deformity such that normal anatomic relationships can be re-established.
  - Linkable designs: Linkable designs have been developed to take advantage of the features of an unlinked implant while capturing the universal applicability of the linked implants. They can be converted from unlinked to linked either at the time of an initial surgery if stability cannot be conferred or remotely if instability becomes an issue postoperatively.

Positioning

- Interposition arthroplasty
  - Supine with the arm across the chest and a bump under the ipsilateral shoulder
  - Alternatively, the lateral decubitus position with the arm over an arm holder
- Total elbow replacement

▪ Patients are placed supine on the operating table with a bump under the ipsilateral shoulder. The arm should be freely mobile through the shoulder to allow manipulation of the joint throughout surgery. The arm can then be placed across the body on a bump or externally rotated through the shoulder and flexed at the elbow (**FIG 3**).

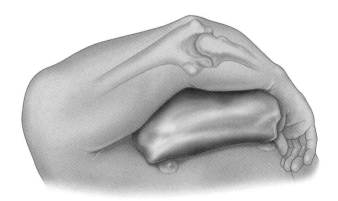

FIG 3 • Patient positioning for total elbow arthroplasty with the arm across the body supported on a bolster.

INTERPOSITION ARTHROPLASTY

▪ Posterior skin incision: Develop medial and lateral subcutaneous flaps.

▪ Isolate and transpose the ulnar nerve.

▪ Perform deep exposure to the elbow through an extensile Köcher approach.[9] The triceps can be partially released from the ulna to allow the triceps–anconeus composite to be mobilized (**TECH FIG 1A**).

▪ Mobilize the common extensor group from the anterior capsule and release it proximally with the extensor carpi radialis longus.

▪ Isolate the lateral ulnar collateral ligament and release it from its humeral origin (**TECH FIG 1B**). Perform an anterior and posterior capsular release. Supination of the forearm allows the ulna to be rotated away from the humerus. Attempt to leave the medial collateral ligament intact as it will improve postoperative stability.

▪ Inspect the cartilage surfaces. If more than 50% of the articular surface is involved, surgery proceeds to interposition.

▪ If extensile exposure is required, the extensile Köcher approach can be expanded to a triceps-reflecting anconeus pedicle (TRAP) approach (**TECH FIG 1C,D**).[13]

▪ Reshape the distal humerus to conform to the olecranon. Remove the cartilage from the distal humerus and smooth the bone, but avoid aggressive resection of bone (**TECH FIG 1E**).

▪ Prepare the interposition tissue. The graft of choice is up to the surgeon, but there is a growing experience with allograft Achilles tendon. In addition to being a robust graft source, it allows for reconstruction of one or both collateral ligaments (**TECH FIG 2A**).

▪ Place drill holes across the supracondylar region from anterior to posterior (**TECH FIG 2B**). These drill holes are placed at the medial aspect of the trochlea, above the trochlear sulcus, at the lateral margin of the trochlea, and at the lateral aspect of the capitellum.

▪ Drape the interposition tissue over the distal humerus and secure it with sutures placed through the graft from front to back. If there is collateral ligament insufficiency, the tails of the graft (especially when using Achilles tendon) can be fashioned to reconstruct the collateral ligaments (**TECH FIG 2C**).

▪ Leave the radial head intact, especially if medial collateral ligament reconstruction is performed, to contribute to the valgus stability of the elbow.

▪ Repair the lateral collateral ligament through drill holes at the center of rotation laterally. Do not tie the ligament until the external fixator is securely applied.

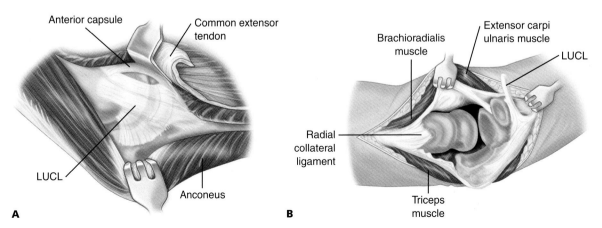

A

Anterior capsule
Common extensor tendon
LUCL
Anconeus

B

Brachioradialis muscle
Extensor carpi ulnaris muscle
LUCL
Radial collateral ligament
Triceps muscle

TECH FIG 1 • **A.** Extensile Köcher approach to the lateral elbow. The anconeus and triceps are elevated off the posterolateral capsule while elbe common extensor group is elevated off the anterior capsule. Exposure can be extended posteriorly with partial release of the triceps from the lateral aspect of the olecranon. **B.** Deep extensile exposure requires release of the lateral collateral ligament and anterior and posterior capsule. *(continued)*

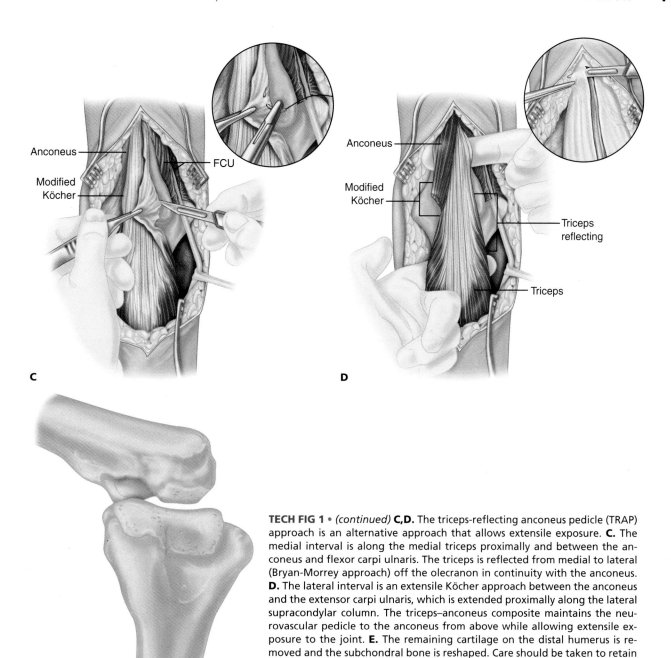

TECH FIG 1 • *(continued)* **C,D.** The triceps-reflecting anconeus pedicle (TRAP) approach is an alternative approach that allows extensile exposure. **C.** The medial interval is along the medial triceps proximally and between the anconeus and flexor carpi ulnaris. The triceps is reflected from medial to lateral (Bryan-Morrey approach) off the olecranon in continuity with the anconeus. **D.** The lateral interval is an extensile Köcher approach between the anconeus and the extensor carpi ulnaris, which is extended proximally along the lateral supracondylar column. The triceps–anconeus composite maintains the neurovascular pedicle to the anconeus from above while allowing extensile exposure to the joint. **E.** The remaining cartilage on the distal humerus is removed and the subchondral bone is reshaped. Care should be taken to retain as much subchondral bone as possible for structural support of the interposition membrane.

Hinged Elbow External Fixator

- Apply a hinged external fixator to protect the interposed graft and to stabilize the joint while soft tissue healing occurs.
- The axis of rotation of the elbow is defined by bony landmarks about the lateral and medial joint (**TECH FIG 3A**).
  - The center of rotation at the lateral elbow is the center point of an arc defined by the articular surface of the capitellum.
  - The center of rotation at the medial elbow is defined by tightly distributed instantaneous centers of rotation approximated by a point at the anterior inferior aspect of the medial epicondyle.
- Establish an axis pin coincident with the lateral and medial centers of rotation. This is the foundation for construction of the fixator.

- The type of fixator used dictates the method of pin insertion relative to the axis pin. Fixator systems that allow the humeral and ulnar pins to be placed independently and than assembled to the axis pin are easiest for the surgeon with limited experience (**TECH FIG 3B**).
- When placing the humeral pin, take care to avoid injury to the neurovascular structures.
  - Pins in the proximal humerus are placed through the anterolateral aspect of the deltoid distal to the axillary nerve.
  - Pins in the midshaft of the humerus are placed in the anterolateral humerus to avoid the radial nerve, which lies posteriorly.
- Ulnar pins are placed along the posterolateral aspect of the ulna.

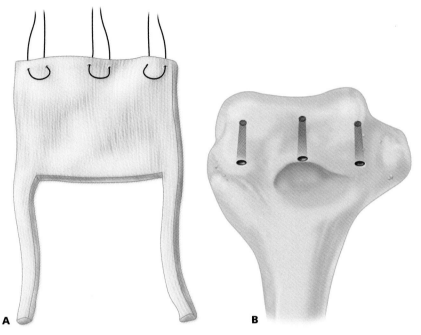

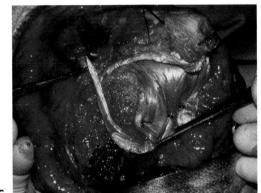

TECH FIG 2 • A. The interposition membrane is prepared with mattress sutures placed distally. The Achilles tendon allograft also permits reconstruction of the collateral ligaments if necessary. **B.** Drill holes are placed from posterior to anterior across the supracondylar region to secure the interposition graft. **C.** The interposition membrane is secured to the distal humerus. If necessary, the graft can be fashioned to reconstruct the collateral ligaments. (From Morrey BF, Larson AN. Interposition arthroplasty of the elbow. In: Morrey BF, Sanchez-Sotelo J, eds. *The Elbow and Its Disorders,* 4th ed. Philadelphia: Elsevier; 2009: Figure 69–6.)

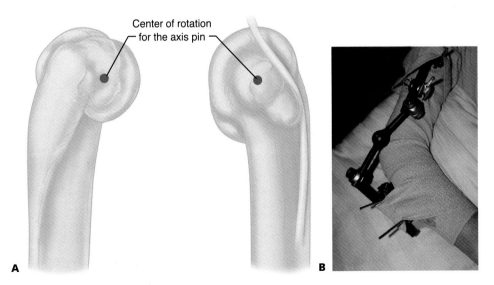

TECH FIG 3 • A. Drawing demonstrating the center of rotation on the lateral and medial side of the elbow. **B.** Photograph demonstrating a hinged external fixator. The humeral and ulnar pins are independently attached to the hinge.

- A bar is fixed to the humeral and another bar is fixed to the ulnar pins.
- The hinge is loosely attached to the humeral and ulnar bars.

- The joint is reduced and ligament reconstruction, if necessary, is completed.
- With the joint reduced, the fixator is tightened. If desired, distraction can be applied.

TOTAL ELBOW REPLACEMENT

Surgical Approach

- A straight posterior skin incision placed off the medial aspect of the olecranon is preferred. Previous incisions may modify the location of the incision. Regardless of the incision used, deep access to the medial and lateral aspect of the joint is essential.
- Identify the ulnar nerve. If not previously handled surgically, the nerve is transposed anteriorly. If the nerve was previously transposed, it only needs to be identified, but not formally dissected unless the position of the nerve places it at risk during surgery.

Triceps Management

- Triceps-reflecting approaches are preferred over triceps-sparing approaches for posttraumatic conditions. Posttraumatic scarring and deformity can make a triceps-sparing approach difficult unless a nonunited distal humeral segment is to be resected.
- A Bryan-Morrey approach is typically performed (**TECH FIG 4A,B**).[9] The medial aspect of the triceps is developed proximally while the interval between the anconeus and flexor carpi ulnaris (FCU) is developed distal to the olecranon. The triceps is reflected from medially to laterally in continuity with the anconeus. Release of the lateral and medial collateral ligaments completes the exposure and allows separation of the ulna from the humerus.

- A modification of the Bryan-Morrey approach involves release of the triceps insertion onto the ulna through an extra-articular osteotomy of the dorsal tip of the ulna (**TECH FIG 4C,D**).[16] The rationale for this modification relates to the recognized complication of triceps insufficiency that occurs with soft tissue release of the triceps. The osteotomy affords several advantages:
  - Bone-to-bone healing of the osteotomy is more reliable than soft tissue healing of the triceps to the ulna.
  - Failure of the osteotomy to heal can be identified radiographically and addressed early.

Deep Dissection

- Release the collateral ligaments and capsule (**TECH FIG 5**). This permits the ulna to be separated from the humerus. If ligamentous integrity is necessary (ie, unlinked arthroplasty) then the lateral ulnar collateral ligament and medial collateral should be tagged with plans at reattachment via bone tunnels in the humerus during closure.
- Release contracted muscles (flexor–pronator and common extensor) to correct deformity, which can result in maltracking of the TEA. Release the scarring about the elbow sufficiently to gain unencumbered access to the humerus and ulna for component implantation.
- The tip of the olecranon can be removed to better visualize the trochlea.

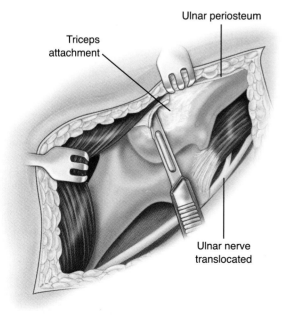

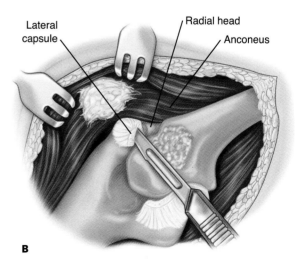

A   **B**

TECH FIG 4 • A,B. Bryan-Morrey triceps-reflecting approach. **A.** The triceps insertion is released in continuity with the anconeus from medial to lateral. **B.** Further dissection allows the collateral ligaments to be released. *(continued)*

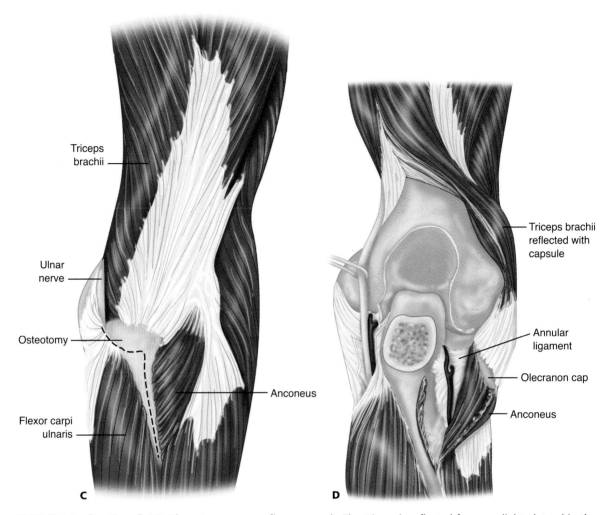

TECH FIG 4 • *(continued)* **C,D.** The osteo-anconeus flap approach. The triceps is reflected from medial to lateral in the distal interval between the flexor carpi ulnaris and anconeus.

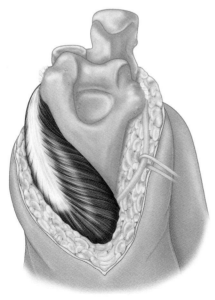

TECH FIG 5 • An extra-articular osteotomy of the tip of the olecranon is performed, leaving the triceps attached to the fragment. The shoulder is externally rotated and the elbow is hyperflexed to allow separation of the ulna from the humerus.

Component Insertion and Completion

- Insertion of total elbow implants is performed in standard fashion and is described in Chapter SE-45.
- After component insertion, the triceps mechanism is repaired through bone tunnels in the ulna. When a sliver of bone is taken with the triceps insertion, transverse tunnels are made. Each limb of nonabsorbable suture is tied over the top of the triceps and bone fragment. An additional cerclage suture is brought through one of the two transverse tunnels and is brought around the tip of the olecranon, incorporating the triceps insertion. This suture counters the pull of the triceps.
- The anconeus is repaired to the flexor carpi ulnaris fascia. Similarly, the medial triceps is repaired to the flexor–pronator group.
- Subcutaneous ulnar nerve transposition is routinely performed.
- A subcutaneous drain is placed and wound closure is performed.

PEARLS AND PITFALLS

Indications	▪ Interposition arthroplasty is considered in patients with a stable elbow and limited, painful ROM. ▪ TEA is considered in carefully selected patients if other nonoperative and operative measures have been exhausted.
Goals of treatment	▪ Regardless of the treatment undertaken, the goal of treatment is a pain-free, functional arc of motion.

Interposition arthroplasty	▪ Predictors of poor outcome:
	  ▪ Painful, mobile elbow
	  ▪ Preoperative instability
	  ▪ Need to reconstruct both the medial and lateral ulnar collateral ligaments at the time of interposition
	▪ Maintain the fixator for at least 4 weeks (preferably 6 weeks).
	▪ Meticulous pin care is required.

TEA	▪ Ulnar nerve transposition in all cases ▪ Triceps-reflecting approach, especially when the joint is very stiff ▪ Release both the medial and lateral collateral ligaments. ▪ Release the flexor–pronator and common extensor, particularly if there is significant preoperative deformity.

POSTOPERATIVE MANAGEMENT

Interposition Arthroplasty

▪ ROM is started as quickly as allowed by the condition of the soft tissues. In general, immediate motion is preferred. However, the prerequisite is a quiet soft tissue envelope. ROM may be assisted with a continuous passive motion machine if desired.

▪ Patients are taught pin care, which is performed daily at home.

▪ Patients are seen at 10 to 14 days postoperatively for staple removal and wound check and every 2 weeks thereafter until pin removal.

▪ The external fixator is left in place for about 4 to 6 weeks and then removed in the operating room with assessment of elbow stability and motion under anesthesia.

  ▪ I prefer to wait 6 weeks to allow collateral ligament healing since instability is the most common complication after fixator removal.

▪ Rehabilitation is continued, focusing on obtaining a functional ROM.

Total Elbow Replacement

▪ The elbow is immobilized in full extension in a well-padded anterior splint.

▪ The arm is elevated on pillows or suspended from an IV pole to reduce swelling.

▪ The splint is removed 24 to 48 hours after surgery.

▪ Gentle active ROM is begun in flexion, pronation, and supination. Active extension is avoided for 6 weeks to protect the triceps repair. However, gravity-assisted extension or passive extension is permitted.

▪ In general, formal physical therapy is rarely required to regain ROM. However, it may be beneficial in patients who struggle to regain their ROM. The general timeline of therapy is:

  ▪ Phase I (0 to 6 weeks): Protect the soft tissue and begin protected active-assistive ROM.

  ▪ Phase II (6 to 12 weeks): Continue to improve ROM. Begin strengthening exercises and encourage functional use of the arm.

  ▪ Phase III (12 to 16 weeks): Return to normal functional activities within the restrictions for TEA.

▪ Postoperative stiffness may be helped with splinting. Static splinting is preferred over dynamic splinting.

▪ Restrictions: Lifetime limitations of the operated extremity include 2- to 5-pound repetitive lifting and 10-lb single-event restriction.

OUTCOMES

Interposition Arthroplasty

▪ The most predictable results for interposition occur in patients presenting with:

  ▪ Stiffness and pain preoperatively

  ▪ Stable elbow

  ▪ One or no ligament reconstruction required at surgery

▪ Poor results are noted when:

  ▪ Pain is the only presenting complaint

  ▪ Elbow is unstable

  ▪ Reconstruction of both the medial and lateral collateral ligaments is needed at the time of interposition

▪ Most studies report a 70% satisfaction rate among patients with respect to pain relief; 80% of patients regain a functional ROM.

▪ Cheng and Morrey[2] found that 67% of patients treated for rheumatoid arthritis had satisfactory relief of pain, and 75% of patients treated for osteoarthritis were satisfied at 5-year follow-up.

Total Elbow Arthroplasty

▪ Patients undergoing TEA for posttraumatic conditions of the elbow tend to be younger and have higher demand.

▪ TEA for posttraumatic conditions of the elbow is associated with improved clinical outcomes.

▪ A higher complication rate is noted for posttraumatic conditions compared to other indications for TEA.

▪ Mechanical complications such as component fracture and increased polyethylene bushing wear are more common. Causes of increased complications include:

  ▪ Multiple previous surgeries

  ▪ Deformity of the elbow requiring realignment of the extremity through the implant

COMPLICATIONS

Interposition Arthroplasty

- Complications of interposition arthroplasty include:
  - Instability
  - Infection
  - Ulnar neuropathy
  - Resorptive bone loss
  - Heterotopic bone formation
- Complications related to the external fixator include:
  - Superficial pin tract infections
  - Deep infection (osteomyelitis)
  - Pin breakage
- In the literature, complications have been reported to occur in up to 25% of patients.

Total Elbow Replacement

- TEA for traumatic conditions is associated with a high complication rate. Major complications include:
  - Infection
    - Current reports indicate an infection rate of 2% to 5% for primary TEA.
    - Higher infection rates are noted with posttraumatic arthritis and a history of prior surgery.
  - Loosening
  - Triceps insufficiency (an underrecognized problem)
  - Neurologic injury (incidence of transient ulnar neuropathy as high as 26% and permanent nerve injury up to 10%)
  - Wound complications
    - Associated with prior surgery
    - Manage wound by immobilizing in extension postoperatively; use a subcutaneous drain to avoid hematoma formation. A significant postoperative hematoma should be evacuated.
  - Periprosthetic fracture (can occur intraoperatively or postoperatively; incidence ranges from 1% to 23%)

REFERENCES

1. Blaine TA, Adams R, Morrey BF. Total elbow arthroplasty after interposition arthroplasty for elbow arthritis. J Bone Joint Surg Am 2005;87A:286–292.
2. Cheng SL, Morrey BF. Treatment of the mobile, painful arthritic elbow by distraction interposition arthroplasty. J Bone Joint Surg Am 2000;82A:233–238.
3. Figgie MP, Inglis AE, Mow CS, et al. Salvage of non-union of supracondylar fracture of the humerus by total elbow arthroplasty. J Bone Joint Surg Am 1989;71A:1058–1065.
4. Figgie HE III, Inglis AE, Ranawat CS, et al. Results of total elbow arthroplasty as a salvage procedure for failed elbow reconstructive operations. Clin Orthop Relat Res 1987;219:185–193.
5. Inglis AE, Inglis AE Jr, Figgie MM, et al. Total elbow arthroplasty for flail and unstable elbows. J Shoulder Elbow Surg 1997;6:29–36.
6. Kamineni S, O'Driscoll SW, Urban M, et al. Intrinsic constraint of unlinked total elbow replacements: the ulnotrochlear joint. J Bone Joint Surg Am 2005;87A:2019–2027.
7. Larson AN, Morrey BF. Interposition arthroplasty with an Achilles tendon allograft as a salvage procedure for the elbow. J Bone Joint Surg Am 2008;90A:2714–2723.
8. Moro JK, King GJ. Total elbow arthroplasty in the treatment of posttraumatic conditions of the elbow. Clin Orthop Relat Res 2000;370:102–114.
9. Morrey BF. Surgical exposures of the elbow. In: Morrey BF, Sanchez-Sotelo J, eds. The Elbow and its Disorders, 4th ed. Philadelphia: Saunders Elsevier, 2009;115–142.
10. Morrey BF, Askew LJ, Chao EY. A biomechanical study of normal functional elbow motion. J Bone Joint Surg Am 1981;63A:872–877.
11. Morrey BF, Schneeberger AG. Total elbow arthroplasty for posttraumatic arthrosis. AAOS Instr Course Lect 2009;58:495–504.
12. Nolla J, Ring D, Lozano-Calderon S, et al. Interposition arthroplasty of the elbow with hinged external fixation for post-traumatic arthritis. J Shoulder Elbow Surg 2008;17:459–464.
13. O'Driscoll SW. The triceps-reflecting anconeus pedicle (TRAP) approach for distal humeral fractures and nonunions. Orthop Clin North Am 2000;31:91–101.
14. Ramsey ML, Adams RA, Morrey BF. Instability of the elbow treated with semiconstrained total elbow arthroplasty. J Bone Joint Surg Am 1999;81A:38–47.
15. Schneeberger AG, Adams R, Morrey BF. Semiconstrained total elbow replacement for the treatment of post-traumatic osteoarthrosis. J Bone Joint Surg Am 1997;79A:1211–1222.
16. Wolfe SW, Ranawat CS. The osteo-anconeus flap: an approach for total elbow arthroplasty. J Bone Joint Surg Am 1990;72A:684–688.

Mark A. Mighell and Thomas J. Kovack

BACKGROUND

- Elbow arthrodesis is a rarely performed orthopaedic procedure.
- It is mainly performed for severe joint destruction due to:
  - Posttraumatic arthrosis
  - Instability
  - Infection
- Historically, it is performed for a tuberculous infection of the elbow.[1]
- Early fusion rates are about 50%.[1]
- With modern techniques, fusion rates approach 50% to 100%.[3,9]
- Arthrodesis of the elbow results in greater functional disability than arthrodesis of the ankle, hip, or knee joints.
- Satisfactory shoulder function is a prerequisite, even though it does not compensate for loss of motion in the elbow.[2]
- Compensatory motion is seen more in the spinal column and wrist.
- A functional hand is also desirable when performing arthrodesis of the elbow.
- No optimal position for arthrodesis exists.
  - The position of fusion is dictated by the needs of the patient.

PATIENT HISTORY AND PHYSICAL FINDINGS

- Skin and soft tissue defects are evaluated.
- The surgeon should evaluate the need for bone graft or soft tissue coverage before arthrodesis.
- If soft tissue coverage is necessary, a plastic surgery consultation is recommended.
- Shoulder, wrist, and spinal column motion is evaluated.
- Neurologic and motor deficits are documented.
- Blood flow to the hand is determined.
- The quality and quantity of bone available for fusion are assessed.

IMAGING AND OTHER DIAGNOSTIC STUDIES

- Standard radiographs of the elbow are obtained.
- Computed tomography (CT) scans of the elbow are obtained for more detailed bony anatomy.
- If infection is suspected:
  - Blood work is obtained for complete blood count, sedimentation rate, and C-reactive protein.
  - The joint is aspirated or an indium scan is performed.

SURGICAL MANAGEMENT

- The elbow is one of the most difficult joints to fuse because of the long lever arm and strong bending forces across the fusion site.
- Arthrodesis should be considered a salvage procedure when no other satisfactory surgical option exists.

Indications

- Septic and tuberculous arthritis
- Sequela of septic arthritis
- Complex war injuries (with large bone and soft tissue defects)
- Young healthy laborers with posttraumatic arthritis who are too young for total elbow arthroplasty
- Posttraumatic arthrosis or severe instability
- Pseudarthrosis
- Severely comminuted intra-articular fractures of the distal humerus with joint destruction
- Chronic osteomyelitis
- Failed elbow arthroplasty
- Failed internal fixation for nonunions

Contraindications

- Massive bone loss preventing successful arthrodesis
- Massive soft tissue loss not amenable to flap reconstruction
- Compromised function of the ipsilateral shoulder, wrist, and spinal column

Preoperative Planning

- The best elbow position is controversial, although the literature suggests between 45 and 110 degrees.
  - Historically, 90 degrees is accepted as the best position.
- Factors for choosing the best position include:
  - Gender
  - Occupation
  - Hand dominance
  - Functional requirements
  - Associated joint involvement
  - Unilateral versus bilateral arthrodesis
  - Patient preference
- One to 3 weeks before surgery, the elbow to be fused is braced or casted in various angles.
  - Generally acceptable angles include:
    - Male: dominant arm at 90 degrees
    - Females seem to prefer lower angles of 40 to 70 degrees.
    - Ninety to 110 degrees is better for personal hygiene.
    - Forty to 70 degrees is better for extrapersonal needs and activities.
    - Bilateral elbow arthrodesis: dominant arm at 110 degrees, nondominant arm at 65 degrees
- Soft tissue coverage is evaluated.
- Flap coverage or skin grafts are performed before arthrodesis.
- If soft tissue coverage is required, the joint is stabilized with an external fixator.
- The surgeon should consider bulk graft with demineralized bone matrix and cancellous allograft or autograft.

- For large bone defects, autograft cancellous bone is preferable.
- Antibiotics are given 30 minutes before the incision.
- General anesthesia is used.
- An axillary or interscalene block can be used.

Special Instruments

- Large fragment locking set (4.5-mm locked narrow plate)
- A 3.5-mm locked plate may be substituted in smaller patients.
- Sterile goniometer
- Plate press

- High-speed burr
- Power drill
- Osteotomes
- Oscillating saw
- Kirschner wire set

Patient Positioning

- A tourniquet is placed as high on the arm as possible. A sterile tourniquet is required to increase the zone of sterility.
- The patient is placed in the lateral decubitus position with the operative arm resting on a padded arm rest.

SURGICAL APPROACH

- Mark existing surgical scars and use prior incisions.
- Use a direct posterior approach for the elbow.
  - An anterior approach may be needed if the tissue is compromised posteriorly.
- If flap coverage is present, a plastic surgeon may be required for exposure.
  - Flaps with vascular pedicles can be located with Doppler.

- Create full-thickness flaps right down to the bone.
  - Split the triceps tendon longitudinally.
  - Carry the triceps split distally in the interval between the flexor carpi ulnaris (FCU) and the anconeus.
- Identify the ulnar nerve and make sure it remains protected.
  - Identify neurovascular structures in known areas before following structures through areas of heavy scar tissue.

ARTHRODESIS

Osteotomy and Fracture Reduction

- Expose the dorsal surface of the distal humerus and proximal ulna.
- Use osteotomes to "fish-scale" the exposed bone.
- Open the medullary canal of the humerus and ulna.
- Perform a step-cut osteotomy of the proximal ulna and distal humerus to increase the surface area for fusion (**TECH FIG 1A**).
- Contour the bone so that it can be reduced at the appropriate angle chosen for arthrodesis.
  - It is often necessary to excise the radial head to allow for adequate reduction of the humerus and ulna.
- Reduce the distal humerus to the proximal ulna.
  - Confirm the fusion angle with a sterile goniometer (**TECH FIG 1B**).
  - Provisionally hold the reduction at the desired angle with 1.6-mm Kirschner wires.

Screw and Plate Fixation

- Drill from distal to proximal for lag screw insertion (**TECH FIG 2A**).
  - Use two or three lag screws whenever possible.

- Apply the 4.5-mm locking plate posteriorly, prebent at the chosen angle of arthrodesis (**TECH FIG 2B**).
  - A long plate should be selected with a minimum of 10 to 14 holes.
  - A plate press is easier to use than bending irons.
- The plate functions as a neutralization device.
  - All compression is achieved with the lag technique employed for screw placement.
- The plate is pulled down to the bone and secured with cortical screws before adding locked screws.
- Use at least one locked screw proximal and distal to the fusion site to increase the torsional strength of the construct (**TECH FIG 2C**).

Completion

- Check the position and fixation of the construct intraoperatively with fluoroscopy.
- The final construct should compress well at the fracture site.
  - The plate should conform securely to the bone at the desired angle of fusion (**TECH FIG 3A**).
- Irrigate and close the wound.
  - Place one or two deep flat drains.
- Final radiographs should be taken intraoperatively (**TECH FIG 3B,C**).

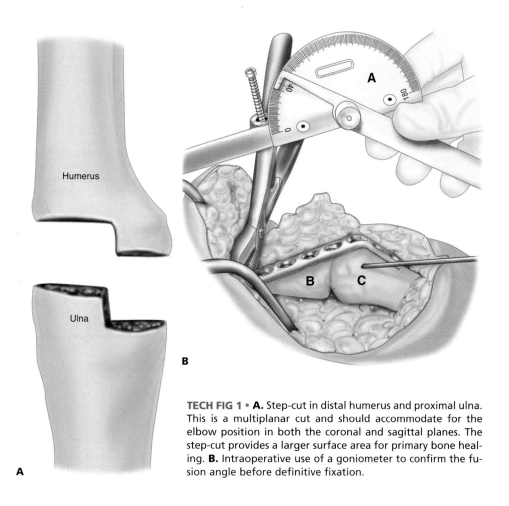

TECH FIG 1 • A. Step-cut in distal humerus and proximal ulna. This is a multiplanar cut and should accommodate for the elbow position in both the coronal and sagittal planes. The step-cut provides a larger surface area for primary bone healing. **B.** Intraoperative use of a goniometer to confirm the fusion angle before definitive fixation.

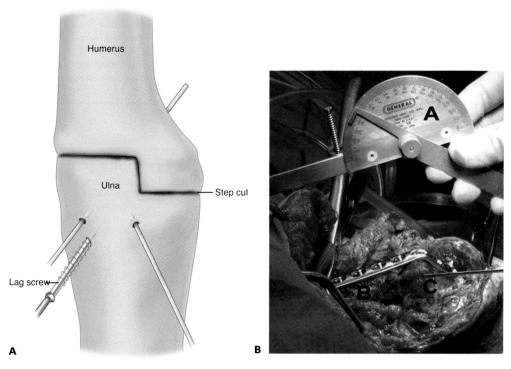

TECH FIG 2 • A. Placement of lag screw. Screws are placed from distal to proximal in a crossed configuration. Two or three lag screws are placed before plate application. Provisional fixation is obtained with Kirschner wires and the fusion position is measured with a goniometer. **B.** Plate placement after the fusion angle has been confirmed. *(continued)*

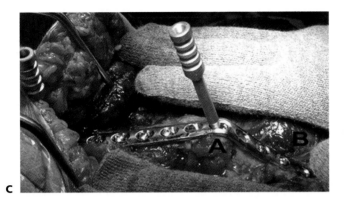

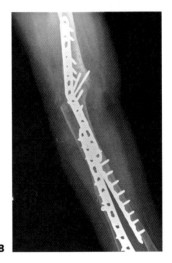

TECH FIG 2 • *(continued)* **C.** A guide for locking the screw through the plate and across the step-cut osteotomy. Compression must be achieved before locking screws are placed. *A,* distal humerus; *B,* proximal ulna.

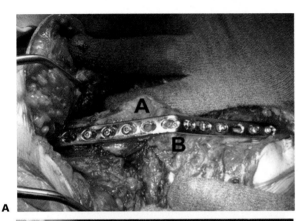

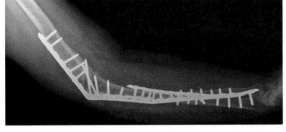

TECH FIG 3 • A. Completed elbow arthrodesis using step-cut osteotomy and 3.5-mm locking plate and lag screw technique. *A,* distal humerus; *B,* proximal ulna. **B,C.** AP and lateral postoperative radiographs of left elbow fusion using step-cut osteotomy and locked plating technique.

PEARLS AND PITFALLS

- Step-cut bone to increase the surface area for healing.
- Place lag screws in both vertical and horizontal planes to increase compression.
- Keep dorsal tissue flaps at full thickness, including the periosteum.
- Use lag technique to compress the bone ends.
- Never identify neurovascular structures in areas of extensive surgical scarring. Work from known to unknown surgical fields.
- Open the medullary canal to facilitate blood flow.
- Select a plate of sufficient length to span the fusion site. Longer plates are desirable.
- Never place locking screws before reduction and compression of the bone ends.
- Keep patients in a cast for at least 4 months, until fusion occurs, depending on radiographs.

POSTOPERATIVE CARE

▪ Drains are removed before hospital discharge.

▪ Intravenous antibiotics are continued for 48 hours or longer, depending on intraoperative cultures.

▪ Sutures or staples are removed at 2 weeks.

▪ The arm is placed in a long-arm cast at the 2-week visit.

▪ The patient is placed in serial casts for at least 4 months.

▪ Cast application is continued until there is radiographic evidence of union.

REFERENCES

1. Arafiles RP. A new technique of fusion for tuberculous arthritis of the elbow. J Bone Joint Surg Am 1981;63A:1396–1400.
2. Beckenbaugh RD. Arthrodesis. In: Morrey BF, ed. The Elbow and its Disorders, ed 3. Philadelphia: WB Saunders, 2000:731–737.
3. Bilic R, Kolundzic R, Bicanic G, et al. Elbow arthrodesis after war injuries. Military Med 2005;170:164–166.
4. Irvine GB, Gregg PJ. A method of elbow arthrodesis: brief report. J Bone Joint Surg Br 1989;71B:145–146.
5. McAuliffe JA, Burkhalter WE, Ouellette EA, et al. Compression plate arthrodesis of the elbow. J Bone Joint Surg Br 1992;74B:300–304.
6. Morrey BF, Askew LJ, Chao EY, et al. A biomechanical study of normal functional elbow motion. J Bone Joint Surg Am 1981;63A:872–877.
7. Nagy SM, Szabo RM, Sharkey NA. Unilateral elbow arthrodesis: the preferred position. J South Orthop Assoc 1999;8:80–85.
8. O'Neill OR, Morrey BG, Tanaka S, et al. Compensatory motion in the upper extremity, after elbow arthrodesis. Clin Orthop Relat Res 1992;281:89–96.
9. Orozco JR. A new technique of elbow arthrodesis. Int Orthop 1996;20:92–93.
10. Presnal BP, Chillaq KJ. Radiohumeral arthrodesis for salvage of failed total elbow arthroplasty. J Arthroplasty 1995;10:699–701.
11. Rashkoff E, Burkhalter WE. Arthrodesis of the salvage elbow. Orthopedics 1986;9:733–738.
12. Tang C, Roidis N, Itamura J, et al. The effect of simulated elbow arthrodesis on the ability to perform activities of daily living. J Hand Surg Am 2001;26A:1146–1150.

Exam Table for Shoulder and Elbow

Examination	Technique	Illustration	Grading & Significance
Shoulder			
Active forward flexion	Patient attempts to actively bring the arm forward above his or her head.		Normal active flexion is 170–180 degrees. Limited active forward flexion is indicative of possible large rotator cuff tear. Patients with function at or above shoulder level are more likely to have improved active forward flexion postoperatively.
Active external rotation	With arms at the patient's side and the elbows flexed to 90 degrees, the patient is asked to maximally externally rotate the arms.		Less active external rotation on the affected side. Decreased external rotation on affected side indicates partial or complete loss of infraspinatus function due to tear involvement or muscle dysfunction.
Abduction strength testing	The arm is placed in 90 degrees abduction in the scapular plane. The patient is asked to resist downward force.		Tests deltoid muscle strength: full strength, decreased strength, or unable to maintain position against gravity. Weak deltoid suggests less postoperative active range of motion secondary to inadequate strength.
External rotation lag sign	Arm is passively placed in maximal external rotation and then released. Patient is asked to maintain the arm in external rotation.		Inability to maintain maximal external rotation ($\geq$20 degree lag sign) suggests the tear extends well into the infraspinatus.

(continued)

Examination	Technique	Illustration	Grading & Significance
External rotation strength testing	Arm is placed in maximal external rotation and patient is asked to resist internal rotation force.		Full-strength resistance suggests no infraspinatus tear involvement. Weakness suggests progressive infraspinatus involvement or dysfunction.
Lift-off test	Patient places the dorsum of the hand against the lumbar region of the back and attempts to lift the hand from the back and hold it.		Inability to lift the hand from the back is a positive result. Indicates subscapularis muscle weakness or tear.
Belly press test (Napoleon test)	The patient is asked to keep the palm of his or her hand on the abdomen with the wrist extended and the shoulder flexed and in maximal internal rotation while the examiner attempts to forcefully pull the patient's hand off the abdomen.		A positive belly-press test occurs when the patient must flex the wrist and extend the arm to maintain the palm on the abdomen. This indicates subscapularis muscle weakness or tear.
Modified belly press	With palm on abdomen, the patient is asked to bring the elbow forward, in front of the plane of the body.		Inability to perform action demonstrates dysfunctional or torn subscapularis tendon and a higher rate of clinical failure with muscle transfer.
Bear hug test	The hand of the affected side is placed on the opposite shoulder with the fingers extended and the elbow elevated forward. The patient resists as the examiner attempts to lift the hand off the shoulder.		If the examiner can lift the hand off the shoulder, then the patient likely has a partial or complete tear of the upper subscapularis tendon. This is perhaps the most sensitive test for a subscapularis tear.
Wall push-up	The patient is asked to perform a wall push-up by placing the hands at shoulder level on a wall and doing a push-up.		The scapula is carefully evaluated for signs and severity of medial or lateral translation.
Impingement sign	With the patient upright, the examiner fixes the scapula to prevent it from moving and then brings the arm into full forward elevation with some force.		A positive test is pain during this maneuver. Forcing the fully forward elevated arm against the fixed scapula helps to localize the finding to the rotator cuff.

Examination	Technique	Illustration	Grading & Significance
Palm-down abduction test	With the scapula stabilized by the examiner, the arm is internally rotated and then elevated forcibly in the plane of the scapula.		A positive test produces pain with the maneuver. By internally rotating the arm, the supra- and anterior infraspinatus tendons are placed directly under the coracoacromial arch. Elevating the arm in the scapular plane when it is in internal rotation compresses these tendons against the undersurface of the acromion.
Coracoid impingement	The arm is forward flexed to 90 degrees, internally rotated, and adducted.		Reproduction of pain or a painful click indicates a positive test. A positive test is indicative of impingement of the coracoid onto the subscapularis.
Apprehension test	The arm is placed in 90 degrees of abduction. The arm is slowly brought into external rotation and extension.		Apprehension, not simply pain, is required for a positive apprehension test. The apprehension test has a sensitivity of 72% and specificity of 96% for anterior instability. Positive anterior apprehension can be associated with anterior labral injuries. Patient feels a sensation of instability with the arm in the at-risk position. Sensation of pain suggests internal impingement, not instability.
Anterior load and shift test	The patient is positioned supine with the arm in 20 degrees abduction, 20 degrees flexion, and neutral rotation. With axial load to reduce the humeral head, an anterior force is applied to the arm.		0 = no translation; 1+ = to the anterior rim; 2+ = over the rim but spontaneously reduces; 3+ = dislocation of the humeral head that locks over the anterior rim. Indicates anterior instability.
Load and shift test	If the right shoulder is examined, the examiner's left hand grasps the humeral shaft with the fingers anterior and the thumb posterior. The examiner's right hand grasps the forearm and positions the arm in the plane of the scapula in 40 to 60 degrees of abduction and neutral rotation. An axial load is applied to the humerus through the forearm and the examiner's left hand displaces the humeral head anteriorly. The degree of displacement of the humeral head on the glenoid rim is noted.		Grade 0: Little or no movement Grade 1: Shift to edge of glenoid Grade 2: Shift over edge of glenoid but spontaneously reduces Grade 3: Shift over edge of glenoid but does not spontaneously relocate This is difficult to perform in the awake patient in clinic but sensitive when the patient is under anesthesia.
Miniaci bony apprehension test	The arm is placed in approximately 45 degrees of abduction. With external rotation, there is development of apprehension.		Apprehension with lower degrees of abduction indicates a significant and symptomatic bony contribution to the instability.

(continued)

Examination	Technique	Illustration	Grading & Significance
Sulcus sign	An inferior force is applied to the arm at the side.		0 = no translation; 1+ = <1 cm; 2+ = 1–2 cm; 3+ = >3 cm. Indicates an inferior component of instability.
Biceps resistance test (Speed's test)	With the patient's arm at 90 degrees of forward elevation, a downward force is applied to the arm while the patient tries to resist that force.		A positive test is pain along the tendon of the long head of the biceps. Pain during this maneuver indicates involvement of the long head of the biceps tendon.
Speed's test	The arm is abducted to 90 degrees and brought forward 45 degrees while the forearm is supinated and the elbow extended. The patient then resists a downward force.		If the maneuver produces pain or tenderness, the test is positive. A positive test may indicate bicipital pathology, although the test is not specific.
Yergason test	The elbow is flexed to 90 degrees. The patient attempts to supinate the arm from a pronated position while the examiner resists.		The patient will experience pain as the biceps tendon subluxes out of the groove with a positive test. A positive test indicates biceps instability.
Scapula stabilization test	When winging is observed, a hand is placed to stabilize the scapula in a reduced position, and the patient then elevates the arm.		The examiner should assess for fixed scapula winging versus reducible winging as well as improvement in arm elevation and comfort with the scapula reduced. This is crucial in determining fixed versus reducible winging.

Examination	Technique	Illustration	Grading & Significance
Selective injection with local anesthetic and corticosteroid	The involved arm is placed on the back to lift the scapula off the chest wall. The injection is given in the scapulothoracic bursa under the superomedial border of the scapula.		Significant pain relief or elimination of the pain confirms the diagnosis.
Elbow			
Range of motion (ROM), elbow	Active and passive ROM (flexion–extension of the elbow, rotation of the forearm) is compared to the uninjured side. Palpable and auditory crepitus should be noted.		Normal values: 0 to 145 degrees of flexion–extension, 85 degrees of supination, and 80 degrees of pronation. The examiner should check for perching on the lateral view. Locking of the elbow could represent loose bodies. Stiffness may indicate intrinsic capsular contracture.
Effusion	The examiner palpates the anconeus triangle (radial head [RH], lateral epicondyle [L], and olecranon tip [O]) and lateral gutter, noting prominence of lateral epicondyle, gutter effusion, or subcutaneous atrophy from prior corticosteroid injections.		It is difficult to estimate the amount of fluid, but the presence of an effusion should be noted and may represent hemarthrosis due to intra-articular fracture, radiocapitellar wear, or ligamentous disruption. In acute injuries an effusion should be present; in more chronic situations it may be absent.

(continued)

Examination	Technique	Illustration	Grading & Significance
Supine lateral pivot-shift test	Patient is supine, with arm extended overhead and supinated. The examiner stabilizes the humerus with one hand and applies a valgus force with the other as the elbow is taken from extension to flexion.		When the elbow is slightly flexed the radial head can be palpated to subluxate or frankly dislocate; as the elbow flexes past 40 degrees, it will relocate, often with a palpable clunk. This test is difficult to perform on an awake patient; often apprehension will be felt and the patient will not allow the test to continue. Examination under anesthesia may be required.
Prone pivot-shift test	Placing the patient prone with the arm hanging over the table stabilizes the humerus and leaves one of the examiner's hands free to palpate the radial head.		A positive test reveals radial head or ulnohumeral subluxation. Same as pivot-shift test.
Elbow drawer test	With the patient in prone position, the humerus is stabilized with one arm while a distraction force is placed on the forearm to sublux the ulnohumeral joint.		A positive test reveals ulnohumeral subluxation.
Push-off test	From a seated position the patient attempts to push off from the armrests. Pain or apprehension is suggestive of lateral ligamentous insufficiency.		A positive test will reproduce the patient's symptoms of apprehension during supination and not pronation. Inability to complete the push-up is a positive test. A positive test indicates a posterolateral rotatory insufficiency.

Examination	Technique	Illustration	Grading & Significance
Table-top relocation test	The symptomatic hand/arm is placed on the lateral edge of a table. The patient is asked to perform push-up with the elbow pointing laterally. The maneuver is repeated with the examiner's thumb stabilizing the radial head during press-up. The maneuver is once again repeated without the examiner's thumb in place.		A positive test elicits pain or apprehension as the elbow reaches 40 degrees.
Varus stress test	Stabilize the humerus and stress the elbow in supination and slight flexion.		A positive test indicates injury to the anterior band of the medial collateral ligament.
Valgus stress test	The examiner stabilizes the humerus and stresses the lateral ulnar collateral ligament in slight flexion.		A positive test indicates injury to the lateral ulnar collateral ligament.
Medial collateral ligament shear test	Patient places the contralateral arm under the injured elbow and grasps the thumb of the symptomatic extremity. With the elbow maximally flexed the patient applies a valgus load to the elbow as he or she brings it out into extension.		A positive test will localize pain to the medial elbow, suggesting an incompetent ulnar collateral ligament.

(continued)

Examination	Technique	Illustration	Grading & Significance
Squeeze test	Deep palpation of interosseous membrane and distal radioulnar joint		This test screens for potential longitudinal instability.
Tinel's test	Percussion of the ulnar nerve proximal to or across the cubital tunnel		A positive test elicits pain at the site of percussion and paresthesias in an ulnar nerve distribution distally, which indicates ulnar neuropathy at the elbow.
Elbow flexion test	With the patient seated, the elbows are maximally flexed and the wrists held in neutral. Reproduction of paresthesias in an ulnar nerve distribution distally within 1 minute is a positive test.		A positive test indicates ulnar neuropathy at the elbow.

Page numbers followed by *f* and *t* indicated figures and tables, respectively.